Gynaecological Cancers Risk: Breast Cancer, Ovarian Cancer and Endometrial Cancer

Gynaecological Cancers Risk: Breast Cancer, Ovarian Cancer and Endometrial Cancer

Editor

Ranjit Manchanda

MDPI • Basel • Beijing • Wuhan • Barcelona • Belgrade • Manchester • Tokyo • Cluj • Tianjin

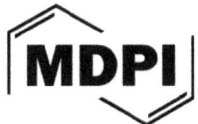

Editor
Ranjit Manchanda
Cancer Research UK,
Barts Centre, Queen Mary
University of London,
Centre for Cancer Prevention,
Wolfson Institute of Preventive
Medicine, Charterhouse Square,
London EC1M 6BQ
UK

Editorial Office
MDPI
St. Alban-Anlage 66
4052 Basel, Switzerland

This is a reprint of articles from the Special Issue published online in the open access journal *Cancers* (ISSN 2072-6694) (available at: https://www.mdpi.com/journal/cancers/special_issues/Gynaecological_Cancers_Risk).

For citation purposes, cite each article independently as indicated on the article page online and as indicated below:

LastName, A.A.; LastName, B.B.; LastName, C.C. Article Title. *Journal Name* **Year**, *Volume Number*, Page Range.

ISBN 978-3-0365-2982-0 (Hbk)
ISBN 978-3-0365-2983-7 (PDF)

© 2022 by the authors. Articles in this book are Open Access and distributed under the Creative Commons Attribution (CC BY) license, which allows users to download, copy and build upon published articles, as long as the author and publisher are properly credited, which ensures maximum dissemination and a wider impact of our publications.
The book as a whole is distributed by MDPI under the terms and conditions of the Creative Commons license CC BY-NC-ND.

Contents

About the Editor ix

Ranjit Manchanda
Special Issue "Gynaecological Cancers Risk: Breast Cancer, Ovarian Cancer and Endometrial Cancer"
Reprinted from: *Cancers* **2022**, *14*, 319, doi:10.3390/cancers14020319 1

Anna Trebo, Nina Ditsch, Christina Kuhn, Helene Hildegard Heidegger, Christine Zeder-Goess, Thomas Kolben, Bastian Czogalla, Elisa Schmoeckel, Sven Mahner, Udo Jeschke and Anna Hester
High Galectin-7 and Low Galectin-8 Expression and the Combination of both are Negative Prognosticators for Breast Cancer Patients
Reprinted from: *Cancers* **2020**, *12*, 953, doi:10.3390/cancers12040953 5

Amanda Dibden, Judith Offman, Stephen W. Duffy and Rhian Gabe
Worldwide Review and Meta-Analysis of Cohort Studies Measuring the Effect of Mammography Screening Programmes on Incidence-Based Breast Cancer Mortality
Reprinted from: *Cancers* **2020**, *12*, 976, doi:10.3390/cancers12040976 27

Faiza Gaba, Oleg Blyuss, Xinting Liu, Shivam Goyal, Nishant Lahoti, Dhivya Chandrasekaran, Margarida Kurzer, Jatinderpal Kalsi, Saskia Sanderson, Anne Lanceley, Munaza Ahmed, Lucy Side, Aleksandra Gentry-Maharaj, Yvonne Wallis, Andrew Wallace, Jo Waller, Craig Luccarini, Xin Yang, Joe Dennis, Alison Dunning, Andrew Lee, Antonis C. Antoniou, Rosa Legood, Usha Menon, Ian Jacobs and Ranjit Manchanda
Population Study of Ovarian Cancer Risk Prediction for Targeted Screening and Prevention
Reprinted from: *Cancers* **2020**, *12*, 1241, doi:10.3390/cancers12051241 43

Ranjit Manchanda, Li Sun, Shreeya Patel, Olivia Evans, Janneke Wilschut, Ana Carolina De Freitas Lopes, Faiza Gaba, Adam Brentnall, Stephen Duffy, Bin Cui, Patricia Coelho De Soarez, Zakir Husain, John Hopper, Zia Sadique, Asima Mukhopadhyay, Li Yang, Johannes Berkhof and Rosa Legood
Economic Evaluation of Population-Based *BRCA1/BRCA2* Mutation Testing across Multiple Countries and Health Systems
Reprinted from: *Cancers* **2020**, *12*, 1929, doi:10.3390/cancers12071929 65

Aleksandra Gentry-Maharaj, Oleg Blyuss, Andy Ryan, Matthew Burnell, Chloe Karpinskyj, Richard Gunu, Jatinderpal K. Kalsi, Anne Dawnay, Ines P. Marino, Ranjit Manchanda, Karen Lu, Wei-Lei Yang, John F. Timms, Max Parmar, Steven J. Skates, Robert C. Bast Jr., Ian J. Jacobs, Alexey Zaikin and Usha Menon
Multi-Marker Longitudinal Algorithms Incorporating HE4 and CA125 in Ovarian Cancer Screening of Postmenopausal Women
Reprinted from: *Cancers* **2020**, *12*, 1931, doi:10.3390/cancers12071931 103

Marina Pavanello, Isaac HY Chan, Amir Ariff, Paul DP Pharoah, Simon A. Gayther and Susan J. Ramus
Rare Germline Genetic Variants and the Risks of Epithelial Ovarian Cancer
Reprinted from: *Cancers* **2020**, *12*, 3046, doi:10.3390/cancers12103046 115

Ailish Gallagher, Jo Waller, Ranjit Manchanda, Ian Jacobs and Saskia Sanderson
Women's Intentions to Engage in Risk-Reducing Behaviours after Receiving Personal Ovarian Cancer Risk Information: An Experimental Survey Study
Reprinted from: *Cancers* **2020**, *12*, 3543, doi:10.3390/cancers12123543 . . . . **139**

Garth Funston, Victoria Hardy, Gary Abel, Emma J. Crosbie, Jon Emery, Willie Hamilton and Fiona M. Walter
Identifying Ovarian Cancer in Symptomatic Women: A Systematic Review of Clinical Tools
Reprinted from: *Cancers* **2020**, *12*, 3686, doi:10.3390/cancers12123686 . . . . **161**

Anthony Howell, Ashu Gandhi, Sacha Howell, Mary Wilson, Anthony Maxwell, Susan Astley, Michelle Harvie, Mary Pegington, Lester Barr, Andrew Baildam, Elaine Harkness, Penelope Hopwood, Julie Wisely, Andrea Wilding, Rosemary Greenhalgh, Jenny Affen, Andrew Maurice, Sally Cole, Julia Wiseman, Fiona Lalloo, David P. French and D. Gareth Evans
Long-Term Evaluation of Women Referred to a Breast Cancer Family History Clinic (Manchester UK 1987–2020)
Reprinted from: *Cancers* **2020**, *12*, 3697, doi:10.3390/cancers12123697 . . . . **183**

Rafah Alnafakh, Gabriele Saretzki, Angela Midgley, James Flynn, Areege M. Kamal, Lucy Dobson, Purushothaman Natarajan, Helen Stringfellow, Pierre Martin-Hirsch, Shandya B. DeCruze, Sarah E. Coupland and Dharani K. Hapangama
Aberrant Dyskerin Expression Is Related to Proliferation and Poor Survival in Endometrial Cancer
Reprinted from: *Cancers* **2021**, *13*, 273, doi:10.3390/cancers13020273 . . . . **203**

Kelechi Njoku, Amy E. Campbell, Bethany Geary, Michelle L. MacKintosh, Abigail E. Derbyshire, Sarah J. Kitson, Vanitha N. Sivalingam, Andrew Pierce, Anthony D. Whetton and Emma J. Crosbie
Metabolomic Biomarkers for the Detection of Obesity-Driven Endometrial Cancer
Reprinted from: *Cancers* **2021**, *13*, 718, doi:10.3390/cancers13040718 . . . . **223**

Jatinderpal Kalsi, Aleksandra Gentry-Maharaj, Andy Ryan, Naveena Singh, Matthew Burnell, Susan Massingham, Sophia Apostolidou, Aarti Sharma, Karin Williamson, Mourad Seif, Tim Mould, Robert Woolas, Stephen Dobbs, Simon Leeson, Lesley Fallowfield, Steven J. Skates, Mahesh Parmar, Stuart Campbell, Ian Jacobs, Alistair McGuire and Usha Menon
Performance Characteristics of the Ultrasound Strategy during Incidence Screening in the UK Collaborative Trial of Ovarian Cancer Screening (UKCTOCS)
Reprinted from: *Cancers* **2021**, *13*, 858, doi:10.3390/ cancers13040858 . . . . **247**

Olga Kondrashova, Jannah Shamsani, Tracy A. O'Mara, Felicity Newell, Amy E. McCart Reed, Sunil R. Lakhani, Judy Kirk, John V. Pearson, Nicola Waddell and Amanda B. Spurdle
Tumor Signature Analysis Implicates Hereditary Cancer Genes in Endometrial Cancer Development
Reprinted from: *Cancers* **2021**, *13*, 1762, doi:10.3390/cancers13081762 . . . . **261**

Eleni Leventea, Elaine F. Harkness, Adam R. Brentnall, Anthony Howell, D. Gareth Evans and Michelle Harvie
Is Breast Cancer Risk Associated with Menopausal Hormone Therapy Modified by Current or Early Adulthood BMI or Age of First Pregnancy?
Reprinted from: *Cancers* **2021**, *13*, 2710, doi:10.3390/cancers13112710 . . . . **277**

Emma C. Atakpa, Adam R. Brentnall, Susan Astley, Jack Cuzick, D. Gareth Evans, Ruth M. L. Warren, Anthony Howell and Michelle Harvie
The Relationship between Body Mass Index and Mammographic Density during a Premenopausal Weight Loss Intervention Study
Reprinted from: *Cancers* **2021**, *13*, 3245, doi:10.3390/cancers13133245 . . . . **293**

Dhivya Chandrasekaran, Monika Sobocan, Oleg Blyuss, Rowan E. Miller, Olivia Evans, Shanthini M. Crusz, Tina Mills-Baldock, Li Sun, Rory F. L. Hammond, Faiza Gaba, Lucy A. Jenkins, Munaza Ahmed, Ajith Kumar, Arjun Jeyarajah, Alexandra C. Lawrence, Elly Brockbank, Saurabh Phadnis, Mary Quigley, Fatima El Khouly, Rekha Wuntakal, Asma Faruqi, Giorgia Trevisan, Laura Casey, George J. Burghel, Helene Schlecht, Michael Bulman, Philip Smith, Naomi L. Bowers, Rosa Legood, Michelle Lockley, Andrew Wallace, Naveena Singh, D. Gareth Evans and Ranjit Manchanda
Implementation of Multigene Germline and Parallel Somatic Genetic Testing in Epithelial Ovarian Cancer: SIGNPOST Study
Reprinted from: *Cancers* **2021**, *13*, 4344, doi:10.3390/cancers13174344 . . . . **309**

About the Editor

Ranjit Manchanda Professor of Gynaecological Oncology and Consultant Gynaecological Oncologist. Co-Lead Cancer Prevention Unit, Director Graduate Studies, Wolfson Institute of Population Health, Queen Mary University of London, London, UK. NHS Innovation Accelerator (NIA) Fellow: Honorary Professor, Department of Health Services Research, Faculty of Public Health & Policy, London School of Hygiene & Tropical Medicine, London, UK; Integrated Academic Training Programme Director, London Specialty School of Obstetrics & Gynaecology, Health Education England, London, UK; Specialty Research Lead for Gynaecological Cancer, NIHR North Thames Clinical Research Network, London, UK; Research interests: focused around Targeted Precision Prevention. This includes population-based germline testing, mainstreaming genetic testing and precision medicine approaches for risk prediction, stratification, targeted screening and cancer prevention along with health economic issues related to these areas.

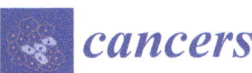

Editorial

Special Issue "Gynaecological Cancers Risk: Breast Cancer, Ovarian Cancer and Endometrial Cancer"

Ranjit Manchanda [1,2,3]

1. Wolfson Institute of Population Health, Queen Mary University of London, London EC1M 6BQ, UK; r.manchanda@qmul.ac.uk
2. Department of Gynaecological Oncology, Barts Health NHS Trust, Whitechapel Road, London E1 1BB, UK
3. Department of Health Services Research, Faculty of Public Health & Policy, London School of Hygiene & Tropical Medicine, London WC1E 7HT, UK

Over the last decade there have been significant advances and developments in our understanding of factors affecting women's cancer risk, our ability to identify individuals at increased risk and risk stratify populations, as well as implement and evaluate strategies for screening and prevention. This special issue of *Cancers (Basel)*, through a series of 13 original articles and three reviews, captures some of the important advances in cancer risk, genetic testing, risk management, screening and prevention of breast, ovarian and endometrial cancers.

Our understanding of the genetic risk of ovarian cancer has significantly improved over the last decade. Pavanello et al. [1] provide an overview of the genetic landscape of ovarian cancer and summarise the evidence and estimates of various rare pathogenic variants (PVs) associated with an increased risk of ovarian cancer. Gaba et al. [2] provide pilot data from the first population-based testing implementation study, providing personalised ovarian cancer risk estimates to general population women. They demonstrate that this approach of personalised population-based OC risk stratification is feasible, acceptable, has high satisfaction, reduces cancer worry/risk perception and does not negatively impact psycho-social well-being or quality of life. This sets the stage for larger implementation studies to follow. In a randomised experimental survey of general population women, Gallagher et al. [3] show that women are willing to undergo risk reducing surgery to reduce their ovarian cancer risk at a range of risk levels and that uptake rates are similar for 5–10% and >10% life time ovarian cancer risks. For the first time, Manchanda et al. [4] demonstrate the cost-effectiveness of population-based *BRCA* testing across multiple high income and upper middle income countries health systems (USA, UK, Netherlands, China and Brazil). This strategy could prevent tens of thousands more breast and ovarian cancers than the current family history-based clinical approach. While this is potentially cost-saving for high income countries, genetic testing costs need to fall further for this to be cost-effective for low income countries. Kalsi et al. [5] show that an annual ultrasound-based screening strategy for ovarian cancer is not suitable as it misses 37.5% of cancers and does not downstage disease. Ovarian cancer screening using the Ca125 biomarker alone also has not demonstrated a mortality benefit [6]. Gentry-Maharaj et al. [7] evaluate the potential for using multi-marker longitudinal algorithms incorporating Ca125, HE4, CA72-4 and anti-TP53 autoantibodies for general population screening for ovarian cancer in post-menopausal women. However, none of the combinations improved the performance of using longitudinal Ca125 alone. Screening for ovarian cancer remains a conundrum which requires further research. Funston et al. [8] systematically evaluate various diagnostic tools used for early diagnosis of ovarian cancer in symptomatic women. Four tools with similar moderate accuracy are described and areas for further research are highlighted. Chandrasekaran et al. [9] demonstrate the importance of implementing parallel panel germline and somatic testing for women at ovarian cancer diagnosis. A panel-based approach increases the yield of PVs

Citation: Manchanda, R. Special Issue "Gynaecological Cancers Risk: Breast Cancer, Ovarian Cancer and Endometrial Cancer". *Cancers* **2022**, *14*, 319. https://doi.org/10.3390/cancers14020319

Received: 29 December 2021
Accepted: 3 January 2022
Published: 10 January 2022

Publisher's Note: MDPI stays neutral with regard to jurisdictional claims in published maps and institutional affiliations.

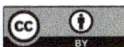

Copyright: © 2022 by the author. Licensee MDPI, Basel, Switzerland. This article is an open access article distributed under the terms and conditions of the Creative Commons Attribution (CC BY) license (https://creativecommons.org/licenses/by/4.0/).

and parallel testing identifies large genomic rearrangements that would have otherwise been missed. Kondrashova et al. [10], using tumor signature analysis, highlighted a number of inheritable cancer susceptibility genes which may be associated with the development of endometrial cancer. Njoku et al. [11] provide initial evidence supporting a potential lipid biomarker-based strategy for endometrial cancer screening in women with elevated body mass index (BMI) who are at an increased risk of this disease. Alnafakh et al. [12] highlight that dyskerrin may be a regulator for endometrial cancer proliferation and a prognostic marker, opening up avenues for further research in this area. Dibden et al. [13] undertook a worldwide review and meta-analysis of cohort studies evaluating mammography-based breast cancer screening programmes, and found a 22% reduction in breast cancer mortality. Atakpa et al. [14] evaluated the association of weight loss (using diet and exercise) for breast cancer risk reduction with changes in breast density in pre-menopausal women. While short-term reduction in BMI is associated with a reduction in fatty breast tissue, it was not associated with changes in glandular or dense breast tissue, indicating that breast density may not capture any weight-loss associated reduction in breast cancer risk. Leventea et al. [15], using data from the PROCAS (Predicting Risk of Cancer at Screening) study, showed that while menopausal hormone therapy was associated with a higher risk of breast cancer, the risk is attenuated by an increase in BMI and adjusting for current BMI, the effect of hormonal therapy was not modified by early BMI or age of first pregnancy. Trebo et al. [16] establish that high Galectin-7 and low Galectin-8 expression are poor prognostic markers for breast cancer, highlighting the need for more research to comprehend the role of galectins in the regulation and interaction of tumor cells and macrophages. Howell et al. [17] describe risk assessment and management outcomes of one of the largest cohorts of women (14,311) seen in a tertiary-level high-risk service for women at increased risk of breast cancer.

GLOBOCAN data predict that breast, ovarian and endometrial cancer cases will increase by 47–53% and deaths by 58–71%, respectively, over the next 20 years [18]. A total of 70–90% of healthcare expenditure is directed at chronic disease management of which cancers is the second most common cause [19,20]. Improving primary and secondary prevention of cancers and other chronic diseases, will be critical for the future viability of our health systems. This issue makes an important contribution to the huge and swiftly advancing knowledge base across the area of ovarian, endometrial and breast cancer risk prediction, screening, prevention and personalised medicine. Greater funding and research efforts need to be directed towards screening and cancer prevention.

Funding: This research received no external funding.

Conflicts of Interest: The author declares no conflict of interest.

References

1. Pavanello, M.; Chan, I.H.; Ariff, A.; Pharoah, P.D.; Gayther, S.A.; Ramus, S.J. Rare Germline Genetic Variants and the Risks of Epithelial Ovarian Cancer. *Cancers* **2020**, *12*, 3046. [CrossRef] [PubMed]
2. Gaba, F.; Blyuss, O.; Liu, X.; Goyal, S.; Lahoti, N.; Chandrasekaran, D.; Kurzer, M.; Kalsi, J.; Sanderson, S.; Lanceley, A.; et al. Population Study of Ovarian Cancer Risk Prediction for Targeted Screening and Prevention. *Cancers* **2020**, *12*, 1241. [CrossRef] [PubMed]
3. Gallagher, A.; Waller, J.; Manchanda, R.; Jacobs, I.; Sanderson, S. Women's Intentions to Engage in Risk-Reducing Behaviours after Receiving Personal Ovarian Cancer Risk Information: An Experimental Survey Study. *Cancers* **2020**, *12*, 3543. [CrossRef] [PubMed]
4. Manchanda, R.; Sun, L.; Patel, S.; Evans, O.; Wilschut, J.; De Freitas Lopes, A.C.; Gaba, F.; Brentnall, A.; Duffy, S.; Cui, B.; et al. Economic Evaluation of Population-Based BRCA1/BRCA2 Mutation Testing across Multiple Countries and Health Systems. *Cancers* **2020**, *12*, 1929. [CrossRef] [PubMed]
5. Kalsi, J.; Gentry-Maharaj, A.; Ryan, A.; Singh, N.; Burnell, M.; Massingham, S.; Apostolidou, S.; Sharma, A.; Williamson, K.; Seif, M.; et al. Performance Characteristics of the Ultrasound Strategy during Incidence Screening in the UK Collaborative Trial of Ovarian Cancer Screening (UKCTOCS). *Cancers* **2021**, *13*, 858. [CrossRef] [PubMed]

6. Menon, U.; Gentry-Maharaj, A.; Burnell, M.; Singh, N.; Ryan, A.; Karpinskyj, C.; Carlino, G.; Taylor, J.; Massingham, S.K.; Raikou, M.; et al. Ovarian cancer population screening and mortality after long-term follow-up in the UK Collaborative Trial of Ovarian Cancer Screening (UKCTOCS): A randomised controlled trial. *Lancet* **2021**, *397*, 2182–2193. [CrossRef]
7. Gentry-Maharaj, A.; Blyuss, O.; Ryan, A.; Burnell, M.; Karpinskyj, C.; Gunu, R.; Kalsi, J.K.; Dawnay, A.; Marino, I.P.; Manchanda, R.; et al. Multi-Marker Longitudinal Algorithms Incorporating HE4 and CA125 in Ovarian Cancer Screening of Postmenopausal Women. *Cancers* **2020**, *12*, 1931. [CrossRef] [PubMed]
8. Funston, G.; Hardy, V.; Abel, G.; Crosbie, E.J.; Emery, J.; Hamilton, W.; Walter, F.M. Identifying Ovarian Cancer in Symptomatic Women: A Systematic Review of Clinical Tools. *Cancers* **2020**, *12*, 3686. [CrossRef] [PubMed]
9. Chandrasekaran, D.; Sobocan, M.; Blyuss, O.; Miller, R.E.; Evans, O.; Crusz, S.M.; Mills-Baldock, T.; Sun, L.; Hammond, R.F.L.; Gaba, F.; et al. Implementation of Multigene Germline and Parallel Somatic Genetic Testing in Epithelial Ovarian Cancer: SIGNPOST Study. *Cancers* **2021**, *13*, 4344. [CrossRef] [PubMed]
10. Kondrashova, O.; Shamsani, J.; O'Mara, T.A.; Newell, F.; McCart Reed, A.E.; Lakhani, S.R.; Kirk, J.; Pearson, J.V.; Waddell, N.; Spurdle, A.B. Tumor Signature Analysis Implicates Hereditary Cancer Genes in Endometrial Cancer Development. *Cancers* **2021**, *13*, 1762. [CrossRef] [PubMed]
11. Njoku, K.; Campbell, A.E.; Geary, B.; MacKintosh, M.L.; Derbyshire, A.E.; Kitson, S.J.; Sivalingam, V.N.; Pierce, A.; Whetton, A.D.; Crosbie, E.J. Metabolomic Biomarkers for the Detection of Obesity-Driven Endometrial Cancer. *Cancers* **2021**, *13*, 718. [CrossRef] [PubMed]
12. Alnafakh, R.; Saretzki, G.; Midgley, A.; Flynn, J.; Kamal, A.M.; Dobson, L.; Natarajan, P.; Stringfellow, H.; Martin-Hirsch, P.; DeCruze, S.B.; et al. Aberrant Dyskerin Expression Is Related to Proliferation and Poor Survival in Endometrial Cancer. *Cancers* **2021**, *13*, 273. [CrossRef] [PubMed]
13. Dibden, A.; Offman, J.; Duffy, S.W.; Gabe, R. Worldwide Review and Meta-Analysis of Cohort Studies Measuring the Effect of Mammography Screening Programmes on Incidence-Based Breast Cancer Mortality. *Cancers* **2020**, *12*, 976. [CrossRef] [PubMed]
14. Atakpa, E.C.; Brentnall, A.R.; Astley, S.; Cuzick, J.; Evans, D.G.; Warren, R.M.L.; Howell, A.; Harvie, M. The Relationship between Body Mass Index and Mammographic Density during a Premenopausal Weight Loss Intervention Study. *Cancers* **2021**, *13*, 3245. [CrossRef] [PubMed]
15. Leventea, E.; Harkness, E.F.; Brentnall, A.R.; Howell, A.; Evans, D.G.; Harvie, M. Is Breast Cancer Risk Associated with Menopausal Hormone Therapy Modified by Current or Early Adulthood BMI or Age of First Pregnancy? *Cancers* **2021**, *13*, 2710. [CrossRef] [PubMed]
16. Trebo, A.; Ditsch, N.; Kuhn, C.; Heidegger, H.H.; Zeder-Goess, C.; Kolben, T.; Czogalla, B.; Schmoeckel, E.; Mahner, S.; Jeschke, U.; et al. High Galectin-7 and Low Galectin-8 Expression and the Combination of both are Negative Prognosticators for Breast Cancer Patients. *Cancers* **2020**, *12*, 953. [CrossRef] [PubMed]
17. Howell, A.; Gandhi, A.; Howell, S.; Wilson, M.; Maxwell, A.; Astley, S.; Harvie, M.; Pegington, M.; Barr, L.; Baildam, A.; et al. Long-Term Evaluation of Women Referred to a Breast Cancer Family History Clinic (Manchester UK 1987–2020). *Cancers* **2020**, *12*, 3697. [CrossRef] [PubMed]
18. International Agency for Research on Cancer. Cancer Tomorrow. In *A Tool That Predicts the Future Cancer Incidence and Mortality Burden Worldwide from the Current Estimates in 2018 Up until 2040*; International Agency for Research on Cancer (IARC): Lyon, France, 2018.
19. Department of Health Long Term Conditions Team. *Long Term Conditions Compendium of Information*, 3rd ed.; Department of Health: Leeds, UK, 2012. Available online: https://www.gov.uk/government/uploads/system/uploads/attachment_data/file/216528/dh_134486.pdf (accessed on 28 December 2021).
20. Murphy, S.L.; Xu, J.Q.; Kochanek, K.D.; Curtin, S.C.; Arias, E. Deaths: Final Data for 2015. *Natl. Vital Stat. Rep.* **2017**, *66*. Available online: https://www.cdc.gov/nchs/data/nvsr/nvsr66/nvsr66_06.pdf (accessed on 28 December 2021).

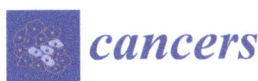

Article

High Galectin-7 and Low Galectin-8 Expression and the Combination of both are Negative Prognosticators for Breast Cancer Patients

Anna Trebo [1,†], Nina Ditsch [1,2,†], Christina Kuhn [1], Helene Hildegard Heidegger [1], Christine Zeder-Goess [1], Thomas Kolben [1], Bastian Czogalla [1], Elisa Schmoeckel [3], Sven Mahner [1], Udo Jeschke [1,2,*] and Anna Hester [1]

1. Department of Obstetrics and Gynecology, University Hospital, Ludwig-Maximilans-Universität (LMU) Munich, 81377 Munich, Germany; Anna.trebo@campus.lmu.de (A.T.); nina.ditsch@uk-augsburg.de (N.D.); christina.kuhn@med.uni-muenchen.de (C.K.); helene.heidegger@med.uni-muenchen.de (H.H.H.); christine.goess@med.uni-muenchen.de (C.Z.-G.); thomas.kolben@med.uni-muenchen.de (T.K.); bastian.czogalla@med.uni-muenchen.de (B.C.); sven.mahner@med.uni-muenchen.de (S.M.); anna.hester@med.uni-muenchen.de (A.H.)
2. Department of Obstetrics and Gynecology, University Hospital Augsburg, 86156 Augsburg, Germany
3. Institute of Pathology, LMU Munich, 81377 Munich, Germany; elisa.schmoeckel@med.uni-muenchen.de
* Correspondence: udo.jeschke@med.uni-muenchen.de; Tel.: +49-89-4400-54240; Fax: +49-89-4400-54916
† These authors contributed equally to this work.

Received: 11 February 2020; Accepted: 8 April 2020; Published: 12 April 2020

Abstract: Galectins are commonly overexpressed in cancer cells and their expression pattern is often associated with the aggressiveness and metastatic phenotype of the tumor. This study investigates the prognostic influence of the expression of galectin-7 (Gal-7) and galectin-8 (Gal-8) in tumor cell cytoplasm, nucleus and on surrounding immune cells. Primary breast cancer tissue of 235 patients was analyzed for the expression of Gal-7 and Gal-8 and correlated with clinical and pathological data and the outcome. To identify immune cell subpopulations, immunofluorescence double staining was performed. Significant correlations of Gal-7 expression in the cytoplasm with HER2-status, PR status, patient age and grading, and of Gal-8 expression in the cytoplasm with HER2-status and patient age and of both galectins between each other were found. A high Gal-7 expression in the cytoplasm was a significant independent prognosticator for an impaired progression free survival (PFS) ($p = 0.017$) and distant disease-free survival (DDFS) ($p = 0.030$). Gal-7 was also expressed by tumor-infiltrating macrophages. High Gal-8 expression in the cytoplasm was associated with a significantly improved overall survival (OS) ($p = 0.032$). Clinical outcome in patients showing both high Gal-7 and with low Gal-8 expression was very poor. Further understanding of the role of galectins in the regulation and interaction of tumor cells and macrophages is essential for finding new therapeutic targets.

Keywords: breast cancer; galectins; galectin-7; galectin-8; prognostic markers; tumor infiltrating macrophages

1. Introduction

Breast cancer is one of the three most prevalent cancers worldwide and the most frequent malignant tumor in women [1]. In 2018, about 2.1 million female patients were diagnosed with breast cancer and it represented the leading cause of tumor-related deaths in over 100 countries [2].

Based on gene profiling studies, breast cancer can be classified into different intrinsic subtypes [3]. In daily clinical practice, a surrogate system based on immunohistochemical and molecular characteristics is generally used: luminal A-like tumors show a strong expression of estrogen (ER) and progesterone (PR) receptors, low proliferation rates and a good prognosis. Luminal B-like human epidermal growth factor receptor 2 (HER2), and negative tumors show a lower hormone receptor expression and higher grading than Luminal A-like tumors and have an intermediate prognosis. Tumors that show an amplification of HER2 can be further classified based on hormone receptor expression in Luminal B-like HER2+ and in HER2+ non-luminal tumors. Triple negative breast cancers (TNBC) lack the expression of both hormone receptors and HER2, and show the worst prognosis of all breast cancer subtypes [3,4]. Even though therapy has improved in recent years, [1] new therapeutic strategies aiming at specific targets are needed [5–7]. This is especially important for TNBC, because patients still have a poor outcome and cannot be treated with endocrine therapy or targeted therapies like anti-HER2-therapy [8].

The discovery of galectins in 1994 [9,10] led to investigations on their impact on tumor development, progression and metastasis [11]. Galectins are a group of proteins able to bind to β-galactoside-binding sugars, either by N-linked or O-linked glycosylation, and they share primary structural homology in their carbohydrate-recognition domains (CRDs) [10]. A total of 12 different human galectin coding genes were found, including two for galectin-9 [12]. Galectins are divided into the subgroups of dimeric galectins (galectin-1,-2,-7,-10,-13,-14) with two identical CRD subunits, tandem galectins (galectin-4,-8,-9,-12) with two distinct CRD subunits, and chimeric galectins (galectin-3) with one or even multiple subunits of the same type [10,12]. Galectins are commonly overexpressed in cancer cells and cancer-associated stromal cells [13]. This altered galectin expression often correlates with the aggressiveness of the tumor and the metastatic phenotype [14]. In breast cancer, a connection between diverse galectin expression patterns and different cancer characteristics—like a correlation of galectin-1 (Gal-1) expression with tumor grading—was found [11,15]. Recently, the role of Gal-1 and galectin-3 (Gal-3) was thoroughly investigated [14]. Silencing Gal-1 led to both impaired tumor growth and reduced metastasis in a breast cancer mouse model [16]. Furthermore, it was found that Gal-1 interacts with E-selectin and influences adhesion [17]. However, targeting Gal-1 still has not come to clinical practice because no strategy of a fully specific Gal-1 blocking has been established yet. Gal-3 was identified as a molecular signature of breast cancer [18] and also as a potential therapeutic target [19]. Galectin-9, however, was described as anti-tumorigenic with possible antimetastatic potential in breast cancer [20]. Galectin-7 (Gal-7), like Gal-1 and Gal-3, seems to have tumor-promoting effects: in a Gal-7 deficient mouse model, a delayed development of HER2+ breast cancer was observed. Further investigations showed a positive correlation of Gal-7 expression with the frequency of HER2+ breast cancer. Furthermore, an association of Gal-7 expression with increased lymph node axillary metastasis in HER2+ tumors was seen [21,22]. Another study revealed an augmented Gal-7 expression in aggressive molecular subtypes, notably in estrogen receptor negative breast cancer and in cell lines with a basal-like phenotype. High expression of Gal-7 caused a higher metastatic risk, rendering cancer cells more resistant to apoptosis in a mouse model. Gal-7 might be part of the p53-promoted cancer progression pathway [23]. It is not known if these effects are specific to Gal-7, as most of the studies focused on one galectin and did not compare all individual galectins with each other. There is no detailed analysis of all galectins and their specific effects in breast cancer and most galectins, like galectin-8 (Gal-8), have not been studied in detail. There are only limited data suggesting that silencing a Gal-8-dependent pathway might lead to impaired tumor growth, especially in TNBC [24].

In this study, the specific role of Gal-7 and Gal-8 in a bigger cohort of human primary non-metastatic breast cancer was evaluated. The analysis included the specific location of galectin expression in the nucleus or cytoplasm and the expression in tumor-surrounding immune cells.

2. Results

2.1. Gal-7 and Gal-8 Expression in Breast Cancer and Correlation to Different Clinical and Pathological Characteristics

2.1.1. Gal-7 and Gal-8 Expression in Breast Cancer Cytoplasm and Nucleus

Expression of both galectins was observed in the cytoplasm as well as in the nucleus, being more pronounced for Gal-7. Gal-7 expression could not be evaluated in 19 sections (due to technical issues). Seven cases showed no Gal-7 expression in the cytoplasm and 35 no staining in the nucleus. For Gal-8, 20 tissue sections could not be analyzed (due to technical issues), and 15 and 63 samples revealed no staining in the cytoplasm and in the nucleus, respectively. The distribution of the immunoreactivity score (IRS) for the staining in the cytoplasm and in the nucleus is shown in Table 1; Table 2. The mean IRS for staining in the cytoplasm was 4.88 for Gal-7 and 4.37 for Gal-8, while it was 2.51 for staining in the nucleus for Gal-7 and 2.56 for Gal-8.

Table 1. Staining results of Gal-7 in the cytoplasm and the nucleus. Gal = galectin; NA = not applicable; IRS = immunoreactivity score.

Gal-7 Cytoplasm			Gal-7 Nucleus		
IRS	n	%	IRS	n	%
0	7	3.0	0	35	14.9
1	2	0.9	1	17	7.2
2	43	18.3	2	64	27.2
3	21	8.9	3	51	21.7
4	40	17.0	4	25	10.6
6	60	25.5	6	24	10.2
8	27	11.5	NA	19	8.1
9	8	3.4	total	235	100.0
12	8	3.4			
NA	19	8.1			
total	235	100.0			

Table 2. Staining results of Gal-8 in the cytoplasm and the nucleus. Gal = galectin; NA = not applicable; IRS = immunoreactivity score.

Gal-8 Cytoplasm			Gal-8 Nucleus		
IRS	n	%	IRS	n	%
0	15	6.4	0	63	26.8
1	12	5.1	1	14	6.0
2	50	21.3	2	55	23.4
3	27	11.5	3	7	3.0
4	18	7.7	4	43	18.3
6	54	23.0	6	22	9.4
8	16	6.8	8	1	0.4
9	18	7.7	9	9	3.8
12	5	2.1	12	1	0.4
NA	20	8.5	NA	20	8.5
total	235	100.0	total	235	100.0

2.1.2. Gal-7 and Gal-8 Expression and Correlation with Clinical Characteristics, Histopathological Breast Cancer Subtypes and Grading

Both Gal-7 and Gal-8 expression in the cytoplasm and in the nucleus did not correlate with the clinical parameters: tumor size and lymph node status. Gal-7 and Gal-8 expression in the cytoplasm correlated negatively with patient age (see Spearman correlation analyses in Supplementary Data: Tables S1 and S2).

The Gal-7 expression correlated negatively with the histopathological subtype. Kruskal–Wallis test and boxplots analysis showed that Gal-7 expression in the cytoplasm was significantly higher in no special type (NST) tumors compared to non-NST tumors (median IRS 6 in NST vs. 4 in non-NST, $p < 0.001$) (Figure 1a). Similarly, Gal-7 expression in the nucleus was significantly higher in NST tumors ($p = 0.042$). The Gal-8 expression did not differ concerning the histological subtype.

Regarding tumor grading, a positive correlation with the cytoplasmic Gal-7 expression was found (Spearman correlation analysis in Table S1). Kruskal–Wallis test showed that Gal-7 expression in the cytoplasm was higher in higher tumor grading (Gal-7 in G1 median IRS 3 and in G2/3 median IRS 6, $p = 0.003$, Figure 1b). The Gal-7 expression in the nucleus and the Gal-8 expression in the cytoplasm were not associated with tumor grading. The Gal-8 expression in the nucleus correlated negatively with the tumor grading and showed a trend towards a lower IRS in higher tumor grading ($p = 0.089$). Exemplary immunohistochemical Gal-7 and Gal-8 staining in tumors with different gradings are shown in Figure 2.

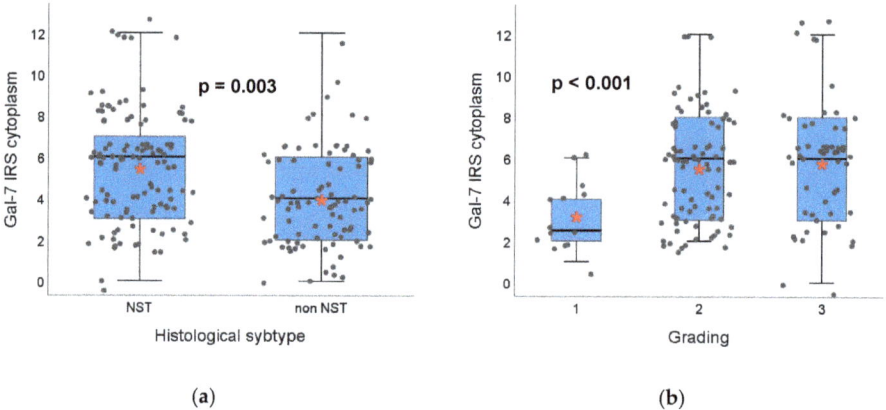

(a) (b)

Figure 1. Association of Gal-7 expression with histological subtype and tumor grading. Boxplots of the median IRS of Gal-7 staining in the cytoplasm dependent on histological subtype (a) and tumor grading (b) of the tumor are shown. (a) In non-NST tumors, Gal-7 expression in the cytoplasm is significantly lower than in NST tumors. (b) Tumors with G2/3 grading show a significantly higher Gal-7 expression in the cytoplasm compared to G1 tumors. Red asterisks indicate means. Please note that individual datapoints have been jittered to avoid overlap.

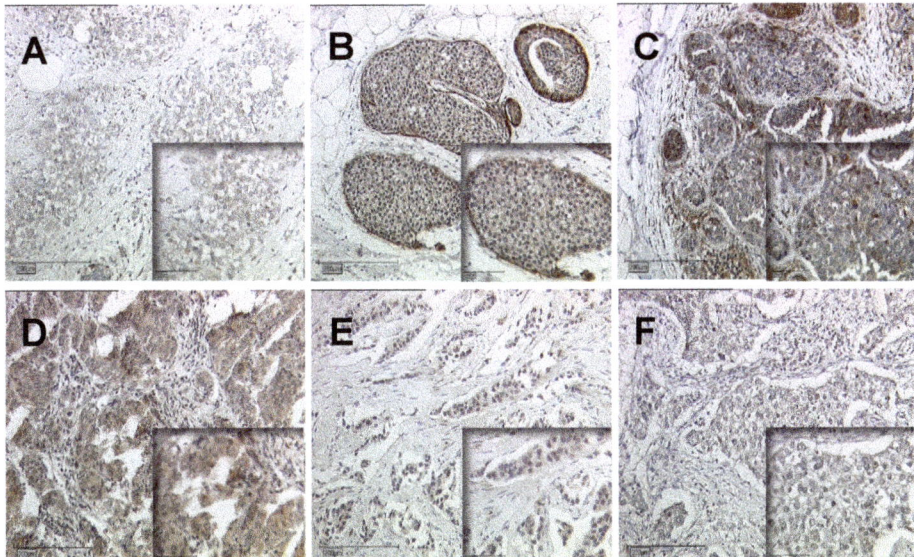

Figure 2. Gal-7 and Gal-8 expression dependent on tumor grading. Exemplary immunohistochemical staining of Gal-7 in grade 1 (**A**), 2 (**B**), and 3 (**C**) tumors and of Gal-8 in grade 1 (**D**), 2 (**E**), 3 (**F**) tumors are shown. Magnification: main images x10, image sections x25.

2.1.3. Gal-7 and Gal-8 Expression and Correlation with Hormone Receptor Status, HER2 Amplification and Surrogate Intrinsic Subtypes

Spearman analysis revealed that Gal-7 expression in the cytoplasm did correlate to PR-status and Gal-8 expression in the nucleus to ER-status (Spearman analysis in Tables S1 and S2). In the Kruskal–Wallis analysis, the Gal-7 staining in the cytoplasm was significantly higher in PR-negative compared to PR-positive tumors (median IRS in PR-positive: 4 vs. in PR-negative: 6, $p = 0.038$, Figure 3b), but was not significantly different concerning ER-status ($p = 0.159$, Figure 3a). The Gal-8 expression in the nucleus was significantly higher in ER-positive tumors ($p = 0.026$, Figure 3c) and a trend towards a higher Gal-8 expression in PR-positive compared to PR-negative tumors was observed ($p = 0.098$, Figure 3d). Both Gal-7 expression in the nucleus and Gal-8 in the cytoplasm did not correlate with the ER- or PR-status.

Both Gal-7 and Gal-8 staining in the cytoplasm correlated significantly with the HER2-status (Spearman analysis in Tables S1 and S2). HER2-positive breast cancer samples showed a distinctly higher Gal-7 expression in the cytoplasm compared to HER2-negative tumor sections (median IRS in HER2+: 8 vs. in HER2-: 4, $p < 0.001$, Figure 3e). Gal-8 expression in the cytoplasm in HER2-positive tissue sections was significantly higher than in HER2-negative samples (median IRS in HER2+: 6 vs. in HER2-: 3, $p = 0.004$, Figure 3f). Gal-7 and Gal-8 staining in the nucleus were not significantly associated with HER2-status (Figure S1).

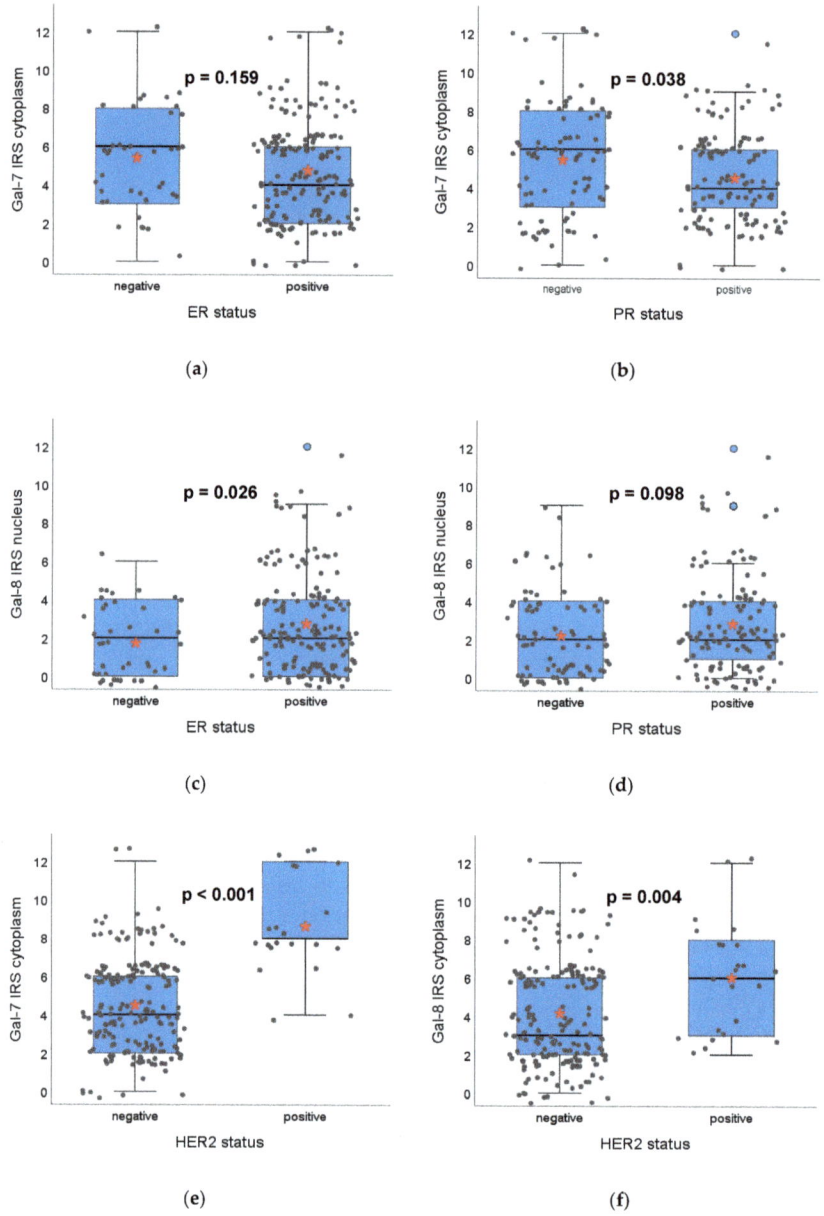

Figure 3. Association of Gal-7 and Gal-8 expression with the ER-, PR- and HER2-status. Boxplots of the median IRS of Gal-7 staining in the cytoplasm dependent on ER-status (**a**), PR-status (**b**) and HER2-status (**e**) and of Gal-8 staining in the nucleus dependent on ER-status (**c**) and PR-status (**d**) as well as Gal-8 staining in the cytoplasm dependent on HER2-status (**f**) are shown. ER-positive tumors do not differ concerning Gal-7 staining but show a higher Gal-8 staining. PR-positive tumors show lower Gal-7 staining and a trend towards higher Gal-8 staining. HER2-positive tumors show a significantly higher Gal-7 and Gal 8 expression in the cytoplasm compared to HER2-negative tumors. Staining in the nucleus does not show significant differences. Red asterisks indicate means. Please note that individual data points have been jittered to avoid overlap.

The Gal-7 expression in the cytoplasm differed significantly regarding the different surrogate intrinsic subtypes ($p < 0.001$) (Figure 4): HER2-positive tumors (both luminal B-like and non-luminal) clearly showed the highest Gal-7 expression in the cytoplasm compared to all other subtypes (Luminal A-like and B-like and TNBC). The distribution of Gal-8 staining, neither in the cytoplasm (Figure S2) nor in the nucleus, and Gal-7 expression in the nucleus in the different surrogate intrinsic subtypes showed no significant differences.

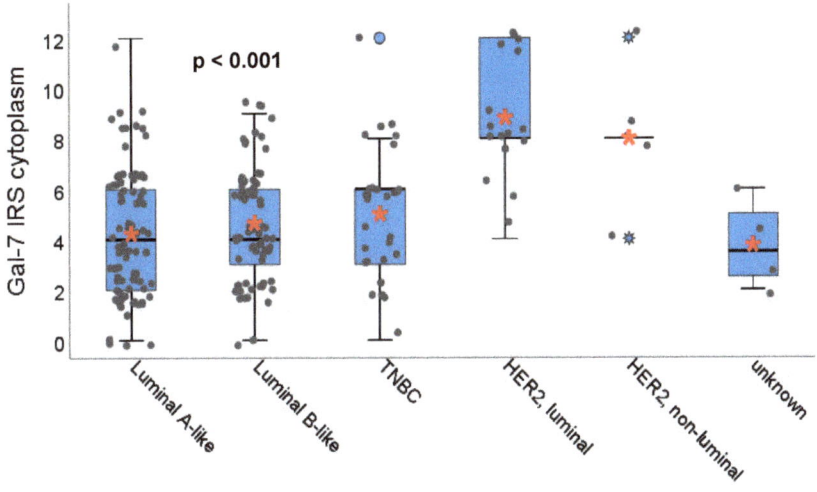

Figure 4. Association of Gal-7 expression with different surrogate intrinsic subtype. Boxplot of the median IRS of Gal-7 staining in the cytoplasm dependent on the surrogate intrinsic subtype of the tumor is shown. HER2-positive, both luminal and non-luminal tumors show a significantly higher Gal-7 expression in the cytoplasm compared to the other subtypes. Red asterisks indicate means. Please note that individual datapoints have been jittered to avoid overlap.

2.1.4. Correlation of Gal-7 and Gal-8 Expression

Gal-7 expression in the nucleus and cytoplasm correlated to each other as well as Gal-8 expression in the nucleus and cytoplasm (Table 3). Gal-7 and Gal-8 expressions in the nucleus and cytoplasm also correlated with each other.

2.2. Correlation of Gal-7 and Gal-8 Expression with Survival in Breast Cancer Patients

Median overall survival (OS), progression-free survival (PFS) and distant disease-free survival (DDFS) in the whole cohort was not reached (NR). The prognostic relevance of Gal-7 and -8 was analyzed concerning PFS, DDFS and OS and tumors were categorized in "high" and "low" expressing tumors using ROC-curve analysis.

2.2.1. High Gal-7 Expression in the Cytoplasm is a Negative Prognosticator for Survival in Breast Cancer Patients

High Gal-7 expression in the cytoplasm (IRS > 6) was associated with a worse outcome: tumors with high Gal-7 expression in the cytoplasm showed a significantly impaired PFS ($p = 0.017$, median PFS in Gal-7 high: 9.7 years, median PFS in Gal-7 low: NR) (Figure 5a) and DDFS ($p = 0.030$, median DDFS in both subgroups NR) (Figure 5b). Concerning OS, no significant difference was detected ($p = 0.927$, median OS in both subgroups NR) (Figure 5c).

Table 3. Spearman correlation analysis of Gal-7 and Gal-8 expression in the nucleus and cytoplasm. Significant correlations are displayed in bold. ** indicates a significance level of $p < 0.01$.

		Gal-7 IRS Cytoplasm	Gal-7 IRS Nucleus	Gal-8 IRS Cytoplasm	Gal-8 IRS Nucleus
Gal-7 IRS cytoplasm	Correlation Coefficient Sig. (2-tailed) N	1.000 216	0.467 ** <0.001 216	0.332 ** <0.001 206	0.188 ** 0.007 206
Gal-7 IRS nucleus	Correlation Coefficient Sig. (2-tailed) N	0.467 ** <0.001 216	1.000 216	0.185 ** 0.008 206	0.301 ** <0.001 206
Gal-8 IRS cytoplasm	Correlation Coefficient Sig. (2-tailed) N	0.332 ** <0.001 206	0.185 ** 0.008 206	1.000 215	0.594 ** 0.000 215
Gal-8 IRS nucleus	Correlation Coefficient Sig. (2-tailed) N	0.188 ** 0.007 206	0.301 ** <0.001 206	0.594 ** <0.001 215	1.000 215

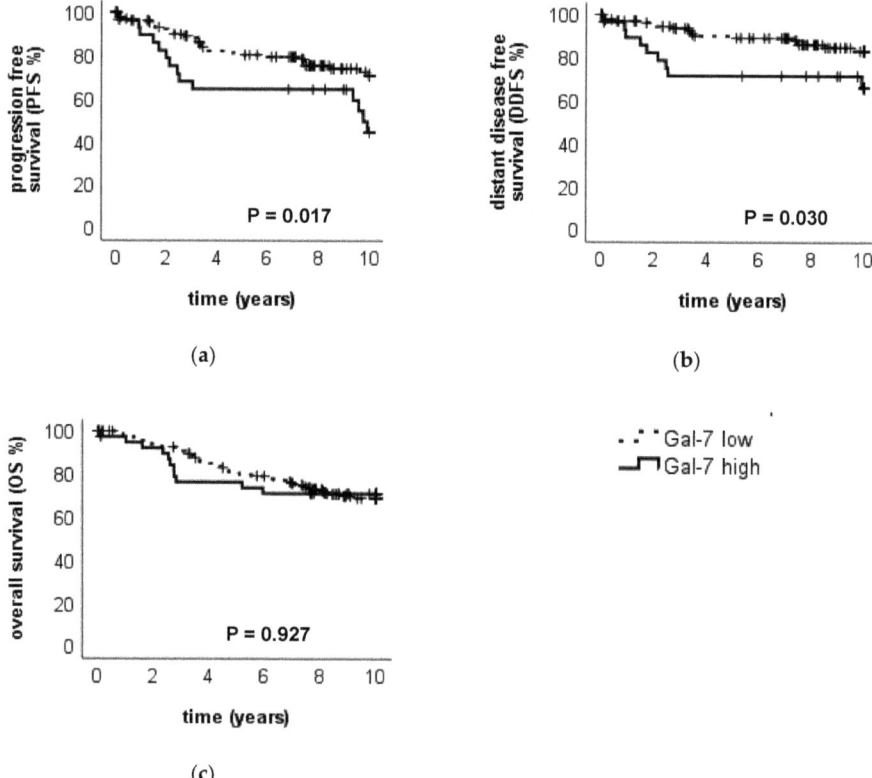

Figure 5. Association of Gal-7 expression in the cytoplasm to the clinical outcome. Kaplan–Meier analysis of PFS (a), DDFS (b) and OS (c) in Gal-7 high- and low-expressing tumors (in the cytoplasm) is shown. Tumors with high Gal-7 expression in the cytoplasm showed a significantly impaired PFS and DDFS.

Multivariate COX regression analysis revealed Gal-7 expression as an independent prognostic factor for PFS (Table 4) but not for DDFS (Table S3). Concerning OS, where Gal-7 was not significant in the univariate analysis, COX regression analysis revealed ER-status, nodal status and age as independent prognosticators (Table S4).

Table 4. Multivariate analysis of PFS concerning Gal 7 expression in the cytoplasm. Significant factors are highlighted in bold.

Prognostic Factor	B	SE	Wald	df	Sig.	Exp(B)	95,0% CI for Exp(B)	
							Lower	Upper
Histological subtype (NST vs. non-NST)	0.245	0.459	0.286	1	0.593	1.278	0.520	3.140
Grading (G1 vs. G2-3)	0.312	0.817	0.146	1	0.702	1.367	0.276	6.773
Tumor size (pT1 vs. pT2-4)	0.284	0.377	0.564	1	0.453	1.328	0.634	2.783
Nodal status (pN0 vs. pN1-3)	0.553	0.397	1.935	1	0.164	1.738	0.798	3.788
HER2 status (positive vs. negative)	−0.161	0.538	0.090	1	0.764	0.851	0.297	2.443
ER (positive vs. negative)	−0.823	0.459	3.219	1	0.073	0.439	0.179	1.079
PR (positive vs. negative)	−0.345	0.460	0.565	1	0.452	0.708	0.288	1.743
Patient age (continuous)	0.010	0.017	0.329	1	0.566	1.010	0.977	1.043
Gal-7 expression in the cytoplasm (high vs. low)	0.806	0.410	3.860	1	**0.049**	2.239	1.002	5.003

Subgroup analysis revealed that Gal-7 expression in the cytoplasm had prognostic relevance for an impaired PFS in the ER-negative (but not in ER-positive) ($p = 0.036$, median PFS in Gal-7 high 2.52 years, Figure S3), in the pT1 (but not in pT > 1) ($p = 0.014$) and in the pN0 (but not in pN > 0) ($p = 0.043$) subgroups. A trend towards an impaired PFS could be observed in PR positive (but not PR negative) ($p = 0.098$) and in HER2 positive (but not in HER2 negative) tumors ($p = 0.084$, Figure S4).

Gal-7 expression in the nucleus did not show prognostic relevance for PFS, DDFS or for the OS (Figure S5). Subgroup analysis did also not show any new prognostic relevance of nuclear Gal-7 expression concerning the subgroups of PR-positive vs. -negative, HER2-positive vs. -negative tumors, grading, tumor size and lymph node status. However, in ER-negative tumors, a high nuclear Gal-7 expression showed an impaired OS while nuclear Gal-7 expression was not relevant in ER-positive tumors even if statistical significance was not reached ($p = 0.082$. Similarly, a worse outcome regarding PFS could be seen in lower grading (G1, $p = 0.058$) (but not in G2-3) when nuclear Gal-7 expression was high.

2.2.2. High Gal-8 Expression in the Cytoplasm is a Positive Prognosticator for Overall Survival in Breast Cancer Patients

High Gal-8 expression in the cytoplasm (IRS > 5) was associated with an improved outcome: Tumors with a high Gal-8 expression in the cytoplasm showed a significantly improved OS compared to tumors with low Gal-8 expression in the cytoplasm ($p = 0.032$, median OS in both subgroups NR) (Figure 6a). No significance in the outcome regarding PFS ($p = 0.974$, median PFS in both subgroups NS, Figure 6b) and DDFS ($p = 0.138$, median DDFS in both subgroups NR, Figure 6c) was found.

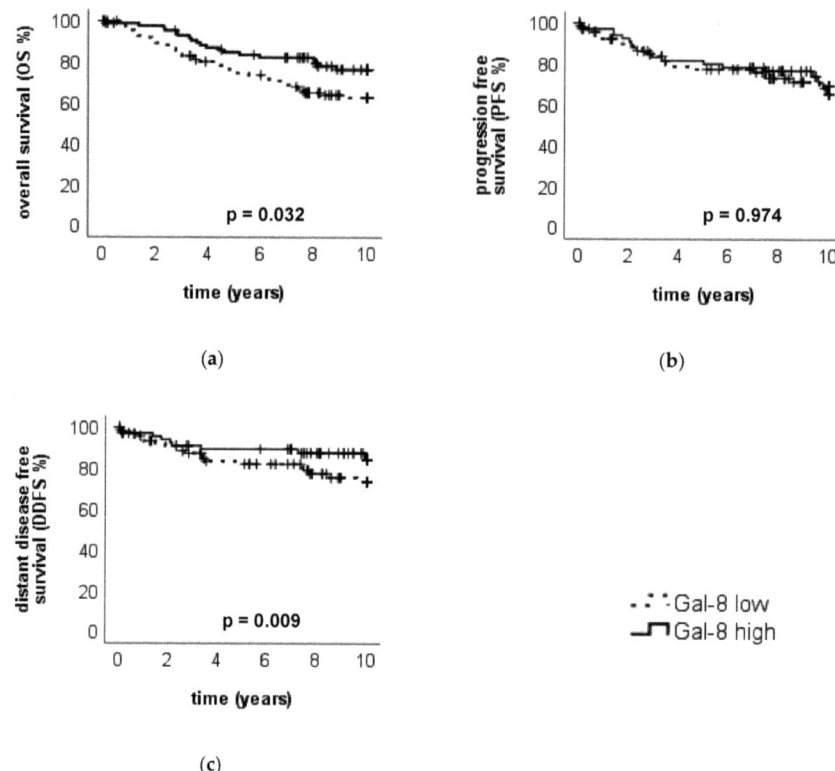

Figure 6. Association of Gal-8 expression in the cytoplasm to the clinical outcome. Kaplan–Meier analysis of OS (**a**), PFS (**b**) and DDFS (**c**) in Gal-8 high- and low-expressing tumors (in the cytoplasm) is shown. Tumors with high Gal-8 expression in the cytoplasm showed a significantly improved OS.

The multivariate COX regression analysis could not confirm Gal-8 expression in the cytoplasm as an independent prognostic factor (Table 5) for OS. In contrast, age at the surgery, ER status and lymph-node status (pN) were detected as independent prognosticators for the OS. Gal-8 was also not prognostically relevant in COX regression for PFS or DDFS.

Table 5. Cox regression analysis of prognostic factors for OS in breast cancer patients. Significant factors are highlighted in bold.

Prognostic Factor	B	SE	Wald	df	Sig.	Exp(B)	95,0% CI for Exp(B)	
							Lower	Upper
Histological subtype (NST vs. non-NST)	0.199	0.456	0.190	1	0.663	1.220	0.499	2.983
Grading (G1 vs. G2-3)	−0.321	0.591	0.295	1	0.587	0.725	0.228	2.311
Tumor size (pT1 vs. pT2-4)	0.237	0.385	0.378	1	0.539	1.267	0.596	2.693
Nodal status (pN0 vs. pN1-3)	1.144	0.406	7.927	1	**0.005**	3.140	1.416	6.964
HER2 status (positive vs. negative)	0.429	0.617	0.483	1	0.487	1.535	0.458	5.143
ER (positive vs. negative)	−1.178	0.504	5.466	1	**0.019**	0.308	0.115	0.827
PR (positive vs. negative)	0.568	0.483	1.381	1	0.240	1.765	0.684	4.551
Patient age (continuous)	0.051	0.017	9.367	1	**0.002**	1.053	1.019	1.088
Gal-8 expression in the cytoplasm (high vs. low)	−0.258	0.372	0.479	1	0.489	0.773	0.372	1.603

Subgroup analysis revealed that Gal-8 expression in the cytoplasm had prognostic relevance with a better outcome for the OS in NST (but not non-NST) tumors ($p = 0.049$), in HER2-negative (but not

HER2-positive) ($p = 0.029$, Figure S6) in ER-positive (but not ER-negative) ($p = 0.055$, Figure S7) and in pT1 (but not in pT2-4) ($p = 0.038$). Concerning PFS and DDFS, no significant prognostic impact could be found for Gal-8 in the different subgroups.

Similar to Gal-7 staining in the nucleus, Gal-8 staining in the nucleus did not show prognostic relevance for neither PFS, DDFS or OS (Figure S8). However, subgroup analysis revealed that high Gal-8 staining in the nucleus was associated with improved PFS in ER-positive patients ($p = 0.041$) but not in ER negative patients and to tendentially ($p = 0.081$) better OS in pT2-4 (but not in pT1) tumors. Regarding the other subgroups (PR-positive vs. -negative, HER2-positive vs. -negative, nodal status, histological subtype), nuclear Gal-8 staining did not show significant prognostic influence, similar to the overall cohort.

2.2.3. Survival Analysis Using Combined Gal-7 and Gal-8 Staining

Survival analysis was also performed in subgroups with high or low Gal-7 expression in the cytoplasm in combination with low or high Gal-8 expression in the cytoplasm, respectively. A high Gal-7 combined with a low Gal-8 expression in the cytoplasm was associated with an impaired OS compared to all other patients ($p = 0.201$, median OS in all subgroups NR, Figure 7a). When Gal-7 expression was high and Gal-8 was low, DDFS was significantly impaired ($p = 0.009$, median DDFS in all subgroups NR, Figure 7b) compared to the rest of the patients, as well as PFS with a borderline significance ($p = 0.067$, median PFS in all subgroups NR, Figure 7c). In summary, two different groups regarding the outcome could be defined: The first group, representing 6.8% of the patients, consisted of tumors expressing Gal-7 high (IRS > 6) and Gal-8 low (IRS ≤ 5) in the cytoplasm. This subgroup showed a poor OS. The second group, formed by 13.6% of the patients with high Gal-8 (IRS > 5) and low Gal-7 (IRS ≤ 6) expression in the cytoplasm, showed good OS (Figure 7a). Comparing the three subgroups concerning PFS and DDFS, the "advantageous" subgroup (high Gal-8, low Gal-7) seems to be less relevant (survival curves similar to the "others" subgroup, Figure S9).

2.2.4. Immune Cell Infiltration Stained with Gal-7

Gal-7 had an interesting expression pattern in the tumor tissue, with staining on only the outer layer of cancer cells and expression in the immune cells next to the tumor cells as well (Figure 8a–d). Gal-7 staining in the immune cells was not included as part of the IRS-scoring for the cancer specimen in the analyses described above. The immune cell staining of Gal-7 correlated significantly with the tumor grading: in tissue sections defined as grade 1 no stained immune cell infiltration was observed, whereas in grade 2 and 3, stained immune cells were detected ($p = 0.008$, Figure S10a). Gal-7-expressing immune cells were furthermore found significantly more often in NST compared to non-NST tumors ($p = 0.001$, Figure S10b) and in tumors with lymph node metastasis ($p = 0.038$, Figure S10c). A double immunofluorescence staining with Gal-7 and CD68 (a macrophage marker) showed that the Gal-7 stained immune cells were macrophages (Figure 8e–g).

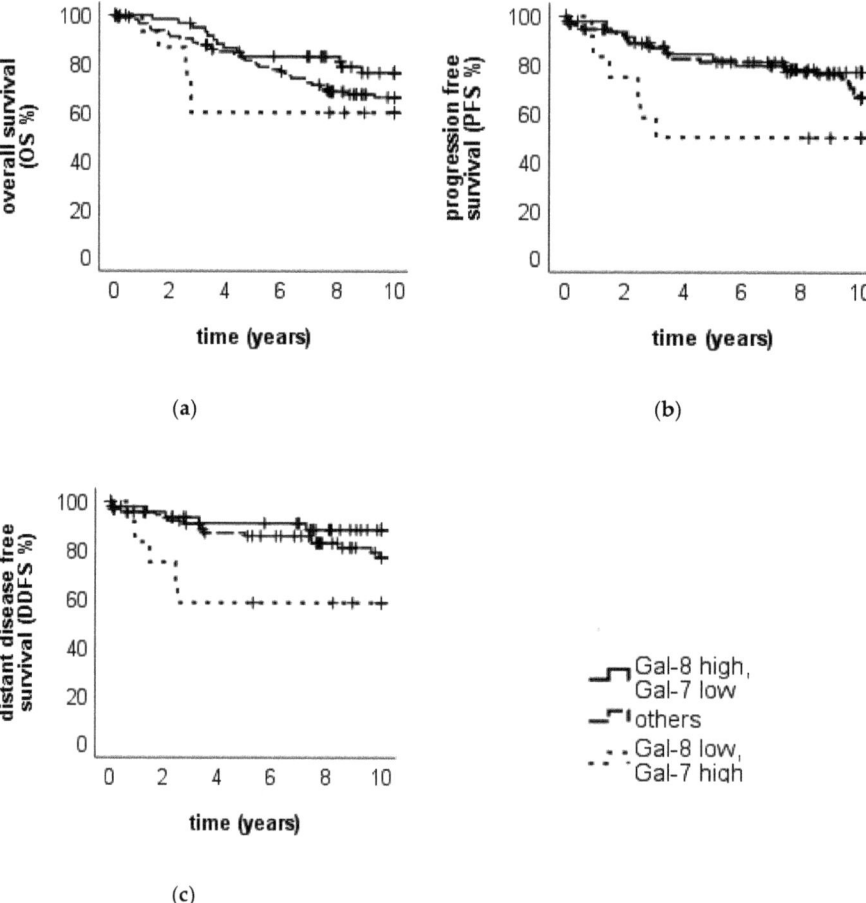

Figure 7. OS, PFS and DDFS for the two groups. Kaplan–Meier analysis of OS (**a**), PFS (**b**) and DDFS (**c**) in tumors with combined high or low Gal-7 expression with low or high Gal-8 expression (in the cytoplasm), respectively, are shown. Tumors with high Gal-7 and low Gal-8 expression in the cytoplasm show the trend of an impaired OS, while tumors with high Gal-8 and low Gal 7 expression show the trend of an improved OS. Tumors with high Gal-7 and low Gal-8 expression in the cytoplasm show the trend of an impaired PFS and a significantly reduced DDFS, while tumors with high Gal-8 and low Gal-7 expression show the trend of an improved PFS and a DDFS.

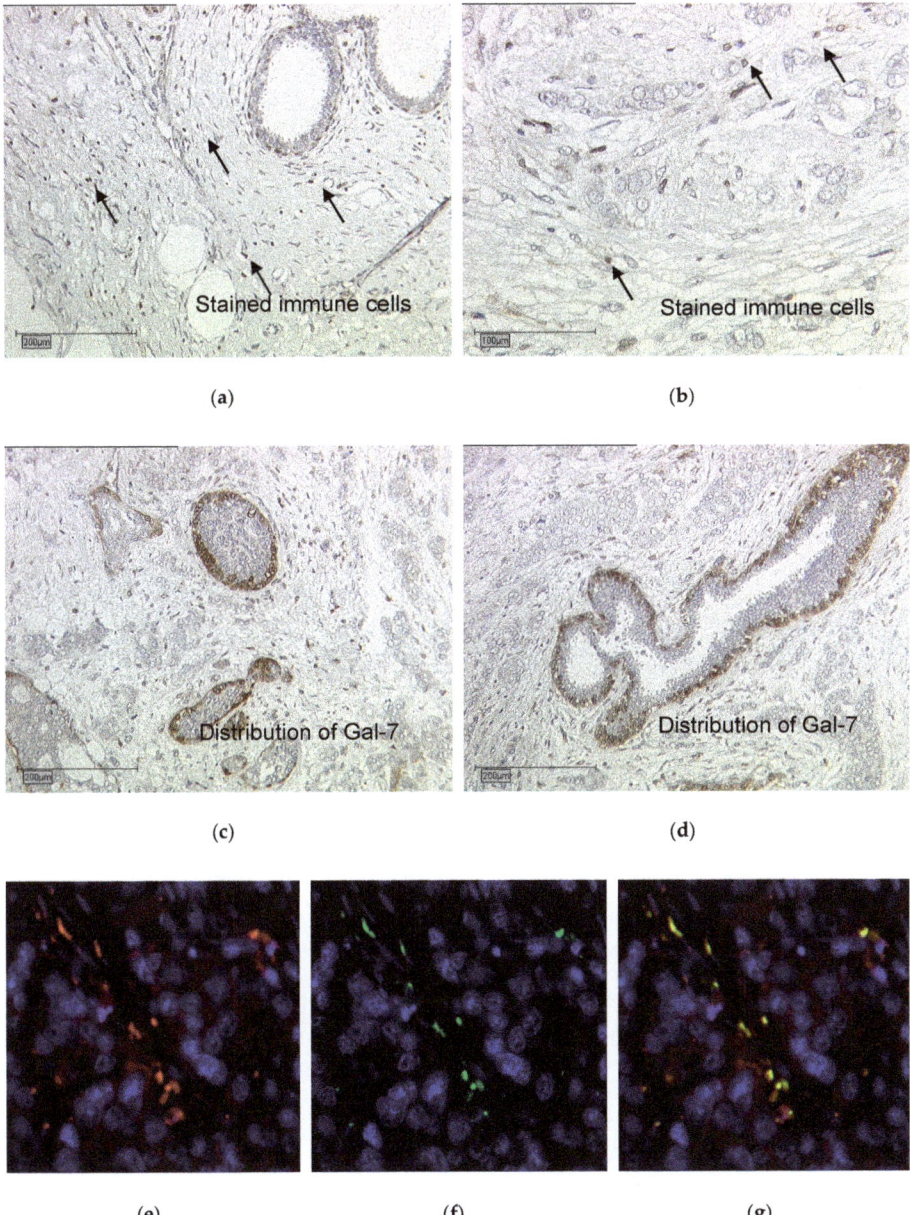

Figure 8. Gal-7-staining results (**a–d**) and double immunofluorescence staining with Gal 7 and CD68 (**e–g**). Exemplary pictures of Gal 7-staining results are shown, revealing the distribution of Gal 7-staining in tumor cells (**a**,**b**). Stained immune cells in Gal 7-expressing tumors are shown in (**c**) and (**d**). Immunofluorescence results: Gal-7 is shown in red (**e**), CD68 in green (**f**) and the nucleus is stained with DAPI in blue. Picture (**g**) shows that Gal 7- and CD8-staining is overlapping in some cells, which appear yellow, showing that these are macrophages. Magnification: Images 8a, 8c and 8d x10, and images 8b, 8e, 8f and 8g x25.

3. Discussion

Galectins have been shown to be a pivotal factor in carcinogenesis. However, data on their relevance in breast cancer are still sparse. As recently proposed [22,25], we could show in our cohort of primary breast cancer patients that Gal-7 was a negative prognosticator for the clinical outcome. Gal-7 expression in the cytoplasm had a negative prognostic impact on PFS and DDFS, a negative trend on OS and was even an independent negative prognosticator for PFS in the multivariate analysis. A strong association between a high Gal-7 expression in the cytoplasm and HER2 amplification was observed, suggesting that HER2-positive tumors might be especially interesting for potentially targeting Gal-7. In HER2-positive tumors—like in the overall cohort—high Gal-7 expression was associated with an impaired prognosis. Gal-8 expression in the cytoplasm, however, was associated with an improved OS.

Our data are in line with Grosset et al., [21,25] who found high Gal-7 expression only in HER2-positive tumors and in TNBC. Recent studies showed Gal-3 as a modifier of the epidermal growth factor receptor (EGFR), which is a regulator of cell growth and survival in normal and cancerous tissues [26–28]. EGFR and HER2 are both known as members of the ErbB receptor family and, when activated, they stimulate the activation of many signaling pathways [29]. Apart from Gal-3, no functional associations between galectins and ErbB receptors have been reported to date. However, these data suggest a functional connection between these two families which might also exist between Gal-7 and HER2.

Other groups showed in an in silico mRNA survival analysis that Gal-7 and Gal-8 did not have a prognostic impact in breast cancer patients. However, regarding protein level—similarly to our data—high Gal-7 expression was associated with an impaired PFS (although not statistically significant), whereas no effect could be shown for Gal-8 (both in the overall cohort) [25].

Our results suggest that combining Gal-7 and Gal-8 expression might further improve prognostic accuracy. Two different groups could be defined: a small group (high Gal-8, low Gal-7) with a very good outcome (6.8% of the patients), compared to a second group (high Gal-7, low Gal-8) with a worse outcome, consisting of 13.6% of the patients. This is especially interesting, as Gal-7 and Gal-8 expressions are strongly correlated. Similar effects have been shown for galectin ligands: in BC patients, high levels of- Gal-1 ligands and low levels of Gal-8 ligands have been observed, making their ratio a strong marker for BC [30]. A similar ratio could be established using the Gal-7/Gal-8 expression for prognostic considerations.

Galectin expression was also associated with tumor cell differentiation: Gal-7 expression was significantly higher in less differentiated cells (reflected by higher grading), whereas Gal-8 expression was highest in highly differentiated cells (reflected by lower grading). This is similar to other data where high Gal-4 (which belongs to the same family as Gal-8) expression in highly differentiated, and low Gal-1 (which belongs to the same family as Gal-7) expression in poorly differentiated, tumors have been shown [31]. Furthermore, in our study, poor tumor cell differentiation was also associated with high Gal-7 expression in tumor-surrounding macrophages, who are known to correlate with poor breast cancer survival rates.

Regarding mechanisms of the regulation of galectin expression and distribution between nucleus and cytoplasm, it is important to consider that Gal-7 is also provided extracellularly: The extracellular Gal-7 controls the intracellular pool of Gal-7, firstly by an increase in the gene transcription, and secondly by a re-entry pathway into the cells [32]. Similarly, for Gal-1 (which belongs to the same group as Gal-7) an extracellular to nucleus transfer has been shown and nuclear Gal-1 accumulation drove epithelial invasiveness. Extracellular glycans that bear N-acetyllactosamins (LacNAc) epitopes bind Gal-1 and trap it extracellularly. An α-2,6-sialylation of these LacNAc epitopes inhibits Gal-1-binding and drives the nuclear transfer of Gal-1 [33]. We could observe in our study that Gal-7 was also present in macrophages next to the tumor cells. Therefore, these macrophages might also provide a source of extracellular Gal-7 for tumor cells and might regulate the intracellular Gal-7 pool. Tumor-associated macrophages are correlated with poor survival rates of breast cancer [34], rendering Gal-7 even more interesting as a therapeutic target. Functional effects that have been described for Gal-8 include the activation of the activated leukocyte cell adhesion molecule (ALCAM) [23,35,36] and the activation of the endothelial nitric oxide synthase (eNOS) pathway on endothelial cells [37]. However, these pathways all describe a tumorigenic potential of Gal-8, while Gal-8 was a positive prognosticator in our study. Therefore, other tumor-suppressing pathways that need further investigation might exist.

First attempts in targeting galectins in breast cancer have already been made: Grosset et al. demonstrated that targeting CRD-independent cytosolic Gal-7 in breast cancer cells, and therefore impairing p53-functions, might be a valuable strategy for the treatment of breast cancer [35]. Targeting Gal-8 has not been performed to date. Gal-3 knockdown enhanced the sensitivity of tumor cells to the apoptotic agent arsenic trioxide (ATO, which is already approved by the US Food and Drug Administration for the treatment of acute myeloid leukemia) [19], making Gal-3 an interesting therapeutic target. An orally applied Gal-3 antagonist was already studied in a mouse model, leading to less lung adenocarcinoma growth [36]. Furthermore, a Gal-1 inhibitor that showed synergistic activity with the chemotherapeutic paclitaxel in BC has been discovered [37]. As Gal-7 belongs to the same family as Gal-1, similar therapeutic potential could exist for Gal-7.

4. Materials and Methods

4.1. Patients

Formalin-fixed, paraffin-embedded (FFPE) primary breast cancer samples of 235 patients were examined in this study (Table 6).

We included in our study all patients that were diagnosed with primary non-metastatic breast cancer and underwent surgery at the Department of Gynaecology and Obstetrics, Ludwig-Maximilians-University Munich, Germany, from the period 1998 to 2000.

Therefore, there was no pre-selection and a complete group of patients attending the clinic was analysed. Only women with benign tumors of the breast were excluded from the study.

Clinical, pathological and follow-up data (up to ten years) were retrieved from patients' charts and from the Munich Cancer Registry. Patient characteristics are displayed in Table 6. In terms of clinical and pathological characteristics and tumor biology, the collective represents the reality of the wide BC spectrum.

Histopathological subtype (no specific type (NST) vs. non-NST), tumor grading (G1-3) according to the Elston and Ellis criteria (1993) [4,38,39], and staging using the TNM-System [40] (T for tumor size, N for the lymph node status and M for metastasis) were determined by a gynecological pathologist. As tumor grading could only be obtained in about 70% of all patients, the results have to be regarded with limited reliability. HER2-positivity is defined by the DAKO Scoring system (DAKO, HER2 FISH pharmDx™ Kit, Agilent Technologies, Waldbronn, Germany). As HER2 status was not determined routinely in Germany before 2001, it was retrospectively assessed. HER2 status was determined as recommended in the national guidelines, i.e., by DAKO Score and FISH analysis in cases of DAKO 2+.

Endpoints regarding the survival data were defined as follows: OS = overall survival, period of time from the date of surgery until the date of death or date of last follow-up; PFS = progression free survival, period of time until local recurrence or metastasis were diagnosed and DDFS = distant disease free survival: period of time until metastasis was diagnosed.

Table 6. Patients' characteristics.

Patients' Characteristics	Median	SD
Age	58.2	13.3
	N	%
Histological subtype		
NST	126	53.6
Non-NST	96	40.9
NA	13	5.5
Intrinsic surrogate subtype		
Luminal A-like	103	43.8
Luminal B-like	73	31.1
HER2-positive, luminal	17	7.2
HER2-positive, non-luminal	7	3.0
TNBC	31	13.2
NA	4	1.7
Grading		
Grade 1	17	7.2
Grade 2	90	38.3
Grade 3	55	23.4
NA	73	31.1
Lymph node involvement (pN)		
pN0	128	54.5
pN1	87	37.0
pN2	10	4.3
NA	10	4.3
Tumor size (pT)		
pT1 (≤2 cm)	160	68.1
pT2 (2–5 cm)	68	28.9
pT3 (>5 cm)	1	0.4
pT4 (with infiltration in the epidermis or the thoracic wall)	5	2.1
NA	1	0.4
HER2 status		
Positive	24	10.2
Negative	208	88.5
NA	3	1.3
ER status		
Positive	192	81.7
Negative	43	18.3
PR status		
Positive	141	60.0
Negative	94	40.0

NST = no special type, NA = not available, ER = estrogen receptor, PR = progesterone receptor, HER2 = human epidermal growth factor receptor 2, TNBC = triple negative breast cancer.

4.2. Immunohistochemistry

Paraffine-embedded breast cancer tissue samples were analyzed by immunohistochemistry. The samples were fixed in neutral buffered formalin and embedded in paraffin after surgery. For histopathological investigations, tissue sections (3 μm) were deparaffinized in Roticlear (Carl Roth GmbH + Co. KG) for 20 min and then the endogenous peroxidase was inactivated with 3% hydrogen peroxide (VWR International GmbH) in methanol. The slides were rehydrated in a descending gradient of ethanol (100%, 75% and 50%) and prepared for epitope retrieval in a pressure cooker for 5 min in sodium citrate buffer (0.1 mol/L citric acid, 0.1 mol/L sodium citrate, pH 6.0). After washing in distilled water and phosphate-buffered saline (PBS), all tissue slides were blocked using a blocking solution (Reagent 1; ZytoChem Plus HRP Polymer System (Mouse/Rabbit); Zytomed Systems GmbH, Berlin,

Germany) for 5 min at room temperature (RT) in order to block non-specific binding of the primary antibodies. Then, a specific procedure followed for each Galectin: the slides were incubated with Gal-7 primary antibody (rabbit, polyclonal; Abcam, ab10482) at a final concentration of 2.5 µg/mL in PBS Dulbecco (Biochrom GmbH) for 16 h at 4 °C. Gal-8 primary antibody (rabbit, monoclonal, Abcam, ab109519) was used for incubation at a final concentration of 3.3 µg/mL in PBS for 1 h at RT. Afterwards, the staining specimens were incubated in post block reagent (Reagent 2) and HRP-polymer (Reagent 3) containing secondary antibodies (anti-mouse/-rabbit) and peroxidase according to the manufacturer's protocol. These antibodies are part of the provided Reagent 3, exact concentrations are not specified by the manufacturer. (Reagent 2 and 3, ZytoChem Plus HRP Polymer System, Mouse/Rabbit). All slides were washed in PBS after every incubation step. The slides were then stained with 3,3′-diaminobenzidine chromogen (DAB; Dako, Glostrup, Denmark) for visualization and counterstained in Mayer acidic hematoxylin. After dehydrating in an ascending ethanol gradient and Roticlear they were cover slipped with Roti-Mount (Carl Roth GmbH + Co. KG). Appropriate tissue slides were used as positive controls (sigma tissue for Gal-7 and placenta for Gal-8). To obtain expression results, the semiquantitative immunoreactive score (IRS, Remmele and Stegner 1987 [41]) was performed using a Leitz Diaplan microscope (Leitz, Wetzlar, Germany). The score was optically obtained by multiplying the predominant staining intensity (0: none; 1: low; 2: moderate; 3: strong) and the percentage of positively stained cancer cells (0 = 0%, 1= 1–10%, 2 = 11–50%, 3 = 51%–80%, and 4 = 81%–100% stained cells). The IRS was determined separately in the cytoplasm and the nucleus of the cancer cells. The staining of other cells, like immune cells, was not included in the IRS. Images were taken with a CCD color camera (JVC, Victor Company of Japan, Japan).

Furthermore, immune cells stained with Gal-7 were analyzed independently of the tumor IRS for Gal-7 and evaluated using following scoring system: 0 = no immune cells were stained, 1 = <50% and 2 = >50% of the immune cells were stained.

4.3. Immunofluorescence

Paraffine-embedded breast cancer tissue samples were also used for immunofluorescence-analyses. The samples were fixed in neutral buffered formalin and embedded in paraffin after surgery. After deparaffinization in Roticlear (Carl Roth GmbH + Co. KG) for 20 min, the slides were rehydrated in a descending gradient of ethanol (100%, 75% and 50%) and prepared for epitope retrieval in a pressure cooker for 5 min in sodium citrate buffer (0.1 mol/L citric acid, 0.1 mol/L sodium citrate, pH 6.0). After washing in distilled water and PBS, all tissue slides were blocked with Ultra V Block (Thermo scientific) for 15 min. The primary antibodies were diluted in Dako Antibody Diluent (Dako North America) incubated with the slides for 16 h at 4 degrees. Gal-7 (rabbit, polyclonal; Abcam, ab10482) was diluted at a final concentration of 2,5 µg/mL and CD68 (mouse, monoclonal, Sigma AldrichAMAb90874) at a concentration of 0.1 µg/mL. Next, the light in the room was dimmed and an incubation with the secondary antibodies for 30 min at RT followed. Secondary antibodies: Goat-Anti Rabbit IgG Cy3 (Dianova/Jackson, 111-165-144) diluted at a concentration of 3 µg/mL and Goat-Anti-Mouse-AlexaFluor488-IgG (Dianova/Jackson, 115-546-062) at a concentration of 15 µg/mL. After the slices were dried in the dark, they were cover slipped with mounting medium for fluorescence with DAPI (Vectashield H-1200). The samples were then analyzed using a Zeiss AxioPhot microscope with an Axiocam MRm within one day.

4.4. Statistical Analysis

Data analyses were performed with SPSS Statistics 25 (Armonk, NY: IBM Corp.). p-values lower than 0.05 were considered as statistically significant. Correlations between staining results and ordinal variables were tested with Spearman's rank correlation coefficient. Group comparisons regarding the IRS of galectins between different clinical and pathological subgroups were tested with Kruskal–Wallis test and displayed as boxplot graphs. Survival times between different groups were compared by Kaplan–Meier analysis, and differences were tested for significance by Log-Rank (Mantel-Cox),

Breslow- and Tarone-Ware-tests. Censored cases are cases for which the second event is not recorded (for example, people still alive at the end of the study). The Kaplan–Meier procedure is a method of estimating time-to-event models in the presence of censored cases. The Kaplan–Meier model is based on estimating conditional probabilities at each time point when an event occurs and taking the product limit of those probabilities to estimate the survival rate at each point in time. Cox-regression analysis was used to determine the independence of prognostic factors.

Concerning survival analysis dependent on Gal-7 and Gal-8 expression, patients were grouped into high and low expression. Cut-off points were selected considering the distribution pattern of IR-scores in the collective. Therefore, the receiver operator curve (ROC curve) was drawn using SPSS software, which is considered as one of the most reliable methods for cut-off point selection. In this context, the ROC curve is a plot representing sensitivity on the y-axis and (1-specificity) the x-axis. Consecutively Youden index, defined as the maximum (sensitivity + specificity−1), was used to find the optimal cut-off maximizing the sum of sensitivity and specificity (exemplary results of the ROC curve analysis in Table S5). Furthermore, the medians of Kruskal–Wallis tests were observed and evaluated in order to find the ideal cutoff. The cytoplasmatic Gal-7 expression was regarded as low with an IRS 0–6 and as high with an IRS > 6. The cytoplasmatic Gal-8 expression was regarded as low with an IRS 0–5 and as high with an IRS > 5.

4.5. Ethics Approval and Consent to Participate

This study has been approved by the Ethics Committee of the Ludwig-Maximilian-University Munich (approval number 048–08). The breast cancer specimens were obtained in clinically indicated surgeries. When the current study was performed, all diagnostic procedures were completed, and the patients' data were anonymized. The ethical principles adopted in the Declaration of Helsinki 1975 have been respected. As per the declaration of our ethics committee, no written informed consent of the participants or permission to publish is needed given the circumstances described above. Researchers were blinded from patient data during experimental and statistical analysis.

5. Conclusions

In summary, our results suggest that Gal-7 might be an independent negative prognostic factor in breast cancer and therapeutic target, especially in HER2-positive breast cancer. Furthermore, Gal-8 was observed to be a positive predictor for overall survival and upregulation should be further investigated. The role of Gal-7 and Gal-8 should be validated in a BC collective treated with today's standard of therapy—even if this might be outdated at the time point of the analysis. Additional studies are required to detect the signaling pathways in which both Gal-7 and Gal-8 are involved, as the combination of both markers showed strong prognostic impact. Gal-7 and Gal-8, as well as the whole group of galectins, seem to be interesting therapeutic and prognostic targets that might help to improve therapies and outcome for breast cancer patients in the future.

Supplementary Materials: The following are available online at http://www.mdpi.com/2072-6694/12/4/953/s1, Figure S1: Association of Gal 7 and Gal¬ 8 expression in the nucleus with HER2 status. Figure S2: Association of Gal-8 expression in the cytoplasm to the different surrogate intrinsic subtypes. Figure S3: Association of Gal-7 expression in the cytoplasm in ER negative tumors to the clinical outcome. Figure S4: Association of Gal-7 expression in the cytoplasm in HER2 positive tumors to the clinical outcome. Figure S5: Association of Gal-7 expression in the nucleus to the clinical outcome. Figure S6: Association of Gal-8 expression in the cytoplasm in HER2 negative tumors to the clinical outcome. Figure S7: Association of Gal-8 expression in the cytoplasm in ER positive tumors to the clinical outcome. Figure S8: Association of Gal-8 expression in the nucleus to the clinical outcome. Figure S9: OS, PFS and DDFS comparing high Gal 7 and low Gal 8 expressing tumors to the rest of the patients. Figure S10: Association of Gal 7 expression in immune cells with tumor grading, histological subtype and lymph node status. Table S1: Correlations of Gal 7 expression with clinical and histological parameters. Table S2: Correlations of Gal 8 expression with clinical and histological parameters. Table S3: Multivariate analysis of DDFS concerning Gal 7 expression in the cytoplasm. Table S4: Multivariate analysis of OS concerning Gal 7 expression in the cytoplasm. Table S5: Coordinates of ROC Curve exemplary for Gal-7 expression in the cytoplasm.

Author Contributions: A.T.: Participated in design and coordination of the study, participated in immunohistochemistry assays and analysis and performed the statistical analysis. C.K. performed technical assistance in immunohistochemistry assays and analysis. A.T. and A.H. wrote the manuscript. N.D.: participated in the design of the study and carefully read the manuscript for important intellectual content. E.S.: supervised immunohistochemistry as a gynecologic pathologist and participated in immunohistochemistry analysis as well as in the design and coordination of the study. C.Z.-G., T.K., B.C., and H.H.H. and S.M. revised the manuscript for important intellectual content. U.J. and A.H.: conceived of the study and participated in its design and coordination, approved the final version of the manuscript. All authors analyzed and interpreted the data and read and approved the final manuscript.

Funding: This research received funding from the "Walter-Schulz-Stiftung".

Acknowledgments: The authors thank Christina Kuhn for her excellent technical assistance. Furthermore, Kerstin Hermelink helped us with the revisions with statistical advice and imaging our data. Thank you very much. We also thank Michael Semmlinger for proofreading of the manuscript.

Conflicts of Interest: Thomas Kolben holds stock of Roche AG and his relative is employed at Roche AG. Anna Hester has received a research grant from the "Walter Schulz" foundation and advisory board, speech honoraria and travel expenses from Roche and Pfizer. Research support, advisory board, honoraria, and travel expenses from AstraZeneca, Clovis, Medac, MSD, Novartis, PharmaMar, Roche, Sensor Kinesis, Tesaro, Teva have been received by Sven Mahner. All other authors declare no conflict of interest. The funders had no role in the design of the study; in the collection, analyses, or interpretation of data; in the writing of the manuscript, or in the decision to publish the results.

References

1. Harbeck, N.; Gnant, M. Breast cancer. *Lancet* **2017**, *389*, 1134–1150. [CrossRef]
2. Bray, F.; Ferlay, J.; Soerjomataram, I.; Siegel, R.L.; Torre, L.A.; Jemal, A. Global cancer statistics 2018: GLOBOCAN estimates of incidence and mortality worldwide for 36 cancers in 185 countries. *CA A Cancer J. Clin.* **2018**, *68*, 394–424. [CrossRef] [PubMed]
3. Sorlie, T.; Tibshirani, R.; Parker, J.; Hastie, T.; Marron, J.S.; Nobel, A.; Deng, S.; Johnsen, H.; Pesich, R.; Geisler, S.; et al. Repeated observation of breast tumor subtypes in independent gene expression data sets. *Proc. Natl. Acad. Sci. USA* **2003**, *100*, 8418–8423. [CrossRef] [PubMed]
4. Perou, C.M.; Sorlie, T.; Eisen, M.B.; van de Rijn, M.; Jeffrey, S.S.; Rees, C.A.; Pollack, J.R.; Ross, D.T.; Johnsen, H.; Akslen, L.A.; et al. Molecular portraits of human breast tumours. *Nature* **2000**, *406*, 747–752. [CrossRef]
5. Cho, S.H.; Jeon, J.; Kim, S.I. Personalized medicine in breast cancer: A systematic review. *J. Breast Cancer* **2012**, *15*, 265–272. [CrossRef]
6. Harris, E.E.R. Precision medicine for breast cancer: The paths to truly individualized diagnosis and treatment. *Int. J. Breast Cancer* **2018**, *2018*, 4809183. [CrossRef]
7. Gaudet, M.M.; Gierach, G.L.; Carter, B.D.; Luo, J.; Milne, R.L.; Weiderpass, E.; Giles, G.G.; Tamimi, R.M.; Eliassen, A.H.; Rosner, B.; et al. Pooled analysis of nine cohorts reveals breast cancer risk factors by tumor molecular subtype. *Cancer Res.* **2018**, *78*, 6011–6021. [CrossRef]
8. Foulkes, W.D.; Smith, I.E.; Reis-Filho, J.S. Triple-negative breast cancer. *N. Engl. J. Med.* **2010**, *363*, 1938–1948. [CrossRef]
9. Barondes, S.H.; Castronovo, V.; Cooper, D.N.W.; Cummings, R.D.; Drickamer, K.; Felzi, T.; Gitt, M.A.; Hirabayashi, J.; Hughes, C.; Kasai, K.-I.; et al. Galectins: A family of animal β-galactoside-binding lectins. *Cell* **1994**, *76*, 597–598. [CrossRef]
10. Barondes, S.H.; Cooper, D.N.; Gitt, M.A.; Leffler, H. Galectins. Structure and function of a large family of animal lectins. *J. Biol. Chem.* **1994**, *269*, 20807–20810.
11. Ebrahim, A.H.; Alalawi, Z.; Mirandola, L.; Rakhshanda, R.; Dahlbeck, S.; Nguyen, D.; Jenkins, M.; Grizzi, F.; Cobos, E.; Figueroa, J.A.; et al. Galectins in cancer: Carcinogenesis, diagnosis and therapy. *Ann. Transl. Med.* **2014**, *2*, 88. [CrossRef] [PubMed]
12. Cummings, R.D.; Liu, F.T. Galectins. In *Essentials of Glycobiology*, 2nd ed.; Varki, A., Cummings, R.D., Esko, J.D., Freeze, H.H., Stanley, P., Bertozzi, C.R., Hart, G.W., Etzler, M.E., Eds.; Cold Spring Harbor Laboratory Press: Cold Spring Harbor, NY, USA; The Consortium of Glycobiology Editors: La Jolla, CA, USA, 2009.
13. Thijssen, V.L.; Heusschen, R.; Caers, J.; Griffioen, A.W. Galectin expression in cancer diagnosis and prognosis: A systematic review. *Biochim. Biophys. Acta* **2015**, *1855*, 235–247. [CrossRef] [PubMed]
14. Liu, F.T.; Rabinovich, G.A. Galectins as modulators of tumour progression. *Nat. Rev. Cancer* **2005**, *5*, 29–41. [CrossRef] [PubMed]

15. Kolbl, A.C.; Andergassen, U.; Jeschke, U. The role of glycosylation in breast cancer metastasis and cancer control. *Front. Oncol.* **2015**, *5*, 219. [CrossRef] [PubMed]
16. Dalotto-Moreno, T.; Croci, D.O.; Cerliani, J.P.; Martinez-Allo, V.C.; Dergan-Dylon, S.; Mendez-Huergo, S.P.; Stupirski, J.C.; Mazal, D.; Osinaga, E.; Toscano, M.A.; et al. Targeting galectin-1 overcomes breast cancer-associated immunosuppression and prevents metastatic disease. *Cancer Res.* **2013**, *73*, 1107–1117. [CrossRef] [PubMed]
17. Reynolds, N.M.; Mohammadalipour, A.; Hall, C.R.; Asghari Adib, A.; Farnoud, A.M.; Burdick, M.M. Galectin-1 influences breast cancer cell adhesion to e-selectin via ligand intermediaries. *Cell Mol. Bioeng.* **2018**, *11*, 37–52. [CrossRef]
18. Simone, G.; Malara, N.; Trunzo, V.; Renne, M.; Perozziello, G.; Di Fabrizio, E.; Manz, A. Galectin-3 coats the membrane of breast cells and makes a signature of tumours. *Mol. Biosyst.* **2014**, *10*, 258–265. [CrossRef]
19. Zhang, H.; Luo, M.; Liang, X.; Wang, D.; Gu, X.; Duan, C.; Gu, H.; Chen, G.; Zhao, X.; Zhao, Z.; et al. Galectin-3 as a marker and potential therapeutic target in breast cancer. *PLoS ONE* **2014**, *9*, e103482. [CrossRef]
20. Irie, A.; Yamauchi, A.; Kontani, K.; Kihara, M.; Liu, D.; Shirato, Y.; Seki, M.; Nishi, N.; Nakamura, T.; Yokomise, H.; et al. Galectin-9 as a prognostic factor with antimetastatic potential in breast cancer. *Clin. Cancer Res.* **2005**, *11*, 2962–2968. [CrossRef]
21. Grosset, A.A.; Poirier, F.; Gaboury, L.; St-Pierre, Y. Galectin-7 expression potentiates her-2-positive phenotype in breast cancer. *PLoS ONE* **2016**, *11*, e0166731. [CrossRef]
22. Demers, M.; Rose, A.A.; Grosset, A.A.; Biron-Pain, K.; Gaboury, L.; Siegel, P.M.; St-Pierre, Y. Overexpression of galectin-7, a myoepithelial cell marker, enhances spontaneous metastasis of breast cancer cells. *Am. J. Pathol.* **2010**, *176*, 3023–3031. [CrossRef] [PubMed]
23. Campion, C.G.; Labrie, M.; Lavoie, G.; St-Pierre, Y. Expression of galectin-7 is induced in breast cancer cells by mutant p53. *PLoS ONE* **2013**, *8*, e72468. [CrossRef] [PubMed]
24. Ferragut, F.; Cagnoni, A.J.; Colombo, L.L.; Sanchez Terrero, C.; Wolfenstein-Todel, C.; Troncoso, M.F.; Vanzulli, S.I.; Rabinovich, G.A.; Marino, K.V.; Elola, M.T. Dual knockdown of Galectin-8 and its glycosylated ligand, the activated leukocyte cell adhesion molecule (ALCAM/CD166), synergistically delays in vivo breast cancer growth. *Biochim. Biophys. Acta Mol. Cell Res.* **2019**, *1866*, 1338–1352. [CrossRef] [PubMed]
25. Grosset, A.A.; Labrie, M.; Vladoiu, M.C.; Yousef, E.M.; Gaboury, L.; St-Pierre, Y. Galectin signatures contribute to the heterogeneity of breast cancer and provide new prognostic information and therapeutic targets. *Oncotarget* **2016**, *7*, 18183–18203. [CrossRef]
26. Piyush, T.; Chacko, A.R.; Sindrewicz, P.; Hilkens, J.; Rhodes, J.M.; Yu, L.G. Interaction of galectin-3 with MUC1 on cell surface promotes EGFR dimerization and activation in human epithelial cancer cells. *Cell Death Differ.* **2017**, *24*, 1937–1947. [CrossRef]
27. Kuo, H.Y.; Hsu, H.T.; Chen, Y.C.; Chang, Y.W.; Liu, F.T.; Wu, C.W. Galectin-3 modulates the EGFR signalling-mediated regulation of Sox2 expression via c-Myc in lung cancer. *Glycobiology* **2016**, *26*, 155–165. [CrossRef]
28. Wu, K.L.; Kuo, C.M.; Huang, E.Y.; Pan, H.M.; Huang, C.C.; Chen, Y.F.; Hsiao, C.C.; Yang, K.D. Extracellular galectin-3 facilitates colon cancer cell migration and is related to the epidermal growth factor receptor. *Am. J. Transl. Res.* **2018**, *10*, 2402–2412.
29. Wang, Z. ErbB receptors and cancer. *Methods Mol. Biol.* **2017**, *1652*, 3–35. [CrossRef]
30. Carlsson, M.C.; Balog, C.I.; Kilsgard, O.; Hellmark, T.; Bakoush, O.; Segelmark, M.; Ferno, M.; Olsson, H.; Malmstrom, J.; Wuhrer, M.; et al. Different fractions of human serum glycoproteins bind galectin-1 or galectin-8, and their ratio may provide a refined biomarker for pathophysiological conditions in cancer and inflammatory disease. *Biochim. Biophys. Acta* **2012**, *1820*, 1366–1372. [CrossRef]
31. Huflejt, M.E.; Leffler, H. Galectin-4 in normal tissues and cancer. *Glycoconj. J.* **2004**, *20*, 247–255. [CrossRef]
32. Bibens-Laulan, N.; St-Pierre, Y. Intracellular galectin-7 expression in cancer cells results from an autocrine transcriptional mechanism and endocytosis of extracellular galectin-7. *PLoS ONE* **2017**, *12*, e0187194. [CrossRef] [PubMed]
33. Bhat, R.; Belardi, B.; Mori, H.; Kuo, P.; Tam, A.; Hines, W.C.; Le, Q.T.; Bertozzi, C.R.; Bissell, M.J. Nuclear repartitioning of galectin-1 by an extracellular glycan switch regulates mammary morphogenesis. *Proc. Natl. Acad. Sci. USA* **2016**, *113*, E4820–E4827. [CrossRef] [PubMed]

34. Zhao, X.; Qu, J.; Sun, Y.; Wang, J.; Liu, X.; Wang, F.; Zhang, H.; Wang, W.; Ma, X.; Gao, X.; et al. Prognostic significance of tumor-associated macrophages in breast cancer: A meta-analysis of the literature. *Oncotarget* **2017**, *8*, 30576–30586. [CrossRef] [PubMed]
35. Grosset, A.A.; Labrie, M.; Gagne, D.; Vladoiu, M.C.; Gaboury, L.; Doucet, N.; St-Pierre, Y. Cytosolic galectin-7 impairs p53 functions and induces chemoresistance in breast cancer cells. *BMC Cancer* **2014**, *14*, 801. [CrossRef]
36. Vuong, L.; Kouverianou, E.; Rooney, C.M.; McHugh, B.J.; Howie, S.E.M.; Gregory, C.D.; Forbes, S.J.; Henderson, N.C.; Zetterberg, F.R.; Nilsson, U.J.; et al. An orally active galectin-3 antagonist inhibits lung adenocarcinoma growth and augments response to pd-l1 blockade. *Cancer Res.* **2019**, *79*, 1480–1492. [CrossRef]
37. Shih, T.C.; Liu, R.; Fung, G.; Bhardwaj, G.; Ghosh, P.M.; Lam, K.S. A novel galectin-1 inhibitor discovered through one-bead two-compound library potentiates the antitumor effects of paclitaxel in vivo. *Mol. Cancer Ther.* **2017**, *16*, 1212–1223. [CrossRef]
38. Elston, C.W.; Ellis, I.O. Pathological prognostic factors in breast cancer. I. The value of histological grade in breast cancer: Experience from a large study with long-term follow-up. *Histopathology* **1991**, *19*, 403–410. [CrossRef]
39. Makki, J. Diversity of breast carcinoma: Histological subtypes and clinical relevance. *Clin. Med. Insights Pathol.* **2015**, *8*, 23–31. [CrossRef]
40. Cserni, G.; Chmielik, E.; Cserni, B.; Tot, T. The new TNM-based staging of breast cancer. *Virchows Arch.* **2018**, *472*, 697–703. [CrossRef]
41. Remmele, W.; Stegner, H.E. Recommendation for uniform definition of an immunoreactive score (IRS) for immunohistochemical estrogen receptor detection (ER-ICA) in breast cancer tissue. *Pathologe* **1987**, *8*, 138–140.

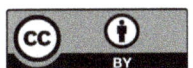

© 2020 by the authors. Licensee MDPI, Basel, Switzerland. This article is an open access article distributed under the terms and conditions of the Creative Commons Attribution (CC BY) license (http://creativecommons.org/licenses/by/4.0/).

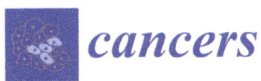

Review

Worldwide Review and Meta-Analysis of Cohort Studies Measuring the Effect of Mammography Screening Programmes on Incidence-Based Breast Cancer Mortality

Amanda Dibden [1], Judith Offman [2], Stephen W. Duffy [1,*] and Rhian Gabe [1]

1. Centre for Cancer Prevention, Wolfson Institute of Preventive Medicine, Queen Mary University of London, Charterhouse Square, London EC1M 6BQ, UK; a.dibden@qmul.ac.uk (A.D.); r.gabe@qmul.ac.uk (R.G.)
2. Comprehensive Cancer Centre, School of Cancer & Pharmaceutical Sciences, Faculty of Life Sciences & Medicine, King's College London, Innovation Hub, Guys Cancer Centre, Guys Hospital, Great Maze Pond, London SE1 9RT, UK; judith.offman@kcl.ac.uk
* Correspondence: s.w.duffy@qmul.ac.uk

Received: 12 March 2020; Accepted: 13 April 2020; Published: 15 April 2020

Abstract: In 2012, the Euroscreen project published a review of incidence-based mortality evaluations of breast cancer screening programmes. In this paper, we update this review to October 2019 and expand its scope from Europe to worldwide. We carried out a systematic review of incidence-based mortality studies of breast cancer screening programmes, and a meta-analysis of the estimated effects of both invitation to screening and attendance at screening, with adjustment for self-selection bias, on incidence-based mortality from breast cancer. We found 27 valid studies. The results of the meta-analysis showed a significant 22% reduction in breast cancer mortality with invitation to screening, with a relative risk of 0.78 (95% CI 0.75–0.82), and a significant 33% reduction with actual attendance at screening (RR 0.67, 95% CI 0.61–0.75). Breast cancer screening in the routine healthcare setting continues to confer a substantial reduction in mortality from breast cancer.

Keywords: breast cancer; screening; mammography; incidence-based mortality

1. Introduction

Reviews of randomised controlled trials (RCTs) of mammography screening estimate that invitation to screening reduces risk of death from breast cancer by around 20% [1,2]. However, as the majority of RCTs were carried out over 30 years ago, they do not take account of changes in breast cancer incidence [3], mortality [4], screening techniques and treatments that have occurred over time. Furthermore, the results may not be representative of the effectiveness of individual population mammography screening programmes [5], which are affected by factors such as varying round lengths, radiographer skill and technology [6]. While RCTs provide reliable evidence and proof of principle that mammography screening is likely to be beneficial, once population screening programmes have been introduced, randomisation to a non-interventional control is no longer ethical and it is necessary to measure the effectiveness of screening in practice through observational studies.

Cohort studies have been used to achieve this objective but there can be important, subtle differences in methods of analysis used. One method is to use incidence-based mortality (IBM) [7], where deaths from breast cancer are only included in women diagnosed after screening has been introduced [8]. This avoids contamination of deaths in the screening period of women who were diagnosed prior to the start of screening, which would bias results against screening [9]. The aim of this review is to provide an overview of all IBM studies evaluating the impact of mammography screening on breast cancer mortality and to establish an up to date estimate of the long term benefit of breast screening.

2. Materials and Methods

2.1. Search Strategy

A systematic search of PubMed was performed in October 2019 with search terms based on those used by Njor et al. in their review of European IBM studies (Euroscreen project) [8]. Inclusion criteria were that (i) the study used IBM in the analysis, (ii) the study outcome was breast cancer mortality and (iii) the paper was in English. No restrictions were placed on age of study participants included to enable the inclusion of as many studies, and hence women, as possible.

2.2. Selection of Sources of Evidence

The titles and abstracts were initially assessed for relevance. A random selection of 100 papers were independently assessed by three reviewers (A.D., S.W.D. and J.O.) for accuracy. Following observation of more than 90% agreement among reviewers, the remainder of the papers were assessed by one reviewer (A.D.). The main text of the potentially eligible papers was then assessed by two reviewers (A.D. and S.W.D.) in order to make a final decision regarding inclusion in the review. We prepared a list of variables to extract from each paper (if available). These included programme characteristics, person years accrued and relative risks associated with invitation and/or exposure to screening as well as the proportion participating in screening (the latter to assist in correction for self-selection bias).

2.3. Statistical Methods

Random effects meta-analyses were undertaken to obtain overall estimates of the effects of (i) invitation to screening and (ii) attendance to screening on risk of breast cancer mortality [10]. It is important to note that when assessing the effect of invitation on mortality, it pertains to populations offered screening and the effect of attendance pertains to women who actually take up the offer of screening and is thus effected by the participation rate. Analyses were repeated stratified by age group (i) 50 and over, (ii) under 50. We chose age 50 to stratify the data as the majority of studies reported on the effects of screening in women aged 50–69, reflecting many national screening programmes, and in order to provide separate evidence in women under 50 years where possible as there has been uncertainty about whether screening younger women is effective and hence, cost-effective. Heterogeneity between studies was assessed using the χ^2 test. Where studies used overlapping data, the largest study was chosen on the basis of better precision with a smaller variance.

Statistical analyses were conducted using Stata Version 13 (StataCorp, College Station, TX, USA) [11].

Adjustment for Self-Selection Bias

Studies have shown that women who do not comply with an invitation to screening usually, but not invariably, have a higher risk of breast cancer mortality than those who choose to attend, resulting in a bias in favour of screening [12]. In order to account for such self-selection bias in studies reporting the effect of attending, we used the statistical adjustment proposed by Duffy et al. [13]. This uses the relative risk of attenders versus non-attenders from the current study, the participation rate, and the risk of death in non-attenders versus uninvited from an appropriate external source (Table 1). The relative risk of non-attenders versus uninvited women of 1.17 (95% CI 1.08–1.26) reported in the Swedish Organised Service Screening Evaluation Group (SOSSEG) study was used in this review as it was a large population based service screening study investigating IBM [14].

Table 1. Statistical adjustments to estimate effect of invitation and attendance to screening.

RR_1: Effect of Invitation to Screening	RR_2: Effect of Attendance Adjusted for Self-Selection
$RR_1 = D_r(pRR_A + 1 - p)$	$RR_2 = \frac{pRR_A D_r}{1-(1-p)D_r}$

RR_A = the relative risk of breast cancer death associated with attending screening versus not attending; p = the proportion of women who attend screening; D_r = the relative risk of breast cancer death for non-attenders versus uninvited = 1.17; Formulae for the variance, and thus the 95% confidence intervals, of these estimates can be found elsewhere [13].

3. Results

3.1. Literature Selection

The literature search identified a total of 5232 titles from three searches performed in PubMed (see Appendix A for details of searches 1, 2 and 3), and 43 were deemed relevant for our review after assessment of abstracts and full text (Figure 1). Of these, four studies assessed the effectiveness of screening programmes outside Europe, one each from Canada [15] and the USA [16], and two from New Zealand [17,18]. The remaining 39 studies were European with twelve from Sweden [14,19–29], nine from Finland [30–38], five from Norway [39–43], four from both Italy [44–47] and Denmark [48–51], two from the Netherlands [52,53] and the UK [54,55] and one from Spain [56].

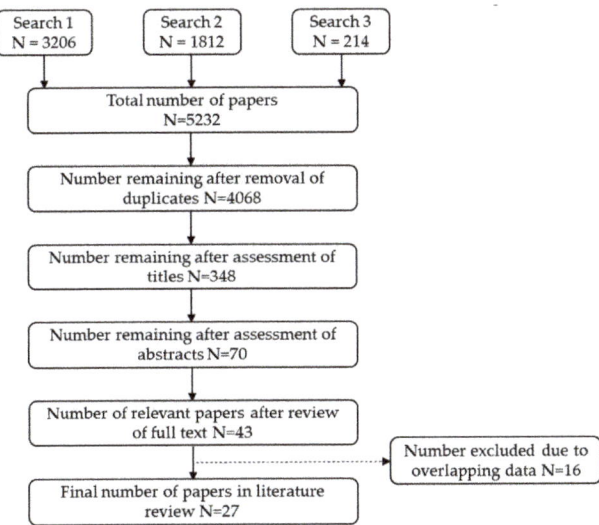

Figure 1. Literature search flow diagram.

There was overlap between some papers, whereby authors used the same data to estimate the effect of different outcomes or updated results with longer follow-up. This resulted in sixteen exclusions (one paper from Denmark [51], four from Finland [31,34,35,37], two from Italy [44,46], three from Norway [39,42,43] and six from Sweden [19,21,22,26,27,29]). The remaining twenty-seven papers included in this review, representing independent populations, are summarized in Table 2.

Table 2. Overview of Studies.

Reference (by Country and Date)	Region	Age Range of Screening	Screening Interval	Comparison Group(s)	Accrual/follow up Period in Screening Group	Accrual/follow up Period in Comparison Group	Person-Years Study/Comparison Groups(Average Population)
Coldman, 2014 [15]	7 provinces, Canada	40–79 depending on province	2 years [1]	Contemporaneous	1990–2009	Same	20,155,000
Beau, 2018 [48]	Copenhagen, Denmark	50–69	2 years	Regional and historical	1991–2007	1977–1991 (pre-screening) 1991–2007 (screening) 1979–1993/95	976,743/17,804,549
Njor, 2015 [49]	Funen, Denmark	50–69	2 years	Regional and historical	1993–2007/09	(pre-screening) 1993–2007/09 (screening) 1981–1991	870,465/ 7,096,056; 828,508; 6,151,011
Olsen, 2005 [50]	Copenhagen, Denmark	50–69	2 years	Regional and historical	1991–2001	(pre-screening) 1991–2001 (screening)	430,823/ 634,224; 4,396,417; 4,055,004
Parvinen, 2015 [30]	Turku, Finland	40–74	2 years [2]	Regional and historical	1987–2009	1976–1986 (pre-screening) 1987–2009 (screening) 1974–1985	853,297/ Helsinki: 2,700,574; Rest of Finland: 21,761,900
Sarkeala, 2008 [33]	8 municipalities, Finland	50–69	2 years	Historical	1992–2003	(pre-screening) 1992–2003 (screening) 1974–1985	228,527
Sarkeala, 2008 [32]	260 municipalities, Finland	50–69	2 years	Historical	1992–2003	(pre-screening) 1992–2003 (screening)	2,731,268
Anttila, 2002 [36] Hakama, 1997 [38]	Helsinki, Finland Finland	50–59 50–64	2 years 2 years	Contemporaneous [3] Contemporaneous	1986–1997 1987–1989/1992	Same Same	161,400/155,400 400,804/299,228
Puliti, 2012 [45]	Florence, Italy	50–69	2 years	Contemporaneous	1991–2007/08	Same	50–59: 270,399/113,409 60–69: 233,543/151,615
Paci, 2002 [47]	Florence, Italy	50–69	2 years	Contemporaneous	1990–1996/99	Same	254,890
Van Dijck, 1997 [52]	Nijmegen, Netherlands	68–83	2 years	Regional	1977–1990	1978–1990	60,313/ 61,832
Peer, 1995 [53]	Nijmegen, Netherlands	35–49	2 years	Regional	1975–1990	1976–1990	166,307/ 154,103
Taylor, 2019 [18]	New Zealand	50–64 45–49/ 65–69	2 years	Historical	2001–03/ 2009–11 2006–08/ 2009–11	1996–98/ 2004–06 2001–03/ 2004–06	930,000/766,000 480,000/409,000 249,000/205,000 [4]

Table 2. Cont.

Study	Location	Age range	Interval	Comparison	Period 1	Period 2	Numbers
Morrell, 2017 [17]	New Zealand	45–69	2 years	Contemporaneous	1999–2011/ 2000–2011	Same	3,707,483/ 5,405,518
Weedon-Fekjær, 2014 [41]	Norway	50–69	2 years	Contemporaneous	1986–2009	Same	2,407,709/ 12,785,325
Hofvind, 2013 [40]	Norway	50–69	2 years	Contemporaneous [5]	1996–2009/10	Same	4,814,060/ 988,641
Ascunce, 2007 [56]	Navarre, Spain	50–69	2 years	Historical	1991–2001/ 1997–2001	1980–1990/ 1986–1990	293,000/ 289,000 [6]
Hellquist, 2011 [20]	Sweden	40–49	1.5–2 years	Regional	1986–2005	Same	7,261,415/ 8,843,852
SOSSEG, 2006 [14]	13 counties, Sweden	40–69 depending on county	2 years	Historical	1980–2001 depending on county	1958–1989	7,542,833/ 7,265,841
Tabár, 2003 [23]	Östergötland and Dalarna, Sweden	40–69	1.5–2 years	Historical	1978–1997	1958–1977	2,399,000/ 2,416,000
Jonsson, 2003 [25]	10 counties, Sweden	70–74	2 years	Regional and historical	1986–1998	1976–1988 (pre-screening) 1986–1998 (screening)	1,251,300/ 580,100; 533,400; 1,162,800
Jonsson, 2003 [24]	Gävleborg, Sweden	40–64	2 years [7]	Regional and historical	1974–1986/1998	1964–1973/1985 (pre-screening) 1974–1986/1998 (screening)	855,000/ 2,581,000; 12,619,000
Jonsson, 2001 [28]	7 counties, Sweden	50–69	2 years	Regional and historical	1986–1994/97	1979–1987/1990 (pre-screening) 1987–1993/97 (screening)	2,0360,00/ 1,265,000; 2,046,000; 1,296,000
Johns, 2017 [54]	England and Wales, UK	49–64	3 years	Contemporaneous	1991–2005 [8]	Same	1,675,356/ 4,719,228
UK Trial of Early Detection of Breast Cancer Group, 1999 [55]	Guildford and Edinburgh, UK	45–64	2 years	Regional	1979–1995	Same	(45,607/ 127,123)
Thompson [16]	Washington, USA	40+ if high risk/50+ if low risk	3 years	Contemporaneous	1982–1988	Same	(94,656)

[1] Two Provinces, British Columbia and Nova Scotia, invited women aged 40–49 annually; [2] Women aged 40–49 were invited yearly for women born in odd years; [3] Invited women born 1935–1939 were compared with uninvited women born in 1930–1934; [4] Estimated from data in the paper; [5] All women followed from 1986 but screening began in 1995; [6] Estimated from data in the paper; [7] The average interval between the first and second, and second and third round was 38 months (range 22–65), but was 23 months between rounds 3 and 4; [8] The 15-year period 1991–2005 was partitioned into observation periods of two years accrual and up to nine years follow-up.

3.2. Study Findings

Whilst the majority of studies included women in the age range 50–64 years, the youngest age of invitation was 35 years and the oldest 83 years. Most countries invite women every two years, with the range between 18 months and three years. Table 3 shows the unadjusted relative risk for the effect of invitation and attendance on the outcome of incidence-based breast cancer mortality as reported in the studies, and corresponding relative risks adjusted for self-selection bias as described above. The effect sizes and the participation rates reported in the studies suggest differences in risk of breast cancer mortality within countries as well as between countries. Participation rates ranged from 44% in Canada to above 90% in Finland.

The studies reviewed used one or more of three types of comparison groups used to estimate breast cancer mortality in an uninvited population: contemporaneous, regional and historical. (i) The contemporaneous comparison group compared women not yet invited, during the same time period and in the same region, as the women invited. (ii) The regional comparison group is often concurrent to the invited women, but in a region not yet invited. (iii) The historical comparison group compares women invited with women from an epoch not yet invited.

Ten studies compared the screening population with a contemporaneous comparison group, five of which estimated the effect of invitation to screening and seven the effect of attending screening. The effect of invitation fell within a narrow range from 0.72 (95% CI 0.64–0.79) [41] to 0.81 (95% CI 0.64–1.01) [47] and the effect of attendance was 0.38 (95% CI 0.30–0.49) [17] to 0.67 (95% CI 0.49–0.97) [38].

A further six studies used a historical comparison group to compare the impact of introducing screening in a particular region or country, the majority of which reported both the effect of invitation and attendance. The range of the respective effect sizes was wider for invitation than the studies that used a contemporaneous comparison group but narrower for attendance at 0.58 (95% CI 0.44–0.75) [56] to 0.83 (95% CI 0.73–0.95) [18] and 0.52 (95% CI 0.46–0.59) [23] to 0.66 (95% CI 0.58–0.75) [32] respectively.

Only four studies used a regional comparison group without any adjustment for differences in underlying cancer incidence between regions. All studies estimated the effect of invitation, with the results ranging from 0.73 (95% CI 0.63–0.84) [55] to 0.94 (95% CI 0.68–1.29) [53]. Just one study reported the effect of attending screening and found a 29% reduction in breast cancer mortality (95% CI 0.62–0.80) [20] in women who attended screening compared to those who did not.

The remaining seven studies used a combination of regional and historical data, and again, all studies estimated the effect of invitation, with effect estimates ranging between 0.75 (95% CI 0.63–0.89) [50] to 0.97 (95% CI 0.73–1.28) [25], which is almost identical to the results of those studies that used a regional control group alone. The two studies that estimated the effect of attendance reported relative risks of 0.60 (95% CI 0.49–0.74) [50] and 0.68 (95% CI 0.59–0.79) [49] respectively.

Table 3. Unadjusted and adjusted relative risks.

Reference (by Country and Date)	Country	Age at Screening	Attendance	RR: Unadjusted Effect on Incidence-Based Breast Cancer Mortality		RR Calculated from Effect of Attendance	RR Adjusted for Self-Selection
				Invited Versus not Invited [1]	Screened Versus not Screened [1]	Invited Versus not Invited(RR_1) [1]	Screened Versus not Screened (RR_2) [1]
Coldman, 2014 [15]	7 provinces, Canada	40-79	0.437	NR	0.60 (0.52-0.67)	0.97 (0.88-1.06)	0.90 (0.68-1.18)
		40-49			0.56 (0.45-0.67) [2]	0.95 (0.85-1.05)	0.84 (0.61-1.16)
		50-59			0.60 (0.49-0.70)	0.97 (0.87-1.07)	0.90 (0.66-1.23)
		60-69			0.58 (0.50-0.67)	0.96 (0.87-1.05)	0.87 (0.69-1.10)
		70-79			0.65 (0.56-0.74) [3]	0.99 (0.90-1.09)	0.97 (0.74-1.29)
Beau, 2018 [48]	Copenhagen, Denmark	50-69	0.71 [4]	0.89 (0.82-0.98)	NR	NA	NA
Njor, 2015 [49]	Funen, Denmark	50-69	0.84	0.78 (0.68-0.89)	0.68 (0.59-0.79)	0.86 (0.75-0.98)	0.82 (0.69-0.98)
Olsen, 2005 [50]	Copenhagen, Denmark	50-69	0.71	0.75 (0.63-0.89) [5]	0.60 (0.49-0.74)	0.84 (0.72-0.97)	0.75 (0.60-0.96)
Parvinen, 2015 [30]	Turku, Finland	40-49	0.867	0.73 (0.50-1.06)	NR	NA	NA
		50-59		0.98 (0.71-1.35)			
		60-74		0.85 (0.66-1.10)			
Sarkeala, 2008 [33]	8 municipalities, Finland	50-59	0.905	0.72 (0.51-0.97)	0.62 (0.43-0.85)	0.77 (0.56-1.06)	0.74 (0.51-1.08)
Sarkeala, 2008 [32]	260 municipalities, Finland	50-69	0.924	0.78 (0.70-0.87)	0.66 (0.58-0.75)	0.80 (0.70-0.92)	0.78 (0.67-0.92)
Anttila, 2002 [36]	Helsinki, Finland	50-59	0.82	0.81 (0.62-1.05)	NR	NA	NA
Hakama, 1997 [38]	Finland	50-64	0.85	0.76 (0.53-1.09)	0.67 (0.46-0.97) [6]	0.84 (0.62-1.15)	0.81 (0.55-1.19)
Puliti, 2012 [45]	Florence, Italy	50-69	0.64	NR	0.44 (0.36-0.54) [7]	0.75 (0.67-0.85)	0.57 (0.45-0.73)
		50-59			0.55 (0.41-0.75)	0.83 (0.71-0.98)	0.71 (0.51-0.98)
		60-69			0.49 (0.38-0.64)	0.79 (0.68-0.91)	0.63 (0.47-0.85)
Paci, 2002 [47]	Florence, Italy	50-69	0.60	0.81 (0.64-1.01)	NR	0.75 (0.67-0.85)	0.57 (0.45-0.73)
Van Dijck, 1997 [52]	Nijmegen, Netherlands	68-83	0.46	0.80 (0.53-1.22)	NR	NA	NA
Peer, 1995 [53]	Nijmegen, Netherlands	35-49	0.65	0.94 (0.68-1.29)	NR	NA	NA
Taylor, 2019 [18]	New Zealand	45-49	0.72	1.00 (0.71-1.42) [8]	NR	NA	NA
		50-64		0.83 (0.73-0.95)			
		65-69		0.81 (0.57-1.16)			
Morrell, 2017 [17]	New Zealand	45-69	0.64	NR	0.38 (0.30-0.49)	0.71 (0.62-0.80)	0.49 (0.37-0.65)
Weedon-Fekjær, 2014 [41]	Norway	50-69	0.76	0.72 (0.64-0.79)	NR	NA	NA
Hofvind, 2013 [40]	Norway	50-69	0.84	NR	0.39 (0.35-0.44)	0.57 (0.51-0.64)	0.47 (0.41-0.55)
Ascunce, 2007 [56]	Navarre, Spain	50-69	0.85	0.58 (0.44-0.75) [9]	NR	NA	NA
Hellquist, 2011 [20]	Sweden	40-49	0.80	0.79 (0.72-0.86)	NR	0.74 (0.66-0.83) [10]	0.71 (0.62-0.80)
SOSSEG, 2006 [14]	13 counties, Sweden	40-69	0.80 [11]	0.73 (0.69-0.77)	0.55 (0.51-0.59)	0.75 (0.68-0.82)	0.66 (0.58-0.74)
Tabar, 2003 [23]	Östergötland and Dalarna, Sweden	40-69	0.85	0.59 (0.53-0.66)	0.52 (0.46-0.59)	0.69 (0.61-0.78)	0.63 (0.54-0.73)
Jonsson, 2003 [25]	10 counties, Sweden	70-74	0.84 [12]	0.97 (0.73-1.28)	NR	NA	NA
Jonsson, 2003 [24]	Gävleborg, Sweden	40-64	0.84	0.86 (0.71-1.05)	NR	NA	NA
Jonsson, 2001 [28]	7 counties, Sweden	50-69	0.80 [11]	0.90 (0.74-1.10)	NR	NA	NA

Table 3. Cont.

Johns, 2017 [54] UK Trial of Early Detection of Breast Cancer Group, 1999 [55]	England and Wales, UK	49–64	0.74	0.79 (0.73–0.84)	0.54 (0.51–0.57)	0.77 (0.71–0.84)	0.67 (0.59–0.76)
	Guildford and Edinburgh, UK	45–64	0.654	0.73 (0.63–0.84)	NR	NA	NA
Thompson, 1994 [16]	Washington, USA	≥50	NR	NR	0.61 (0.23–1.62)	NA	NA
Pooled RR from all studies			Random effects	0.78 (0.75–0.82)	0.54 (0.49–0.59)	0.76 (0.71–0.83)	0.67 (0.61–0.75)
			Heterogeneity p-value	<0.001	<0.001	<0.001	<0.001
Pooled RR from studies inviting women aged 50 and over			Random effects	0.80 (0.77–0.84)	0.57 (0.51–0.64)	0.82 (0.74–0.92)	0.74 (0.64–0.85)
			Heterogeneity p-value	0.175	<0.001	<0.001	<0.001
Pooled RR from studies inviting women under 50 years			Random effects	0.81 (0.74–0.87)	0.56 (0.45–0.67) [13]	0.84 (0.66–1.06)	0.73 (0.65–0.82)
			Heterogeneity p-value	0.418		0.002	0.343

[1] RR, relative risk (95% confidence interval), NR, not reported, NA, not applicable; [2] Pooled RR of three provinces; [3] Pooled RR of four provinces; [4] Participation rate not reported so taken from Olsen AH, Njor SH, Vejborg I, Schwartz W, Dalgaard P, Jensen, M.B; et al. Breast cancer mortality in Copenhagen after introduction of mammography screening: cohort study. *BMJ* **2005**, *330*, 220. [50]; [5] Not included in meta-analysis due to later paper by Beau et al.; [6] Calculated from data in the paper; [7] Unadjusted RR calculated from data in the paper; [8] RR calculated from data in the paper. The accrual period for women aged 50–64 was 2001–2003 and for women aged 45–49 and 65–69 was 2006–2008; [9] Excludes prevalent cases; [10] RR1 and RR2 are as reported by authors in the paper; [11] Attendance rate not reported so taken from Giordano L, von Karsa L, Tomatis M, Majek O, de Wolf C, Lancucki L, et al. Mammographic screening programmes in Europe: organization, coverage and participation. *J. Med Screen.* **2012**, *19*, 72–82. [57] as region reported invites women until the age of 74; [12] Attendance rate not reported so taken from Swedish Organised Service Screening Evaluation Group. Reduction in breast cancer mortality from the organised service screening with mammography: 2. Validation with alternative analytic methods. *Cancer Epidemiol Biomark. Prev.* **2006**, *15*, 52–56. [58]; [13] One study only.

3.3. Meta-Analysis by Age-Group of Women

There were twenty-two studies that assessed the effect of invitation to screening (Table 3 and Figure 2). All studies had a relative risk of less than or equal to 1, with the largest studies achieving statistical significance. The largest studies were those by SOSSEG [14] and Johns et al. [54] who found a 20–30% reduction in breast cancer mortality. The pooled rate ratio was 0.78 (95% CI 0.75–0.82) with significant heterogeneity ($p < 0.001$).

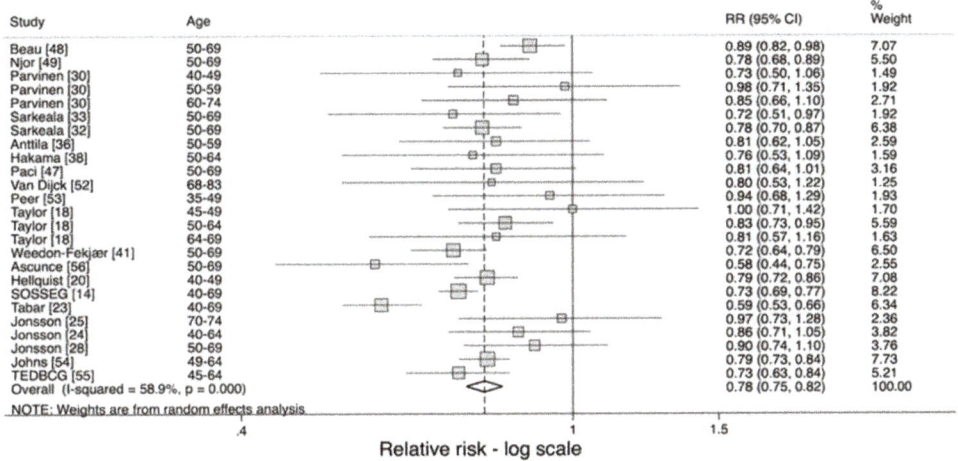

Figure 2. Effect of invitation on risk of breast cancer mortality [14,18,20,23–25,28,30,32,33,36,38,41,47–49,52–56].

Fourteen studies reported on the effect of being screened, eight of which also reported on the effect of being invited. All but one study reported a statistically significant result with the largest studies again by SOSSEG [14] and Johns et al. [54] with relative risks of 0.54 and 0.55 respectively. This therefore led to a pooled estimate of 0.54 (95% CI 0.49–0.59) with significant heterogeneity at $p < 0.001$. However, as discussed previously, the effect estimate of being screened is likely to be subject to self-selection bias. Therefore, an adjustment was made to account for this.

To be able to calculate the adjustments for self-selection suggested by Duffy et al. [13], it is necessary to know the proportion of women attending screening. This is not reported in the paper by Thompson et al. [16] and so the adjusted relative risks cannot be estimated. However, this study is small and therefore omission of this study in the calculation of the pooled relative risk would not have a substantial effect.

The intention to treat estimate, RR_1, was 0.76 (95% CI 0.71–0.83) with significant heterogeneity ($p < 0.001$). This estimate is almost identical to the effect size presented in Figure 2 (RR 0.78). The adjusted pooled relative risk for the effect of being screened, RR_2, was 0.67 (95% CI 0.61–0.75) and again there was significant heterogeneity between studies with $p < 0.001$ (Figure 3).

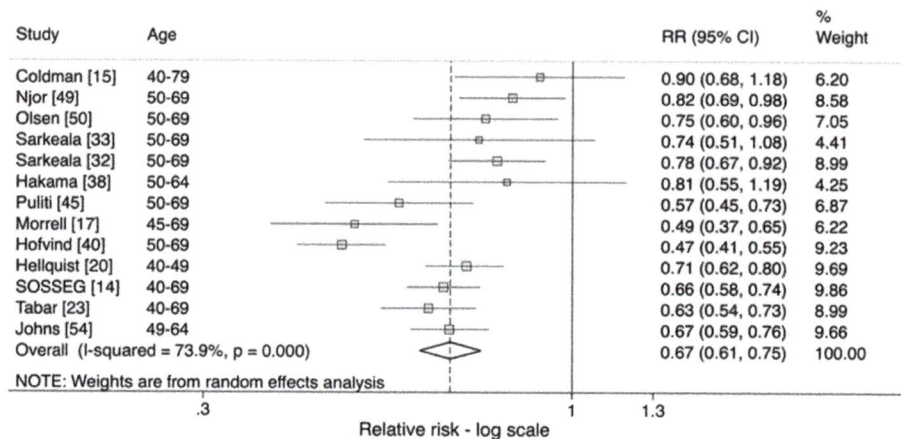

Figure 3. Estimated effect of attendance adjusted for self-selection on risk of breast cancer mortality (RR_2) [14,15,17,20,23,32,33,38,40,45,49,50,54].

When assessing the effect of invitation in women aged 50 and over (Figure 4), whilst the pooled relative risk was similar to that in women of all ages, the p-value was 0.175, suggesting no heterogeneity between studies. However, there was still evidence of heterogeneity when assessing the effect of attendance with a relative risk, adjusted for self-selection, of 0.74 (95% CI 0.64–0.85) and a p-value of <0.001 (Figure 5).

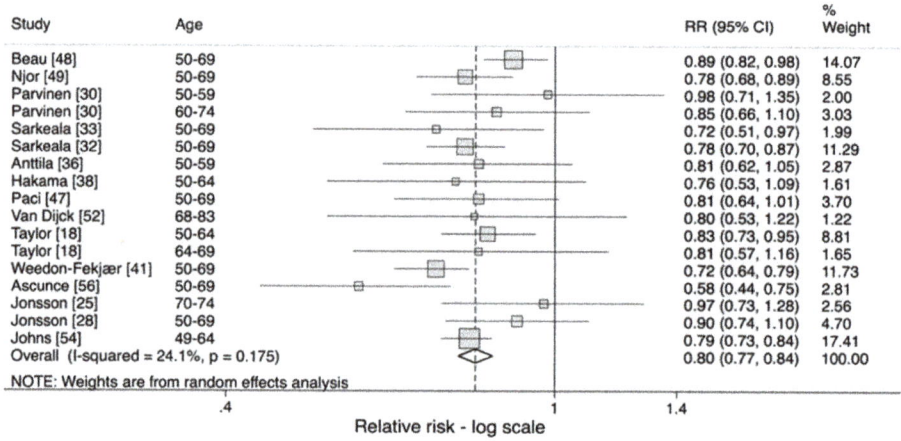

Figure 4. Effect of invitation on risk of breast cancer mortality in women aged 50 and over [18,25,28,30,32,33,36,38,41,47–49,52,54,56].

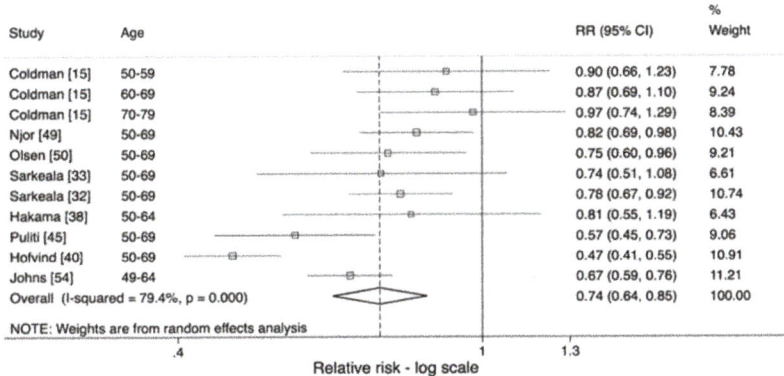

Figure 5. Estimated effect of attendance adjusted for self-selection on risk of breast cancer mortality (RR_2) in women aged 50 and over [15,32,33,38,40,45,49,50,54].

There were five studies that reported on the effect of screening in women under 50 years. Four studies [18,20,30,53] report the effect of invitation with a pooled relative risk of 0.81 (95% CI 0.74–0.87) and no evidence of heterogeneity ($p = 0.418$). Two studies [15,20] reported the effect of attendance to screening and the adjusted relative risk was 0.73 (95% CI 0.65–0.82).

4. Discussion

This systematic review and meta-analysis of IBM studies estimates that the risk of death from breast cancer in women invited for screening is reduced by 22% compared to women not invited (RR 0.78, 95% CI 0.75–0.82), with similar results across age groups. This result is consistent with earlier overviews of cohort studies [5,6] and from the RCTs in breast cancer screening, which suggest invitation to screening reduces mortality by approximately 20% [1].

The studies with contemporaneous control groups are likely to be least biased, with the regional and historical comparison groups potentially affected by differences in the underlying risk of breast cancer mortality between regions or across time periods respectively. When assessing the effect of invitation, the results of studies with contemporaneous control groups ranged from 0.72 (95% CI 0.64–0.79) in the Norwegian study by Weedon-Fekjær [41] to 0.81 (95% CI 0.64–1.01) in the Italian study by Paci [47].

The relative risk, RR_2, estimates the effect of attendance adjusted for self-selection bias. Using population specific attendance rates and $D_r = 1.17$ from the SOSSEG study [14] results in a mortality decrease of 33% (RR: 0.67, 95% CI 0.61–0.75). This is slightly more conservative than the relative risk estimated by Broeders et al. [5] although it is unclear whether their result is adjusted for self-selection bias.

The relative risk, RR_1, estimating the effect of invitation to screening from the relative risk of attendance adjusting for potential self-selection bias, is almost identical to the pooled effect estimated directly. The agreement between the two measures suggests that the adjustment method is valid.

There appears to be significant heterogeneity of the effect of invitation in the meta-analysis of all studies, which disappears when the analysis is stratified by the age. This suggests that there is a difference in the effect of invitation in differing age groups, and that the varying distributions by age among studies is contributing to the heterogeneity of the effect for all ages combined. The heterogeneity of the effect of attendance adjusted for self-selection bias (RR_2), however, is present for women screened at any age and in women screened over the age of 50 years, suggesting that variation in age distributions is not entirely responsible for heterogeneity among studies. It is likely that this is partly due to differing screening regimens and practices.

Attendance rates varied between studies, from 0.44 in the Canadian study [15] to 0.92 in the study by Sarkeala et al. [32]. Canada differs from other countries in respect of protocol for call and recall, requiring women to self-refer in some provinces. When this opportunistic screening is taken into account, the attendance rate is estimated to be 63.1% [59]. Additionally, the screening programme has a high retention rate, with nearly 80% of previous participants attending a subsequent screen within 36 months.

IBM studies have been the focus of this review but they are not without their limitations. The main limitation is the identification of an appropriate comparison group in the absence of screening [8]. In addition, they are prospective studies and require a long follow-up period to accumulate enough deaths to achieve statistical power [60] and to see the full benefit of screening. Results from the Swedish Two-County Trial suggest that the full benefit of screening requires follow-up of at least 20 years [61]. The majority of studies included in this review had at least 10 years follow-up, with some having over 20 years. In addition, the length of the accrual period should be equal in comparison groups and should be equal to the length of the follow-up period. The effect of screening will be underestimated if the accrual period is shorter than the follow-up period, as more cases will accrue in the screened population than the non-screened population. Seventeen studies in this review had equal accrual and follow-up periods, with ten studies having a shorter accrual period.

Our results update and confirm those of the Euroscreen project for IBM studies [5,8]. Case-control studies reviewed in the Euroscreen project tended to find rather stronger effects than the IBM studies with the effect of invitation 0.69 (95% CI 0.57–0.83) and the effect of attendance adjusted for self-selection bias 0.52 (95% CI 0.42–0.65). This may be due to ascertainment biases in the case-control approach [12]. In addition, the Euroscreen project estimated the effect from trend studies to be between 28–36%, which is comparable to the results in this review [62].

There have been suggestions of alternative analysis methods using the IBM approach. Tabar et al. [63] suggest using as the endpoint the incidence of breast cancers subsequently proving fatal, within ten or twenty years. This method links exposure to endpoint more accurately, but requires a long follow-up period. Sasieni et al. [64] propose a method for estimating the expected number of deaths in the population without screening, which can be used when there is no contemporaneous comparison group. Neither of these methods have been used extensively up to now.

5. Conclusions

IBM studies yield estimates uncontaminated by pre-screening cancers. Results from these international studies indicate that inviting women to screening results in a 22% reduction in breast cancer mortality and that the effect of attending screening reduces the risk of death by around 30%. Breast cancer screening in the routine healthcare setting continues to confer a substantial reduction in mortality from breast cancer.

Author Contributions: Conceptualization, S.D. and A.D.; methodology, A.D., J.O., S.W.D. and R.G.; data extraction A.D.; writing—original draft preparation, A.D., S.W.D. and R.G.; writing—review and editing, A.D., J.O., S.W.D. and R.G. All authors have read and agree to the published version of the manuscript.

Funding: This research is funded by the National Institute for Health Research (NIHR) Policy Research Programme, conducted through the Policy Research Unit in Cancer Awareness, Screening and Early Diagnosis, 106/0001. The views expressed are those of the author(s) and not necessarily those of the NIHR or the Department of Health and Social Care.

Conflicts of Interest: The authors declare no conflict of interest.

Appendix A

Search Strategy

The following search terms were used to conduct the review of the literature in PubMed. These search terms were taken from previous review by Njor et al. [8], however our search was restricted to three out of the four searches performed by Njor et al. and papers in English only.

(1) ("breast neoplasms/mortality*" [MeSH Terms] OR breast cancer mortality OR "mortality" [MeSH Terms]) AND (("mass screening" [MeSH Terms] OR screening) AND ("mammography" [MeSH Terms] OR mammography) AND English [lang] [8]
(2) (effect* OR evaluation OR impact OR trend) AND (service screening OR programme screening OR mass screening) AND breast cancer AND (mortality OR survival) AND English [lang]
(3) "Breast neoplasm/mortality*" [MeSH Terms] AND "mass screening" [MeSH Terms] AND ("mortality/trends" [MeSH Terms] OR "survival analysis" [MeSH Terms] OR "survival rate/trends" [MeSH Terms]) AND English [lang]

References

1. Independent UK Panel on Breast Cancer Screening. The benefits and harms of breast cancer screening: An independent review. *Lancet (Lond. Engl.)* **2012**, *380*, 1778–1786. [CrossRef]
2. Gotzsche, P.C.; Jorgensen, K.J. Screening for breast cancer with mammography. *Cochrane Database Syst. Rev.* **2013**. [CrossRef] [PubMed]
3. Cancer Research UK. Breast Cancer Incidence Statistics. Available online: https://www.cancerresearchuk.org/health-professional/cancer-statistics/statistics-by-cancer-type/breast-cancer/incidence-invasive#heading-Two (accessed on 24 April 2019).
4. Cancer Research UK. Breast Cancer Mortality Statistics. Available online: https://www.cancerresearchuk.org/health-professional/cancer-statistics/statistics-by-cancer-type/breast-cancer/mortality#heading-Two (accessed on 24 April 2019).
5. Broeders, M.; Moss, S.; Nystrom, L.; Njor, S.; Jonsson, H.; Paap, E.; Massat, N.; Duffy, S.; Lynge, E.; Paci, E. The impact of mammographic screening on breast cancer mortality in Europe: A review of observational studies. *J. Med. Screen.* **2012**, *19*, 14–25. [CrossRef] [PubMed]
6. Gabe, R.; Duffy, S.W. Evaluation of service screening mammography in practice: The impact on breast cancer mortality. *Ann. Oncol. Off. J. Eur. Soc. Med. Oncol.* **2005**, *16*, ii153–ii162. [CrossRef]
7. Chu, K.C.; Miller, B.A.; Feuer, E.J.; Hankey, B.F. A method for partitioning cancer mortality trends by factors associated with diagnosis: An application to female breast cancer. *J. Clin. Epidemiol.* **1994**, *47*, 1451–1461. [CrossRef]
8. Njor, S.; Nystrom, L.; Moss, S.; Paci, E.; Broeders, M.; Segnan, N.; Lynge, E. Breast cancer mortality in mammographic screening in Europe: A review of incidence-based mortality studies. *J. Med. Screen.* **2012**, *19*, 33–41. [CrossRef]
9. Duffy, S.W.; Chen, T.H.H.; Yen, A.M.F.; Tabar, L.; Gabe, R.; Smith, R.A. Methodologic Issues in the Evaluation of Service Screening. *Semin. Breast Dis.* **2007**, *10*, 68–71. [CrossRef]
10. Egger, M.; Davey Smith, G.; Schneider, M. *Systematic Reviews in Health Care: Meta-Analysis in Context*, 2nd ed.; BMJ Publishing Group: London, UK, 2008; Volume 2, pp. 211–227.
11. StataCorp. *Stata Statistical Software: Release 13*; StataCorp LP: College Station, TX, USA, 2013.
12. Duffy, S.W. Case-Control Studies to Evaluate the Effect of Mammographic Service Screening on Mortality from Breast Cancer. *Semin. Breast Dis.* **2007**, *10*, 61–63. [CrossRef]
13. Duffy, S.W.; Cuzick, J.; Tabar, L.; Vitak, B.; Hsiu-Hsi Chen, T.; Yen, M.-F.; Smith, R.A. Correcting for non-compliance bias in case–control studies to evaluate cancer screening programmes. *J. R. Stat. Soc. Ser. C (Appl. Stat.)* **2002**, *51*, 235–243. [CrossRef]
14. Swedish Organised Service Screening Evaluation Group. Reduction in breast cancer mortality from organized service screening with mammography: 1. Further confirmation with extended data. *Cancer Epidemiol. Biomark. Prev.* **2006**, *15*, 45–51. [CrossRef]

15. Coldman, A.; Phillips, N.; Wilson, C.; Decker, K.; Chiarelli, A.M.; Brisson, J.; Zhang, B.; Payne, J.; Doyle, G.; Ahmad, R. Pan-Canadian study of mammography screening and mortality from breast cancer. *J. Natl. Cancer Inst.* **2014**, *106*. [CrossRef] [PubMed]
16. Thompson, R.S.; Barlow, W.E.; Taplin, S.H.; Grothaus, L.; Immanuel, V.; Salazar, A.; Wagner, E.H. A population-based case-cohort evaluation of the efficacy of mammographic screening for breast cancer. *Am. J. Epidemiol.* **1994**, *140*, 889–901. [CrossRef] [PubMed]
17. Morrell, S.; Taylor, R.; Roder, D.; Robson, B.; Gregory, M.; Craig, K. Mammography service screening and breast cancer mortality in New Zealand: A National Cohort Study 1999–2011. *Br. J. Cancer* **2017**, *116*, 828–839. [CrossRef] [PubMed]
18. Taylor, R.; Gregory, M.; Sexton, K.; Wharton, J.; Sharma, N.; Amoyal, G.; Morrell, S. Breast cancer mortality and screening mammography in New Zealand: Incidence-based and aggregate analyses. *J. Med. Screen.* **2019**, *26*, 35–43. [CrossRef]
19. Hellquist, B.N.; Czene, K.; Hjalm, A.; Nystrom, L.; Jonsson, H. Effectiveness of population-based service screening with mammography for women ages 40 to 49 years with a high or low risk of breast cancer: Socioeconomic status, parity, and age at birth of first child. *Cancer* **2015**, *121*, 251–258. [CrossRef]
20. Hellquist, B.N.; Duffy, S.W.; Abdsaleh, S.; Bjorneld, L.; Bordas, P.; Tabar, L.; Vitak, B.; Zackrisson, S.; Nystrom, L.; Jonsson, H. Effectiveness of population-based service screening with mammography for women ages 40 to 49 years: Evaluation of the Swedish Mammography Screening in Young Women (SCRY) cohort. *Cancer* **2011**, *117*, 714–722. [CrossRef]
21. Jonsson, H.; Bordas, P.; Wallin, H.; Nystrom, L.; Lenner, P. Service screening with mammography in Northern Sweden: Effects on breast cancer mortality—An update. *J. Med. Screen.* **2007**, *14*, 87–93. [CrossRef]
22. Baker, S.G.; Kramer, B.S.; Prorok, P.C. Comparing breast cancer mortality rates before-and-after a change in availability of screening in different regions: Extension of the paired availability design. *BMC Med. Res. Methodol.* **2004**, *4*, 12. [CrossRef]
23. Tabar, L.; Yen, M.F.; Vitak, B.; Chen, H.H.; Smith, R.A.; Duffy, S.W. Mammography service screening and mortality in breast cancer patients: 20-year follow-up before and after introduction of screening. *Lancet (Lond. Engl.)* **2003**, *361*, 1405–1410. [CrossRef]
24. Jonsson, H.; Nystrom, L.; Tornberg, S.; Lundgren, B.; Lenner, P. Service screening with mammography. Long-term effects on breast cancer mortality in the county of Gavleborg, Sweden. *Breast (Edinb. Scotl.)* **2003**, *12*, 183–193. [CrossRef]
25. Jonsson, H.; Tornberg, S.; Nystrom, L.; Lenner, P. Service screening with mammography of women aged 70–74 years in Sweden. Effects on breast cancer mortality. *Cancer Detect. Prev.* **2003**, *27*, 360–369. [CrossRef]
26. Duffy, S.W.; Tabar, L.; Chen, H.H.; Holmqvist, M.; Yen, M.F.; Abdsalah, S.; Epstein, B.; Frodis, E.; Ljungberg, E.; Hedborg-Melander, C.; et al. The impact of organized mammography service screening on breast carcinoma mortality in seven Swedish counties. *Cancer* **2002**, *95*, 458–469. [CrossRef] [PubMed]
27. Tabar, L.; Vitak, B.; Chen, H.H.; Yen, M.F.; Duffy, S.W.; Smith, R.A. Beyond randomized controlled trials: Organized mammographic screening substantially reduces breast carcinoma mortality. *Cancer* **2001**, *91*, 1724–1731. [CrossRef]
28. Jonsson, H.; Nystrom, L.; Tornberg, S.; Lenner, P. Service screening with mammography of women aged 50–69 years in Sweden: Effects on mortality from breast cancer. *J. Med. Screen.* **2001**, *8*, 152–160. [CrossRef]
29. Jonsson, H.; Tornberg, S.; Nystrom, L.; Lenner, P. Service screening with mammography in Sweden–evaluation of effects of screening on breast cancer mortality in age group 40–49 years. *Acta Oncol. (Stockh. Swed.)* **2000**, *39*, 617–623.
30. Parvinen, I.; Heinavaara, S.; Anttila, A.; Helenius, H.; Klemi, P.; Pylkkanen, L. Mammography screening in three Finnish residential areas: Comprehensive population-based study of breast cancer incidence and incidence-based mortality 1976–2009. *Br. J. Cancer* **2015**, *112*, 918–924. [CrossRef]
31. Wu, J.C.-Y.; Anttila, A.; Yen, A.M.-F.; Hakama, M.; Saarenmaa, I.; Sarkeala, T.; Malila, N.; Auvinen, A.; Chiu, S.Y.-H.; Chen, T.H.-H. Evaluation of breast cancer service screening programme with a Bayesian approach: Mortality analysis in a Finnish region. *Breast Cancer Res. Treat.* **2010**, *121*, 671–678. [CrossRef]
32. Sarkeala, T.; Heinavaara, S.; Anttila, A. Organised mammography screening reduces breast cancer mortality: A cohort study from Finland. *Int. J. Cancer* **2008**, *122*, 614–619. [CrossRef]
33. Sarkeala, T.; Heinavaara, S.; Anttila, A. Breast cancer mortality with varying invitational policies in organised mammography. *Br. J. Cancer* **2008**, *98*, 641–645. [CrossRef]

34. Anttila, A.; Sarkeala, T.; Hakulinen, T.; Heinavaara, S. Impacts of the Finnish service screening programme on breast cancer rates. *BMC Public Health* **2008**, *8*, 38. [CrossRef]
35. Parvinen, I.; Helenius, H.; Pylkkanen, L.; Anttila, A.; Immonen-Raiha, P.; Kauhava, L.; Rasanen, O.; Klemi, P.J. Service screening mammography reduces breast cancer mortality among elderly women in Turku. *J. Med. Screen.* **2006**, *13*, 34–40. [CrossRef] [PubMed]
36. Anttila, A.; Koskela, J.; Hakama, M. Programme sensitivity and effectiveness of mammography service screening in Helsinki, Finland. *J. Med. Screen.* **2002**, *9*, 153–158. [CrossRef] [PubMed]
37. Hakama, M.; Pukkala, E.; Soderman, B.; Day, N. Implementation of screening as a public health policy: Issues in design and evaluation. *J. Med. Screen.* **1999**, *6*, 209–216. [CrossRef] [PubMed]
38. Hakama, M.; Pukkala, E.; Heikkila, M.; Kallio, M. Effectiveness of the public health policy for breast cancer screening in Finland: Population based cohort study. *BMJ (Clin. Res. Ed.)* **1997**, *314*, 864–867. [CrossRef]
39. Moller, M.H.; Lousdal, M.L.; Kristiansen, I.S.; Stovring, H. Effect of organized mammography screening on breast cancer mortality: A population-based cohort study in Norway. *Int. J. Cancer* **2019**, *144*, 697–706. [CrossRef]
40. Hofvind, S.; Ursin, G.; Tretli, S.; Sebuodegard, S.; Moller, B. Breast cancer mortality in participants of the Norwegian Breast Cancer Screening Program. *Cancer* **2013**, *119*, 3106–3112. [CrossRef]
41. Weedon-Fekjaer, H.; Romundstad, P.R.; Vatten, L.J. Modern mammography screening and breast cancer mortality: Population study. *BMJ (Clin. Res. Ed.)* **2014**, *348*, g3701. [CrossRef]
42. Olsen, A.H.; Lynge, E.; Njor, S.H.; Kumle, M.; Waaseth, M.; Braaten, T.; Lund, E. Breast cancer mortality in Norway after the introduction of mammography screening. *Int. J. Cancer* **2013**, *132*, 208–214. [CrossRef]
43. Kalager, M.; Zelen, M.; Langmark, F.; Adami, H.O. Effect of screening mammography on breast-cancer mortality in Norway. *N. Engl. J. Med.* **2010**, *363*, 1203–1210. [CrossRef]
44. Capodaglio, G.; Zorzi, M.; Tognazzo, S.; Greco, A.; Michieletto, F.; Fedato, C.; Montaguti, A.; Turrin, A.; Ferro, A.; Cinquetti, S.; et al. Impact of breast cancer screening in a population with high spontaneous coverage with mammography. *Tumori* **2018**, *104*, 258–265. [CrossRef]
45. Puliti, D.; Miccinesi, G.; Zappa, M.; Manneschi, G.; Crocetti, E.; Paci, E. Balancing harms and benefits of service mammography screening programs: A cohort study. *Breast Cancer Res. BCR* **2012**, *14*, R9. [CrossRef] [PubMed]
46. Paci, E.; Duffy, S.W.; Giorgi, D.; Zappa, M.; Crocetti, E.; Vezzosi, V.; Bianchi, S.; del Turco, M.R. Quantification of the effect of mammographic screening on fatal breast cancers: The Florence Programme 1990–1996. *Br. J. Cancer* **2002**, *87*, 65–69. [CrossRef] [PubMed]
47. Paci, E.; Giorgi, D.; Bianchi, S.; Vezzosi, V.; Zappa, M.; Crocetti, E.; Rosselli del Turco, M. Assessment of the early impact of the population-based breast cancer screening programme in Florence (Italy) using mortality and surrogate measures. *Eur. J. Cancer (Oxf. Engl. 1990)* **2002**, *38*, 568–573. [CrossRef]
48. Beau, A.B.; Andersen, P.K.; Vejborg, I.; Lynge, E. Limitations in the Effect of Screening on Breast Cancer Mortality. *J. Clin. Oncol. Off. J. Am. Soc. Clin. Oncol.* **2018**, *36*, 2988–2994. [CrossRef] [PubMed]
49. Njor, S.H.; Schwartz, W.; Blichert-Toft, M.; Lynge, E. Decline in breast cancer mortality: How much is attributable to screening? *J. Med. Screen.* **2015**, *22*, 20–27. [CrossRef] [PubMed]
50. Olsen, A.H.; Njor, S.H.; Vejborg, I.; Schwartz, W.; Dalgaard, P.; Jensen, M.B.; Tange, U.B.; Blichert-Toft, M.; Rank, F.; Mouridsen, H.; et al. Breast cancer mortality in Copenhagen after introduction of mammography screening: Cohort study. *BMJ (Clin. Res. Ed.)* **2005**, *330*, 220. [CrossRef]
51. Olsen, A.H.; Njor, S.H.; Lynge, E. Estimating the benefits of mammography screening: The impact of study design. *Epidemiology (Camb. Mass.)* **2007**, *18*, 487–492. [CrossRef]
52. Van Dijck, J.A.; Verbeek, A.L.; Beex, L.V.; Hendriks, J.H.; Holland, R.; Mravunac, M.; Straatman, H.; Werre, J.M. Breast-cancer mortality in a non-randomized trial on mammographic screening in women over age 65. *Int. J. Cancer* **1997**, *70*, 164–168. [CrossRef]
53. Peer, P.G.; Werre, J.M.; Mravunac, M.; Hendriks, J.H.; Holland, R.; Verbeek, A.L. Effect on breast cancer mortality of biennial mammographic screening of women under age 50. *Int. J. Cancer* **1995**, *60*, 808–811. [CrossRef]
54. Johns, L.E.; Coleman, D.A.; Swerdlow, A.J.; Moss, S.M. Effect of population breast screening on breast cancer mortality up to 2005 in England and Wales: An individual-level cohort study. *Br. J. Cancer* **2017**, *116*, 246–252. [CrossRef]

55. UK Trial of Early Detection of Breast Cancer Group. 16-year mortality from breast cancer in the UK Trial of Early Detection of Breast Cancer. *Lancet (Lond. Engl.)* **1999**, *353*, 1909–1914. [CrossRef]
56. Ascunce, E.N.; Moreno-Iribas, C.; Barcos Urtiaga, A.; Ardanaz, E.; Ederra Sanz, M.; Castilla, J.; Egues, N. Changes in breast cancer mortality in Navarre (Spain) after introduction of a screening programme. *J. Med. Screen.* **2007**, *14*, 14–20. [CrossRef] [PubMed]
57. Giordano, L.; von Karsa, L.; Tomatis, M.; Majek, O.; de Wolf, C.; Lancucki, L.; Hofvind, S.; Nyström, L.; Segnan, N.; Ponti, A. Mammographic screening programmes in Europe: Organization, coverage and participation. *J. Med. Screen.* **2012**, *19*, 72–82. [CrossRef] [PubMed]
58. Swedish Organised Service Screening Evaluation Group. Reduction in breast cancer mortality from the organised service screening with mammography: 2. Validation with alternative analytic methods. *Cancer Epidemiol. Biomark. Prev.* **2006**, *15*, 52–56. [CrossRef]
59. Doyle, G.P.; Major, D.; Chu, C.; Stankiewicz, A.; Harrison, M.L.; Pogany, L.; Mai, V.M.; Onysko, J. A review of screening mammography participation and utilization in Canada. *Chronic Dis. Inj. Can.* **2011**, *31*, 152–156.
60. Breslow, N.E.; Day, N.E. *Statistical Methods in Cancer Research. Vol II. The Deisgn and Analysis of Cohort Studies*; International Agency for Cancer Research: Lyon, France, 1987.
61. Tabár, L.; Vitak, B.; Chen, T.H.-H.; Yen, A.M.-F.; Cohen, A.; Tot, T.; Chiu, S.Y.-H.; Chen, S.L.-S.; Fann, J.C.-Y.; Rosell, J.; et al. Swedish Two-County Trial: Impact of Mammographic Screening on Breast Cancer Mortality during 3 Decades. *Radiology* **2011**, *260*, 658–663. [CrossRef]
62. Moss, S.M.; Nystrom, L.; Jonsson, H.; Paci, E.; Lynge, E.; Njor, S.; Broeders, M. The impact of mammographic screening on breast cancer mortality in Europe: A review of trend studies. *J. Med. Screen.* **2012**, *19*, 26–32. [CrossRef]
63. Tabar, L.; Dean, P.B.; Chen, T.H.; Yen, A.M.; Chen, S.L.; Fann, J.C.; Chiu, S.Y.; Ku, M.M.; Wu, W.Y.; Hsu, C.Y.; et al. The incidence of fatal breast cancer measures the increased effectiveness of therapy in women participating in mammography screening. *Cancer* **2019**, *125*, 515–523. [CrossRef]
64. Sasieni, P. On the expected number of cancer deaths during follow-up of an initially cancer-free cohort. *Epidemiology (Camb. Mass.)* **2003**, *14*, 108–110. [CrossRef]

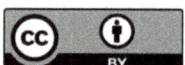

© 2020 by the authors. Licensee MDPI, Basel, Switzerland. This article is an open access article distributed under the terms and conditions of the Creative Commons Attribution (CC BY) license (http://creativecommons.org/licenses/by/4.0/).

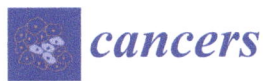

Article

Population Study of Ovarian Cancer Risk Prediction for Targeted Screening and Prevention

Faiza Gaba [1,2], Oleg Blyuss [3,4,5], Xinting Liu [1], Shivam Goyal [1], Nishant Lahoti [1], Dhivya Chandrasekaran [1,2], Margarida Kurzer [2], Jatinderpal Kalsi [6], Saskia Sanderson [7], Anne Lanceley [6], Munaza Ahmed [8], Lucy Side [9], Aleksandra Gentry-Maharaj [10], Yvonne Wallis [11], Andrew Wallace [12], Jo Waller [13], Craig Luccarini [14], Xin Yang [14], Joe Dennis [14], Alison Dunning [14], Andrew Lee [14], Antonis C. Antoniou [14], Rosa Legood [15], Usha Menon [10], Ian Jacobs [16] and Ranjit Manchanda [1,2,10,*]

[1] Wolfson Institute of Preventative Medicine, Barts CRUK Cancer Centre, Queen Mary University of London, Charterhouse Square, London EC1M 6BQ, UK; f.gaba@qmul.ac.uk (F.G.); xintingliu@yahoo.co.uk (X.L.); s.goyal@smd15.qmul.ac.uk (S.G.); n.lahoti@smd15.qmul.ac.uk (N.L.); d.chandrasekaran@qmul.ac.uk (D.C.)
[2] Department of Gynaecological Oncology, St Bartholomew's Hospital, Barts Health NHS Trust, London EC1A 7BE, UK; m.kurzer@nhs.net
[3] School of Physics, Astronomy and Mathematics, University of Hertfordshire, College Lane, Hatfield AL10 9AB, UK; o.blyuss@qmul.ac.uk
[4] Department of Paediatrics and Paediatric Infectious Diseases, Sechenov First Moscow State Medical University, Moscow 119146, Russia
[5] Department of Applied Mathematics, Lobachevsky State University of Nizhny Novgorod, Nizhny Novgorod 603098, Russia
[6] Department of Women's Cancer, Elizabeth Garrett Anderson Institute for Women's Health, University College London, London WC1E 6AU, UK; j.k.kalsi@ucl.ac.uk (J.K.); a.lanceley@ucl.ac.uk (A.L.)
[7] Department of Behavioural Science and Health, University College London, 1-19 Torrington Place, London WC1E 6BT, UK; saskia.sanderson@ucl.ac.uk
[8] Department Clinical Genetics, North East Thames Regional Genetics Unit, Great Ormond Street Hospital, London WC1N 3JH, UK; munaza.ahmed@gosh.nhs.uk
[9] Department of Clinical Genetics, University Hospital Southampton NHS Foundation Trust, Southampton SO16 6YD, UK; Lucy.Side@uhs.nhs.uk
[10] Medical Research Council Clinical Trials Unit at UCL, Institute of Clinical Trials and Methodology, University College London, 90 High Holborn, London WC1V 6LJ, UK; a.gentry-maharaj@ucl.ac.uk (A.G.-M.); u.menon@ucl.ac.uk (U.M.)
[11] West Midlands Regional Genetics Laboratory, Birmingham Women's NHS Foundation Trust, Birmingham B15 2TG, UK; y.wallis@nhs.net
[12] Manchester Centre for Genomic Medicine, 6th Floor Saint Marys Hospital, Oxford Rd, Manchester M13 9WL, UK; Andrew.Wallace@mft.nhs.uk
[13] Cancer Prevention Group, King's College London, Great Maze Pond, London SE1 9RT, UK; jo.waller@kcl.ac.uk
[14] Centre for Cancer Genetic Epidemiology, Department of Public Health and Primary Care, University of Cambridge, Strangeways Laboratory, Worts Causeway, Cambridge CB1 8RN, UK; craig@srl.cam.ac.uk (C.L.); xy249@medschl.cam.ac.uk (X.Y.); jgd29@cam.ac.uk (J.D.); amd24@medschl.cam.ac.uk (A.D.); ajl65@medschl.cam.ac.uk (A.L.); aca20@medschl.cam.ac.uk (A.C.A.)
[15] Department of Health Services Research and Policy, London School of Hygiene and Tropical Medicine, London WC1E 7HT, UK; Rosa.Legood@lshtm.ac.uk
[16] Department of Women's Health, University of New South Wales, Australia, Level 1, Chancellery Building, Sydney 2052, Australia; i.jacobs@unsw.edu.au
* Correspondence: r.manchanda@qmul.ac.uk

Received: 1 April 2020; Accepted: 6 May 2020; Published: 15 May 2020

Abstract: Unselected population-based personalised ovarian cancer (OC) risk assessment combining genetic/epidemiology/hormonal data has not previously been undertaken. We aimed to perform a feasibility study of OC risk stratification of general population women using a personalised OC risk tool followed by risk management. Volunteers were recruited through London primary care networks. Inclusion criteria: women ≥18 years. Exclusion criteria: prior ovarian/tubal/peritoneal cancer, previous genetic testing for OC genes. Participants accessed an online/web-based decision aid along with optional telephone helpline use. Consenting individuals completed risk assessment and underwent genetic testing (*BRCA1/BRCA2/RAD51C/RAD51D/BRIP1*, OC susceptibility single-nucleotide polymorphisms). A validated OC risk prediction algorithm provided a personalised OC risk estimate using genetic/lifestyle/hormonal OC risk factors. Population genetic testing (PGT)/OC risk stratification uptake/acceptability, satisfaction, decision aid/telephone helpline use, psychological health and quality of life were assessed using validated/customised questionnaires over six months. Linear-mixed models/contrast tests analysed impact on study outcomes. Main outcomes: feasibility/acceptability, uptake, decision aid/telephone helpline use, satisfaction/regret, and impact on psychological health/quality of life. In total, 123 volunteers (mean age = 48.5 (SD = 15.4) years) used the decision aid, 105 (85%) consented. None fulfilled NHS genetic testing clinical criteria. OC risk stratification revealed 1/103 at ≥10% (high), 0/103 at ≥5%–<10% (intermediate), and 100/103 at <5% (low) lifetime OC risk. Decision aid satisfaction was 92.2%. The telephone helpline use rate was 13% and the questionnaire response rate at six months was 75%. Contrast tests indicated that overall depression ($p = 0.30$), anxiety ($p = 0.10$), quality-of-life ($p = 0.99$), and distress ($p = 0.25$) levels did not jointly change, while OC worry ($p = 0.021$) and general cancer risk perception ($p = 0.015$) decreased over six months. In total, 85.5–98.7% were satisfied with their decision. Findings suggest population-based personalised OC risk stratification is feasible and acceptable, has high satisfaction, reduces cancer worry/risk perception, and does not negatively impact psychological health/quality of life.

Keywords: population genetic testing; ovarian cancer risk; risk stratification; *BRCA1*; BRCA2; RAD51C; RAD51D; BRIP1; SNP; risk modelling

1. Introduction

BRCA1/BRCA2 pathogenic variants have a 17–44% ovarian cancer (OC) risk until age 80 years [1]. Testing for OC susceptibility genes (CSGs)—*RAD51C* (lifetime OC risk = 11%) [2], *RAD51D* (lifetime OC risk = 13%) [2] and *BRIP1* (lifetime OC risk = 5.8%) [3]—is now part of clinical practice. Genome-wide association studies (GWAS) have discovered ~30 validated single-nucleotide polymorphisms (SNPs) which modify OC risk [4,5]. Newer risk prediction models incorporating validated SNPs as a polygenic risk score with epidemiologic/family history(FH)/hormonal data and moderate–high-penetrance CSGs can be used to predict lifetime OC risk, improving the precision of risk estimation and allowing population division into risk strata, enabling targeted downstream risk-stratified prevention/screening for those at increased risk [4,6].

The current practice of identifying high-risk women uses clinical criteria/FH-based testing for CSGs, misses >50% CSG carriers who do not fulfil genetic testing criteria and requires people to get cancer before identifying unaffected family members who can benefit from prevention [7–10]. Given the effective cancer risk management/prevention options available, the adequacy of current practice, representing massive missed opportunities for risk-stratified prevention, is questionable. Unselected population genetic testing (PGT) overcomes these limitations and identifies many more individuals at increased OC risk. PGT can be cost effective and prevent thousands of more OC/BC cases than clinical criteria/FH-based genetic testing [11].

Most PGT evidence comes from UK/Israeli/Canadian studies in Ashkenazi Jewish (AJ) populations [9,10,12]. These show that AJ population-based *BRCA* testing is acceptable, feasible, can be community based, doubles the *BRCA* pathogenic variant individuals identified, does not harm psychological health/quality of life (QoL), reduces long-term anxiety, has high satisfaction rates (90–95%) [9,10,13], and is extremely cost effective (potentially cost saving) for the UK/US health systems [14]. However, prospective/unbiased PGT data and model-based OC risk stratification for a general (non-Jewish) low-risk population are lacking.

We describe results from a feasibility study in order to stratify a general population using predicted lifetime OC risk and offer risk management options of screening and prevention, within the Predicting Risk of Ovarian Malignancy Improved Screening and Early detection programme (PROMISE-FS, ISRCTN54246466). This article reports on (1) the acceptability, feasibility, and uptake of PGT/OC risk stratification; (2) perceived risks/limitations; (3) decision aid (DA)/telephone helpline use; (4) satisfaction; (5) cancer worry/risk perception; (6) impact on psychological health/QoL.

2. Results

Between June 2017 and August 2017, 218 women registered and 123 viewed the online DA. In total, 105/123 (85%) DA users consented to genetic testing/risk assessment, and two withdrew. In total, 103 were eligible for analysis (Figure 1). In total, 2/103 were excluded from RPA assessment (Figure 1). Women who chose not to participate declined providing information on factors affecting decision making. The follow-up questionnaire response rate was 94%, 84%, and 75% at seven days, three months and six months post results, respectively.

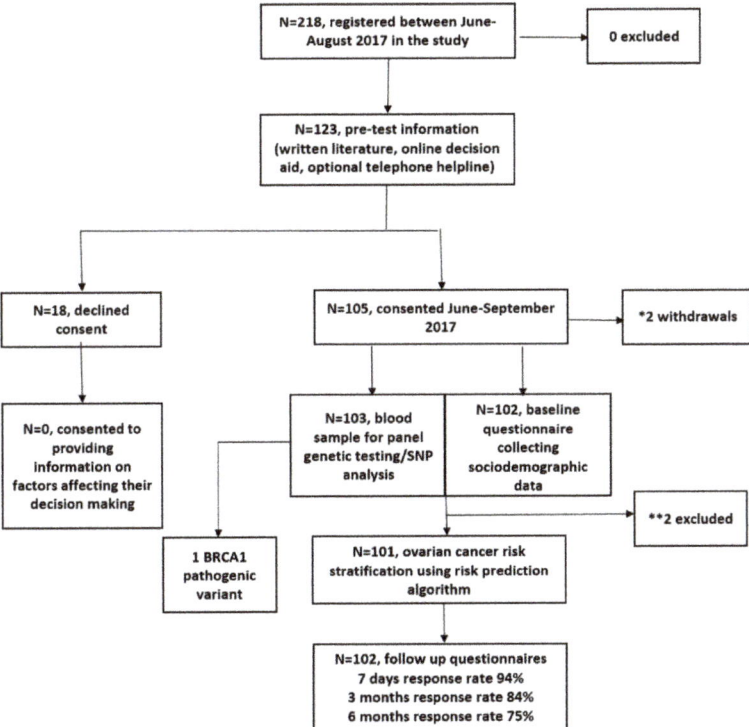

Figure 1. Study flow chart. * Reasons for withdrawal: miscarriage (*n* = 1) and inability to use public transport to attend an outpatient blood test appointment for genetic testing (*n* = 1). ** Reasons for exclusion: one participant was excluded because she entered this study at age 84 and the model predicts risks to age 80; the second participant did not provide the baseline demographic information required to run the algorithm.

Table 1 summarises cohort baseline characteristics. The mean age of participants was 48.5 (SD = 15.4; range = 18–85) years; 44.6% (n = 45) had university level education; 55.7% (n = 54) had a household income >£40,000; 74.5% (n = 76) were Caucasian; 7% (n = 7) were smokers; 64% (n = 63) ate >5 portions of fruit/vegetables daily; 78% (n = 80) were physically active over the last month. None had a clinically significant FH of cancer (fulfilling NHS genetic testing criteria). RPA revealed 1/103 at ≥10%, 0/103 at ≥5%–<10% and 100/103 at <5% lifetime OC risk. As expected using the algorithm, the epidemiological risk factors alone provide a greater level of OC risk stratification among the participants compared to the polygenic risk score (PRS) alone (Figure S1). However, risk stratification is further improved when the full model incorporating both epidemiological risk factors and PRS is considered. One high-risk participant, aged 35 years, had a lifetime OC risk of 42%. She had a pathogenic duplication of exon-13 in BRCA1. History included one second-degree relative with OC—parity = 1, 10 years oral contraceptive pill (OCP) use, endometriosis, BMI = 30.4, and no tubal ligation/hormone-replacement therapy (HRT) use. Following results, the participant opted for Risk of Ovarian Cancer Algorithm (ROCA)-based screening (24) within a research study (ALDO, https://www.uclh.nhs.uk/OurServices/ServiceA-Z/Cancer/NCV/Pages/TheALDOproject.aspx) and for risk-reducing early salpingectomy within a clinical trial (PROTECTOR, ISRCTN25173360, http://www.protector.org.uk/). She underwent MRI screening for BC risk. Four Class-3 variants of uncertain significance (VUS) were detected (BRCA1:c.3328_3330delAAG, c.2998_3003del; BRCA2:c.1438T>G; RAD51D:c.482T>C).

Table 1. Baseline characteristics of cohort.

Characteristic	%	N
Mean age, years (SD, range)		48.54 (15.42, 18–85)
Marital status		
Single	20	20/100
Married	52	52/100
Cohabiting/living with partner	15	15/100
Divorced/separated	11	11/100
Widowed	2	2/100
Children		
Have children	65.69	67/102
Mean number of children (SD, range)		1.34 (1.23, 0–5)
Education		
No formal qualification	5.94	6/101
GCSE/O-level/CSE	17.82	18/101
NVQ1/NVQ2	0.99	1/101
A-level/NVQ3	26.73	27/101
NVQ4	3.96	4/101
Bachelors	26.73	27/101
Masters	13.86	14/101
PhD	3.96	4/101
Income (£)		
<10,000	13.4	13/97
10,000–19,000	7.22	7/97
20,000–29,000	13.4	13/97
30,000–39,900	10.31	10/97
40,000–49,900	11.34	11/97
>50,000	44.33	43/97

Table 1. Cont.

Characteristic	%	N
Ethnicity		
White	74.51	76/102
Asian	13.73	14/102
Black/Afro-Caribbean	2.94	3/102
Mixed	6.86	7/102
Other	1.96	2/102
Religion		
Christian	59.41	60/101
Muslim	6.93	7/101
Jewish	4.95	5/101
Buddhist	0.99	1/101
Hindu	1.98	2/101
Sikh	1.98	2/101
No religion	22.77	23/101
Other	0.99	1/101
FH/clinical criteria positive	0	0/102
FH of cancer		
Total number of participants with any FH of ovarian cancer	11.76	12/102
Number of participants with a FDR with ovarian cancer	5.88	6/102
Number of participants with a SDR with ovarian cancer	5.88	6/102
Number of participants with a TDR with ovarian cancer	0	0/102
Total number of participants with any FH of breast cancer	44.12	45/102
Number of participants with a FDR with breast cancer	14.71	15/102
Number of participants with a SDR with breast cancer	23.53	24/102
Number of participants with a TDR with breast cancer	5.88	6/102
Total number of participants with a FH of breast and ovarian cancer	0.98	1/102
Total number of participants with any FH of prostate cancer	17.65	18/102
Number of participants with a FDR with prostate cancer	7.84	8/102
Number of participants with a SDR with prostate cancer	7.84	8/102
Number of participants with a TDR with prostate cancer	1.96	2/102
Total number of participants with any FH of pancreatic cancer	4.9	5/102
Number of participants with a FDR with pancreatic cancer	0.00	0/102
Number of participants with a SDR with pancreatic cancer	3.92	4/102
Number of participants with a TDR with pancreatic cancer	0.98	1/102
Psychiatric history		
Depression	9	9/100
Other psychiatric condition	5	5/100
Current medication for psychiatric condition	5	5/100
Personal history of non-ovarian cancer		
Breast cancer	0	0/102
Other cancers	3.92	4/102
Previous genetic testing unrelated to HBOC	1.98	2/101
Breast self-examination in the last 12 months		
Never	29.41	30/102
<once a month	48.04	49/102
once a month	14.71	15/102
>once a month	7.84	8/102
Clinical screening for breast cancer		
Ever had a clinical breast exam	56.57	56/99
Ever had a MRI	4	4/100
Ever had a mammogram	54.46	55/101

Table 1. Cont.

Characteristic	%	N
Ovarian cancer screening		
Currently undergoing screening	1.96	2/102
Have previously undergone screening	11.11	11/99
Previous surgical prevention to prevent ovarian cancer	0	0/102
Health behaviour and lifestyle		
Smoking		
Ever smokers	25.49	26/102
Current smokers	7.07	7/99
Alcohol consumption in the past 12 months		
Every week	48.04	49/102
Every month	14.71	15/102
Less frequently than once a month	21.57	22/102
Not at all	15.69	16/102
Median alcohol consumption on a typical day in units (IQR)		2 (1–2)
≥5 portions of fruit and vegetables	63.64	63/99
Number of participants who consume red meat	81.37	83/102
Number of participants currently using vitamin supplements	51.51	51/99
Physical exercise (past month)	78.43	80/102
Risk prediction algorithm results		
High lifetime ovarian cancer risk	0.97	1/103
Intermediate ovarian cancer risk	0	0/103
Low lifetime ovarian cancer risk	97.09	100/103
Excluded *	1.94	2/103
Mean lifetime risk prediction score (excluding the high-risk participant (SD, range))		1.39 (0.69, 0.56–4.38)
Mean lifetime risk prediction score (including the high-risk participant (SD, range))		1.80 (4.10, 0.56–41.98)

FH: family history; FDR: first-degree relative; SDR: second-degree relative; TDR: third-degree relative; HBOC: hereditary breast and ovarian cancer; SD: standard deviation. * One participant was excluded because she entered this study at age 84 and the model predicts risks to age 80. A second participant was excluded because she did not provide any baseline demographic information. Both participants were provided with their high-penetrance gene results, but personalised risk scores were not provided.

Key perceived benefits/risks of PGT/OC risk assessment are shown in Table S1. Need for reassurance, reduction in uncertainty, enhancing cancer prevention, benefiting research, knowledge about enhanced screening/prevention and children's risks were rated somewhat/very important by ~70–98% women. Important risks/limitations of PGT/OC risk assessment rated somewhat/very important included concern about effect on family (56.4%) and being unable to handle it emotionally (38.6%). A minority felt stigmatization (9%) or targeting of an ethnic group (11%) was a somewhat/very important risk. Insurance and confidentiality were highlighted as somewhat/very important by 28% and 24.7% respectively.

Participant responses to the ten DA items are shown in Table S2. The mean number of times DA was viewed was non-significantly higher in consenters versus decliners (1.61 vs. 1.05; $p = 0.06$). The mean DA score was not significantly different between consenters and decliners (8.1 vs. 7.4; $p = 0.14$). Consenters were older than decliners (48.5 vs. 40, $p = 0.016$). The mean age of volunteers who registered but did not view the DA was 45.5 years and not significantly different from consenters ($p = 0.16$) or decliners ($p = 0.24$). There was no statistically significant difference in 9/10 DA item responses between consenters and decliners. (Table S2). In total, 88.3% of consenters versus 75% of decliners ($p = 0.036$) would regret not participating if they developed OC in the future. In total, 23/123 viewed the DA on multiple occasions, and DA scores increased on repeat attempts (Tables S3 and S4). For 122/123 participants, there was concordance between participant decision making and

DA outcome category. One participant (85 years, Caucasian, no OC-FH) consented to PGT/OC risk stratification despite DA advice to the contrary (DA score = −1). Table 2 summarises responses to the DA evaluation questionnaire. In total, 92.2% (94/102) were very satisfied/satisfied and 82.2% (83/101) would recommend the DA. The amount of information provided, length of time taken to view and level of detail available was deemed just right by 98% (100/102), 97.1% (99/102), and 97% (98/101), respectively. No part of the DA needed omitting.

Table 2. Decision aid evaluation questionnaire responses.

Satisfaction	%		N						
Very satisfied	47.06		48/102						
Satisfied	45.1		46/102						
Neither satisfied nor dissatisfied	5.88		6/102						
Dissatisfied	0.98		1/102						
Very dissatisfied	0.98		1/102						
Amount of information provided									
Too little	1.96		2/102						
About right	98.04		100/102						
Too much	0		0/102						
Length of time taken to view DA									
Too short	0		0/102						
About right	97.06		99/102						
Too long	2.94		3/102						
Do any parts of the DA require more detail?									
Yes	2.97		3/101						
No	97.03		98/101						
Are there any parts of the DA that should be left out?									
Yes	0		0/99						
No	100		99/99						
Would you recommend DA use?									
Yes	82.18		83/101						
No	0.99		1/101						
Not sure	16.83		17/101						
How much the DA improved understanding of:	Not at all		Not very much		Somewhat		Quite a bit		A lot	
	%	N	%	N	%	N	%	N	%	N
OC	7.92	8/101	12.87	13/101	34.65	35/101	28.71	29/101	15.84	16/101
Disadvantages of discovering OC risk (%)	3.96	4/101	6.93	7/101	40.59	41/101	28.71	29/101	19.8	20/101
Advantages of discovering OC risk	2.97	3/101	7.92	8/101	26.73	27/101	36.63	37/101	25.74	26/101
Genetic testing for OC genes	1.98	2/101	8.91	9/101	29.7	30/101	33.66	34/101	25.74	26/101
Implications of carrying OC gene alteration	3.96	4/101	5.94	6/101	36.63	37/101	28.71	29/101	24.75	25/101
Emotional response to DA										
Worried/concerned	56.44	57/101	27.72	28/101	13.86	14/101	1.98	2/101	0	0/101
Reassured	6.86	7/102	12.75	13/102	35.29	36/102	25.49	26/102	19.61	20/102
Upset	80.2	81/101	14.85	15/101	3.96	4/101	0	0/101	0.99	1/101

In total, 13% (13/103) of consenters used the optional telephone helpline (Table 3), and 8/13 filled in an evaluation questionnaire. No decliner used the telephone helpline. The mean number of calls to the telephone helpline was 1.38 (SD = 1.12; range = 1–5). In total, 12.5% (1/8) used the telephone helpline to aid decision making and 75% (6/8) had study specific queries—of which, DA technical assistance queries (4/8) were the most common. All helpline users were very satisfied/satisfied with their experience and 75% (6/8) would recommend the helpline. In total, 37.5% (3/8) felt that the helpline aided decision making. There was no difference in baseline characteristics between helpline users and non-users. When comparing how much the DA improved understanding of OC/gene testing/advantages and disadvantages of discovering personalised OC risk or DA satisfaction, there was no statistically significant difference between helpline users/non-users. Helpline users had a significantly greater degree of worry (2/13 vs. 0/89; $p = 0.02$) and upset (1/13 vs. 0/89; $p = 0.003$) when viewing the DA in comparison to non-users. Helpline users had a higher DA mean score than non-users (9.123 vs. 8.019; $p = 0.032$)

Table 3. Telephone helpline evaluation questionnaire responses.

Telephone Helpline Evaluation Questionnaire	%	N
Total number of women using the helpline	12.62	13/103
Number of participants using helpline who consented to this study	100	13/13
Mean number of times used (SD, range)		1.38 (1.12, 1–5)
Reason for helpline use		
To help decide whether to take part in this study	12.5	1/8
To ask a study specific question not related to decision making	75	6/8
Technical assistance with the decision aid	50	4/8
Pregnancy related query	25	2/8
Results query	12.5	1/8
Satisfaction with helpline		
Very satisfied	75	6/8
Satisfied	25	2/8
Neither satisfied nor dissatisfied	0	0/8
Dissatisfied	0	0/8
Very dissatisfied	0	0/8
Did the helpline help with decision making?		
Yes	37.5	3/8
No	50	4/8
Not sure	12.5	1/8
Would you recommend helpline use?		
Yes	75	6/8
No	0	0/8
Not sure	25	2/8

SD: standard deviation; 8/13 participants who used the telephone helpline completed the telephone helpline questionnaire. Data are presented for these eight participants.

Mean Hospital Anxiety and Depression Scale (HADS)/EuroQol-5D-5L (EQ-5D-5L)/Impact of Events Scale (IES)/Cancer Risk Perception questionnaire (CRP)/Cancer Worry Scale questionnaire (CWS)/Decision Regret Satisfaction questionnaire (DRS) questionnaire scores at baseline and at seven days/three months/six months follow up are shown in Table 4.

Table 4. Mean questionnaire scores at baseline and at seven days, three months and six months follow up.

Validated Questionnaire	Baseline	7 Days Post Results	3 Months Post Results	6 Months Post Results
HADS				
Total	9.06 (SD = 6.11, range 0–23)	10.43 (SD = 6.26, range 0–30)	9.78 (SD = 7.1, range 0–31)	9.64 (SD = 7.06, range 0–28)
Anxiety	6.11 (SD = 4.05, range 0–17)	7.02 (SD = 4.02, range 0–18)	6.35 (SD = 3.97, range 0–16)	6.1 (SD = 4.06, range 0–15)
Depression	2.92 (SD = 2.9, range 0–11)	3.41 (SD = 3.07, range 0–14)	3.36 (SD = 3.71, range 0–16)	3.55 (SD = 3.62, range 0–14)

Table 4. Cont.

Validated Questionnaire	Baseline	7 Days Post Results	3 Months Post Results	6 Months Post Results
EQ-5D-5L				
Total	0.86 (SD = 0.14, range 0.382–1)	0.84 (SD = 0.17, range 0.259–1)	0.83 (SD = 0.21, range 0.051–1)	0.84 (SD = 0.17, range –0.035–1)
VAS	81.27 (SD = 13.9, range 35–100)	80.61 (SD = 16.11, range 4–100)	80.45 (SD = 18.81, range 15–100)	80.76 (SD = 15.3, range 20–100)
Mobility	1.25 (SD = 0.57, range 1–3)	1.26 (SD = 0.55, range 1–3)	1.35 (SD = 0.8, range 1–5)	1.47 (SD = 0.92, range 1–5)
Self-care	1.08 (SD = 0.39, range 1–4)	1.04 (SD = 0.2, range 1–2)	1.12 (SD = 0.57, range 1–5)	1.21 (SD = 0.82, range 1–5)
Usual activities	1.25 (SD = 0.57, range 1–4)	1.24 (SD = 0.52, range 1–3)	1.38 (SD = 0.77, range 1–5)	1.42 (SD = 0.94, range 1–5)
Pain/discomfort	1.55 (SD = 0.71, range 1–4)	1.65 (SD = 0.8, range 1–4)	1.68 (SD = 0.95, range 1–5)	1.71 (SD = 0.82, range 1–5)
Anxiety/depression	1.43 (SD = 0.69, range 1–4)	1.58 (SD = 0.88, range 1–5)	1.58 (SD = 0.88, range 1–5)	1.53 (SD = 0.71, range 1–3)
IES		7.93 (SD = 15.06, range 0–67)	7.57 (SD = 17.07, range 0–73)	4.95 (SD = 10.61, range 0–48)
CWS	5.8 (SD = 1.96, range 4–14)	5.13 (SD = 1.61, range 4–12)	5.04 (SD = 1.51, range 4–11)	5.17 (SD = 1.61, range 4–11)
CRP				
CRP Likert scale	2.93 (SD = 0.78, range 1–5)	2.72 (SD = 0.83, range 1–5)	2.86 (SD = 0.66, range 1–5)	2.93 (SD = 0.74, range 1–5)
CRP VAS	46.05 (SD = 22.1, range 0–90)	44.51 (SD = 24.61, range 2–90)	47.43 (SD = 21.81, range 0–90)	49.67 (SD = 22.84, 1–90)
DRS				
DRS scale			27 (SD = 52.11, range 0–250)	
DRS Madalinska			1.16 (SD = 0.4, range 1–3)	

HADS: Hospital Anxiety and Depression Scale questionnaire; IES: Impact of Events Scale questionnaire; CRP: Cancer Risk Perception questionnaire; CWS: Cancer Worry Scale questionnaire; DRS: Decision Regret Satisfaction questionnaire; VAS: Visual Analogue Scale. HADS: 14 item questionnaire, with 7 items pertaining to anxiety and 7 to depression. Each item is scored on a 4-point Likert scale, from 0 to 3, with total scores ranging from 0 to 42. Higher scores indicate higher levels of anxiety/depression. EQ-5D-5L: EuroQol-5D-5L 5 item questionnaire. Each item (mobility, self-care, usual activities, pain/discomfort, and anxiety/depression) is scored on a 5-point Likert scale, from 1 to 5. Higher scores indicate poorer health. Total scores are then converted into a utility value using published reference values for the UK by the EuroQol Research Foundation. Utility values range from 0 to 1, with 0 indicating the worst health and 1 the best health. In addition, participants are asked to state "how good or bad your health is today" using a Visual Analogue Scale ranging from 0 (worst health) to 100 (best health). IES: 15 item questionnaire. Each item is scored on a 4-point Likert scale, from 0 to 5, with total scores ranging from 0 to 75. Higher scores indicate higher distress levels. CWS: 4 item questionnaire. Each item is scored on a 4-point Likert scale, from 1 to 4, with total scores ranging from 4 to 16. Higher scores indicate greater worry of developing ovarian cancer. CRP: 1 item questionnaire. The item is scored on a 5-point Likert scale, from 1 to 5. A higher score indicates that the individual perceives that they are at greater risk of developing cancer of any type at some point in their life compared to other women of the same age. In addition, participants are asked to state "on a scale from 0 to 100, where 0 is no chance at all, and 100 is absolutely certain, what do you think are the chances that you will get cancer (of any type) sometime during your lifetime?" DRS: First part consists of a 5 item questionnaire (Decision Satisfaction Regret Scale. Each item is scored on a 5-point Likert scale, from 0 to 100, with total scores ranging from 0 to 500. Higher scores indicate less satisfaction/more regret. Second part consists of a 1 item questionnaire (Madalinska). The item is scored on a 5-point Likert scale, from 0 to 100. Higher scores indicate less satisfaction/more regret.

Linear random-effects mixed-model outputs showing the association of covariates with different outcomes are shown in Table 5. There was a transient increase in HADS anxiety at seven days ($p = 0.048$), returning to baseline by three months ($p = 0.318$). Compared to baseline, there was a small increase in HADS depression scores at individual time points of 3 months ($p = 0.027$) and

6 months ($p \leq 0.001$), while QoL scores were marginally lower at three ($p = 0.025$) and six months ($p = 0.036$). However, the absolute level of change from baseline in all these scores was extremely small (HADS depression = 2.92 to 3.55; HADS anxiety = 6.11 to 7.02; EQ-5D-5L = 0.86 to 0.84) and not clinically meaningful. Additionally, contrast tests evaluating whether overall mean values at seven days, three months and six months were jointly different from the baseline suggested that anxiety, depression and QoL at these time points were not jointly different from the baseline value for the cohort (Table 5). Distress scores decreased with time and were significantly lower at six months versus 7 days ($p = 0.042$). Compared to baseline, OC worry was significantly lower at 7 days ($p \leq 0.001$), 3 months ($p \leq 0.001$) and 6 months ($p \leq 0.001$). Contrast tests evaluating the overall time effect showed a significant decrease in OC worry scores ($p = 0.02$) but not distress scores ($p = 0.25$) over time (Table 5). General cancer risk perception showed a decrease at 7 days ($p = 0.012$), returning to baseline by 6 months ($p = 0.45$).

Table 5. Linear random-effects mixed models and overall contrast tests for study outcomes.

Model and Variable	Coef.	Std. Err	$p > |z|$	95% CI
HADS Total				
FH Breast Cancer	1.66	1.334	0.217	−0.782 to 4.3
FH Ovarian Cancer	0.426	2.146	0.843	−3.766 to 4.616
* 7 Days	1.068	0.513	0.039	0.159 to 2.071
3 Months	0.986	0.537	0.068	−0.094 to 2.148
* 6 Months	1.268	0.557	0.024	0.215 to 2.385
Age	−0.015	0.046	0.742	−0.101 to 0.078
Income	−0.633	0.411	0.127	−1.452 to 0.178
Marital Status	1.321	1.424	0.356	−1.608 to 4.675
Ethnicity	3.349	1.899	0.081	−0.716 to 7.141
Religion: Jewish	−1.715	3.116	0.584	−7.559 to 4.456
Religion: Muslim	−6.223	3.228	0.057	−12.655 to 0.751
Religion: Atheist	−0.736	1.582	0.643	−3.893 to 2.478
Religion: Other	−3.759	2.848	0.19	−9.587 to 2.509
HADS Total	**df**	**Chi-sq**	**p-value**	
# BL vs. Overall (joint)	3	5.2	0.158	
HADS Anxiety				
FH Breast Cancer	0.933	0.801	0.248	−0.63 to 2.625
FH Ovarian Cancer	−0.142	1.285	0.912	−2.552 to 2.373
* 7 Days	0.649	0.326	0.048	0.006 to 1.278
3 Months	0.339	0.339	0.318	−0.377 to 1.022
6 Months	0.172	0.353	0.628	−0.498 to 0.88
Age	−0.026	0.028	0.346	−0.083 to 0.028
Income	−0.216	0.247	0.383	−0.66 to 0.255
Marital Status	0.505	0.856	0.557	−1.285 to 2.123
Ethnicity	1.688	1.143	0.143	−0.433 to 3.799
Religion: Jewish	0.039	1.871	0.984	−3.838 to 3.558
* Religion: Muslim	−4.136	1.941	0.036	−7.79 to −0.387
Religion: Atheist	−0.89	0.951	0.352	−2.71 to 1.051
Religion: Other	−1.975	1.707	0.251	−5.541 to 1.271
HADS Anxiety	**df**	**Chi-sq**	**p-value**	
# BL vs. Overall (joint)	3	6.22	0.102	
HADS Depression				
FH Breast Cancer	0.778	0.655	0.238	−0.55 to 2.141
FH Ovarian Cancer	0.942	1.086	0.387	−1.201 to 3.16
7 Days	0.481	0.292	0.101	−0.03 to 1.048
* 3 Months	0.68	0.304	0.027	0.062 to 1.257
* 6 Months	1.155	0.317	<0.001	0.54 to 1.772
Age	0.012	0.022	0.586	−0.033 to 0.054

Table 5. Cont.

* Income	−0.403	0.2	0.047	−0.805 to −0.031
Marital Status	0.8	0.702	0.258	−0.579 to 2.132
Ethnicity	1.642	0.925	0.079	−0.249 to 3.377
Religion: Jewish	−1.782	1.53	0.248	−5.021 to 1.214
Religion: Muslim	−1.996	1.562	0.205	−5.08 to 1.209
Religion: Atheist	0.148	0.776	0.85	−1.312 to 1.787
Religion: Other	−1.769	1.388	0.206	−4.607 to 1.095
HADS Depression	**df**	**Chi-sq**	***p*-value**	
# BL vs. Overall (joint)	3	3.7	0.296	
EQ-5D-5L Total				
FH Breast Cancer	−0.068	0.031	0.034	−0.135 to −0.008
FH Ovarian Cancer	−0.066	0.052	0.204	−0.171 to 0.028
7 Days	−0.026	0.015	0.082	−0.056 to 0.003
* 3 Months	−0.034	0.015	0.025	−0.062 to −0.004
6 Months	−0.033	0.016	0.036	−0.069 to −0.005
Age	−0.002	0.001	0.138	−0.004 to 0.001
Income	0.013	0.01	0.19	−0.007 to 0.032
Marital Status	−0.01	0.034	0.756	−0.076 to 0.061
Ethnicity	−0.05	0.044	0.262	−0.136 to 0.038
Religion: Jewish	−0.011	0.073	0.885	−0.155 to 0.136
Religion: Muslim	0.059	0.075	0.435	−0.106 to 0.209
Religion: Atheist	0.058	0.037	0.12	−0.012 to 0.136
Religion: Other	0.078	0.066	0.242	−0.058 to 0.202
EQ-5D-5L Total	**df**	**Chi-sq**	***p*-value**	
# BL vs. Overall (joint)	3	0.14	0.987	
EQ-5D-5L VAS				
FH Breast Cancer	−4.74	2.792	0.093	−10.024 to 0.915
FH Ovarian Cancer	−6.613	4.908	0.18	−16.246 to 3.636
7 Days	−1.537	1.68	0.361	−5.063 to 2.159
3 Months	−3.244	1.749	0.065	−6.533 to 0.491
6 Months	−2.492	1.798	0.167	−6.161 to 1.046
Age	0.048	0.097	0.621	−0.143 to 0.243
* Income	1.819	0.859	0.037	0.267 to 3.524
Marital Status	−0.386	2.997	0.898	−6.607 to 5.465
Ethnicity	−7.129	4.004	0.078	−15.297 to −0.015
Religion: Jewish	−1.73	6.474	0.79	−14.671 to 10.225
Religion: Muslim	10.205	6.774	0.136	−3.622 to 25.287
Religion: Atheist	0.921	3.322	0.782	−6.351 to 7.29
Religion: Other	2.139	5.9	0.718	−9.416 to 14.159
EQ-5D-5L VAS	**df**	**Chi-sq**	***p*-value**	
# BL vs. Overall (joint)	3	1.63	0.654	
IES				
FH Breast	−2.691	2.783	0.337	−8.768 to 2.934
FH Ovarian	−2.838	4.625	0.541	−11.282 to 6.296
3 Months	0.541	1.688	0.749	−2.841 to 3.86
* 6 Months	−3.533	1.724	0.042	−6.764 to −0.456
Age	−0.009	0.1	0.93	−0.183 to 0.178
Income	−1.53	0.895	0.091	−3.193 to 0.129
Marital Status	−1.252	3.005	0.678	−7.493 to 4.494
Ethnicity	1.551	4.379	0.724	−6.956 to 10.635
Religion: Jewish	7.084	6.242	0.26	−5.696 to 18.636
Religion: Muslim	−12.871	7.211	0.078	−25.685 to 2.043
* Religion: Atheist	−8.159	3.377	0.018	−15.396 to −1.292
Religion: Other	−3.833	6.028	0.527	−16.369 to 8.471

Table 5. Cont.

IES	df	Chi-sq	p-value	
# BL vs. Overall (joint)	2	2.78	0.249	
CWS				
FH Breast Cancer	0.019	0.306	0.952	−0.616 to 0.639
FH Ovarian Cancer	−0.138	0.535	0.797	−1.316 to 1.001
* 7 Days	−0.73	0.182	<0.001	−1.096 to −0.399
* 3 Months	−0.802	0.189	<0.001	−1.173 to −0.448
* 6 Months	−0.775	0.195	<0.001	−1.16 to −0.358
Age	−0.013	0.011	0.215	−0.035 to 0.009
Income	−0.126	0.094	0.186	−0.325 to 0.065
Marital Status	0.335	0.329	0.311	−0.374 to 0.973
Ethnicity	0.585	0.44	0.187	−0.264 to 1.439
Religion: Jewish	1.375	0.71	0.056	−0.091 to 2.772
Religion: Muslim	−1.073	0.737	0.149	−2.593 to 0.455
Religion: Atheist	−0.491	0.365	0.182	−1.224 to 0.247
Religion: Other	1.157	0.647	0.078	−0.035 to 2.428
CWS	df	Chi-sq	p-value	
# BL vs. Overall (joint)	3	9.7	0.021	
CRP Likert Scale				
FH Breast Cancer	0.436	0.138	0.002	0.135 to 0.696
FH Ovarian Cancer	0.248	0.238	0.299	−0.207 to 0.748
* 7 Days	−0.195	0.077	0.012	−0.349 to −0.041
3 Months	−0.093	0.079	0.241	−0.251 to 0.068
6 Months	−0.062	0.083	0.454	−0.237 to 0.111
Age	−0.007	0.005	0.131	−0.017 to 0.002
Income	0.024	0.042	0.58	−0.071 to 0.107
Marital Status	−0.032	0.148	0.83	−0.308 to 0.269
Ethnicity	−0.089	0.197	0.654	−0.475 to 0.309
Religion: Jewish	0.173	0.321	0.592	−0.475 to 0.73
Religion: Muslim	−0.179	0.332	0.59	−0.89 to 0.524
Religion: Atheist	−0.115	0.164	0.486	−0.44 to 0.196
Religion: Other	0.127	0.292	0.665	−0.459 to 0.714
CRP Likert Scale	df	Chi-sq	p-value	
# BL vs. Overall (joint)	3	10.44	0.015	
CRP VAS				
FH Breast Cancer	6.455	4.416	0.148	−2.004 to 15.098
FH Ovarian Cancer	−4.31	7.495	0.566	−19.607 to 9.766
7 Days	−2.985	2.441	0.223	−7.692 to 2.013
3 Months	0.579	2.675	0.829	−4.12 to 5.918
6 Months	−0.093	2.77	0.973	−5.488 to 5.632
Age	−0.194	0.153	0.207	−0.487 to 0.084
Income	1.471	1.353	0.28	−1.386 to 4.059
Marital Status	0.794	4.727	0.867	−9.788 to 9.475
Ethnicity	−9.792	6.261	0.121	−22.644 to 3.523
Religion: Jewish	3.429	10.238	0.739	−15.525 to 24.542
Religion: Muslim	−0.805	10.561	0.939	−22.586 to 20.999
Religion: Atheist	−6.437	5.263	0.225	−16.92 to 3.543
Religion: Other	1.36	9.434	0.886	−17.183 to 21.316
CRP VAS	df	Chi-sq	p-value	
# BL vs. Overall (joint)	3	2.51	0.474	
DRS scale				
FH Breast Cancer	1.741	12.287	0.888	−22.846 to 26.328
FH Ovarian Cancer	11.808	17.974	0.514	−24.157 to 47.773

Table 5. Cont.

	Coef	Std. Err	p	95% CI
Age	0.208	0.437	0.636	−0.667 to 1.083
Income	−0.001	<0.001	0.216	−0.001 to 0
Marital Status	24.362	14.121	0.09	−3.894 to 52.617
* Ethnicity	47.091	20.396	0.024	6.28 to 87.902
Religion: Jewish	24.538	25.272	0.336	−26.031 to 75.108
Religion: Muslim	−11.145	32.366	0.732	−75.909 to 53.62
Religion: Atheist	10.411	16.022	0.518	−21.65 to 42.471
* Religion: Other	62.958	25.021	0.015	12.891 to 113.024
DRS Madalinska				
FH Breast Cancer	0.118	0.093	0.21	−0.068 to 0.303
FH Ovarian Cancer	0.022	0.136	0.871	−0.25 to 0.294
Age	0.001	0.003	0.849	−0.006 to 0.007
* Income	<0.001	<0.001	0.045	0 to 0
* Marital Status	0.247	0.107	0.025	0.033 to 0.46
Ethnicity	0.18	0.154	0.248	−0.129 to 0.488
Religion: Jewish	0.145	0.191	0.451	−0.238 to 0.528
Religion: Muslim	−0.151	0.245	0.541	−0.641 to 0.34
Religion: Atheist	0.068	0.121	0.573	−0.173 to 0.31
* Religion: Other	0.642	0.189	0.001	0.263 to 1.021

HADS: Hospital Anxiety and Depression Scale questionnaire; IES: Impact of Events Scale questionnaire; CRP: Cancer Risk Perception questionnaire; CWS: Cancer Worry Scale questionnaire; DRS: Decision Regret Satisfaction questionnaire; VAS: Visual Analogue Scale; FH: family history; Coef: coefficient; Std. Err: standard error. FH of breast cancer: positive versus negative (reference category); FH of ovarian cancer: positive versus negative (reference category); 7 days: questionnaire scores at 7 days versus baseline (reference category); 3 months: questionnaire scores at 3 months versus baseline (reference category); 6 months: questionnaire scores at 6 months versus baseline (reference category); age: age in years (continuous variable); income: as a continuous variable, but measured in £10,000 increments; marital status: cohabiting/living with partner/married (reference category) versus divorced/separated/single/widowed; ethnicity: Caucasian (reference category) versus non-Caucasian; religion Jewish: Christian (reference category) versus Jewish; religion Muslim: Christian (reference category) versus Muslim; Atheist: Christian (reference category) versus atheist; religion other (Hindu, Buddhist, Sikh): Christian (reference category) versus other. # BL vs. Overall (joint): Overall contrast test reflecting whether the mean outcome scale values at each time point (7 days, 3 months, or 6 months) were jointly different from the baseline for the whole group. This showed a significant decrease for CWS and CRP (Likert), but no significant change for HADS, HADS anxiety, HADS depression, EQ-5D-5L, IES and CRP (VAS) outcomes jointly over time. * Variables of statistical significance ($p < 0.05$).

In total, 85.5% strongly agreed and 13.2% agreed that their decision to undergo PGT/OC risk stratification was the right decision and that they were satisfied with it. In total, 95% would make the same choice again. Only 1.3% regretted their decision. Table 6 summarises responses to the DRS questionnaire.

Table 6. Decision Regret Satisfaction questionnaire responses according to individual questionnaire items.

Questionnaire Items	Questionnaire Responses									
	Strongly Disagree		Disagree		Neither Agree nor Disagree		Agree		Strongly Agree	
	%	N	%	N	%	N	%	N	%	N
It was the right decision	0	0/76	0	0/76	1.32	1/76	13.16	10/76	85.53	65/76
I regret the choice that was made	80.26	61/76	14.47	11/76	2.63	2/76	1.32	1/76	1.32	1/76
I would go for the same choice if I had to do it over again	0	0/76	1.32	1/76	3.95	3/76	13.16	10/76	81.58	62/76
The choice did me a lot of harm	89.33	67/75	8	6/75	2.67	2/75	0	0/75	0	0/75
The decision was a wise one	1.32	1/76	0	0/76	2.63	2/76	13.16	10/76	82.89	63/76
I am satisfied with the decision I have made	0	0/76	0	0/76	1.32	1/76	13.16	10/76	85.53	65/76

A FH of BC ($p = 0.034$) but not OC ($p = 0.20$) was negatively associated with QOL. Having a FH of OC was not associated with an increase in OC worry or general cancer risk perception.

However, women with a FH of BC perceived themselves to be at higher cancer risk ($p = 0.002$) but did not have increased OC worry.

Results from contrast tests assessing the joint effect of between-group and within-group differences in various outcomes over six months compared to baseline are shown in Table 7. There was no statistically significant between-group difference for groups 'with' and 'without' a FH of OC for HADS total/HADS depression/HADS anxiety/QoL/distress/OC worry/general cancer risk perception over time. There was no statistically significant within-group difference for groups 'with' and 'without' a FH of OC for HADS total/HADS anxiety/QoL/general cancer risk perception over six months. However, there was a statistically significant within-group difference for individuals 'without' a FH of OC but not 'with' a FH of OC for HADS depression ($p = 0.003$, $p = 0.866$, respectively), distress ($p = 0.043$, $p = 0.524$ respectively) and OC worry ($p \leq 0.001$, $p = 0.582$, respectively) over six months. Viewing the contrast tests together in combination with the linear random-effects mixed-model outputs would suggest a small increase in HADS depression scores not of clinical significance and a decrease in distress and OC worry over six months for the 'without' a FH of OC group.

Table 7. Contrast tests for between-group and within-group analyses over time.

HADS total	df	Chi-sq	p-value	CRP Likert scale	df	Chi-sq	p-value
Event#Group				Event#Group			
BL vs. 7 Days (joint)	1	0.43	0.51	BL vs. 7 Days (joint)	1	1.16	0.281
BL vs. 3 Months (joint)	1	0.07	0.797	BL vs. 3 Months (joint)	1	2.7	0.101
BL vs. 6 Months (joint)	1	0.13	0.719	BL vs. 6 Months (joint)	1	0.78	0.378
BL vs. Overall (joint)	3	1.05	0.788	BL vs. Overall (joint)	3	2.8	0.423
Event|Group				Event|Group			
BL vs. Joint|OC FH−	3	7.08	0.07	BL vs. Joint|OC FH−	3	6.69	0.083
BL vs. Joint|OC FH+	3	2.57	0.463	BL vs. Joint|OC FH+	3	6.59	0.086
HADS anxiety	df	Chi-sq	p-value	**CRP VAS**	df	Chi-sq	p-value
Event#Group				Event#Group			
BL vs. 7 Days (joint)	1	0.62	0.431	BL vs. 7 Days (joint)	1	2.23	0.135
BL vs. 3 Months (joint)	1	<0.01	0.972	BL vs. 3 Months (joint)	1	0.51	0.477
BL vs. 6 Months (joint)	1	0.04	0.849	BL vs. 6 Months (joint)	1	1.1	0.294
BL vs. Overall (joint)	3	1.05	0.79	BL vs. Overall (joint)	3	5.63	0.131
Event|Group				Event|Group			
BL vs. Joint|OC FH−	3	4.39	0.222	BL vs. Joint|OC FH−	3	2.37	0.5
BL vs. Joint|OC FH+	3	3.51	0.319	BL vs. Joint|OC FH+	3	4.37	0.224
HADS depression	df	Chi-sq	p-value	**EQ-5D-5L UK score**	df	Chi-sq	p-value
Event#Group				Event#Group			
BL vs. 7 Days (joint)	1	0.03	0.869	BL vs. 7 Days (joint)	1	2.36	0.125
BL vs. 3 Months (joint)	1	<0.01	0.971	BL vs. 3 Months (joint)	1	2.44	0.118
BL vs. 6 Months (joint)	1	0.91	0.339	BL vs. 6 Months (joint)	1	2.25	0.133
BL vs. Overall (joint)	3	1.18	0.759	BL vs. Overall (joint)	3	3.66	0.3
Event|Group				Event|Group			
* BL vs. Joint|OC FH−	3	14.18	0.003	BL vs. Joint|OC FH−	3	7	0.072
BL vs. Joint|OC FH+	3	0.73	0.866	BL vs. Joint|OC FH+	3	1.11	0.774
IES Score	df	Chi-sq	p-value	**EQ-5D-5L VAS**	df	Chi-sq	p-value
Event#Group				Event#Group			
BL vs. 3 Months (joint)	1	1.09	0.297	BL vs. 7 Days (joint)	1	0.64	0.425
BL vs. 6 Months (joint)	1	0.01	0.93	* BL vs. 3 Months (joint)	1	6.47	0.011
BL vs. Overall (joint)	2	1.3	0.523	BL vs. 6 Months (joint)	1	1.4	0.237

Table 7. Cont.

	df	Chi-sq	p-value		df	Chi-sq	p-value
Event|Group				BL vs. Overall (joint)	3	6.74	0.081
* BL vs. Joint|OC FH−	2	6.31	0.043	Event|Group			
BL vs. Joint|OC FH+	2	1.29	0.524	BL vs. Joint|OC FH−	3	3.89	0.273
CWS Score	df	Chi-sq	p-value				
Event#Group							
BL vs. 7 Days (joint)	1	0.99	0.32				
BL vs. 3 Months (joint)	1	0.25	0.615				
BL vs. 6 Months (joint)	1	0.18	0.675				
BL vs. Overall (joint)	3	1	0.802				
Event|Group							
* BL vs. Joint|OC FH−	3	26.92	<0.001				
BL vs. Joint|OC FH+	3	1.95	0.582				

BL: baseline; FH: family history; HADS: Hospital Anxiety and Depression Scale questionnaire; IES: Impact of Events Scale questionnaire; CRP: Cancer Risk Perception questionnaire; CWS: Cancer Worry Scale questionnaire; VAS: Visual Analogue Scale. 'Group' refers to either participants with a family history of ovarian cancer (OC FH+ group) or no family history of ovarian cancer (OC FH− group). 'Event#Group' refers to the group–time interaction, which reflects the 'between-group' (OC FH+ vs. OC FH−) difference over time. BL vs. 7 days (joint), BL vs. 3 months (joint), and BL vs. 6 months (joint) reflect whether the mean between-group difference at each time point (7 days, 3 months, or 6 months) was different from baseline. BL vs. Overall (joint) reflects whether the mean between-group differences at each time point (7 days, 3 months, or 6 months) were jointly different from the baseline between-group difference. Event\|Group refers to the group–time interaction, which reflects the 'within-group' difference over time. BL vs. Joint |OC FH− reflects whether the mean outcome scale value at each time point (7 days, 3 months, or 6 months) was jointly different from the baseline within the ovarian cancer family history negative group. BL vs. Joint |OC FH+ reflects whether the mean outcome scale value at each time point (7 days, 3 months, or 6 months) was jointly different from the baseline within the ovarian cancer family history positive group. * Statistical significance ($p < 0.05$).

3. Discussion

This is the first unselected population-based, prospective cohort study recruiting participants without cancer history in self/family, evaluating the feasibility of personalised lifetime OC risk stratification followed by offering risk management options. Data suggest that OC risk stratification using genetic/non-genetic (epidemiological/hormonal) factors in general population women is feasible and acceptable.

The 85% uptake of PGT and OC risk stratification suggests high acceptability, similar to previously published data indicating putative 85% uptake of PGT (n = 734/829 in a survey study assessing attitudes of a general population of women to unselected PGT and risk-stratified OC screening [15,16]. Findings are also similar to data showing the high acceptability of unselected BRCA testing in AJ populations (up to 88% uptake) [17]. The 85%–98% overall satisfaction we found with PGT is similar to rates reported with population-based BRCA testing in AJ populations [9,12].

Data from unselected BRCA testing in the AJ population [9,10,14,18,19] show acceptability/feasibility/effectiveness/cost effectiveness/lack of detrimental impact on psychological health/QoL, and support the concept of population-based BRCA testing in Jewish populations. However, these inferences cannot be directly generalized to a non-Jewish general population. Our findings of overall time effect contrast tests showing levels of anxiety/depression/QoL/distress not being jointly different from baseline values but a significant reduction in OC-specific worry/general cancer risk perception following OC risk stratification are reassuring. Small changes in scores observed in some outcomes at individual time points were not clinically meaningful. While larger studies are warranted, these initial findings concur with short-/long-term outcome data following unselected BRCA testing in AJ populations [9,13] and are similar to findings amongst high-risk individuals undergoing clinical criteria-based genetic testing [20–22]. In total, 25.5% of our cohort was non-Caucasian (13.7% Asian). We found no difference in psychological health/QoL outcomes amongst non-Caucasians versus Caucasians. More research is required for understanding the role of various risk factors in non-Europeans.

Our online DA was successfully completed by women from a wide range of ages (18–85), education levels, and ethnicities, with high levels (92.2%) of satisfaction. Women who used the optional telephone helpline reported higher levels of worry/upset when viewing the DA. In total, 75% of women using the telephone helpline did so for technical DA assistance. All went on to successfully view the online DA. The telephone helpline appears to have been used as a source of emotional/technical support, emphasising the importance/need for a telephone helpline as an adjunct to online web applications to facilitate access/decision making for PGT/OC risk stratification. That one volunteer consented despite her DA score (−1) indicating she was "leaning against taking part", highlights that whilst decision aids are adjuncts aiding decision making, individuals retain ultimate autonomy. While we showed the feasibility of using an online DA and helpline approach for PGT, this has not been compared in randomised trials to more standard/established methods (face-to-face/telephone-based/DVD-assisted counselling).

Our study strengths include population-based recruitment in a non-Jewish, ethnically diverse general population. We engaged and worked with primary care networks prior to study commencement. They helped increase awareness of this study, identify eligible women and facilitate recruitment. Engagement with primary care would be vital for the implementation of any national population-based model for PGT/OC risk stratification. Other advantages include a good questionnaire response rate, ranging from 99% (baseline) to 75% (six months follow up).

Limitations include the small sample size, lack of long-term follow up on QoL/psychological health/health behaviours. Additionally, this study was non-randomised and a control arm (without genetic testing) to compare any change in outcomes was lacking. However, the high-risk individual identified did opt for appropriate screening and preventive interventions to reduce OC/BC risk. Lack of intermediate-risk women identified probably reflects the small sample size.

In our cohort, 45% vs. 40% [23] of the UK general population had a university level education; 7% vs. 15% [23] were current smokers; 64% vs. 32% [23] ate the recommended ≥5 portions of fruit/vegetables daily; 78% vs. 64% [23] were physically active over the last month; median total household income was >£50,000 vs. £29,000 in the UK general population [23]. Higher income, education levels and healthy lifestyle behaviour in our study participants compared to the UK's general population may indicate a London bias. The income/education levels/lifestyle choices are similar to those of the UK Jewish population [9,17]. Significant associations of some study outcome variables seen with demographic variables of income/age are consistent with observations from population-based data reported in other population cohorts.

Precision prevention is a prevention strategy incorporating individual variation in genetic, epi-genetic and non-genetic (e.g., environment, hormonal, lifestyle, behavioural) risk factors. This comprises primary prevention to prevent occurrence of disease and, secondary prevention for screening/early detection of pre-symptomatic disease. Next-generation sequencing technologies, falling costs and advances in computational bioinformatics makes personalised risk-stratified prevention feasible. Improvements in the precision of risk estimation, genetic understanding of disease and increasing awareness offers an opportunity to apply this knowledge and technology at a broad population scale to make an important shift in health care towards disease prevention. Over 50% of OCs occur in 9% of the population, which is at >5% OC risk [4]. This provides a huge opportunity for population stratification for precision prevention. Identification of unaffected women at increased risk offers opportunities for risk-stratified prevention to reduce cancer burden. Women at increased OC risk can opt for risk-reducing salpingo-oophorectomy (RRSO) to prevent tubal cancer/OC [24], now advocated at >4–5% lifetime OC risk [25–27].

Access to and uptake of testing for CSGs remains restricted. Only a small proportion of at-risk *BRCA* carriers have been identified [7,8]. Our approach offers opportunities to maximise pathogenic variant identification and population stratification for OC prevention. While recent data suggest that population-based genetic testing for OC/BC gene pathogenic variants could be cost effective in general population women [11], additional research including general population implementation studies are needed to address knowledge gaps before considering this. Additional looked for findings have recently been offered and returned following post hoc sequencing and/or analysis of some large genomic study cohorts. These studies would enable evaluation of CSG pathogenic variant carriage rates. However, this would not address in a prospective unbiased fashion key questions around the (i) logistics of population testing; (ii) information giving, a priori informed consent, and uptake of testing; (iii) uptake of preventive options. This 'bolt-on' paradigm of returning additional 'secondary findings' cannot be equated to prospective uptake of testing CSGs in an unselected unaffected population.

A prospective, Canadian cohort study offering *BRCA1/BRCA2* testing to unselected men/women (The Screen Project) is ongoing. The study is evaluating the feasibility of a direct-to-consumer approach, satisfaction, OC worry, prevalence of *BRCA1/BRCA2* pathogenic variants and the number of OCs/BCs prevented. Results from our feasibility study would inform the development of a larger UK-wide study that implements PGT/OC risk-stratified prevention. An important challenge is identifying optimum implementation pathways. It is likely that different context-specific models are needed for various health care systems internationally. Risk assessment pathways could be established through a community/primary care-based approach outside the traditional hospital-based genetics clinic model. A key issue that needs resolving is a system for monitoring/managing VUS. Commissioning/funding of a system where laboratory reports can be reviewed and re-issued in light of new evidence is needed. A framework/structure for data management and legal and regulatory protections will also need to be established.

4. Materials and Methods

4.1. Design

A multicentre, prospective cohort, feasibility study (ISRCTN:54246466). Inclusion criteria: women ≥18 years. Exclusion criteria: history of ovarian/tubal/primary peritoneal cancer or previous genetic testing for OC CSGs.

4.2. Recruitment

Recruitment was by self-referral. Study information/leaflets were made available through North-East London primary care practices. Interested volunteers received a detailed participant information sheet and access to an online DA prior to consent to genetic testing/participation. All had access to use an 'optional' telephone helpline for support/advice/queries. The helpline was manned by a doctor/research nurse experienced in cancer genetic risk assessment/management. Individuals deciding to undergo PGT/OC risk assessment consented. Decliners were asked to provide information on factors affecting decision making.

4.3. Decision Aid (DA)

A bespoke web-based DA was developed, enabling potential participants to make an informed decision on whether they wish to determine their OC risk and undergo PGT/OC risk assessment [16,28]. The DA (Table S2) included information on OC, genetic testing and the PROMISE programme, followed by ten questions/items on potential advantages/disadvantages of learning about OC risk. Responses were rated according to two different 3-point Likert scales. Individual questions were scored according to responses ((a) 1 = in favour of taking part, −1 = against taking part, 0 = neither in-favour or against taking part; or (b) 1 = agree, −1 = disagree, 0 = unsure). Sum of all questions/items scores taken together ranged from −10 to 10. Women with total scores between −10 and −1 were considered "leaning against taking part", 0–5 "undecided", and 6–10 "leaning towards taking part".

4.4. Genetic Analysis

Genetic testing involved next-generation sequencing of *BRCA1/BRCA2/RAD51C/RAD51D/BRIP1* genes and 30 GWAS-validated OC SNPs. Pathogenic variants detected were reconfirmed in an NHS laboratory.

4.5. Risk Model

Epidemiological/hormonal/reproductive data affecting OC risk collected at baseline (age/OC-FH/body mass index (BMI)/tubal ligation/hormone-replacement therapy (HRT)/oral contraceptive pill (OCP) use/endometriosis/parity) were combined with genetic information in a risk prediction algorithm (RPA) to provide a personalised predicted lifetime OC risk (till 80 years). Model validation (personal communication) [5] was undertaken in prospective datasets and cancers accrued in the UK OC screening trial cohorts [5,29,30]. Following RPA assessment, all participants were stratified into risk categories by lifetime OC risk (low risk: <5%; intermediate risk: ≥5%–<10%; high risk: ≥10%).

4.6. Test Result Management

High/intermediate-risk (and an equivalent number of randomly selected low-risk) individuals received their result at a face-to-face post test risk stratification counselling appointment. Identified pathogenic/likely pathogenic variant heterozygotes were referred to an NHS regional genetics clinic for confirmatory testing and to established NHS risk management services. Other low-risk individuals received results via post. Variants of uncertain significance (VUS) results were not returned.

4.7. Assessment of Demographics, Outcomes and Follow Up

Sociodemographic, family history, perceived risk/limitation (4-point Likert scale), telephone helpline and DA evaluation data were collected using customised questionnaires. Anxiety and depression were assessed with the Hospital Anxiety and Depression Scale (HADS) [31]. Distress was assessed using the Impact of Events Scale (IES) [32]. General cancer risk perception was measured by two items. Comparative risk: 'Compared with other people of your age/sex, do you think your chances of getting cancer in your life are: much-lower, lower, about-the-same, higher, much-higher?' An additional risk item: 'On a scale from 0 to 100, where 0 is no chance at all and 100 is absolutely certain, what are the chances you will get cancer sometime during your lifetime?'. OC worry was assessed by the Cancer Worry Scale (CWS) [33]. Generic QoL was measured with the EQ-5D-5L questionnaire [34]. Satisfaction and regret were measured by the Decision Regret Satisfaction Scale (DRS) and one additional 5-point Likert scale item, 'I am satisfied with the decision I have made' [35]. Smoking, diet and physical activity were evaluated. Data were gathered at baseline following consent and post results delivery (seven days/three months/six months).

4.8. Statistical Analysis

Descriptive statistics were used for baseline characteristics/telephone helpline/DA/follow-up questionnaire data. The Wilcoxon rank sum test and Fisher's exact test evaluated differences in means and proportions correspondingly.

As outcome data from the HADS/EQ-5D-5L/IES/CWS/CRP/DRS questionnaires were collected over multiple time points, linear random-effects mixed models were used to allow for individual baseline-level variability. Each scale was analysed, with the outcome as a continuous response variable. Models included a group effect and time effect. Models were adjusted for FH of OC/BC (positive/negative), age, income (in £10,000 increments), marital status (cohabiting/living with partner/married versus divorced/separated/single/widowed), ethnicity (Caucasian versus non-Caucasian) and religion (Muslim/Christian/Jewish/no religion/other (Hindu/Buddhist/Sikh)). Linear random-effects mixed models were used to model trends in DA scores for participants viewing the DA on multiple occasions.

Post modelling, three contrast tests were considered (each on three degrees of freedom). We assessed (a) overall time effects, i.e., whether the overall mean values at seven days, three months and six months from baseline were jointly different from the baseline level, (b) between-group differences over time (whether the mean group differences between those 'with' and 'without' a FH of OC at seven days, three months and six months from baseline were jointly different from the baseline level) and (c) within-group differences over time (whether mean values at seven days, three months and six months from baseline were jointly different from the baseline level within the groups 'with' and 'without' FH of OC). Statistical analysis used Stata-13.0 (Stata-Corp-LP, TX, https://www.stata.com/) and R version 3.5.1 (https://www.r-project.org/).

5. Conclusions

Our current health care systems remain primarily centred on improving disease diagnosis and treatment rather than prevention. Prevention of chronic disease, cancer being the second most common cause, is a major challenge for our health systems. PGT and personalised OC risk stratification can spur CSG detection and maximise precision prevention to reduce OC burden. We have shown that population-based personalised OC risk stratification is feasible and acceptable, has high satisfaction, reduces cancer worry/risk perception, and does not negatively impact on psychological health/quality of life. Further research and implementation studies evaluating the impact, clinical efficacy, long-term psychological, and socioethical consequences and cost effectiveness of this strategy are needed. This includes evaluation through large implementation studies of real-world health outcomes. Future implementation of such a strategy will require varying levels of workforce expansion/upskilling and reorganisation of health service infrastructure covering aspects of genetic testing and downstream care including screening and prevention pathways. PGT is an exciting and evolving field and personalised OC risk stratification offers a new paradigm for precision prevention in OC.

Supplementary Materials: The following are available online at http://www.mdpi.com/2072-6694/12/5/1241/s1, Table S1: Perceived benefits, risks, limitations or panel genetic testing/ovarian cancer risk assessment measured at baseline; Table S2: Decision aid question responses for women who consented and who did not consent to this study; Table S3: Mean scores at repeat viewings for participants who viewed the decision aid on multiple occasions; Table S4: Linear random-effects mixed models for trends in decision aid scores in participants viewing the decision aid on multiple occasions; Figure S1: Distributions of the remaining lifetime ovarian cancer risks given by different model versions.

Author Contributions: All authors have read and agree to the published version of the manuscript. Conception of study: I.J. and R.M. Design and development: R.M. and I.J. Trial management: R.M., F.G., I.J., U.M., L.S., M.A., M.K., J.K., and A.G.-M. Genetic testing: A.W., Y.W., C.L., J.D., A.D., and A.L. (Andrew Lee). Decision aid development: S.S., A.L. (Anne Lanceley), J.W., L.S., and R.M. Risk modelling: A.C.A., X.Y., U.M., R.M., and F.G. Data acquisition: F.G., R.M., X.L., S.G., N.L., D.C., and M.K. Data analysis: F.G., O.B., and R.M. Preparation of tables: F.G., O.B., and R.M. Initial draft of manuscript: F.G., R.M., O.B., and R.L.

Funding: This study was funded by Cancer Research UK and The Eve-Appeal Charity (C16420/A18066). U.M. received support from the National Institute for Health Research University College London Hospitals Biomedical Research Centre. A.A. is supported by Cancer Research UK (grant number C12292/A20861). The funding bodies had no role in the study design, data collection, analysis, interpretation or writing of the report or decision to submit for publication. The research team was independent of funders.

Acknowledgments: This study is supported by researchers at the Cancer Research UK Barts Centre, Queen Mary University of London (C16420/A18066). We are particularly grateful to the women who participated in this study. We are grateful to the entire medical, nursing, and administrative staff who work on the PROMISE Feasibility Study.

Conflicts of Interest: Ranjit Manchanda declares research funding from Barts and the London Charity and Rosetrees Trust outside this work, an honorarium for grant review from the Israel National Institute for Health Policy Research and an honorarium for advisory board membership from Astrazeneca/MSD. Ranjit Manchanda is supported by an NHS Innovation Accelerator (NIA) Fellowship for population testing. Ian Jacobs and Usha Menon have a financial interest in Abcodia, Ltd., a company formed to develop academic and commercial development of biomarkers for early detection of cancer. Ian Jacobs is a member of the board of Abcodia Ltd., a Director of Women's Health Specialists Ltd. and received consultancy from Beckton Dickinson. The other authors declare no conflict of interest. The funders had no role in the design of the study; in the collection, analyses, or interpretation of data; in the writing of the manuscript, or in the decision to publish the results.

References

1. Kuchenbaecker, K.B.; Hopper, J.L.; Barnes, D.R.; Phillips, K.A.; Mooij, T.M.; Roos-Blom, M.J.; Jervis, S.; van Leeuwen, F.E.; Milne, R.L.; Andrieu, N.; et al. Risks of Breast, Ovarian, and Contralateral Breast Cancer for BRCA1 and BRCA2 Mutation Carriers. *JAMA* **2017**, *317*, 2402–2416. [CrossRef] [PubMed]

2. Yang, X.; Song, H.; Leslie, G.; Engel, C.; Hahnen, E.; Auber, B.; Horváth, J.; Kast, K.; Niederacher, D.; Turnbull, C.; et al. Ovarian and breast cancer risks associated with pathogenic variants in RAD51C and RAD51D. *JNCI: J. Natl. Cancer Inst.* **2020**. [CrossRef] [PubMed]
3. Ramus, S.J.; Song, H.; Dicks, E.; Tyrer, J.P.; Rosenthal, A.N.; Intermaggio, M.P.; Fraser, L.; Gentry-Maharaj, A.; Hayward, J.; Philpott, S.; et al. Germline Mutations in the BRIP1, BARD1, PALB2, and NBN Genes in Women With Ovarian Cancer. *J. Natl. Cancer Inst.* **2015**, *107*. [CrossRef] [PubMed]
4. Jervis, S.; Song, H.; Lee, A.; Dicks, E.; Harrington, P.; Baynes, C.; Manchanda, R.; Easton, D.F.; Jacobs, I.; Pharoah, P.P.; et al. A risk prediction algorithm for ovarian cancer incorporating BRCA1, BRCA2, common alleles and other familial effects. *J. Med. Genet.* **2015**. [CrossRef]
5. Yang, X.; Leslie, G.; Gentry-Maharaj, A.; Ryan, A.; Intermaggio, M.; Lee, A.; Kalsi, J.K.; Tyrer, J.; Gaba, F.; Manchanda, R.; et al. Evaluation of polygenic risk scores for ovarian cancer risk prediction in a prospective cohort study. *J. Med. Genet.* **2018**. [CrossRef]
6. Pearce, C.L.; Stram, D.O.; Ness, R.B.; Stram, D.A.; Roman, L.D.; Templeman, C.; Lee, A.W.; Menon, U.; Fasching, P.A.; McAlpine, J.N.; et al. Population distribution of lifetime risk of ovarian cancer in the United States. *Cancer Epidemiol. Biomark. Prev.* **2015**, *24*, 671–676. [CrossRef]
7. Childers, C.P.; Childers, K.K.; Maggard-Gibbons, M.; Macinko, J. National Estimates of Genetic Testing in Women With a History of Breast or Ovarian Cancer. *J. Clin. Oncol.* **2017**, *35*, 3800–3806. [CrossRef]
8. Manchanda, R.; Blyuss, O.; Gaba, F.; Gordeev, V.S.; Jacobs, C.; Burnell, M.; Gan, C.; Taylor, R.; Turnbull, C.; Legood, R.; et al. Current detection rates and time-to-detection of all identifiable BRCA carriers in the Greater London population. *J. Med Genet.* **2018**. [CrossRef]
9. Manchanda, R.; Loggenberg, K.; Sanderson, S.; Burnell, M.; Wardle, J.; Gessler, S.; Side, L.; Balogun, N.; Desai, R.; Kumar, A.; et al. Population testing for cancer predisposing BRCA1/BRCA2 mutations in the Ashkenazi-Jewish community: A randomized controlled trial. *J. Natl. Cancer Inst.* **2015**, *107*, 379. [CrossRef]
10. Gabai-Kapara, E.; Lahad, A.; Kaufman, B.; Friedman, E.; Segev, S.; Renbaum, P.; Beeri, R.; Gal, M.; Grinshpun-Cohen, J.; Djemal, K.; et al. Population-based screening for breast and ovarian cancer risk due to BRCA1 and BRCA2. *Proc. Natl. Acad. Sci. USA* **2014**, *111*, 14205–14210. [CrossRef]
11. Manchanda, R.; Patel, S.; Gordeev, V.S.; Antoniou, A.C.; Smith, S.; Lee, A.; Hopper, J.L.; MacInnis, R.J.; Turnbull, C.; Ramus, S.J.; et al. Cost-effectiveness of Population-Based BRCA1, BRCA2, RAD51C, RAD51D, BRIP1, PALB2 Mutation Testing in Unselected General Population Women. *J. Natl. Cancer Inst.* **2018**, *110*, 714–725. [CrossRef] [PubMed]
12. Manchanda, R.; Gaba, F. Population Based Testing for Primary Prevention: A Systematic Review. *Cancers* **2018**, *10*, 424. [CrossRef] [PubMed]
13. Manchanda, R.; Burnell, M.; Gaba, F.; Desai, R.; Wardle, J.; Gessler, S.; Side, L.; Sanderson, S.; Loggenberg, K.; Brady, A.F.; et al. Randomised trial of population-based BRCA testing in Ashkenazi Jews: Long-term outcomes. *BJOG* **2019**. [CrossRef] [PubMed]
14. Manchanda, R.; Legood, R.; Burnell, M.; McGuire, A.; Raikou, M.; Loggenberg, K.; Wardle, J.; Sanderson, S.; Gessler, S.; Side, L.; et al. Cost-effectiveness of population screening for BRCA mutations in Ashkenazi jewish women compared with family history-based testing. *J. Natl. Cancer Inst.* **2015**, *107*, 380. [CrossRef] [PubMed]
15. Meisel, S.F.; Fraser, L.S.M.; Side, L.; Gessler, S.; Hann, K.E.J.; Wardle, J.; Lanceley, A.; PROMISE Study Team. Anticipated health behaviour changes and perceived control in response to disclosure of genetic risk of breast and ovarian cancer: A quantitative survey study among women in the UK. *BMJ Open* **2017**, *7*, e017675. [CrossRef] [PubMed]
16. Meisel, S.F.; Freeman, M.; Waller, J.; Fraser, L.; Gessler, S.; Jacobs, I.; Kalsi, J.; Manchanda, R.; Rahman, B.; Side, L.; et al. Impact of a decision aid about stratified ovarian cancer risk-management on women's knowledge and intentions: A randomised online experimental survey study. *BMC Public Health* **2017**, *17*, 882. [CrossRef] [PubMed]
17. Manchanda, R.; Burnell, M.; Gaba, F.; Sanderson, S.; Loggenberg, K.; Gessler, S.; Wardle, J.; Side, L.; Desai, R.; Brady, A.F.; et al. Attitude towards and factors affecting uptake of population-based BRCA testing in the Ashkenazi Jewish population: A cohort study. *BJOG* **2019**, *126*, 784–794. [CrossRef]
18. Manchanda, R.; Burnell, M.; Loggenberg, K.; Desai, R.; Wardle, J.; Sanderson, S.C.; Gessler, S.; Side, L.; Balogun, N.; Kumar, A.; et al. Cluster-randomised non-inferiority trial comparing DVD-assisted and traditional genetic counselling in systematic population testing for BRCA1/2 mutations. *J. Med. Genet.* **2016**, *53*, 472–480. [CrossRef]

19. Manchanda, R.; Patel, S.; Antoniou, A.C.; Levy-Lahad, E.; Turnbull, C.; Evans, D.G.; Hopper, J.L.; Macinnis, R.J.; Menon, U.; Jacobs, I.; et al. Cost-effectiveness of population based BRCA testing with varying Ashkenazi Jewish ancestry. *Am. J. Obstet. Gynecol.* **2017**, *217*. [CrossRef]
20. Nelson, H.D.; Fu, R.; Goddard, K.; Mitchell, J.P.; Okinaka-Hu, L.; Pappas, M.; Zakher, B. *Risk Assessment, Genetic Counseling, and Genetic Testing for BRCA-Related Cancer: Systematic Review to Update the U.S. Preventive Services Task Force Recommendation*; Agency for Healthcare Research and Quality: Rockville, MD, USA, 2013.
21. Metcalfe, K.A.; Poll, A.; Llacuachaqui, M.; Nanda, S.; Tulman, A.; Mian, N.; Sun, P.; Narod, S.A. Patient satisfaction and cancer-related distress among unselected Jewish women undergoing genetic testing for BRCA1 and BRCA2. *Clin. Genet.* **2010**, *78*, 411–417. [CrossRef]
22. Sivell, S.; Iredale, R.; Gray, J.; Coles, B. Cancer genetic risk assessment for individuals at risk of familial breast cancer. *Cochrane Database Syst. Rev.* **2007**, Cd003721. [CrossRef]
23. Kerber, R.A.; Slattery, M.L. Comparison of self-reported and database-linked family history of cancer data in a case-control study. *Am. J. Epidemiol.* **1997**, *146*, 244–248. [CrossRef] [PubMed]
24. Rebbeck, T.R.; Kauff, N.D.; Domchek, S.M. Meta-analysis of risk reduction estimates associated with risk-reducing salpingo-oophorectomy in BRCA1 or BRCA2 mutation carriers. *J. Natl. Cancer Inst.* **2009**, *101*, 80–87. [CrossRef] [PubMed]
25. Manchanda, R.; Legood, R.; Antoniou, A.C.; Gordeev, V.S.; Menon, U. Specifying the ovarian cancer risk threshold of 'premenopausal risk-reducing salpingo-oophorectomy' for ovarian cancer prevention: A cost-effectiveness analysis. *J. Med. Genet.* **2016**, *53*, 591–599. [CrossRef]
26. Manchanda, R.; Legood, R.; Antoniou, A.C.; Pearce, L.; Menon, U. Commentary on changing the risk threshold for surgical prevention of ovarian cancer. *BJOG* **2018**. [CrossRef]
27. Manchanda, R.; Legood, R.; Pearce, L.; Menon, U. Defining the risk threshold for risk reducing salpingo-oophorectomy for ovarian cancer prevention in low risk postmenopausal women. *Gynecol. Oncol.* **2015**, *139*, 487–494. [CrossRef]
28. Meisel, S.F.; Side, L.; Fraser, L.; Gessler, S.; Wardle, J.; Lanceley, A. Population-based, risk-stratified genetic testing for ovarian cancer risk: A focus group study. *Public Health Genom.* **2013**, *16*, 184–191. [CrossRef]
29. Jacobs, I.J.; Menon, U.; Ryan, A.; Gentry-Maharaj, A.; Burnell, M.; Kalsi, J.K.; Amso, N.N.; Apostolidou, S.; Benjamin, E.; Cruickshank, D.; et al. Ovarian cancer screening and mortality in the UK Collaborative Trial of Ovarian Cancer Screening (UKCTOCS): A randomised controlled trial. *Lancet* **2016**. [CrossRef]
30. Rosenthal, A.N.; Fraser, L.S.M.; Philpott, S.; Manchanda, R.; Burnell, M.; Badman, P.; Hadwin, R.; Rizzuto, I.; Benjamin, E.; Singh, N.; et al. Evidence of Stage Shift in Women Diagnosed With Ovarian Cancer During Phase II of the United Kingdom Familial Ovarian Cancer Screening Study. *J. Clin. Oncol.* **2017**, *35*, 1411–1420. [CrossRef]
31. Zigmond, A.S.; Snaith, R.P. The hospital anxiety and depression scale. *Acta Psychiatr. Scand.* **1983**, *67*, 361–370. [CrossRef]
32. Horowitz, M.; Wilner, N.; Alvarez, W. Impact of Event Scale: A measure of subjective stress. *Psychosom. Med.* **1979**, *41*, 209–218. [CrossRef] [PubMed]
33. Lerman, C.; Daly, M.; Masny, A.; Balshem, A. Attitudes about genetic testing for breast-ovarian cancer susceptibility. *J. Clin. Oncol.* **1994**, *12*, 843–850. [CrossRef] [PubMed]
34. Herdman, M.; Gudex, C.; Lloyd, A.; Janssen, M.; Kind, P.; Parkin, D.; Bonsel, G.; Badia, X. Development and preliminary testing of the new five-level version of EQ-5D (EQ-5D-5L). *Qual. Life Res.* **2011**, *20*, 1727–1736. [CrossRef] [PubMed]
35. Madalinska, J.B.; Hollenstein, J.; Bleiker, E.; van Beurden, M.; Valdimarsdottir, H.B.; Massuger, L.F.; Gaarenstroom, K.N.; Mourits, M.J.; Verheijen, R.H.; van Dorst, E.B.; et al. Quality-of-life effects of prophylactic salpingo-oophorectomy versus gynecologic screening among women at increased risk of hereditary ovarian cancer. *J. Clin. Oncol.* **2005**, *23*, 6890–6898. [CrossRef] [PubMed]

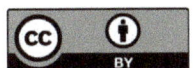

© 2020 by the authors. Licensee MDPI, Basel, Switzerland. This article is an open access article distributed under the terms and conditions of the Creative Commons Attribution (CC BY) license (http://creativecommons.org/licenses/by/4.0/).

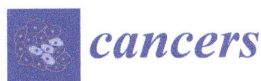

Article

Economic Evaluation of Population-Based *BRCA1/BRCA2* Mutation Testing across Multiple Countries and Health Systems

Ranjit Manchanda [1,2,3,*], Li Sun [1,4], Shreeya Patel [1], Olivia Evans [1,2], Janneke Wilschut [5], Ana Carolina De Freitas Lopes [6], Faiza Gaba [1,2], Adam Brentnall [7], Stephen Duffy [7], Bin Cui [8], Patricia Coelho De Soarez [6], Zakir Husain [9,10], John Hopper [11], Zia Sadique [4], Asima Mukhopadhyay [12,13], Li Yang [8], Johannes Berkhof [5] and Rosa Legood [4]

1. Wolfson Institute for Preventive Medicine, CRUK Barts Cancer Centre, Queen Mary University of London, London EC1M 6BQ, UK; li.sun1@lshtm.ac.uk (L.S.); shreeyapatel09@hotmail.co.uk (S.P.); o.evans@qmul.ac.uk (O.E.); f.gaba@qmul.ac.uk (F.G.)
2. Department of Gynaecological Oncology, Barts Health NHS Trust, Royal London Hospital, London E1 1BB, UK
3. MRC Clinical Trials Unit at UCL, Institute of Clinical Trials & Methodology, Faculty of Population Health Sciences, University College London, London WC1V 6LJ, UK
4. Department of Health Services Research and Policy, London School of Hygiene & Tropical Medicine, London WC1H 9SH, UK; Zia.Sadique@lshtm.ac.uk (Z.S.); Rosa.Legood@lshtm.ac.uk (R.L.)
5. Department of Epidemiology and Biostatistics, Amsterdam UMC, Vrije Universiteit Amsterdam, 1081 HV Amsterdam, Netherlands; j.wilschut@amsterdamumc.nl (J.W.); h.berkhof@amsterdamumc.nl (J.B.)
6. Departamento de Medicina Preventiva, Faculdade de Medicina FMUSP, Universidade de Sao Paulo, 01246903 Sao Paulo, Brazil; acflopes@usp.br (A.C.D.F.L.); patricia.soarez@usp.br (P.C.D.S.)
7. Centre for Cancer Prevention, Wolfson Institute of Preventive Medicine, Queen Mary University of London, London EC1M 6BQ, UK; a.brentnall@qmul.ac.uk (A.B.); s.w.duffy@qmul.ac.uk (S.D.)
8. School of Public Health, Peking University, Beijing 100191, China; cuibin@bjmu.edu.cn (B.C.); lyang@bjmu.edu.cn (L.Y.)
9. Department of Humanities & Social Sciences, Indian Institute of Technology, Kharagpur, West Bengal 721302, India; dzhusain@gmail.com
10. Department of Economics, Presidency University, Kolkata 700073, India
11. Centre for Epidemiology & Biostatistics, Melbourne School of Population & Global Health, Faculty of Medicine, Dentistry & Health Sciences, University of Melbourne, Victoria 3010, Australia; j.hopper@unimelb.edu.au
12. Tata Medical Centre, Kolkata, West Bengal 700160, India; asima7@yahoo.co.in
13. Northern Institute for Cancer Research, Newcastle University, Newcastle upon Tyne NE2 4HH, UK
* Correspondence: r.manchanda@qmul.ac.uk

Received: 7 June 2020; Accepted: 13 July 2020; Published: 17 July 2020

Abstract: Clinical criteria/Family history-based *BRCA* testing misses a large proportion of *BRCA* carriers who can benefit from screening/prevention. We estimate the cost-effectiveness of population-based *BRCA* testing in general population women across different countries/health systems. A Markov model comparing the lifetime costs and effects of *BRCA1/BRCA2* testing all general population women ≥30 years compared with clinical criteria/FH-based testing. Separate analyses are undertaken for the UK/USA/Netherlands (high-income countries/HIC), China/Brazil (upper–middle income countries/UMIC) and India (low–middle income countries/LMIC) using both health system/payer and societal perspectives. *BRCA* carriers undergo appropriate screening/prevention interventions to reduce breast cancer (BC) and ovarian cancer (OC) risk. Outcomes include OC, BC, and additional heart disease deaths and incremental cost-effectiveness ratio (ICER)/quality-adjusted life year (QALY). Probabilistic/one-way sensitivity analyses evaluate model uncertainty. For the base case, from a societal perspective, we found that population-based *BRCA* testing is cost-saving in HIC (UK-ICER = $−5639/QALY; USA-ICER = $−4018/QALY; Netherlands-ICER = $−11,433/QALY), and it appears cost-effective in UMIC (China-ICER = $18,066/QALY; Brazil-ICER = $13,579/QALY), but it is not cost-effective in LMIC (India-ICER = $23,031/QALY). From a payer perspective, population-based *BRCA* testing is highly cost-effective in HIC (UK-ICER = $21,191/QALY, USA-ICER = $16,552/QALY, Netherlands-ICER = $25,215/QALY), and it is cost-effective in UMIC (China-ICER = $23,485/QALY, Brazil–ICER = $20,995/QALY), but it is not cost-effective in LMIC (India-ICER = $32,217/QALY). *BRCA* testing costs below $172/test (ICER = $19,685/QALY), which makes it cost-effective (from a societal perspective) for LMIC/India. Population-based *BRCA* testing can prevent an additional 2319 to 2666 BC and 327 to 449 OC cases per million women than the current clinical strategy. Findings suggest that population-based *BRCA* testing for countries evaluated is extremely cost-effective across HIC/UMIC health systems, is cost-saving for HIC health systems from a societal perspective, and can prevent tens of thousands more BC/OC cases.

Keywords: BRCA; population testing; cost-effectiveness; ovarian cancer; breast cancer; cancer prevention

1. Introduction

Around 10–20% of ovarian cancer (OC) [1] and 6% breast cancer (BC) [2] overall are caused by inheritable *BRCA1/BRCA2* mutations. Women carrying *BRCA1/BRCA2* mutations have a 17–44% risk of OC and 69–72% risk of BC until age 80 years [3]. Most of these cancers can be prevented in unaffected *BRCA1/BRCA2* women carriers. Women can opt for risk-reducing salpingo-oophorectomy (RRSO), to reduce OC risk [4]. In *BRCA* women, RRSO reduces OC risk by 79–96% [4–6]. Additionally, they can opt for MRI/mammography screening, chemoprevention with selective estrogen-receptor modulators (SERM) or aromatase inhibitors [7]; or risk-reducing mastectomy (RRM) [8,9] to reduce their BC risk [10]. RRM reduces BC risk by 90–95% [8,9]. Mutation identification also enables women to make timely, informed reproductive/lifestyle choices and consider prenatal/pre-implantation genetic diagnosis.

Despite 25 years of *BRCA* testing and effective mechanisms for prevention, current guidelines and access to testing/treatment pathways remain complex and associated with a massive under-utilisation of genetic testing [11]. Only 20% of eligible US women have accessed/undergone genetic testing [11]. A UK analysis shows the huge majority (>97%) of *BRCA* carriers in the population remain unidentified [12]. This highlights substantial missed opportunities for early detection and primary prevention. The current approach uses established clinical-criteria/family-history (FH) based *a priori* *BRCA* probability thresholds to identify high-risk individuals eligible for *BRCA* testing. These clinical criteria/FH-based criteria are used to calculate mutation probability and have been loosened over the years. Earlier, the threshold for offering *BRCA* testing used to be 20% probability. Most countries/health systems now offer *BRCA* testing at a *BRCA* mutation probability of around 10% [13]. A number of different strategies ranging from standardised criteria to complex mathematical (Empirical/Mendelian) models have been used to calculate mutation probability and are used in clinical practice. However, this requires individuals and health practitioners to recognise and act on a significant FH. *BRCA* carriers, who are unaware of their FH, unappreciative of its risk/significance, not proactive in seeking advice, or lack a strong FH (small families/paternal inheritance/chance) get excluded. Over 50% *BRCA* carriers do not fulfil clinical criteria and are missed [14–20]. Current detection rates are inadequate to identify all *BRCA* carriers and even doubling detection rates will need 165 years to ascertain the 'clinically detectable' proportion of *BRCA* carriers [12]. Why should we wait for decades for people to develop cancer before identifying *BRCA* carriers and unaffected at-risk family members to offer prevention?

These limitations can be overcome through unrestricted/unselected population based *BRCA* testing. Falling *BRCA* testing costs, advances in computing/bioinformatics, and next-generation sequencing has made this possible. Jewish population studies show this is feasible, acceptable, has high satisfaction (91–95%), significantly reduces anxiety, doesn't harm psychological well-being or quality of life, and is extremely cost-effective [15,16,21,22]. Pilot general population studies are ongoing in the UK/Canada [23]. However, the potential applicability and scope for primary prevention transcends continents and countries. Health systems, infrastructure, costs, environment, contexts, opportunities, and capacity along with health sector priorities vary considerably across different countries, [24]. Economic evaluations of health interventions, health perspectives and cost-effectiveness thresholds differ amongst countries. Nevertheless, economic evaluation is important to weigh up costs and health effects of alternative health strategies, to help health policy decision making with respect to cost efficiency and resource allocation. For interventions to be sustainable, they need to be cost-effective and affordable. The World Bank separates countries into four income categories using Gross National Income (GNI) per capita (USA dollars): Low-income (LIC: ≤$1025), Lower–Middle Income (LMIC: $1026–$4035), Upper–Middle Income (UMIC: $4036–$12,475), and High Income (HIC: ≥$12,476). In settings of state funded universal health care coverage, the difference between government and societal perspectives is narrower than countries with a limited social security structure/net, where this gap can be significantly larger and consequences considerable. We for the first time evaluate the cost-effectiveness of population-based *BRCA*-testing (compared to clinical-criteria/family-history testing) across multiple countries/health systems: India (LMIC), Brazil (UMIC), China (UMIC), the USA (HIC), the UK (HIC), and the Netherlands (HIC). We present analyses from both health system or payer (here forth called 'payer') and societal perspectives.

2. Results

The comparison of lifetime costs and quality-adjusted life year (QALYs) of population testing and clinical-criteria/FH testing for women in different countries along with the country-specific incremental cost-effectiveness ratios (ICERs) and willingness-to-pay (WTP) thresholds are given in Table 1. Our results show that from a 'societal perspective' (using WHO guidelines), population-based *BRCA* testing is actually 'cost-saving' and contributes to better health in HIC of the UK (ICER = $−5,639/QALY; life expectancy gained = 3.0 days), USA (ICER = $−4018/QALY; life expectancy gained = 2.2 days), and The Netherlands (ICER = $−11,433/QALY; life expectancy gained = 2.8 days). It appears potentially cost-effective in UMICs of China (ICER = $18,066/QALY; life expectancy gained = 1.8 days) and cost-effective in Brazil (ICER = $13,579/QALY; life expectancy gained = 3.7 days), but it is not cost-effective in India (ICER = $23,031/QALY; life expectancy gained = 2.5 days) (LMIC) for the base case.

From a 'payer perspective' (using WHO guidelines), population-based *BRCA* testing is 'highly' cost-effective compared with clinical criteria/FH-based testing in HIC, with UK-ICER = $21,191/QALY (life expectancy gained = 3.0 days), USA-ICER = $16,552/QALY (life expectancy gained = 2.2 days), and Netherlands-ICER = $25,215/QALY (life expectancy gained = 2.8 days). In UMIC population-based *BRCA* testing is cost-effective with ICER = $23,485/QALY in China (life expectancy gained = 1.8 days) and ICER = $20,995/QALY in Brazil (life expectancy gained = 3.7 days). Population-based *BRCA* testing is not cost-effective in LMIC with ICER = $32,217/QALY in India (life expectancy gained = 2.5 days).

If we consider local, country-specific guidelines for the UK, USA, and the Netherlands, then population-based *BRCA* testing is cost-effective from the payer perspective (UK-ICER = $24,066/QALY; USA-ICER = $16,552/QALY; Netherlands-ICER = $17655/QALY), and cost-saving from the societal perspective (UK-ICER = −$3543/QALY; USA-ICER = −$4018/QALY; Netherlands ICER = −$3185/QALY). The corresponding values for life expectancy gained are 2.6 days (UK), 2.2 days (USA) and 4.2 days Netherlands. Figure 1a,b plot change in ICER/QALY with varying *BRCA* testing costs in Brazil, China and India for payer and societal perspectives. Population testing becomes potentially cost-effective (from a societal perspective) in India if the *BRCA* testing cost falls to $172/test (ICER = $19,685/QALY) (Figure 1a; Appendix D). *BRCA* testing costs need to reach $95/test (ICER = $19,670/QALY) for cost-effective population testing in India from the payer perspective (Figure 1b; Appendix D).

The lifetime population impact (reduction in BC and OC cases and deaths; and excess coronary heart disease (CHD)) of offering population *BRCA* testing for the six countries is detailed in Table 2. A population-based *BRCA* testing approach can potentially prevent an additional 2319 to 2666 BC and 327 to 449 OC cases per million women, translating to tens of thousands more BC/OC prevented across the population than the current clinical strategy.

Table 1. Baseline analysis.

Baseline Analysis Based on WHO Guidelines, Using GDP-Based Thresholds

	Population-Based Testing								#FH-Based Testing								ICER		WTP Threshold ($/QALY)	
	Health Effects		Costs		Cost/LY		Cost/QALY (95% Credible Intervals)		Health Effects		Costs		Cost/LY		Cost/QALY (95% Credible Intervals)					
	LY	QALY	Payer	Societal					LY	QALY	Payer	Societal	Payer	Societal	Payer	Societal	1*GDP per Capita	3*GDP per Capita		
UK	25.67	25.62	2543	18,568					25.66	25.61	2336	18,623	25,530	−6794	21,191 (14,857, 29,619)	−5639 (−11,880, 1895)	42,656	127,969		
USA	25.23	25.18	7250	21,951					25.22	25.18	7122	21,982	20,997	−5097	16,552 (4435, 30,280)	−4018 (−15,947, 8764)	57,589	172,766		
Netherlands	25.86	25.81	2478	24,642					25.85	25.80	2239	24,750	30,587	−13,868	25,215 (18,193, 34,069)	−11,433 (−18,054, −3689)	50,539	151,616		
China	20.70	20.69	820	7687					20.70	20.68	665	7568	30,788	23,684	23,485 (13,947, 36,162)	18066 (8683, 30,653)	15,531	46,592		
Brazil	24.54	24.51	834	6314					24.53	24.49	586	6153	24,496	15,844	20,995 (15,707, 27,953)	13,579 (8561, 20,180)	15,182	45,545		
India	18.17	18.16	634	30,968					18.17	18.15	369	30,779	39,473	28,218	32,217 (23,982, 42,786)	23,031 (15,107, 22,112)	6574	19,722		

Country-Specific Analysis Based on Local Health Economic Guidelines Where they Exist

	Population-Based Testing								#FH-Based Testing								ICER		WTP Threshold ($/QALY)
	Health effects		Costs		Cost/LY		Cost/QALY (95% Credible Intervals)		Health effects		Costs		Cost/LY		Cost/QALY (95% Credible Intervals)				
	LY	QALY	Payer	Societal					LY	QALY	Payer	Societal	Payer	Societal	Payer	Societal			
UK ‖	23.55	23.51	2263	16,570					23.55	23.50	2053	16,601	29,273	−4309	24,066 (16,407, 33,590)	−3543 (−10452, 4901)	28,471	42,857
USA	25.23	25.18	7250	21,951					25.22	25.17	7122	21,982	20,997	−5097	16,552 (4435, 30,280)	−4018 (−15947, 8764)	50,000	100,000
Netherlands ∫	34.58	34.51	1968	19,109					34.57	34.49	1725	19,153	20,796	−3752	17,655 (12,948, 23,766)	−3185 (−7568, 2319)	24,390	60,976

ICER: incremental cost-effectiveness ratio, LY—life years, QALY—quality-adjusted life years, FH—family history, GDP—gross domestic product. # Reference Strategy. Costs are given in $ WTP: willingness to pay. This reflects the different cost-effective thresholds for different countries. For GDP-based thresholds: Three times GDP per capita is the threshold for being cost-effective and one time GDP per capita is the threshold for being highly cost-effective. Discount rate is 3% for costs and health effects (LYs and QALYs). For country-specific thresholds: For the UK, this is £20,000 to £30,000 [25]; For the USA, this is: $50,000 to $100,000 [26]; For the Netherlands, this is: €20,000 to €50,000 [27]. Values in £s and €s have been converted to $ using PPP (purchasing power parity) [28]. ‖ For the UK, the discount rate is 3.5% for costs and health effects as per National Institute of Health and Care Excellence (NICE) economic evaluation guidelines [25]. ∫ For the Netherlands, the discount rate is 4% for costs and 1.5% for QALYs as per Dutch health economic analysis guidelines. Perspective: Dutch guidelines recommend a societal perspective. UK NICE guidelines recommend a payer perspective [25]. (See Appendix D for details and references). 1*GDP means 1 × GDP; 3*GDP means 3 × GDP

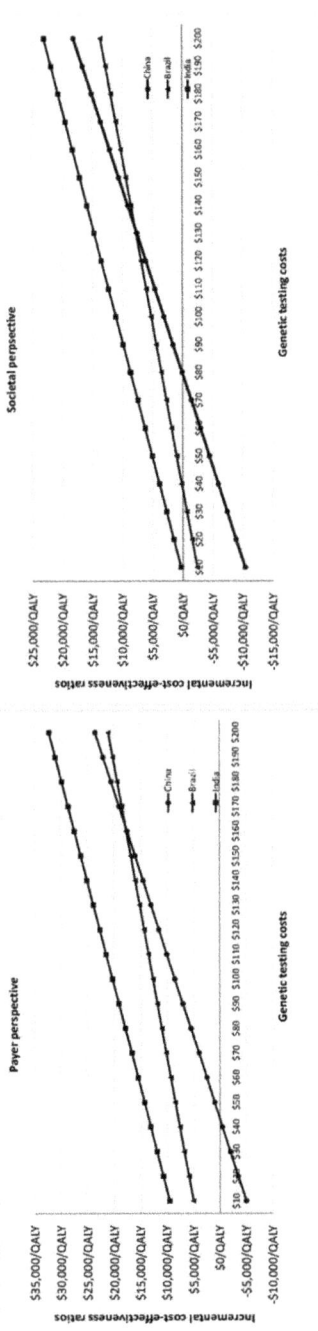

Figure 1. Change in ICER/QALY with varying *BRCA* testing costs in Brazil, China, and India. (**a**) Change in ICER/QALY with varying *BRCA* testing costs in Brazil, China and India from a payer/healthcare perspective. (**b**) Change in ICER/QALY with varying *BRCA* testing costs in Brazil, China, and India from a societal perspective. The graphs depict the change in ICER/QALY at varying costs of BRCA testing for Brazil, China, and India from payer (Figure 1a) and societal (Figure 1b) perspectives. **X axis:** BRCA testing costs in US$; **Y axis:** ICER/QALY.

Table 2. Lifetime population impact of offering genetic testing for the population.

	Population-Based Testing		FH-Based Testing		Difference	
	Per Million	Actual	Per Million	Actual	Per Million	Actual
	UK (female population over 30 years = 21,760,299)					
BC cases	112,014	2,437,458	114,666	2,495,166	−2652	−57,708
OC cases	15,822	344,291	16,269	354,018	−447	−9727
BC deaths	12,985	282,557	13,258	288,498	−273	−5941
OC deaths	278	6049	550	11,968	−272	−5919
Excess CHD deaths	17	370	0	0	17	370
	USA (female population over 30 years = 101,428,241)					
BC cases	106,431	10,795,109	109,084	11,064,198	−2653	−269,089
OC cases	9985	1,012,761	10,417	1,056,578	−432	−43,817
BC deaths	8113	822,887	8285	840,333	−172	−17,446
OC deaths	235	23,836	475	48,178	−240	−24,343
Excess CHD deaths	17	1724	0	0	17	1724
	Netherlands (female population over 30 years = 5,694,479)					
BC cases	111,732	636,256	114,398	651,437	−2666	−15,181
OC cases	10,964	62,434	11,413	64,991	−449	−2557
BC deaths	11,822	67,320	12,072	68,744	−250	−1424
OC deaths	277	1577	542	3086	−265	−1509
Excess CHD deaths	17	97	0	0	17	97
	China (female population over 30 years = 422,831,894)					
BC cases	27,062	11,442,677	29,546	12,492,991	−2484	−1,050,314
OC cases	3862	1,632,977	4228	1,787,733	−366	−154,756
BC deaths	3728	1576317	4015	1,697,670	−287	−121,353
OC deaths	163	68922	369	156,025	−206	−87,103
Excess CHD deaths	12	5074	0	0	12	5074
	Brazil (female population over 30 years = 58,670,634)					
BC cases	66,227	3,885,580	68,891	4,041,879	−2664	−156,299
OC cases	5358	314,357	5787	339,527	−429	−25,170
BC deaths	12,901	756,910	13,421	787,419	−520	−30,509
OC deaths	271	15,900	539	31,623	−268	−15,724
Excess CHD deaths	17	997	0	0	17	997
	India (female population over 30 years = 298,650,697)					
BC cases	13,713	4,095,397	16,032	4,787,968	−2319	−692,571
OC cases	2826	843,987	3153	941,646	−327	−97,659
BC deaths	3796	1,133,678	4391	1,311,375	−595	−177,697
OC deaths	168	50,173	429	128,121	−261	−77,948
Excess CHD deaths	8	2389	0	0	8	2389

BC—breast cancer, CHD—coronary heart disease, FH—family history, OC—ovarian cancer. The female population data is obtained from the World Bank [29]. We used the modelling to estimate the number of BC cases, OC cases, BC deaths, OC deaths, and excess CHD deaths per million women aged 30 years in the six countries and calculated the number of cases prevented and deaths prevented. The actual numbers of cases prevented and deaths prevented were estimated based on the number of female population aged over 30 years in the six countries [29].

Scenario analyses results are given in Table 3. Different scenarios analysed include no reduction in BC risk from RRSO, nil compliance with hormone replacement therapy (HRT), reduction in RRM and RRSO rates by half, and reduced genetic testing costs of $100. Population-based *BRCA* testing remains cost-effective from payer and societal perspectives in each HIC and UMIC country at their respective WTP thresholds, even without reduction in BC risk from RRSO, no HRT uptake after RRSO, and 50% lower RRM and RRSO uptake rates (Table 3). If the *BRCA* testing costs fell to $100/test, it would be highly cost-effective from the payer perspective and cost-saving (negative ICERs) from the societal perspective for HIC; highly cost-effective from payer/societal perspectives for UMIC, and cost-effective from the societal perspective for India (LMIC). The maximum *BRCA* testing costs for population testing to remain cost-effective from the payer/societal perspectives respectively are in Appendix E. At the 3*GDP WTP threshold, these are: UK = $1254/$1520; USA = $1417/$1577; Netherlands = $1407/$1758; China = $354/$390; Brazil = $493/$582; and India = $95/$172. Using UK/USA/Netherlands guideline-based WTP thresholds, these maximum *BRCA* testing costs are UK = $365, USA = $850–$1010, and Netherlands = $800.

Results of the one-way sensitivity analysis indicate that model outcomes are not impacted much by treatment costs, utility scores, mutation prevalence, and probabilities (Appendix E). The variable with the maximum effect on ICERs is the cost of *BRCA* testing. Probabilistic sensitivity analysis (PSA) results (Figure 2) show that at the WTP thresholds in each country, a population-testing strategy is cost-effective compared to clinical-criteria/FH-testing strategy from both the payer and societal perspectives for HIC and UMIC but not LMIC countries evaluated. The PSAs were highly cost-effective for the evaluated HIC and UMIC countries. All (100%) simulations are cost-effective at the guideline-specific thresholds for the UK/USA/Netherlands from payer and societal perspectives. For the 3*GDP-based WTP threshold for China/Brazil/India, 100%/100%/22.2% for the societal perspective and 100%/100%/0% simulations for the payer perspective were cost-effective (Figure 2a,b). However, a population strategy becomes cost-effective in India (LMIC) at $172/test. At the country-specific WTP thresholds for UK/USA/Netherlands, 84.9%/100%/98.5% of simulations for the payer perspective were cost-effective, and 100% simulations for the societal perspective were cost-effective for all three countries).

Table 3. Scenario analysis.

	Population-Based Testing					FH-Based Testing						ICER				WTP	
	Health Effects		Costs			Health Effects		Costs		Cost/LY		Cost/QALY			GDP per Capita	3*GDP per Capita
	LY	QALY	Payer	Societal		LY	QALY	Payer	Societal	Payer	Societal	Payer	Societal			
					Scenario: No reduction in breast cancer risk from RRSO (P9 = 1)											
UK †	25.67	25.62	2550	18,589		25.66	25.61	2336	18,626	27,692	−4729	23,188	−3960		42,656	127,969
USA ‡	25.22	25.18	7273	21,982		25.22	25.17	7125	21,986	25,474	−565	20,318	−450		57,589	172,766
Netherlands ʃ	25.86	25.81	2483	24,668		25.85	25.80	2240	24,754	32,834	−11,559	27,318	−9617		50,539	151,616
China	20.69	20.69	825	7693		20.70	20.68	666	7569	32,874	25,745	25,401	19,892		15,531	46,592
Brazil	24.54	24.51	837	6321		24.53	24.49	586	6154	26,175	17,447	22,577	15,049		15,182	45,545
India	18.17	18.16	637	30,974		18.17	18.15	370	30,779	41,333	30,125	34,019	24,795		6574	19,722
					Scenario: No compliance with HRT (P13 = 0)											
UK †	25.67	25.62	2542	18,569		25.66	25.61	2335	18,623	26,315	−6954	21,707	−5736		42,656	127,969
USA ‡	25.22	25.18	7250	21,951		25.22	25.17	7122	21,982	21,997	−5280	17,173	−4122		57,589	172,766
Netherlands ʃ	25.86	25.81	2477	24,647		25.85	25.80	2239	24,751	31,629	−13,869	25,897	−11,356		50,539	151,616
China	20.69	20.69	812	7678		20.70	20.68	664	7566	29,975	22,722	22,750	17,246		15,531	46,592
Brazil	24.54	24.51	833	6312		24.53	24.49	586	6153	24,932	16,077	21,296	13,732		15,182	45,545
India	18.17	18.16	623	30,957		18.17	18.15	367	30,777	38,327	26,995	31,242	22,005		6574	19,722
					Scenario: Half RRM uptake (p2 = 0.235) *											
UK †	25.67	25.62	2545	18,590		25.66	25.61	2336	18,627	27,301	−4834	22,648	−4010		42,656	127,969
USA ‡	25.22	25.18	7265	21,978		25.22	25.17	7125	21,987	24,248	−1503	19,122	−1185		57,589	172,766
Netherlands ʃ	25.86	25.81	2480	24,671		25.85	25.80	2240	24,755	32,616	−11,449	26,879	−9435		50,539	151,616
China	20.69	20.69	826	7695		20.70	20.68	666	7569	33,440	26,362	25,453	20,066		15,531	46,592
Brazil	24.54	24.51	838	6324		24.53	24.49	587	6155	26,622	17,938	22,762	15,337		15,182	45,545
India	18.17	18.16	620	30,959		18.17	18.15	367	30,777	39,820	28,637	32,377	23,285		6574	19,722
					Scenario: Half RRSO uptake (p8 = 0.275)											
UK †	25.67	25.62	2546	18,589		25.66	25.61	2336	18,628	28,209	−5272	23,325	−4359		42,656	127,969
USA ‡	25.22	25.18	7271	21,982		25.22	25.17	7127	21,989	25,917	−1205	20,308	−944		57,589	172,766
Netherlands ʃ	25.86	25.81	2482	24,675		25.85	25.80	2241	24,758	33,868	−11,681	27,799	−9588		50,539	151,616
China	20.69	20.69	820	7688		20.70	20.68	665	7568	32,321	25,018	24,651	19,081		15,531	46,592
Brazil	24.54	24.51	835	6319		24.53	24.49	586	6154	26,241	17,341	22,475	14,852		15,182	45,545
India	18.17	18.16	630	30,967		18.17	18.15	369	30,779	40,490	29,175	33,037	23,805		6574	19,722

Table 3. Cont.

	Population-Based Testing					FH-Based Testing					ICER				WTP	
	Health Effects		Costs			Health Effects		Costs			Cost/LY		Cost/QALY		GDP per Capita	3*GDP per Capita
	LY	QALY	Payer	Societal		LY	QALY	Payer	Societal		Payer	Societal	Payer	Societal		
					Scenario: Genetic testing cost of $100											
UK [†]	25.67	25.62	2443	18,468		25.66	25.61	2335	18,622		13,337	−18,988	11,070	−15,761	42,656	127,969
USA [‡]	25.23	25.18	7150	21,851		25.22	25.17	7121	21,981		4717	−21,377	3718	−16,852	57,589	172,766
Netherlands [∫]	25.86	25.81	2378	24,542		25.85	25.80	2238	24,749		17,893	−26,562	14,750	−21,897	50,539	151,616
China	20.70	20.69	721	7587		20.70	20.68	664	7567		11,165	4061	8517	3098	15,531	46,592
Brazil	24.54	24.51	735	6214		24.53	24.49	585	6152		14,741	6089	12,635	5219	15,182	45,545
India	18.17	18.16	535	30,869		18.17	18.15	368	30,778		24,832	13,577	20,267	11,081	6574	19,722

LY—life years, QALY—quality-adjusted life year, FH—family history, GDP—gross domestic product, HRT—hormone replacement therapy, ICER—incremental cost-effectiveness ratio, RRM—risk-reducing mastectomy, RRSO—risk-reducing salpingo-oophorectomy, WTP—willingness to pay. * Half the RRM uptake rate of the baseline case analysis. Baseline uptake = 47%, Half the baseline = 23.5%. # Half the RRSO uptake rate of the baseline case analysis. Baseline uptake = 55%, Half the baseline = 27.5%. [†] UK health-economic guideline based threshold is $28,471–$42,857/QALY. £s have been converted to $ using PPP (purchasing power parity) [28]. [‡] USA health-economic guideline based WTP threshold is $50,000–$100,000/QALY. [∫] Netherlands health-economic guideline based WTP threshold is $24,390–$60,976/QALY. €s have been converted to $ using PPP (purchasing power parity).

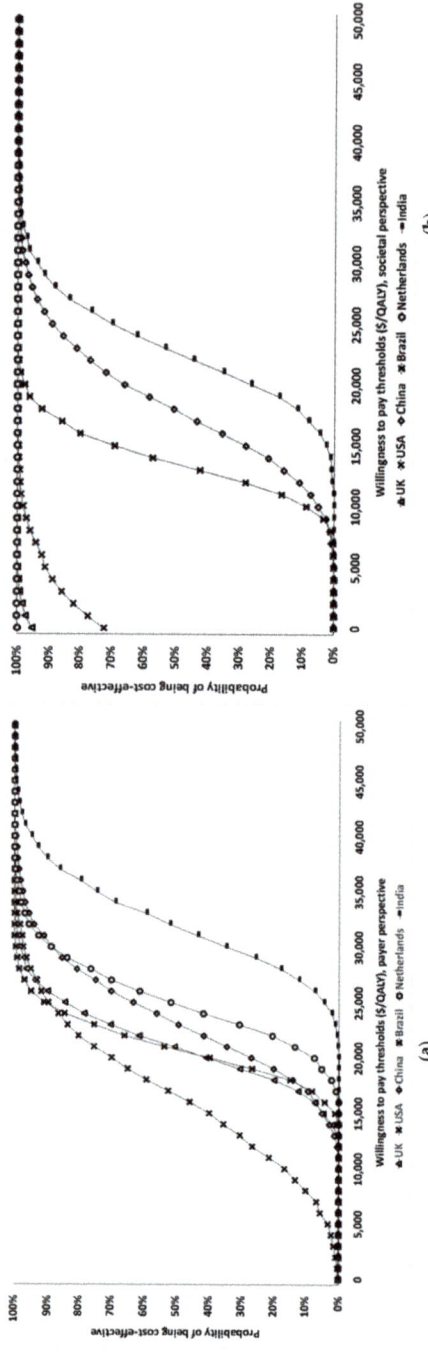

Figure 2. Cost-effectiveness acceptability curves. (**a**) Cost-effectiveness acceptability curve—payer perspective. (**b**) Cost-effectiveness acceptability curve—societal perspective. * The GDP-based (WHO) willingness-to-pay thresholds are $127,969/QALY in the UK, $172,766/QALY in the US, $151,616/QALY in the Netherlands, $46,592/QALY in China, $45,545/QALY in Brazil, and $19,722/QALY in India (Table 2). The country guideline-specific willingness-to-pay thresholds are $42,857/QALY in the UK, $100,000 in the US, and $60,976 in the Netherlands (Table 2). Probabilistic sensitivity analysis in which all model parameters/variables are varied simultaneously across their distributions to further explore model uncertainty. X-axis: Willingness-to-pay thresholds in terms of Cost ($s)/QALY; Y-axis: Proportion of simulations. The results of 1000 simulations were plotted on a cost-effectiveness acceptability curve showing the proportion of simulations (Y-axis) that indicated that the intervention was cost-effective at different willingness-to-pay thresholds (X-axis). Separate curves are plotted for the UK, USA, Netherlands, China, Brazil, and India, with different analyses provided for both payer (Figure 2a) and societal (Figure 2b) perspectives.

3. Discussion

For the first time, we explore the cost-effectiveness of population-based *BRCA* testing across countries from HIC, UMIC and LMIC health systems. We show that population-based *BRCA* testing is extremely cost-effective across HIC/UMIC health systems assessed and is potentially cost-saving for HIC health systems (UK/USA/Netherlands) if analysed from a societal perspective. Societal perspective analyses are associated with lower ICER/QALY than the payer perspective, as it incorporates additional costs linked to productivity loss. There is increasing recognition of the importance and need for economic cost-effectiveness evaluations to conform to the societal perspective and is recommended by WHO/international bodies. This is particularly important in middle/lower–income countries that lack a robust/comprehensive state-funded social security system. However, some countries such as the UK only consider a payer perspective when making health policy.

A population-based *BRCA* testing approach can potentially prevent an additional 57,708/269,089/15,181/1,050,314/156,299/692,571 BC cases and 9727/43,817/2557/154,756/25,170/97,659 OC cases in the UK/USA/Netherlands/China/Brazil/India respectively (Table 2) compared to the current clinical strategy. Given the huge under-utilisation of *BRCA* testing along with limited access and uptake associated with current treatment pathways [11,12], one could postulate that the benefit could be even higher. Our findings are important, as we show that a new population-based approach can have much broader global applicability and a far greater impact on BC/OC burden in the population than current treatment strategies. Cost-effectiveness analyses are necessary to guide policy decisions on healthcare resource allocation. Our findings support a change in paradigm toward population testing to maximise OC/BC prevention and highlights a need for further implementation research in this area.

Our results are sensitive to the cost of testing, particularly in LMIC countries. *BRCA* testing costs need to fall further for population testing to be cost-effective in LMIC countries. In India, it would become potentially cost-effective at $172/test. Although our base case analysis uses costs higher than this, we are aware of Indian providers who offer *BRCA* testing for around $140/test. Genetic testing costs have fallen considerably over the last 5 years and remain on a downward trajectory. While we have used a standard cost for *BRCA* testing that is currently available across countries, some providers may charge more than this. Our analysis of maximum cost(s) of *BRCA* testing for a population testing strategy remaining cost-effective (Appendix D) shows that these lie above what is charged by a number of providers today.

The precise definition of an appropriate cost-effectiveness threshold remains an important issue of ongoing debate. While this has been clearly defined in some (particularly HIC) health systems, a WHO-CHOICE 3*GDP threshold is considered too high by some, as it ignores opportunity costs [30]. Additionally, whilst cost-effectiveness is a key factor for allocating health budgets, it needs to be considered along with context-specific local issues, affordability, budget impact, fairness, and feasibility [31]. Some advocate against a single fixed threshold and recommend a range of thresholds for different contexts. The Norwegian health system prioritises interventions based on health benefit, resource implications, and health loss to the beneficiary if the intervention was absent (higher priority for higher health loss to the beneficiary) [32]. We provide a range of cost estimates for *BRCA* testing linked to varying potential cost-effectiveness thresholds (ICER/QALY) from payer and societal perspectives to help decision makers in UMIC and LIC. This is important, as the main model parameter impacting the overall result is the cost of *BRCA* testing (Figure 1a,b).

Our analysis has several advantages. We follow the transparency principle to facilitate the interpretation of methodology and results and use current standard of care or best practice as the comparator for measuring costs and effects. As per NICE recommendations, we use QALYs to measure health outcomes, which captures both length of life and quality of life and is generalisable across disease states. Our economic evaluation uses a lifetime horizon that is long enough to capture all costs and effects relevant to the decision problem. Additionally, costs and effects are discounted to reflect their value at the time of decision making, ensuring that the potential time preferences of the relevant population are accounted for. Our base case reflects direct health-care costs and health outcomes, and our analysis includes a societal perspective. We explore heterogeneity through scenario analyses and uncertainty and variability through extensive one-way/PSA analyses, as recommended. Our results remain robust at parameter extremes on one-way analysis (Appendix E) and with PSA (Figure 2). Our analysis uses PPP (purchasing power parity), which is a mechanism for accounting for different relative costs of goods when undertaking a comparative analysis of expenditures and incomes in different countries. Besides OC/BC outcomes, we also included excess CHD deaths from premenopausal oophorectomy [33] and incorporate costs for HRT, excess heart disease, bone health monitoring, and treatment. Our costs also include pre-test counselling for all and post-test genetic counselling for pathogenic mutations and VUS.

Similar to other modelling studies, our study has some limitations. In line with earlier analyses in high-risk and low-risk women, our base case analysis assumes a reduction in BC risk with premenopausal oophorectomy. However, recently, there has been uncertainty around the benefit of BC risk reduction from RRSO. Nonetheless, our scenario analysis shows cost-effectiveness in HIC/UMIC even without BC risk reduction (Table 3). We use established surgical prevention rates from HIC in the base-case analysis (Table 4). However, RRM/RRSO rates vary, and lower rates are reported in some populations [34]. The uptake of breast screening, chemoprevention, and risk-reducing surgery may also be influenced by socioeconomic, demographic, and cultural factors and may vary across populations [34]. Rates of screening and preventive interventions have also increased with time. Higher rates are reported in the last 10 years compared to earlier decades, as knowledge and awareness of these issues has improved. Rates could be lower in carriers ascertained from population testing, particularly in the absence of cancer burden in the family. More prospective data on the uptake of surgical prevention following population-based testing will be needed. Our scenario analyses confirm cost-effectiveness for both payer and societal perspectives, even at half of standard surgical prevention rates (Table 3). Although we incorporate a disutility for RRSO and RRM in the analysis, these procedures have potential complication rates of around 3–4% and 21%, respectively [35,36]. This needs to be part of the informed consent and decision-making process. While RRSO has been reported to have high satisfaction rates, less cancer worry, and no detriment in generic quality of life; poorer sexual function despite HRT use has been found [37]. RRM has an adverse association with body image and sexual pleasure but not with sexual activity/habit/discomfort, anxiety/depression, or generic quality of life, and overall satisfaction rates are good. Countries such as India and China lack established national breast cancer screening programmes. The uptake of mammograms is much lower in these countries. The cost-effectiveness of population testing may be higher for these countries than estimated, as the implementation of these interventions in BRCA carriers are likely to be more beneficial in the absence of routine mammograms in the population. In our analysis, while we included productivity loss, we did not include all indirect costs in the analysis. This may be a limitation. However, including additional indirect costs would improve cost-effectiveness, so our analysis is conservative in that respect. While our analysis covers some important/key countries across different income groups, it does not cover most countries, and therefore, these results are not generalisable globally to all countries across different (HIC/UMIC/LMIC) income groups. While the countries represented in this analysis are from four continents—North America, South America, Europe, and Asia—we do not have representation from Africa or Australia. The populations of countries in our analysis contribute approximately 45% to the global population.

Population-based *BRCA* testing implementation studies have been completed in the Jewish population [15,21,22,38], and pilot ones are being undertaken in the UK and Canadian general populations [23]. For population testing to be feasible, newer approaches for delivering pre-test information will be needed to facilitate informed decision-making. These will need to be country/region or context-specific. The best modality to deliver pre-test education within the population testing setting remains unresolved. We do not feel there will eventually be a one-size-fits-all model. Although we have costed for pre-test counselling for all in our analyses, whether formal pre-test counselling will be needed for all in the future remains uncertain. Israeli and Canadian Jewish population studies provided only 'pre-test information' and post-test genetic counselling for BRCA carriers, with >90% satisfaction rates [39,40]. An Australian Jewish population [41] and a UK general population study have demonstrated the feasibility of an online web-based decision aid (along with an optional telephone helpline) pre-test education and consent process [42].

A strategy for the management of variants of unknown significance (VUS) is important and will need developing. People have raised concerns at unnecessary treatment or screening/preventive intervention(s) being undertaken for VUS alone. However, VUS are currently identified through routine clinical testing, too. There is clear acceptance in clinical practice that for a VUS (class-3 variant), no clinical action should be taken based on that variant alone [43]. A key presumption inherent in a public health screening strategy is that it is not designed to identify 'all' individuals with disease, but the large/significant proportion of individuals in a clinically efficient and cost-effective manner. Therefore, some suggest an alternative option of not providing VUS results within a population-testing context [14]. We incorporate a cost for VUS counselling and management in our analysis.

Chronic disease accounts for 90% US Medicare and 70% UK health care expenditure and is a major challenge facing most health systems, with cancer being its second commonest cause. Between 2006 and 2016, the average annual age-standardised incidence rates for all cancers increased in 130 of 195 countries [44]. The leading cause for women is BC: 1.7 million cases, 535,000 deaths, 14.9 million disability adjusted life-years (DALYs) [44]. Globally breast/ovarian cancers in women are predicted to increase by 46.5%/47% and cancer deaths are predicted to increase by 58.3%/58.6% respectively over the next 20 years [45]. Population testing for BRCA genes can significantly increase BRCA carrier detection rates for maximising prevention and reducing cancer burden. It can also serve as an initial model, which subsequently informs the potential applicability of a population testing risk-stratification strategy for other cancer genes and other chronic diseases.

While developing an approach towards implementing population-based BRCA-testing, it is important to bear in mind the principles of population testing of disease. These were initially proposed by Wilson and Jungner [46]. Updated criteria have been suggested by the UK National Screening Committee [47], Khoury [48], the CDC (ACCE model) [49], and Burke and Zimmerman (Public Health Foundation) [50]. Analytic validity, clinical validity, clinical utility, and associated ethical, legal, and social implications remain key principles of the ACCE model, providing a framework for evaluating the applicability of a genetic test [49]. In our study, we focussed on BRCA testing, as testing for these genes has well-established clinical utility fulfilling the ACCE principles. Multigene panel testing is widely available in current clinical practice. We are against indiscriminate large-scale commercial panel testing without well-established clinical benefit/utility in the population-testing context. The low incidence of moderate penetrance genes, poor precision, and wide confidence intervals around prevalence and penetrance estimates require more data on the clinical significance of pathogenic variants in multigene panels, and these are reasons against currently implementing large multigene panel testing in the general population [51,52]. The USPSTF currently recommends against population testing in the general population [51]. More data are needed on the 'E' (Ethical, legal, and social implications) of a population-based BRCA testing approach across different populations and health systems. There is an urgent need for multiple implementation studies across countries for evaluating general population BRCA testing and to develop local/regional and context-specific implementation pathways. These studies will need to provide prospective data on the impact of population testing on psychological well-being, quality of life, long-term health behaviour, socio-ethics, and lifestyle outcomes. A number of challenges and logistic hurdles will need to be overcome, including varying levels of workforce expansion/upskilling and the reorganisation of health services infrastructure. These include increasing public and health-professional awareness, establishing/expanding laboratory testing infrastructure, expanding downstream management pathways, and involving general practitioners, genetics services, gynaecologists, and breast clinicians/services. A framework/structure for data management and legal and regulatory protections will need to be established. These changes will need to be system/country and context-specific.

4. Materials and Methods

We developed a Markov model (Figure 3) (TreeAge-Pro-2018 Williamson, MA, USA) to compare the lifetime costs and effects of *BRCA1/BRCA2* testing all general population women ≥30 years compared with clinical-criteria/FH-based testing. We describe separate analyses for populations in the UK, USA, Netherlands, China, Brazil, and India using both payer and societal perspectives. While some countries only consider a payer perspective, a societal perspective is recommended by the WHO and other international bodies [53]. In the model, all women ≥30 years in the Population testing arm and only those fulfilling clinical/FH criteria in the Clinical-Criteria/FH-based testing arm undergo genetic testing for *BRCA* mutations. We include pre-test counselling for all and assume a 70% uptake of genetic testing (from the published literature) [22]. We include the cost of post-test counselling for mutation carriers as well as the cost of post-test counselling for those with variants of uncertain significance (VUS). We assume a VUS prevalence of 2% [54]. Model probabilities are described in Table 4, Appendix A, and costs are outlined in Appendix B. *BRCA* carriers identified are offered RRSO to reduce OC risk [4] and MRI/mammography screening, chemoprevention with SERM or RRM [8] to reduce their BC risk [10]. OC screening is excluded given the lack of mortality benefit. Women undergoing RRSO receive hormone replacement therapy (HRT) until 51 years. We include the costs of bone health monitoring and dual energy X-ray scans. We incorporate the excess risk and mortality from coronary heart disease (CHD) after premenopausal RRSO for women who do not take HRT (absolute mortality increase = 3.03%) [33]. Associated costs are modelled over an individual's lifetime. The Markov cycles' run depends on life expectancy and these are different across countries (starting from age 30): UK = 53 cycles, US = 52 cycles, Netherlands = 53 cycles, China = 48 cycles, Brazil = 49 cycles, and India = 38 cycles. Cancer incidence is estimated by summing the probabilities of pathways ending in OC or BC.

4.1. Probabilities

The model probabilities for different pathways are given in Table 4, and a detailed explanation is given in Appendix A. The age-specific incidence of BC and OC among general population women is obtained from Cancer Research UK [55,56], USA Cancer Statistics [57], and the International Agency for Research on Cancer (GLOBOCAN-2018) [58]. The BC/OC incidence for *BRCA1/BRCA2* carriers is obtained from the literature [3].

Figure 3 is a schematic diagram showing the Markov model structure for population and clinical-criteria/family-history (FH)-based *BRCA1/BRCA2* testing. In the Population testing arm, all women ≥30 years old are offered *BRCA1/BRCA2* testing and get classified as *BRCA*-positive and *BRCA*-negative. *BRCA* mutation carriers identified are offered options of risk-reducing mastectomy (RRM) and risk-reducing salpingo-oophorectomy (RRSO). Depending on the probability of *BRCA* women undertaking RRM and/or RRSO (+/− chemoprevention), they are placed into different health states and then progress to either *BRCA*-associated breast cancer (BC) or *BRCA*-associated ovarian cancer (OC). All women undergoing RRSO have an increased risk of fatal coronary heart disease (CHD). In addition, they have a probability of dying from the background all-cause mortality. Hence, patients in the model can go from intervention to death without ever developing breast cancer, ovarian cancer, or coronary artery disease. Patients can move from healthy state to death as they have a probability of dying from the background all-cause mortality. *BRCA*-positive women who do not progress or die would stay in the health states and undertake the next cycle. *BRCA1/BRCA2*-negative women progress to sporadic non-*BRCA* OC or non-*BRCA* BC based on the age-dependent probabilities. They also have a probability of dying from the background all-cause mortality. Women do not progress or die would stay in the health states to undertake the next cycle.

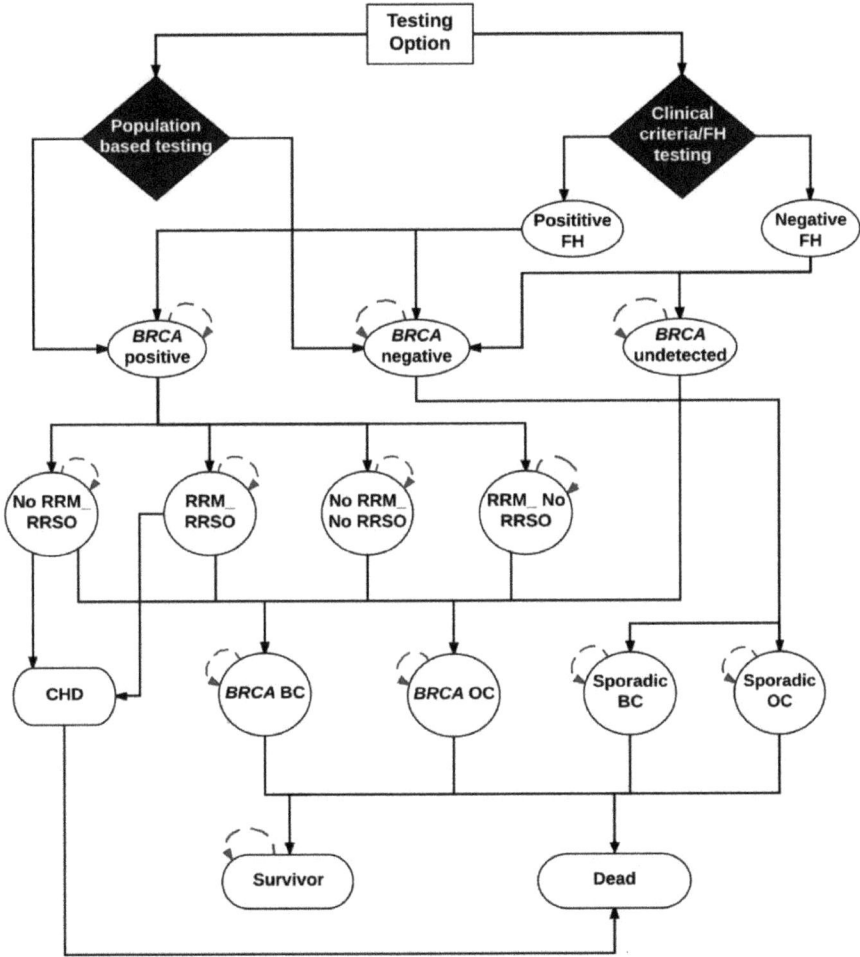

Figure 3. BC, breast cancer; CHD, coronary heart disease; FH, family history; OC, ovarian cancer; RRM, risk-reducing mastectomy; RRSO, risk-reducing salpingo-oophorectomy.

In the Clinical criteria/FH arm, only women whose FH fulfil current clinical criteria (based on current guidelines) undergo *BRCA1/BRCA2* genetic testing and get classified as *BRCA*-positive and *BRCA*-negative. Women with a negative FH are either *BRCA* negative or have an undetected *BRCA* mutation. Options of RRM and RRSO and disease progression for identified *BRCA* mutation carriers and disease progression for *BRCA* negative women are the same as those in the population testing arm and are described above. All women undergoing RRSO have an increased risk of fatal coronary heart disease (CHD). Undetected *BRCA* women are not offered RRM or RRSO. Depending on the baseline risk (no risk-reducing options), they progress to *BRCA*-associated BC or *BRCA*-associated OC. In addition, they have a probability of dying from the background all-cause mortality. Hence, patients in the model can go from intervention to death without developing breast cancer, ovarian cancer, or coronary artery disease. Patients can move from healthy state to death as they may die from the background all-cause mortality. Women who do not progress or die stay in the health state of *BRCA* undetected and undertake the next cycle.

Progression through the model is dependent on the probabilities provided in Table 4.

Table 4. Probability Values.

Probability	Description	Value	(95% CI) (Range)	Source
P1	BRCA1/2 mutation prevalence in general population	0.0067	(0.0059, 0.0077)	[59]
P2	Probability that carriers will undergo RRM	0.47	(0.34, 0.56)	[60]
P3	Reduction in ovarian cancer risk from RRSO	0.96	[0.8, 0.96]	[4,6]
P4	Probability of having a positive FH	0.0098	(0.0047, 0.0179)	ABCFS
P5	BRCA1/2 mutation prevalence in FH-positive individuals	0.1		[10]
P6	BRCA1/2 mutation prevalence in FH-negative individuals	0.0058	(0.0051, 0.0068)	[59], ABCFS
P7	Reduction in breast cancer risk from RRM without RRSO in BRCA1/2 carriers	0.91	(0.62, 0.98)	[8]
P8	Probability that carriers will undergo RRSO	0.55	(0.45, 0.64)	[61]
P9	Hazard ratio in breast cancer risk from RRSO alone	0.49	(0.37, 0.65)	[4]
P10	Reduction in risk of breast cancer from RRM with RRSO	0.95	(0.78, 0.99)	[8]
P11	Excess CHD risk	0.0072	(0.0068, 0.0076)	[33]
P12	Fatal CHD risk	0.0303	(0.011, 0.043)	[33]
P13	Compliance with HRT	0.8	(0.76, 0.83)	[62]
P14	HR of breast cancer risk from breast cancer chemoprevention	0.71	(0.6, 0.83)	[63]
P15	Uptake of breast cancer chemoprevention	0.163	(0.136, 0.19)	[64]

95%CI—95% confidence interval, ABCFS—Australia Breast Cancer Family Study, CHD—coronary heart disease, FH—family history, RRM—risk-reducing mastectomy, RRSO—risk-reducing salpingo-oophorectomy. A detailed explanation of probabilities is given in Appendix A.

4.2. Costs

The analysis was conducted from both a payer perspective and societal perspective. All costs are reported at 2016 USA dollars, which was converted by purchasing power parity (PPP) factor [28]. PPP reflects the value of a country's currency required to purchase equivalent amounts of goods and services in the domestic market as the USA dollar would buy in the USA. Thus, it is used to translate and compare costs of goods/services between countries using the USA dollar as a common reference point. For comparison, we convert values in all other country currencies (£s, €s, ¥, ₹, R$) to $ (USA) using the purchasing power parity (PPP) factor [28]. In line with the National Institute of Health and Care Excellence (NICE) recommendations, future healthcare costs not associated with BC/OC/heart disease were not considered [25]. We collected primary data on relevant direct medical costs from the Urban Basic Medical Insurance Database in China [65]; the Dutch Healthcare Authority (NZA) in Netherlands; Management System of Procedures/Medical drugs/Orthotics/Prosthetics/Special Materials (SIGTAP) [66], the Health Price Bank (BPS) [67], and Chamber of Regulation of the Market of Medicines (CMED) [68] in Brazil; and an accredited cancer centre (Tata Medical Centre) in India (details in Appendix B). Costing data were obtained from published national health service (NHS) reference costs for the UK [69,70] and published literature for the USA (details in Appendix B). We adopted a standard internationally available *BRCA* testing cost (US $200) for our base case and explored the impact of change in testing costs on the overall results in the sensitivity analyses.

The retirement ages for females are 65 in the UK, 62 in the USA, 50–55 in China, 60 in Brazil, 68 in Netherlands, and 60–65 in India. We used the lower values of the retirement age ranges in China and India to get the conservative estimates of productivity loss. The female labour force participation rates are 56.77% in the UK, 55.99% in the USA, 62.03% in China, 53.32% in Brazil, 58.02% in the Netherlands, and 27.45% in India, which were obtained from the World Bank [71]. For the hourly wage rates across countries, see Appendix C. Additionally, we categorised costs due to productivity loss (for details: see Appendix C) as three subcomponents: (1) temporary disability due to short-term work absences following diagnosis, (2) permanent disability from reduced working hours following return to work or workforce departure; and (3) premature mortality due to death before retirement [72]. We estimated temporary disability as time absent from work multiplied by age-specific gross earnings. We calculated productivity costs due to permanent disability by applying age-specific gross earnings to the reduction in working hours, or the number of working hours in cases of permanent workforce departure, until retirement age. Regarding productivity loss from premature mortality, we assumed that without cancer, the productive capacity of an individual would continue from the age of diagnosis until the age of retirement. We multiplied the projected years of life lost by the age-specific gross earnings for the remainder of the working life to generate monetary estimates (see Appendix C). While we included productivity loss, we did not include all indirect costs in the analysis.

4.3. Life Years

Lifetime tables from each country were used to model the lifetime health outcomes, and these were obtained from the World Health Organisation (WHO) [73]. The median ages for RRM and RRSO in unaffected *BRCA* carriers were assumed to be 37 and 40 years [60]. BC and OC survival were modelled using five-year survival data from the CONCORD global surveillance of cancer survival [74]. No significant overall long-term survival differences between germ-line and sporadic BC/OC have been found [75–77]. After five years, the probability of death was assumed to be the same as that of the general population. Modelling estimated the number of BC cases, OC cases, BC deaths, OC deaths, and excess CHD deaths per million women aged 30 years in the six countries, and it calculated the number of cases prevented and deaths prevented. The actual numbers of cases prevented and deaths prevented were estimated based on the number of female population aged over 30 years in the six countries [29].

4.4. Quality-Adjusted Life Years (QALY)

QALYs are recommended by NICE as the appropriate summary measure of health effects for economic evaluation. Utility scores multiplied by life years provides QALYs. QALY = (survival in life years) x (utility score). Utility score is an adjustment for quality of life. It is an indication of individual preferences for specific health states where 1 = perfect health and 0 = death. The utility scores for early, advanced, recurrent, and end-stage breast cancer are 0.71, 0.65, 0.45, and 0.16 [78]. The utility scores used for early, advanced, recurrent, and end-stage OC are 0.81, 0.55, 0.61, and 0.16, respectively [79]. Additionally, utility scores used for RRM is 0.88 (SD = 0.22) and RRSO is 0.95 (SD = 0.10) [80].

4.5. Analysis

The Markov model is illustrated in Figure 3. Model outcomes include OC, BC, and excess deaths from CHD. Future costs and health effects are discounted at WHO-recommended 3% rate for the WHO analyses [81] and at country-recommended rates for country-specific analyses (see Table 1). The lifetime costs and QALYs were estimated in both population-testing and clinical-criteria/FH-testing arms. The incremental cost-effectiveness ratio (ICER) was calculated by dividing the difference in cost by the difference in health effects between these two strategies. ICER = (Cost$^{\text{Population-Testing}}$−Cost$^{\text{Criteria/FH-testing}}$)/(Effect$^{\text{Population-Testing}}$−Effect$^{\text{Criteria/FH-testing}}$). The potential population impact was estimated by calculating the additional reduction in BC and OC incidence/deaths obtained through *BRCA* testing women aged >30 years. We present analyses using a range of cost-effectiveness thresholds. For all countries, we present the initial WHO recommendation of three times gross domestic product (GDP) per capita (threshold of being cost-effective) and one-time GDP per capita (threshold for being highly cost-effective) [82]. For countries (UK [25], USA [26], Netherlands [27]) with specific health economic willingness-to-pay (WTP) threshold guidelines, we also present analysis using those guidelines: UK = £20,000–30,000 [25]; USA = $50,000–100,000 [26]; Netherlands = €20,000–50,000. [27] Additionally, given the lack of a clear established threshold, we evaluate changes in ICER/QALY with *BRCA* testing costs for China, Brazil, and India to identify the *BRCA* testing cost threshold for a given economic cost-effectiveness threshold. We use $ (USA) conversion with PPP for comparison [28].

We also explored a number of scenario analyses, including: (1) no BC risk reduction from RRSO (p9 = 1); (2) no HRT uptake (p13 = 0); (3) 50% reduction in RRM uptake; (4) 50% reduction in RRSO uptake; (5) lower *BRCA*-testing costs of $100; and (6) the maximum genetic testing costs at which population *BRCA* testing remains cost-effective (see Table 3, Appendix D). In the one-way sensitivity analysis, each parameter is varied to evaluate their individual impact on results. Probabilities and utility scores were varied according to 95% confidence intervals or ranges where available or by +/−10%.

Costs were varied by +/−30%. Probabilistic sensitivity analysis (PSA) was undertaken, and parameters varied simultaneously across their distributions. Costs were specified as having a Gamma distribution, quality of life was specified as having a log-normal distribution, and probability was specified as having a beta distribution, as recommended [83]. A cost-effectiveness acceptability curve was used to plot the results of 1000 simulations for each country, showing the probability of population-based *BRCA* testing being cost-effective at different WTP thresholds. Different curves were generated for payer and societal perspectives.

5. Conclusions

The increasing societal awareness and acceptability of genetic testing, falling costs, computational advancements, and technological advancements provides the ability to implement large-scale population testing. We have demonstrated the potential cost-effectiveness of *BRCA* testing on a much broader scale in the general population and across a number of health systems. This is cost-effective for HIC and UMIC health systems and can prevent tens of thousands more BC and OC than the current clinical strategy. Such an approach can bring about a new paradigm for improving global cancer prevention. Context-specific implementation strategies and pathways for population testing need to be developed. A number of implementation studies providing data on the impact of population *BRCA* testing on real-world outcomes are needed. All this is essential for population genomics to achieve its potential for maximising early detection and cancer prevention.

Author Contributions: Conceptualisation, R.M.; methodology, L.S., S.P., R.M. and R.L. software, L.S.; validation, L.S., S.P., R.M., and R.L.; formal analysis, L.S., R.M., S.P., R.L., A.B., S.D., and Z.S.; data curation, J.W., H.B., A.M., Z.H., L.S., L.Y., B.C., P.C.D.S., J.H., F.G., and O.E.; writing—original draft preparation, R.M., L.S., and R.L.; writing—review and editing, all authors.; visualisation, L.S., R.M., R.L., F.G., and O.E.; All authors have read and agreed to the published version of the manuscript.

Funding: R.L., L.Y. and L.S. are supported by travel costs funded by the Royal Society UK and National Natural Science Foundation of China (7181101283). R.M. is supported through an NHS Innovation Accelerator Fellowship and by The Eve Appeal. A.B. is supported by C569/A16891 grant from Cancer Research UK.

Acknowledgments: We are grateful to Melissa Southey (Monash University, Australia) for her support of this work. The study is supported by researchers at the Barts Cancer Research UK Centre for Excellence, Queen Mary University of London (C16420/A18066). This study/analysis received full ethics approval from the Institute of Child Health/ Great Ormond Street Hospital Research Ethics Committee on (REC Reference number 08/H0713/44, Substantial Amendment 3/7/2018).

Conflicts of Interest: R.M. is supported by a NHS Innovation Accelerator Fellowship. R.M. declares research funding from The Eve Appeal and Cancer Research UK into population testing and funding from Barts & the London Charity and Rosetree Trust outside this work, as well as an honorarium for grant review from Israel National Institute for Health Policy Research and honorarium for advisory board meeting for MSD and Astrazeneca. The study is supported by researchers at the Barts Cancer Institute Cancer Research UK Centre for Excellence, Queen Mary University of London (C16420/A18066). A.B. is supported by a Cancer Research UK Grant (C569/A16891). The other authors declare no conflict of interest. The funders had no role in the design of the study; in the collection, analyses, or interpretation of data; in the writing of the manuscript, or in the decision to publish the results.

Appendix A. Probability Values and Explanation

Table A1. Probability Values.

Probability	Description	Value	(95% CI) (Range)	Source
P1	BRCA1/2 mutation prevalence in general population	0.0067	(0.0059, 0.0077)	[59]
P2	Probability that carriers will undergo RRM	0.47	(0.34, 0.56)	[60]
P3	Reduction in ovarian cancer risk from RRSO	0.96	(0.8, 0.96)	[4,6]
P4	Probability of having a positive FH	0.0098	(0.0047, 0.0179)	ABCFS
P5	BRCA1/2 mutation prevalence in FH positive individuals	0.1		[84]
P6	BRCA1/2 mutation prevalence in FH negative individuals	0.0058	(0.0051, 0.0068)	[59], ABCFS
P7	Reduction in breast cancer risk from RRM without RRSO in BRCA1/2 carriers	0.91	(0.62, 0.98)	[8]
P8	Probability that carriers will undergo RRSO	0.55	(0.45, 0.64)	[61]
P9	Hazard ratio in breast cancer risk from RRSO alone	0.49	(0.37, 0.65)	[4]

Table A1. Cont.

Probability	Description	Value	(95% CI) (Range)	Source
P10	Reduction in risk of breast cancer from RRM with RRSO	0.95	(0.78, 0.99)	[8]
P11	Excess CHD risk	0.0072	(0.0068, 0.0076)	[33]
P12	Fatal CHD risk	0.0303	(0.011, 0.043)	[33]
P13	Compliance with HRT	0.8	(0.76, 0.83)	[62]
P14	HR of breast cancer risk from breast cancer chemoprevention	0.71	(0.6, 0.83)	[63]
P15	Uptake of breast cancer chemoprevention	0.163	(0.136, 0.19)	[64]

95%CI—95% confidence interval, ABCFS—Australia Breast Cancer Family Study, CHD—coronary heart disease, FH—family history, RRM—risk-reducing mastectomy, RRSO—risk-reducing salpingo-oophorectomy.

Explanations

P1: *BRCA1/2* mutation prevalence in the general population is calculated based on Jervis 2015 [59].

P2: The probability that unaffected carriers will undergo RRM is taken from an analysis of UK *BRCA1/2* carriers by Evans et al. 2009 [60]. A composite uptake rate for *BRCA1* (60% RRM rate) and *BRCA2* (43% RRM rate) carriers weighted for the relative prevalence of *BRCA1* and *BRCA2* mutations was computed [60].

P3: The reduction in ovarian cancer risk obtained from RRSO is taken from previous studies which report a 4% residual risk of primary peritoneal cancer following RRSO [6].

P4: The probability of having a positive family history in general population is obtained from the Australia Breast Cancer Family Study (ABCFS).

P5: The overall *BRCA1/BRCA2* mutation prevalence (10%) among FH-positive breast cancer patients is based on the current testing guideline.

P6: The *BRCA1/2* mutation prevalence in FH negative individuals is calculated based on the BRCA1/2 mutation prevalence in the general population, the BRCA1/2 mutation prevalence in FH-positive individuals, and the probability of having a positive FH.

P7: The reduction in breast cancer risk from RRM in *BRCA1/BRCA2* mutation carriers not undergoing RRSO is taken from the PROSE study data by Rebbeck et al. 2004 [8].

P8: The uptake of RRSO in unaffected *BRCA1/BRCA2* carriers is taken from a study among high-risk UK women [7].

P9: The hazard ratio for breast cancer in premenopausal unaffected *BRCA1/BRCA2* women undergoing RRSO alone is taken from a meta-analysis by Rebbeck et al. 2009 [4].

P10: The reduction in breast cancer risk in *BRCA1/BRCA2* mutation carriers undergoing RRM and RRSO is taken from the PROSE study data by Rebbeck et al. 2004 [8].

P11: Excess risk of CHD after RRSO is estimated using data from Parker 2013 [33]. The absolute excess CHD incidence is obtained by subtracting CHD incidence in women undergoing RRSO from those who have not.

P12: The risk of CHD mortality is obtained from the Nurses Health Study (Parker et al. 2013) [33]. Death from CHD is reported in 1 in 33 premenopausal women undergoing RRSO and not taking HRT [33].

P13: HRT compliance rate is obtained from a UK cohort (Read et al., 2010) [62].

P14: The Hazard Ratio for breast cancer risk from chemoprevention in high-risk women is obtained from the extended long-term follow-up of the IBIS-I breast cancer prevention trial (Cuzick et al. 2015) [63].

P15: The uptake of breast cancer chemoprevention is obtained from a recent meta-analysis by Smith et al. 2016 [64].

Appendix B. Medical Costs in 2016 Values (USA Dollars Converted by PPP)

Table A2. Medical costs in 2016 values (USA dollars converted by PPP).

Cost descriptions	UK GBP	UK USD	US USD	Netherlands EUR	Netherlands USD	China RMB	China USD	Brazil BRL	Brazil USD	India INR	India USD
Cost of genetic testing	29	200	200	55	200	0	200	135	200	733	200
Cost of genetic counselling	29	42	42	55	67	4525	1308	957	483	82,368	4712
Cost of prophylactic bilateral salpingo-oophorectomy	2799	3999	7904	3713	4584	12,991	3755	12,564	6345	613,662	35,107
Cost of ovarian cancer diagnosis and treatment	14,268	20,383	133,121	23,238	28,689	48,495	14,016	4442	2244	290,086	16,595
Annual cost of ovarian cancer in years 1 to 2	5433	7761	14,635	10,865	13,413	48,021	13,879	4278	2161	280,720	16,059
Annual cost of ovarian cancer in years 3 to 5	5090	7271	14,635	10,480	12,939	10,060	2907	1358	686	80,623	4612
Terminal care cost with ovarian cancer	16,452	23,503	93,005	11,325	13,981	2634	761	867	438	278,474	15,931
Cost of risk reducing mastectomy	4143	5919	13,101	2950	3642	2148	621	217	110	15,595	892
Annual cost of hormone replacement therapy	60	86	52	61	76	82	24	42	21	2051	117
Cost of mammography	60	85	156	95	117	605	175	252	127	7222	413
Cost of MRI	203	290	1477	215	265	74,959	21,664	23,218	11,726	226,451	12,955
Cost of breast cancer diagnosis and treatment in general population	18,148	25,926	85,372	11,977	14,786	12,360	3572	2328	1176	55,519	3176
Annual cost of breast cancer in general population	1388	1982	8048	2718	3355	68,476	19,791	20,861	10,536	200,902	11,493
Cost of breast cancer diagnosis and treatment in BRCA1/2 carriers	16,499	23,570	78,964	10,780	13,309	10,827	3129	1999	1009	53,959	3087
Annual cost of breast cancer in BRCA1/2 carriers	1400	2000	8048	2656	3279	10,060	2907	1358	686	80,623	4612
Terminal care cost with breast cancer	16,452	23,503	68,022	11,325	13,981	11,972	3460	2953	1491	47,673	2727
Cost of fatal coronary heart disease	3387	4839	23,934	3008	3714	526	152	124	63	3708	212
Annual cost of excess coronary heart disease	122	175	7277	109	134	93	27	499	252	62	4
Annual cost of chemoprevention	19	27	899	36	45						

CHD—coronary heart disease, HRT—hormone replacement therapy, MRI—magnetic resonance imaging, RRM—risk-reducing mastectomy, RRSO—risk-reducing salpingo-oophorectomy, PPP—purchasing power parity.

Appendix B.1. Explanations

All costs are adjusted for 2016 consumer price index.

For comparison, we convert values in all other country currencies (£s, €s, ¥, ₹, R$) to $ (USA) using purchasing power parity (PPP) factor [28].

We collected primary data on relevant direct medical costs from the Urban Basic Medical Insurance Database in China [65]; the Dutch Healthcare Authority (NZA) in Netherlands; Management System of Procedures/Medical drugs/Orthotics/Prosthetics/Special Materials (SIGTAP) [66], the Health Price Bank (BPS) [67] and Chamber of Regulation of the Market of Medicines (CMED) [68] in Brazil; and an accredited Cancer Centre (Tata Medical Centre) in India. UK costing data were obtained from published NHS reference costs for the UK [69,70].

Appendix B.2. Cost of Genetic Testing/Counselling

We use a standard international cost for genetic testing for all countries (US$ 200 in 2016). We assume a 71% uptake of genetic testing (based on our previous population based research studies) [22]. All participants have pre-test counselling and post-test counselling is received by those testing positive (pathogenic/likely pathogenic carriers). We assume a VUS prevalence of 2% and include the cost of post-test counselling for VUS in these 2% cases [54].

The cost of BRCA1/BRCA2 testing is based on testing costs for these genes in our population testing research programme as well as confirmatory testing costs in an accredited national genetics laboratory for those testing positive. The UK national unit cost assumed for genetic counselling is £44 per hour of client contact from PSSRU Unit costs of Health and Social Care 2010 [22,85,86]. The US genetic counselling costs are obtained from Schwartz 2014 and include ancillary preparation (scheduling/administration), counsellor preparation, and counselling [87]. The genetic counselling costs in the Netherlands, Brazil, and India were obtained from primary data. There is no additional physician genetic counselling cost charged from patients in China; hence, this was not incorporated for Chinese analysis.

Appendix B.3. RRSO Costs

The UK RRSO costs are obtained from NHS reference costs [88], and the US costs are from Grann 2011 [89] inflated using the medical component of the USA consumer price index to 2016 US$. Costs of HRT for the UK are taken from BNF [90] and for the USA from William-Frame 2009 [91]. The costs of RRSO and HRT in Netherlands, China, Brazil, and India are obtained from primary data. Costs assume HRT is given from average age of RRSO to the average age of menopause (51 years). These costs are calculated for the 80% assumed to be compliant with HRT. Costs include the cost of three follow-up DEXA scans for monitoring bone health and calcium and vitamin-D3 for additional osteo-protection.

Appendix B.4. RRM

The UK RRM costs are obtained from NHS reference costs [88], and the USA costs are from Grann 2011 [89] inflated using the medical component of the US consumer price index to 2016 US$. The RRM costs in Netherlands, China, Brazil and India are obtained from primary data.

Appendix B.5. Costs of Ovarian Cancer

We assume that the costs of ovarian cancer diagnosis include a pelvic examination, ultrasound scan, CA125 test, CT scan, percutaneous biopsy, and peritoneal cytology. The costs of ovarian cancer treatment include the reference cost for a lower and upper genital tract very complex major procedure and administration of chemotherapy based on 6 cycles of carboplatin and paclitaxel treatment. It is assumed that in the first and second years, treated survivors would have a further three consultant visits, a CT scan, and four CA125 tests each year. In the third to fifth years post-surgery, it is assumed that survivors would have two consultant visits and two CA125 tests.

Costs for ovarian cancer diagnosis and treatment in the UK are derived from national reference costs and a recent ovarian cancer guideline developed by NICE [88,92]. Annual costs of ovarian cancer treatment in the USA are taken from Grann et al. 2011 [89] and inflated using the medical component of the USA consumer price index to 2016 US$. We include the costs of treatment of recurrence taken from Cancer Research UK [93] and Grann 2011 [89]. The costs of ovarian cancer diagnosis and treatment in Netherlands, China, Brazil, and India are obtained from primary data.

The costs of ovarian cancer terminal care are derived from end-of-life costs for cancer patients based on a report from the National Audit office UK [94]. For the USA, the terminal care costs for ovarian cancer are obtained from Grann 2011 [89], which were inflated using the medical component of the USA consumer price index to 2016 US$. The costs of ovarian cancer terminal care are obtained from primary data in the Netherlands, China, Brazil and India. In line with NICE recommendations, future healthcare costs not associated with ovarian cancer are not considered [95].

Appendix B.6. Costs of Breast Cancer

In the general population, 10% breast cancer is non-invasive DCIS and 90% is invasive. 95% of invasive breast cancer is early and locally advanced (stages 1–3), and 5% of invasive breast cancer is advanced breast cancer (stage 4) [96]. In *BRCA1/2* carriers, 20% of cancers are DCIS and 80% are invasive [9,97].

Seventy percent of invasive breast cancers are ER-positive [98,99], among which 49% are premenopausal; 15% of early/locally advanced breast cancers and 25% of advanced breast cancers are HER2-positive; 27% *BRCA1* and 67% *BRCA2* breast cancers are ER-positive; 5% *BRCA1* and 14% *BRCA2* breast cancers are HER2-positive [100–105]. All costs are adjusted for *BRCA1/BRCA2* breast cancers for differences in stage at presentation, the proportion of being non-invasive, and the proportion of being ER-positive or HER2-positive.

Annual breast cancer treatment costs in the USA are obtained from Grann et al. 2011 [89] and inflated using the medical component of the USA consumer price index to 2016 US$. In the UK, Netherlands, China, Brazil, and India, breast cancer treatment costs are estimated based on clinical guidelines and unit costs are detailed as below.

Diagnosis costs: Whether suspected at breast screening or through presentation to the GP, diagnosis in the breast clinic is made by triple assessment (clinical assessment, mammography, and ultrasound imaging with core biopsy and/or fine needle aspiration cytology) [98]. Clinical examination and mammography costs are from the paper by Robertson C et al. [106]. Breast ultrasound and biopsy costs are obtained from NHS reference costs [88] in the UK and from primary data in Netherlands, China, Brazil, and India. For all patients presented with suspected advanced breast cancer, MRI should be offered to assess for bone metastases [99].

Sentinel lymph node biopsy (SLNB) costs: SLNB is used for staging axilla for early invasive breast cancer and no evidence of lymph node involvement on ultrasound or a negative ultrasound-guided needle biopsy (73% of early and locally advanced invasive cancers). The SLNB costs in the UK are obtained from NHS reference costs including sentinel lymph node scan and unilateral intermediate breast procedures [88]. The SLNB costs in Netherlands, China, Brazil, and India are obtained from the primary data sources described above.

Pretreatment axilla ultrasound costs: Pretreatment ultrasound evaluation of the axilla should be performed for all patients being investigated for early invasive breast cancer and, if morphologically abnormal lymph nodes are identified, ultrasound-guided needle sampling should be offered [96]. The commissioning cost of pretreatment ultrasound evaluation of the breast and axilla is the same as that of the breast only [88]. The costing model considers the cost of ultrasound-guided needle sampling only, obtained from NHS reference costs (UK) [24] and primary data (Netherlands, China, Brazil, and India).

Axillary lymph node dissection (ALND) costs: ALNB is undertaken for lymph node positive cancers (approximately 31% early and locally advanced invasive cancers—NICE guideline and

BCCOM project [96,98,107]; 30% node positive for BRCA1/2 breast cancer—familial breast cancer screening studies, breast cancer case series and Early Breast Cancer Trialists' Collaborative Group data) [97,100–102,108]. The cost of ALND is assumed to be 25% of the cost of breast surgery as per NICE guideline development group recommendations [96].

Breast surgery costs include costs of breast-conserving surgery (assumed for all non-invasive cancers and 75% of early/locally advanced invasive cancers) and costs of mastectomy with reconstruction (for 25% early/locally advanced and all advanced cancers). Costs are obtained from the national NHS reference costs (UK) [88] and primary data (Netherlands, China, Brazil, and India).

Chemotherapy and radiotherapy costs: Invasive breast cancers who are not at low risk [107,109,110] receive adjuvant treatment in line with NICE guidelines. Costs include radiotherapy costs for 60% of early invasive/locally advanced, radiotherapy, and chemotherapy costs for 40% early invasive/locally advanced, and chemotherapy for all advanced cancers. Radiotherapy costs include planning and 40Gy in 15 fractions over 3 weeks [98] or palliative treatment; these were taken from national NHS reference costs [88]. Chemotherapy costs based on polychemotherapy [108] include administration costs, the costs of first and second-line therapy and toxicity from NICE guidelines [96,99]. In the Netherlands, China, Brazil, and India, radiotherapy costs and chemotherapy costs are obtained from the primary data sources described above.

Endocrine therapy costs: As per NICE guidelines [96,98], ER-positive invasive breast cancers receive Tamoxifen 20 mg/day (premenopausal) or Anastrazole 1mg/day (postmenopausal). Seventy percent of invasive breast cancers are ER-positive [98,99], among which 49% are premenopausal. We assume that the length of endocrine therapy is 5 years. The drug costs are obtained from the BNF [26] in the UK. ER testing costs are obtained from a local NHS trust and included for all invasive breast cancers. The costs of drugs and ER testing are obtained from primary data sources in the Netherlands, China, Brazil, and India described above.

Target therapy costs: HER2-positive breast cancer patients can be given at 3-week intervals for 1 year or until disease recurrence as per NICE guidelines. Breast cancer patients with positive HER2 are eligible for treatment with trastuzumab [98,99]. Ten percent of the eligible patients are intolerant of trastuzumab. Among women suitable for this treatment, 80% receive trastuzumab [96]. HER2 testing costs are obtained from a local NHS trust and included for all invasive breast cancers. The trastuzumab cost per patient including the administration of treatment and cardiac monitoring is £15080, which was obtained from the NICE costing report [96]. In the Netherlands, China, Brazil, and India, the costs of HER2 testing and trastuzumab are obtained from the primary data sources described above.

Follow-up costs: Breast cancer patients are offered mammographic surveillance and clinical follow up, with the screening cost of £141.45 per women in 2011 [106]. We assume that patients are followed up every four months in the first two years, every six months from the third to the fifth year, and every year from the sixth to the 10th year.

Bisphosphonate costs: Bisphosphonates is considered to be offered to patients newly diagnosed with bone metastases to prevent skeletal-related events and reduce pain [99]. Seventy-four percent of patients with advanced breast cancer will develop bone metastases, and 65% of patients with bone metastases are offered bisphosphonates [96,111]. Bisphosphonates that are currently offered include oral sodium clodronate, ibandronic acid, zoledronic acid, and pamidronate. The proportions of patients receiving the four drugs are 20%, 30%, 25%, and 25%, respectively. The annual costs including administration for the four drugs are £1971, £2541.96, £3208, and £3208 respectively, which were obtained from the NICE costing report [96]. We assume that the average length of bisphosphonates treatment is 2.7 years, which is the life expectancy of advanced breast cancers based on one-year survival rate (63.2%) [112]. The bisphosphonate costs in the Netherlands, China, Brazil, and India are obtained from the primary data sources described above.

Recurrence costs: For non-invasive breast cancers, the non-invasive and invasive relapse rates are both 12.5%. Thirty-five percent of early and locally advanced invasive breast cancers progress to advanced disease [96]. The recurrence rates for early and locally advanced breast cancer are 15.9% for node-positive [113] and 11% for node-negative disease [114]. Weighted for 31% node positive and 69% node negative, the composite recurrence rate for early and locally advanced breast cancer is 12.5%. The recurrence rate for the advanced disease is 66% (34% relapse-free five-year survival) [115].

Terminal care costs: The costs of terminal care for breast cancer are derived from end-of-life costs for cancer patients based on a report from the National Audit office UK [30]. For the US, the terminal care costs for breast cancer are obtained from Grann 2011 [89], and these were inflated using the medical component of the US consumer price index to 2016 US$. The costs of breast cancer terminal care are obtained from primary data sources in the Netherlands, China, Brazil, and India. In line with NICE recommendations, future healthcare costs not associated with breast cancer were not considered [95].

Appendix B.7. Cost of Breast Cancer Screening

For non-carriers, we assume routine triennial mammography between 50 and 70 years as per the UK NHS breast cancer screening programme [116] (seven mammograms on average). Breast screening in the USA assumes mammography every two years starting at 50 years [117]. In the Netherlands, the National Breast Cancer Screening Programme is designed for women between 50 and 75 years of age. Once every 2 years, women in this age group are invited for a mammogram. The guidelines from the Brazilian Ministry of Health is for all women aged 50–69 years to be screened with mammography only every 2 years. The coverage in the target age group remains low ranging from 27% to 51% [118]. To obtain a conservative estimate of the cost-effectiveness of population-based genetic testing, we adopted the highest value of uptake (51%) in Brazil. There is no national breast cancer screening programme in China or India.

For BRCA1/BRCA2 mutation carriers, we assume an annual mammogram from 40 to 69 years and annual MRI from 30–49 years as per NICE guidelines for familial breast cancer [119] (30 mammograms and 20 MRIs on average). We assume that breast cancer screening policies for BRCA1/2 carriers in the Netherlands, China, Brazil, and India, are the same as that in the UK. For the USA, it is based on annual mammography and MRI starting at 30 years, and annual mammography only from age 50 years [117].

Appendix B.8. Cost of Chemoprevention

BRCA1/BRCA2 mutation carriers are offered tamoxifen (premenopausal) or raloxifene (postmenopausal) for 5 years [119,120] to reduce breast cancer risk. The drug costs are obtained from the BNF (UK) [90], Grann 2011 (US) [89], and primary data (Netherlands, China, Brazil, and India). A 16.3% uptake is assumed for chemoprevention [64].

Appendix B.9. Cost of CHD

Cost of excess CHD: British Heart Foundation statistics reports costs per capita across four commissioning regions in England (London, Midlands and East, North, and South) [121].

The costs of CHD and stroke are averaged across the four regions. The prevalence of CHD is estimated at 12.0% in the UK [121] and 11.7% in the USA [122], with the onset of CHD estimated at 55 years of age [33,123].

The yearly cost of CHD in the UK is obtained by dividing the per capita cost by the population prevalence of CHD [121]. Using the report published by the American Heart Association [124], the total cost of CHD, CHF, and stroke were divided by the population with CHD [122,125], giving the yearly cost of CHD in the USA. This yearly cost is multiplied by the number of years between onset of CHD and average life expectancy to provide the cost attributed to excess CHD.

Cost of fatal CHD: This is costed on the basis of a fatal myocardial infarction using NHS reference costs [88]. USA costs are obtained from Afana et al. 2015 [126], and these are inflated using the medical component of the US consumer price index to 2016 US$.

We used the ratio of breast cancer treatment costs in the Netherlands, China, Brazil, and India compared to treatment costs in the UK to impute the costs of excess CHD and fatal CHD in each of these countries (Netherlands, China, Brazil, and India) based on the cost of CHD in the UK.

Appendix C. Estimation of Productivity Loss

The retirement ages for females are 65 in the UK, 62 in the USA, 50–55 in China, 60 in Brazil, 68 in Netherlands, and 60–65 in India. We used the lower values of the retirement age ranges in China and India to get the conservative estimates of productivity loss. The female labour force participation rates are 56.77% in the UK, 55.99% in the USA, 62.03% in China, 53.32% in Brazil, 58.02% in Netherlands, and 27.45% in India, which were obtained from the World Bank [71]. The hourly wage rage across countries are presented in Table A3.

Table A3. Hourly wage rage across countries (USA dollars in 2016).

Age	UK	USA	Netherlands	China	Brazil	India
30–34	19.47	13.08	16.85	5	5.54	4.77
35–39	19.47	14.75	22.37	5	5.54	4.58
40–44	19.33	14.75	22.37	5	5.54	4.58
45–49	19.33	14.97	24.11	5	5.54	6.56
50–54	17.42	14.97	24.11		5.54	6.56
55–59	17.42	15.10	24.19		5.54	3.71
60–64	15.08	15.10	24.19			
65–69			21.32			
Source	[127]	[128]	[129]	[130]	[131]	[132]

We categorised the productivity costs as three subcomponents: (1) temporary disability due to short-term work absences following diagnosis, (2) permanent disability due to reduced working hours following a return to work or workforce departure; and (3) premature mortality due to death before retirement [72], as detailed in Table A4.

Table A4. Descriptive statistics for productivity loss in breast and ovarian cancer patients.

Variables	Breast Cancer	Ovarian Cancer
(1) Temporary disability		
Percentage of temporary disability cases	94.0%	98% [1]
Average time taken off work following diagnosis (weeks)	44.9	47.22 [2]
(2) Permanent disability		
Percentage of permanent disability: reduced hours	26%	40% [3]
Reduced hours per week after returning to work (hours)	5.5	5.5
(3) Premature mortality (before retirement)		
Percentage of permanent disability: workforce departure	12.9%	30% [3]

Source: Hanly P, et al., 2012 [72]. [1] We assume 98% ovarian cancer patients have cancer-related short-term work absences after diagnosis. [2] We assume ovarian cancer patients experience four weeks for surgery, 24 weeks for chemotherapy, and 24 weeks for recurrence treatment with the recurrence rate of 80% [133]. [3] We assume the percentages of permanent disability for ovarian cancer are 40% for reduced working hours and 30% for workforce departure.

We estimated temporary disability as time absent from work multiplied by age-specific gross earnings.

We calculated productivity costs due to permanent disability by applying age-specific gross earnings to the reduction in working hours, or the number of working hours if permanent workforce departure, until retirement age. Regarding productivity loss from premature mortality, we assumed that without cancer, the productive capacity of an individual would continue from the age of diagnosis until age of retirement. We multiplied the projected years of life lost by the age-specific gross earnings for the remainder of the working life to generate monetary estimates.

Appendix D. Maximum Values of Genetic Testing Costs at Which Offering Genetic Testing for the Population Remains Cost-Effective.

Table A5. Maximum values of genetic testing costs at which offering genetic testing for the population remains cost-effective.

	Payer Perspective		Societal Perspective	
	Lower WTP [#]	Higher WTP [##]	Lower WTP [#]	Higher WTP [##]
Thresholds based on GDP				
UK	$412 ($42,648/QALY)	$1254 ($127,869/QALY)	$677 ($42,639/QALY)	$1520 ($127,960/QALY)
USA	$519 ($57,490/QALY)	$1417 ($172,735/QALY)	$680 ($57,582/QALY)	$1577 ($172,698/QALY)
Netherlands	$442 ($50,539/QALY)	$1407 ($151,520/QALY)	$792 ($50,517/QALY)	$1758 ($151,603/QALY)
China	$146 ($15,402/QALY)	$354 ($46,536/QALY)	$183 ($15,522/QALY)	$390 ($46,506/QALY)
Brazil	$130 ($15,143/QALY)	$493 ($45,490/QALY)	$219 ($15,168/QALY)	$582 ($45,515/QALY)
India	Not cost-effective	$95 ($19,670/QALY)	$62 ($6,540/QALY)	$172 ($19,685/QALY)
Thresholds based on local economic evaluation guidelines				
UK	$238 ($28,386/QALY)	$365 ($42,826/QALY)	$481 ($28,406/QALY)	$608 ($42,845/QALY)
USA	$460 ($49,919/QALY)	$850 ($99,969/QALY)	$620 ($49,882/QALY)	$1010 ($99,933/QALY)
Netherlands∫	$293 ($24,364/QALY)	$800 ($60,934/QALY)	$582 ($24,369/QALY)	$1089 ($60,939/QALY)

[#] 1*GDP per capita, [##] 3*GDP per capita, WTP—willingness to pay (threshold), GDP—gross domestic product.

90

The appendix describes the maximum genetic testing costs and corresponding ICER/QALY (in brackets) at which offering *BRCA* testing for the population will remain cost-effective. Results are presented for both the payer and societal perspectives.

For GDP-based thresholds: This is cost-effective at the standard 3*GDP per capita WTP threshold and highly cost-effective at the 1*GDP per capita WTP threshold [82]. The discount rate is 3% for costs and health effects (LYs and QALYs) [81].

For country-specific thresholds:

For the UK, this is £20,000 to £30,000 [25,134]; for the USA, this is $50,000 to $100,000 [26,135]; for the Netherlands, this is: €20,000 to €50,000 [27]. Values in £s and €s have been converted to $ using PPP (purchasing power parity) [28].

For country-specific thresholds:

For the UK, the discount rate is 3.5% discount for costs and QALYs [25,134]; for the USA, this is 3% discount for costs and QALYs [53]; for the Netherlands, this is 4% discount for costs and 1.5% discount for QALYs [136].

Perspective:

WHO guidelines recommend a societal perspective [81,82].

Dutch guidelines recommend a societal perspective [136]. UK NICE guidelines recommend a payer perspective [25]. US guidelines recommend presentation of both societal and payer perspectives [53].

Appendix E. One-Way Sensitivity Analyses

One-way sensitivity analysis for all probabilities, costs, and utilities in terms of ICER of population-based BRCA testing compared to a clinical-criteria/FH-based approach in the UK, USA, Netherlands, China, Brazil, and India from both the payer perspective and the societal perspective.

X-axis: Incremental cost-effectiveness ratio (ICER): cost (£s or $s) per quality-adjusted life year (QALY) (discounted).

Y-axis: Probability, cost, and utility parameters in the model. The model is run at both lower and upper values/limits of the 95% confidence interval or range of all probability parameters described in Table 1, and both lower and upper values/limits of the cost and utility-score parameters given in the methods and Table 2.

'Upper value' represents outcomes for the upper limit of the parameter, and 'Lower value' represents outcomes for lower limit of the parameter.

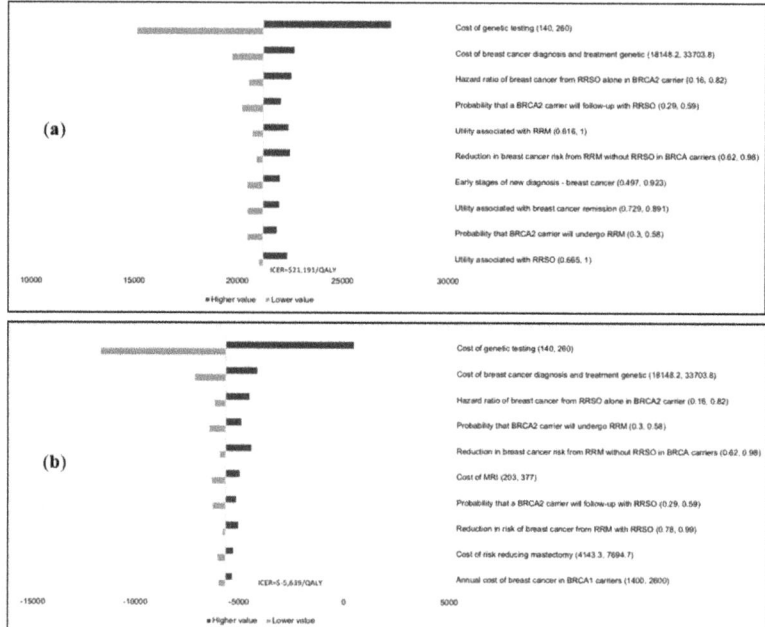

Figure A1. Tornado Diagram in the UK (**a**) from the healthcare payer perspective. (**b**) from the societal perspective.

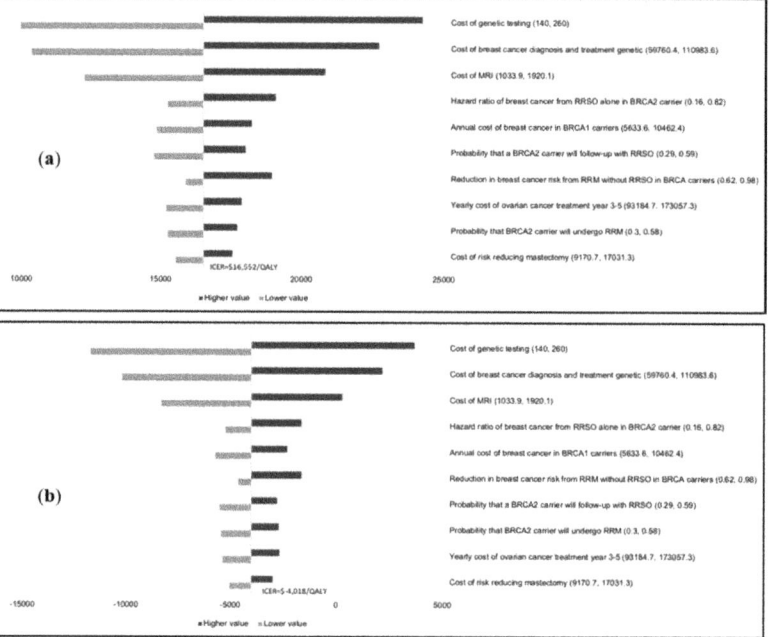

Figure A2. Tornado Diagram in the USA (**a**) from the healthcare payer perspective. (**b**) from the societal perspective.

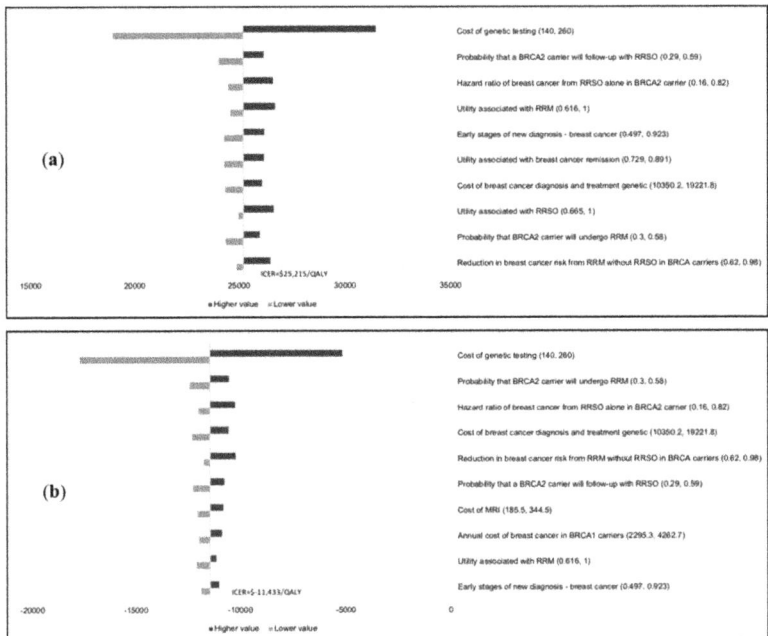

Figure A3. Tornado Diagram in the Netherlands (**a**) from the healthcare payer perspective. (**b**) from the societal perspective.

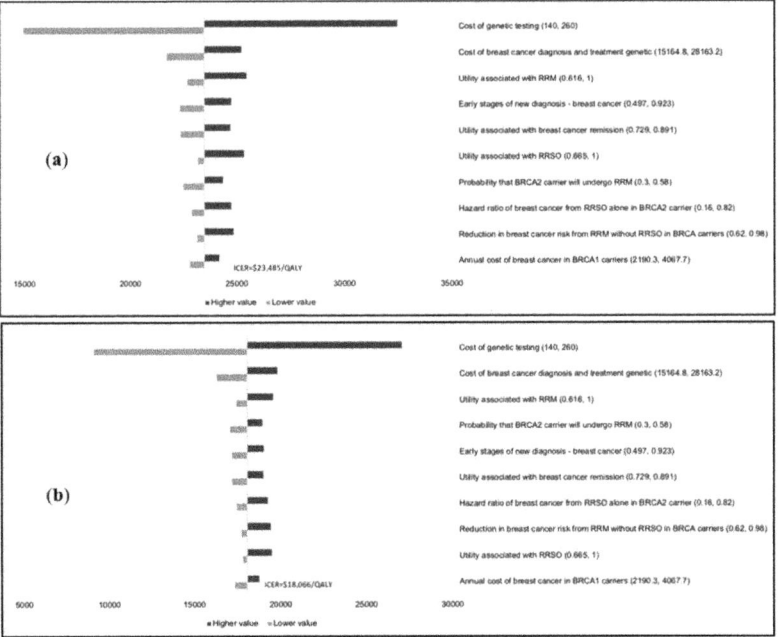

Figure A4. Tornado Diagram in China (**a**) from the healthcare payer perspective. (**b**) from the societal perspective.

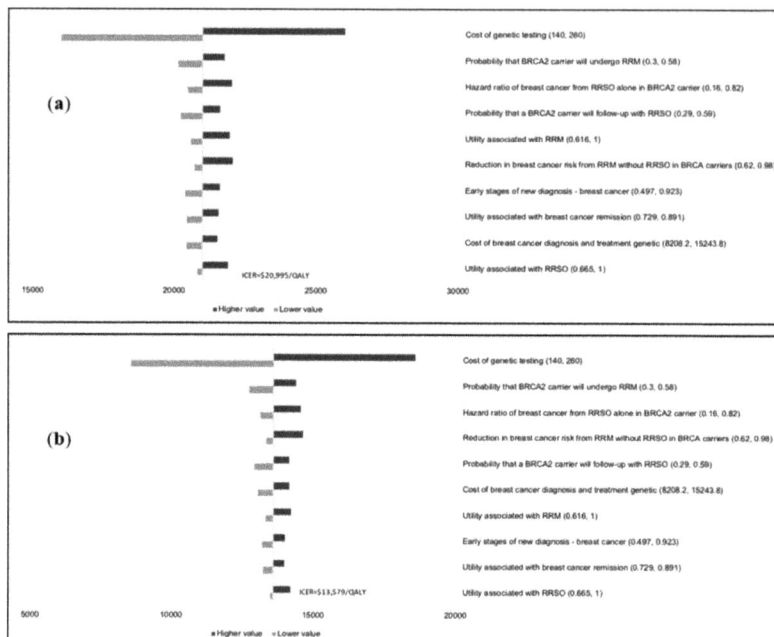

Figure A5. Tornado Diagram in Brazil (**a**) from the healthcare payer perspective. (**b**) from the societal perspective.

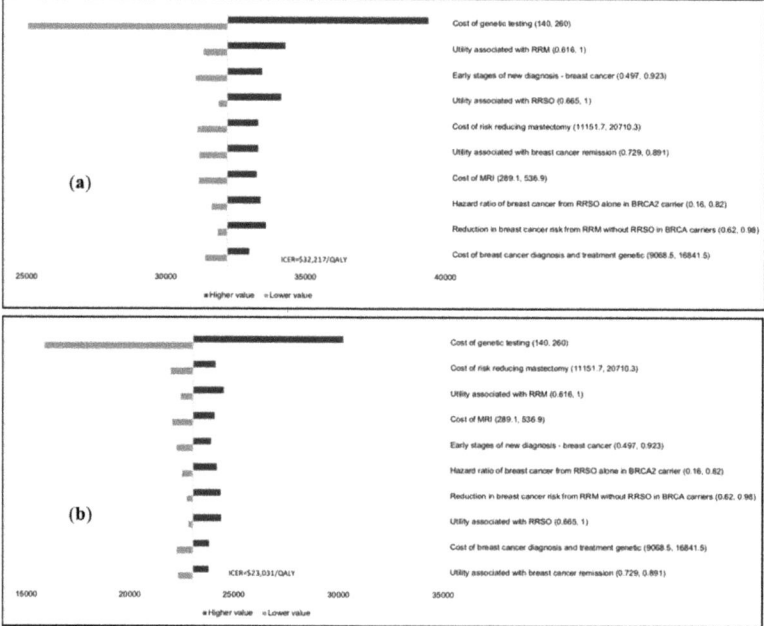

Figure A6. Tornado Diagram in India (**a**) from the healthcare payer perspective. (**b**) from the societal perspective.

References

1. Harter, P.; Hauke, J.; Heitz, F.; Reuss, A.; Kommoss, S.; Marme, F.; Heimbach, A.; Prieske, K.; Richters, L.; Burges, A.; et al. Prevalence of deleterious germline variants in risk genes including BRCA1/2 in consecutive ovarian cancer patients (AGO-TR-1). *PLoS ONE* **2017**, *12*, e0186043. [CrossRef]
2. Buys, S.S.; Sandbach, J.F.; Gammon, A.; Patel, G.; Kidd, J.; Brown, K.L.; Sharma, L.; Saam, J.; Lancaster, J.; Daly, M.B. A study of over 35,000 women with breast cancer tested with a 25-gene panel of hereditary cancer genes. *Cancer* **2017**, *123*, 1721–1730. [CrossRef] [PubMed]
3. Kuchenbaecker, K.B.; Hopper, J.L.; Barnes, D.R.; Phillips, K.A.; Mooij, T.M.; Roos-Blom, M.J.; Jervis, S.; Van Leeuwen, F.E.; Milne, R.L.; Andrieu, N.; et al. Risks of Breast, Ovarian, and Contralateral Breast Cancer for BRCA1 and BRCA2 Mutation Carriers. *JAMA* **2017**, *317*, 2402–2416. [CrossRef] [PubMed]
4. Rebbeck, T.R.; Kauff, N.D.; Domchek, S.M. Meta-analysis of risk reduction estimates associated with risk-reducing salpingo-oophorectomy in BRCA1 or BRCA2 mutation carriers. *J. Natl. Cancer Inst.* **2009**, *101*, 80–87. [CrossRef] [PubMed]
5. Kauff, N.D.; Domchek, S.M.; Friebel, T.M.; Robson, M.E.; Lee, J.; Garber, J.E.; Isaacs, C.; Evans, D.G.; Lynch, H.; Eeles, R.A.; et al. Risk-reducing salpingo-oophorectomy for the prevention of BRCA1- and BRCA2-associated breast and gynecologic cancer: A multicenter, prospective study. *J. Clin. Oncol.* **2008**, *26*, 1331–1337. [CrossRef]
6. Finch, A.; Beiner, M.; Lubinski, J.; Lynch, H.T.; Moller, P.; Rosen, B.; Murphy, J.; Ghadirian, P.; Friedman, E.; Foulkes, W.D.; et al. Salpingo-oophorectomy and the risk of ovarian, fallopian tube, and peritoneal cancers in women with a BRCA1 or BRCA2 Mutation. *JAMA* **2006**, *296*, 185–192. [CrossRef]
7. Nelson, H.D.; Fu, R.; Zakher, B.; Pappas, M.; McDonagh, M. Medication Use for the Risk Reduction of Primary Breast Cancer in Women: Updated Evidence Report and Systematic Review for the US Preventive Services Task Force. *JAMA* **2019**, *322*, 868–886. [CrossRef]
8. Rebbeck, T.R.; Friebel, T.; Lynch, H.T.; Neuhausen, S.L.; Van't Veer, L.; Garber, J.E.; Evans, G.R.; Narod, S.A.; Isaacs, C.; Matloff, E.; et al. Bilateral prophylactic mastectomy reduces breast cancer risk in BRCA1 and BRCA2 mutation carriers: The PROSE Study Group. *J. Clin. Oncol.* **2004**, *22*, 1055–1062. [CrossRef] [PubMed]
9. Nelson, H.D.; Pappas, M.; Zakher, B.; Mitchell, J.P.; Okinaka-Hu, L.; Fu, R. Risk assessment, genetic counseling, and genetic testing for BRCA-related cancer in women: A systematic review to update the U.S. Preventive Services Task Force recommendation. *Ann. Intern. Med.* **2014**, *160*, 255–266. [CrossRef] [PubMed]
10. NICE. *Familial Breast Cancer: Classification and Care of People at Risk of Familial Breast Cancer and Management of Breast Cancer and Related Risks in People with a Family History of Breast Cancer.* In *NICE Clinical Guideline CG164*; National Institute for Health and Care Excellence: London, UK, 2013.
11. Childers, C.P.; Childers, K.K.; Maggard-Gibbons, M.; Macinko, J. National Estimates of Genetic Testing in Women With a History of Breast or Ovarian Cancer. *J. Clin. Oncol.* **2017**, *35*, 3800–3806. [CrossRef] [PubMed]
12. Manchanda, R.; Blyuss, O.; Gaba, F.; Gordeev, V.S.; Jacobs, C.; Burnell, M.; Gan, C.; Taylor, R.; Turnbull, C.; Legood, R.; et al. Current detection rates and time-to-detection of all identifiable BRCA carriers in the Greater London population. *J. Med. Genet.* **2018**, *55*. [CrossRef] [PubMed]
13. NHS England. *Clinical Commissioning Policy: Genetic Testing for BRCA1 and BRCA2 Mutations*; NHS England Specialised Services Clinical Reference Group for Medical Genetics: London, UK, 2015.
14. Manchanda, R.; Lieberman, S.; Gaba, F.; Lahad, A.; Levy-Lahad, E. Population Screening for Inherited Predisposition to Breast and Ovarian Cancer. *Annu. Rev. Genom. Hum. Genet.* **2020**. [CrossRef] [PubMed]
15. Gabai-Kapara, E.; Lahad, A.; Kaufman, B.; Friedman, E.; Segev, S.; Renbaum, P.; Beeri, R.; Gal, M.; Grinshpun-Cohen, J.; Djemal, K.; et al. Population-based screening for breast and ovarian cancer risk due to BRCA1 and BRCA2. *Proc. Natl. Acad. Sci. USA* **2014**, *111*, 14205–14210. [CrossRef] [PubMed]
16. Manchanda, R.; Burnell, M.; Gaba, F.; Desai, R.; Wardle, J.; Gessler, S.; Side, L.; Sanderson, S.; Loggenberg, K.; Brady, A.F.; et al. Randomised trial of population-based BRCA testing in Ashkenazi Jews: Long-term outcomes. *BJOG* **2020**, *127*, 364–375. [CrossRef]
17. George, A.; Riddell, D.; Seal, S.; Talukdar, S.; Mahamdallie, S.; Ruark, E.; Cloke, V.; Slade, I.; Kemp, Z.; Gore, M.; et al. Implementing rapid, robust, cost-effective, patient-centred, routine genetic testing in ovarian cancer patients. *Sci. Rep.* **2016**, *6*, 29506. [CrossRef]

18. Moller, P.; Hagen, A.I.; Apold, J.; Maehle, L.; Clark, N.; Fiane, B.; Lovslett, K.; Hovig, E.; Vabo, A. Genetic epidemiology of BRCA mutations—Family history detects less than 50% of the mutation carriers. *Eur. J. Cancer* **2007**, *43*, 1713–1717. [CrossRef] [PubMed]
19. Norum, J.; Grindedal, E.M.; Heramb, C.; Karsrud, I.; Ariansen, S.L.; Undlien, D.E.; Schlichting, E.; Maehle, L. BRCA mutation carrier detection. A model-based cost-effectiveness analysis comparing the traditional family history approach and the testing of all patients with breast cancer. *ESMO Open* **2018**, *3*, e000328. [CrossRef]
20. Beitsch, P.D.; Whitworth, P.W.; Hughes, K.; Patel, R.; Rosen, B.; Compagnoni, G.; Baron, P.; Simmons, R.; Smith, L.A.; Grady, I.; et al. Underdiagnosis of Hereditary Breast Cancer: Are Genetic Testing Guidelines a Tool or an Obstacle? *J. Clin. Oncol.* **2018**, *37*. [CrossRef]
21. Manchanda, R.; Legood, R.; Burnell, M.; McGuire, A.; Raikou, M.; Loggenberg, K.; Wardle, J.; Sanderson, S.; Gessler, S.; Side, L.; et al. Cost-effectiveness of population screening for BRCA mutations in Ashkenazi jewish women compared with family history-based testing. *J. Natl. Cancer Inst.* **2015**, *107*, 380. [CrossRef]
22. Manchanda, R.; Loggenberg, K.; Sanderson, S.; Burnell, M.; Wardle, J.; Gessler, S.; Side, L.; Balogun, N.; Desai, R.; Kumar, A.; et al. Population testing for cancer predisposing BRCA1/BRCA2 mutations in the Ashkenazi-Jewish community: A randomized controlled trial. *J. Natl. Cancer Inst.* **2015**, *107*, 379. [CrossRef]
23. Manchanda, R.; Gaba, F. Population Based Testing for Primary Prevention: A Systematic Review. *Cancers* **2018**, *10*, 424. [CrossRef]
24. Griffiths, U.K.; Legood, R.; Pitt, C. Comparison of Economic Evaluation Methods Across Low-income, Middle-income and High-income Countries: What are the Differences and Why? *Health Econ.* **2016**, *25* (Suppl. 1), 29–41. [CrossRef] [PubMed]
25. NICE. *Guide to the Methods of Technology Appraisal*; National Institute of Health and Care Excellence: London, UK, 2013.
26. Neumann, P.J.; Cohen, J.T.; Weinstein, M.C. Updating cost-effectiveness—The curious resilience of the $50,000-per-QALY threshold. *N. Engl. J. Med.* **2014**, *371*, 796–797. [CrossRef]
27. *Kosteneffectiviteit in de Praktijk*; Zorginstituut Nederland (National Health Care Institute, Netherlands): Diemen, The Netherlands, 2015.
28. The World Bank. PPP Conversion Factor, GDP. Available online: http://data.worldbank.org/indicator/PA.NUS.PPP (accessed on 9 August 2019).
29. World Bank. Population, Female. Available online: https://data.worldbank.org/indicator/SP.POP.TOTL.FE.IN?year_high_desc=true (accessed on 29 January 2019).
30. Woods, B.; Revill, P.; Sculpher, M.; Claxton, K. Country-Level Cost-Effectiveness Thresholds: Initial Estimates and the Need for Further Research. *Value Health* **2016**, *19*, 929–935. [CrossRef] [PubMed]
31. Bertram, M.Y.; Lauer, J.A.; De Joncheere, K.; Edejer, T.; Hutubessy, R.; Kieny, M.P.; Hill, S.R. Cost-effectiveness thresholds: Pros and cons. *Bull. World Health Organ.* **2016**, *94*, 925–930. [CrossRef]
32. Ottersen, T.; Forde, R.; Kakad, M.; Kjellevold, A.; Melberg, H.O.; Moen, A.; Ringard, A.; Norheim, O.F. A new proposal for priority setting in Norway: Open and fair. *Health Policy* **2016**, *120*, 246–251. [CrossRef]
33. Parker, W.H.; Feskanich, D.; Broder, M.S.; Chang, E.; Shoupe, D.; Farquhar, C.M.; Berek, J.S.; Manson, J.E. Long-term mortality associated with oophorectomy compared with ovarian conservation in the nurses' health study. *Obstet. Gynecol.* **2013**, *121*, 709–716. [CrossRef]
34. Metcalfe, K.; Eisen, A.; Senter, L.; Armel, S.; Bordeleau, L.; Meschino, W.S.; Pal, T.; Lynch, H.T.; Tung, N.M.; Kwong, A.; et al. International trends in the uptake of cancer risk reduction strategies in women with a BRCA1 or BRCA2 mutation. *Br. J. Cancer* **2019**, *121*. [CrossRef] [PubMed]
35. Manchanda, R.; Abdelraheim, A.; Johnson, M.; Rosenthal, A.N.; Benjamin, E.; Brunell, C.; Burnell, M.; Side, L.; Gessler, S.; Saridogan, E.; et al. Outcome of risk-reducing salpingo-oophorectomy in BRCA carriers and women of unknown mutation status. *BJOG* **2011**, *118*, 814–824. [CrossRef]
36. Miller, M.E.; Czechura, T.; Martz, B.; Hall, M.E.; Pesce, C.; Jaskowiak, N.; Winchester, D.J.; Yao, K. Operative risks associated with contralateral prophylactic mastectomy: A single institution experience. *Ann. Surg. Oncol.* **2013**, *20*, 4113–4120. [CrossRef] [PubMed]
37. Gaba, F.; Manchanda, R. Systematic review of acceptability, cardiovascular, neurological, bone health and HRT outcomes following risk reducing surgery in BRCA carriers. *Best Pract. Res. Clin. Obstet. Gynaecol.* **2020**, *65*. [CrossRef] [PubMed]

38. Metcalfe, K.A.; Poll, A.; Royer, R.; Llacuachaqui, M.; Tulman, A.; Sun, P.; Narod, S.A. Screening for founder mutations in BRCA1 and BRCA2 in unselected Jewish women. *J. Clin. Oncol.* **2010**, *28*, 387–391. [CrossRef] [PubMed]
39. Lieberman, S.; Tomer, A.; Ben-Chetrit, A.; Olsha, O.; Strano, S.; Beeri, R.; Koka, S.; Fridman, H.; Djemal, K.; Glick, I.; et al. Population screening for BRCA1/BRCA2 founder mutations in Ashkenazi Jews: Proactive recruitment compared with self-referral. *Genet. Med.* **2016**, *19*. [CrossRef]
40. Metcalfe, K.A.; Poll, A.; Llacuachaqui, M.; Nanda, S.; Tulman, A.; Mian, N.; Sun, P.; Narod, S.A. Patient satisfaction and cancer-related distress among unselected Jewish women undergoing genetic testing for BRCA1 and BRCA2. *Clin. Genet.* **2010**, *78*, 411–417. [CrossRef] [PubMed]
41. Yuen, J.; Cousens, N.; Barlow-Stewart, K.; O'Shea, R.; Andrews, L. Online BRCA1/2 screening in the Australian Jewish community: A qualitative study. *J. Community Genet.* **2019**, *11*. [CrossRef] [PubMed]
42. Manchanda, R. Predicting risk of ovarian malignancy improved screening and early detection feasibility study. In *ISRCTN Registry: ISRCTN54246466*; BioMed Central: London, UK, 2017.
43. Plon, S.E.; Eccles, D.M.; Easton, D.; Foulkes, W.D.; Genuardi, M.; Greenblatt, M.S.; Hogervorst, F.B.; Hoogerbrugge, N.; Spurdle, A.B.; Tavtigian, S.V.; et al. Sequence variant classification and reporting: Recommendations for improving the interpretation of cancer susceptibility genetic test results. *Hum. Mutat.* **2008**, *29*, 1282–1291. [CrossRef] [PubMed]
44. Global Burden of Disease Cancer, C.; Fitzmaurice, C.; Akinyemiju, T.F.; Al Lami, F.H.; Alam, T.; Alizadeh-Navaei, R.; Allen, C.; Alsharif, U.; Alvis-Guzman, N.; Amini, E.; et al. Global, Regional, and National Cancer Incidence, Mortality, Years of Life Lost, Years Lived With Disability, and Disability-Adjusted Life-Years for 29 Cancer Groups, 1990 to 2016: A Systematic Analysis for the Global Burden of Disease Study. *JAMA Oncol.* **2018**, *4*, 1553–1568. [CrossRef]
45. International Agency for Research on Cancer. Cancer Tomorrow. In *A Tool That Predicts the Future Cancer Incidence and Mortality Burden Worldwide from the Current Estimates in 2018 up until 2040*; International Agency for Research on Cancer (IARC): Lyon, France, 2018.
46. Wilson, J.; Jungner, G. *Principles and Practice of Screening for Disease*; 34; World Health Organisation: Geneva, Switzerland, 1968.
47. UK, N.S.C. Criteria for Appraising the Viability, Effectiveness and Appropriateness of a Screening Programme. Available online: https://www.gov.uk/government/publications/evidence-review-criteria-national-screening-programmes/criteria-for-appraising-the-viability-effectiveness-and-appropriateness-of-a-screening-programme (accessed on 1 December 2019).
48. Khoury, M.J.; McCabe, L.L.; McCabe, E.R. Population screening in the age of genomic medicine. *N. Engl. J. Med.* **2003**, *348*, 50–58. [CrossRef]
49. CDC. ACCE Model Process for Evaluating Genetic Tests. In *Genomic Testing*; The Office of Public Health Genomics (OPHG), Centers for Disease Control and Prevention (CDC): Atlanta, GA, USA, 2010.
50. Burke, W.; Zimmerman, R. *Moving Beyond ACCE: An Expanded Framework for Genetic Test Evaluation*; PHG Foundation: London, UK, 2007.
51. Force, U.S.P.S.T.; Owens, D.K.; Davidson, K.W.; Krist, A.H.; Barry, M.J.; Cabana, M.; Caughey, A.B.; Doubeni, C.A.; Epling, J.W., Jr.; Kubik, M.; et al. Risk Assessment, Genetic Counseling, and Genetic Testing for BRCA-Related Cancer: US Preventive Services Task Force Recommendation Statement. *JAMA* **2019**, *322*, 652–665. [CrossRef]
52. Nelson, H.D.; Pappas, M.; Cantor, A.; Haney, E.; Holmes, R. Risk Assessment, Genetic Counseling, and Genetic Testing for BRCA-Related Cancer in Women: Updated Evidence Report and Systematic Review for the US Preventive Services Task Force. *JAMA* **2019**, *322*, 666–685. [CrossRef]
53. Sanders, G.D.; Neumann, P.J.; Basu, A.; Brock, D.W.; Feeny, D.; Krahn, M.; Kuntz, K.M.; Meltzer, D.O.; Owens, D.K.; Prosser, L.A.; et al. Recommendations for Conduct, Methodological Practices, and Reporting of Cost-effectiveness Analyses: Second Panel on Cost-Effectiveness in Health and Medicine. *JAMA* **2016**, *316*, 1093–1103. [CrossRef] [PubMed]
54. Eggington, J.M.; Bowles, K.R.; Moyes, K.; Manley, S.; Esterling, L.; Sizemore, S.; Rosenthal, E.; Theisen, A.; Saam, J.; Arnell, C.; et al. A comprehensive laboratory-based program for classification of variants of uncertain significance in hereditary cancer genes. *Clin. Genet.* **2014**, *86*, 229–237. [CrossRef] [PubMed]

55. Cancer Research UK. Breast Cancer Incidence (Invasive) Statistics. Available online: http://www.cancerresearchuk.org/health-professional/cancer-statistics/statistics-by-cancer-type/breast-cancer/incidence-invasive#collapseOne (accessed on 14 March 2019).
56. Cancer Research UK. Ovarian Cancer Incidence Statistics. Available online: http://www.cancerresearchuk.org/health-professional/cancer-statistics/statistics-by-cancer-type/ovarian-cancer/incidence#heading-One (accessed on 14 March 2019).
57. United States Cancer Statistics. Rate of New Cancers by Age Group, All Races, Female. Available online: https://gis.cdc.gov/Cancer/USCS/DataViz.html (accessed on 19 November 2019).
58. International Agency for Research on Cancer. Estimated Number of New Cases in 2018, Worldwide, Females, All Ages. Available online: http://gco.iarc.fr/today/online-analysis-table (accessed on 21 November 2019).
59. Jervis, S.; Song, H.; Lee, A.; Dicks, E.; Harrington, P.; Baynes, C.; Manchanda, R.; Easton, D.F.; Jacobs, I.; Pharoah, P.P.; et al. A risk prediction algorithm for ovarian cancer incorporating BRCA1, BRCA2, common alleles and other familial effects. *J. Med. Genet.* **2015**, *52*, 465–475. [CrossRef] [PubMed]
60. Evans, D.G.; Lalloo, F.; Ashcroft, L.; Shenton, A.; Clancy, T.; Baildam, A.D.; Brain, A.; Hopwood, P.; Howell, A. Uptake of risk-reducing surgery in unaffected women at high risk of breast and ovarian cancer is risk, age, and time dependent. *Cancer Epidemiol. Biomark. Prev.* **2009**, *18*, 2318–2324. [CrossRef]
61. Manchanda, R.; Burnell, M.; Abdelraheim, A.; Johnson, M.; Sharma, A.; Benjamin, E.; Brunell, C.; Saridogan, E.; Gessler, S.; Oram, D.; et al. Factors influencing uptake and timing of risk reducing salpingo-oophorectomy in women at risk of familial ovarian cancer: A competing risk time to event analysis. *BJOG* **2012**, *119*, 527–536. [CrossRef] [PubMed]
62. Read, M.D.; Edey, K.A.; Hapeshi, J.; Foy, C. Compliance with estrogen hormone replacement therapy after oophorectomy: A prospective study. *Menopause Int.* **2010**, *16*, 60–64. [CrossRef]
63. Cuzick, J.; Sestak, I.; Cawthorn, S.; Hamed, H.; Holli, K.; Howell, A.; Forbes, J.F.; Investigators, I.-I. Tamoxifen for prevention of breast cancer: Extended long-term follow-up of the IBIS-I breast cancer prevention trial. *Lancet Oncol.* **2015**, *16*, 67–75. [CrossRef]
64. Smith, S.G.; Sestak, I.; Forster, A.; Partridge, A.; Side, L.; Wolf, M.S.; Horne, R.; Wardle, J.; Cuzick, J. Factors affecting uptake and adherence to breast cancer chemoprevention: A systematic review and meta-analysis. *Ann. Oncol.* **2016**, *27*, 575–590. [CrossRef]
65. Chen, H.; Chen, Y.; Cui, B. The association of multimorbidity with healthcare expenditure among the elderly patients in Beijing, China. *Arch. Gerontol. Geriatr.* **2018**, *79*, 32–38. [CrossRef] [PubMed]
66. SIGTAP. *Sistema de Gerenciamento da Tabela de Procedimentos, Medicamentos e OPM do SUS*; Ministry of Health, Brazil: Brasilia, Brazil, 2020.
67. BPS. *Banco de Preços em Saúde*; Health Price Bank; Ministry of Health, Brazil: Brasilia, Brazil, 2019.
68. CMED. *Câmara de Regulação do Mercado de Medicamentos*; ANVISA, Barzilian Health Regulatory Agency: Brasilia, Brazil, 2016.
69. Curtis, L.; Burns, A. *Unit Costs of Health and Social Care 2016*; Personal Social Services Research Unit (PSSRU): Canterbury, Kent, UK, 2016.
70. NHS Improvement. *NHS Reference Costs 2016/17*; NHS Improvement: London, UK, 2017.
71. The World Bank. Labor Force Participation Rate, Female (% of Female Population Ages 15+) (Modeled ILO Estimate). Available online: https://data.worldbank.org/indicator/SL.TLF.CACT.FE.ZS (accessed on 7 November 2019).
72. Hanly, P.; Timmons, A.; Walsh, P.M.; Sharp, L. Breast and prostate cancer productivity costs: A comparison of the human capital approach and the friction cost approach. *Value Health* **2012**, *15*, 429–436. [CrossRef]
73. World Health Organisation. Life Tables. Available online: http://apps.who.int/gho/data/node.main.687?lang=en (accessed on 27 January 2020).
74. Allemani, C.; Matsuda, T.; Di Carlo, V.; Harewood, R.; Matz, M.; Niksic, M.; Bonaventure, A.; Valkov, M.; Johnson, C.J.; Esteve, J.; et al. Global surveillance of trends in cancer survival 2000-14 (CONCORD-3): Analysis of individual records for 37,513,025 patients diagnosed with one of 18 cancers from 322 population-based registries in 71 countries. *Lancet* **2018**, *391*, 1023–1075. [CrossRef]
75. Bordeleau, L.; Panchal, S.; Goodwin, P. Prognosis of BRCA-associated breast cancer: A summary of evidence. *Breast Cancer Res. Treat.* **2010**, *119*, 13–24. [CrossRef] [PubMed]

76. Rennert, G.; Bisland-Naggan, S.; Barnett-Griness, O.; Bar-Joseph, N.; Zhang, S.; Rennert, H.S.; Narod, S.A. Clinical outcomes of breast cancer in carriers of BRCA1 and BRCA2 mutations. *N. Engl. J. Med.* **2007**, *357*, 115–123. [CrossRef] [PubMed]
77. McLaughlin, J.R.; Rosen, B.; Moody, J.; Pal, T.; Fan, I.; Shaw, P.A.; Risch, H.A.; Sellers, T.A.; Sun, P.; Narod, S.A. Long-term ovarian cancer survival associated with mutation in BRCA1 or BRCA2. *J. Natl. Cancer Inst.* **2013**, *105*, 141–148. [CrossRef] [PubMed]
78. National Institue for Health and Care Excellence (NICE). *Clinical Guideline (CG81)—Advanced Breast Cancer: Diagnosis and Treatment*; National Collaborating Centre for Cancer, National Institute for Health and Clinical Excellence: Cardiff, UK, 2009.
79. Havrilesky, L.J.; Broadwater, G.; Davis, D.M.; Nolte, K.C.; Barnett, J.C.; Myers, E.R.; Kulasingam, S. Determination of quality of life-related utilities for health states relevant to ovarian cancer diagnosis and treatment. *Gynecol. Oncol.* **2009**, *113*, 216–220. [CrossRef]
80. Grann, V.R.; Patel, P.; Bharthuar, A.; Jacobson, J.S.; Warner, E.; Anderson, K.; Tsai, W.Y.; Hill, K.A.; Neugut, A.I.; Hershman, D. Breast cancer-related preferences among women with and without BRCA mutations. *Breast Cancer Res. Treat.* **2010**, *119*, 177–184. [CrossRef]
81. Edejer, T.; Baltussen, R.; Adam, T.; Hutubessy, R.; Acharya, A.; Evans, D.; Murray, C. *WHO Guide to Cost-Effectiveness Analysis*; World Health Organisation: Geneva, Switzerland, 2003.
82. Hutubessy, R.; Chisholm, D.; Edejer, T.T. Generalized cost-effectiveness analysis for national-level priority-setting in the health sector. *Cost Eff. Resour. Alloc.* **2003**, *1*, 8. [CrossRef]
83. Briggs, A. Probabilistic analysis of cost-effectiveness models: Statistical representation of parameter uncertainty. *Value Health* **2005**, *8*, 1–2. [CrossRef]
84. National Institute for Health and Care Excellence (NICE). *Familial Breast Cancer: Classification, Care and Managing Breast Cancer and Related Risks in People with a Family History of Breast Cancer*; National Institute for Health and Clinical Excellence: Cardiff, UK, 2013.
85. Manchanda, R.; Burnell, M.; Loggenberg, K.; Desai, R.; Wardle, J.; Sanderson, S.C.; Gessler, S.; Side, L.; Balogun, N.; Kumar, A.; et al. Cluster-randomised non-inferiority trial comparing DVD-assisted and traditional genetic counselling in systematic population testing for BRCA1/2 mutations. *J. Med. Genet.* **2016**, *53*, 472–480. [CrossRef]
86. Curtis, L. *Unit Costs of Health and Social Care 2011*; Personal Social Services Research Unit (PSSRU): Canterbury, UK, 2011.
87. Schwartz, M.D.; Valdimarsdottir, H.B.; Peshkin, B.N.; Mandelblatt, J.; Nusbaum, R.; Huang, A.T.; Chang, Y.; Graves, K.; Isaacs, C.; Wood, M.; et al. Randomized noninferiority trial of telephone versus in-person genetic counseling for hereditary breast and ovarian cancer. *J. Clin. Oncol.* **2014**, *32*, 618–626. [CrossRef]
88. NHS Reference Costs 2015 to 2016. Available online: https://assets.publishing.service.gov.uk/government/uploads/system/uploads/attachment_data/file/577083/Reference_Costs_2015-16.pdf (accessed on 1 March 2019).
89. Grann, V.R.; Patel, P.R.; Jacobson, J.S.; Warner, E.; Heitjan, D.F.; Ashby-Thompson, M.; Hershman, D.L.; Neugut, A.I. Comparative effectiveness of screening and prevention strategies among BRCA1/2-affected mutation carriers. *Breast Cancer Res. Treat.* **2011**, *125*, 837–847. [CrossRef] [PubMed]
90. British National Formulary. *British National Formulary*; BMJ Group and Pharmaceutical Press (Royal Pharmaceutical Society of Great Britain): London, UK, 2018.
91. Williams-Frame, A.; Carpenter, J.S. Costs of hormonal and nonhormonal prescription medications for hot flashes. *Womens Health (Lond)* **2009**, *5*, 497–502. [CrossRef]
92. National Institue for Health and Care Excellence (NICE). *Ovarian Cancer: The Recognition and initial Management of Ovarian Cancer*; National Institute for Health and Clinical Excellence (NICE): Cardiff, UK, 2011.
93. Cancer Research UK. *Saving Lives, Averting Costs. an Analysis of the Financial Implications of Achieving Earlier Diagnosis of Colorectal, Lung and Ovarian Cancer*; CRUK: London, UK, 2014.
94. National Audit Office. *End of Life Care*; National Audit Office (NAO), House of Commons: London, UK, 2008.
95. National Institute of Health and Clinical Excellence. *Guide to the Methods of Technology Appraisal*; National Institute for Health and Clinical Excellence (NICE): London, UK, 2013.

96. National Institute for Health and Clinical Excellence. *National Costing Report: Early and Locally Advanced Breast Cancer/Advanced Breast Cancer*; National Institute for Health and Clinical Excellence: London, UK, 2009.
97. Heijnsdijk, E.A.; Warner, E.; Gilbert, F.J.; Tilanus-Linthorst, M.M.; Evans, G.; Causer, P.A.; Eeles, R.A.; Kaas, R.; Draisma, G.; Ramsay, E.A.; et al. Differences in natural history between breast cancers in BRCA1 and BRCA2 mutation carriers and effects of MRI screening-MRISC, MARIBS, and Canadian studies combined. *Cancer Epidemiol. Biomarkers Prev.* 2012, *21*, 1458–1468. [CrossRef] [PubMed]
98. National Institue for Health and Care Excellence (NICE). *Early and Locally Advanced Breast Cancer: Diagnosis and Treatment*; National Collaborating Centre for Cancer, National Institute for Health and Clinical Excellence: Cardiff, UK, 2009.
99. National Institute for Health and Care Excellence (NICE). *Advanced Breast Cancer: Diagnosis and Treatment*; National Institute for Health and Clinical Excellence: London, UK, 2009.
100. Cortesi, L.; Turchetti, D.; Marchi, I.; Fracca, A.; Canossi, B.; Battista, R.; Ruscelli, S.; Pecchi, A.R.; Torricelli, P.; Federico, M. Breast cancer screening in women at increased risk according to different family histories: An update of the Modena Study Group experience. *BMC Cancer* 2006, *6*, 210. [CrossRef] [PubMed]
101. MARIBS Study Group. Screening with magnetic resonance imaging and mammography of a UK population at high familial risk of breast cancer: A prospective multicentre cohort study (MARIBS). *Lancet* 2005, *365*, 1769–1778. [CrossRef]
102. Robson, M.E.; Chappuis, P.O.; Satagopan, J.; Wong, N.; Boyd, J.; Goffin, J.R.; Hudis, C.; Roberge, D.; Norton, L.; Begin, L.R.; et al. A combined analysis of outcome following breast cancer: Differences in survival based on BRCA1/BRCA2 mutation status and administration of adjuvant treatment. *Breast Cancer Res.* 2003, *6*, R8–R17. [CrossRef]
103. Comen, E.; Davids, M.; Kirchhoff, T.; Hudis, C.; Offit, K.; Robson, M. Relative contributions of BRCA1 and BRCA2 mutations to "triple-negative" breast cancer in Ashkenazi Women. *Breast Cancer Res. Treat.* 2011, *129*, 185–190. [CrossRef] [PubMed]
104. Tung, N.; Garber, J.E.; Lincoln, A.; Domchek, S.M. Frequency of triple-negative breast cancer in BRCA1 mutation carriers: Comparison between common Ashkenazi Jewish and other mutations. *J. Clin. Oncol.* 2012, *30*, 4447–4448. [CrossRef]
105. Chappuis, P.O.; Nethercot, V.; Foulkes, W.D. Clinico-pathological characteristics of BRCA1- and BRCA2-related breast cancer. In *Seminars in Surgical Oncology*; John Wiley & Sons: Hoboken, NJ, USA, 2000; Volume 18, pp. 287–295.
106. Robertson, C.; Arcot Ragupathy, S.K.; Boachie, C.; Dixon, J.M.; Fraser, C.; Hernandez, R.; Heys, S.; Jack, W.; Kerr, G.R.; Lawrence, G.; et al. The clinical effectiveness and cost-effectiveness of different surveillance mammography regimens after the treatment for primary breast cancer: Systematic reviews registry database analyses and economic evaluation. *Health Technol. Assess* 2011, *15*, i–vi. [CrossRef]
107. Bates, T.; Kearins, O.; Monypenny, I.; Lagord, C.; Lawrence, G. Clinical outcome data for symptomatic breast cancer: The Breast Cancer Clinical Outcome Measures (BCCOM) Project. *Br. J. Cancer* 2009, *101*, 395–402. [CrossRef]
108. Breast, E.; Trialist, C. Group C. Effects of chemotherapy and hormonal therapy for early breast cancer on recurrence and 15-year survival: An overview of the randomised trials. *Lancet* 2005, *365*, 1687–1717. [CrossRef]
109. Blamey, R.W.; Ellis, I.O.; Pinder, S.E.; Lee, A.H.; Macmillan, R.D.; Morgan, D.A.L.; Robertson, J.F.R.; Mitchell, M.J.; Ball, G.R.; Haybittle, J.L.; et al. Survival of invasive breast cancer according to the Nottingham Prognostic Index in cases diagnosed in 1990–1999. *Eur. J. Cancer* 2007, *43*, 1548–1555. [CrossRef] [PubMed]
110. Gribbin, J.; Dewis, R. *Adjuvant! Online: Review of Evidence Concerning Its Validity, and Other Considerations Relating to Its Use in the NHS*; National Institute for Health and Clinical Excellence: Cardiff, UK, 2009.
111. Kozlow, W.; Guise, T.A. Breast cancer metastasis to bone: Mechanisms of osteolysis and implications for therapy. *J. Mammary Gland Biol.* 2005, *10*, 169–180. [CrossRef] [PubMed]
112. Breast cancer survival statistics. Available online: https://www.cancerresearchuk.org/health-professional/cancer-statistics/statistics-by-cancer-type/breast-cancer/survival (accessed on 1 April 2018).

113. Wapnir, I.L.; Anderson, S.J.; Mamounas, E.P.; Geyer, C.E., Jr.; Jeong, J.H.; Tan-Chiu, E.; Fisher, B.; Wolmark, N. Prognosis after ipsilateral breast tumor recurrence and locoregional recurrences in five National Surgical Adjuvant Breast and Bowel Project node-positive adjuvant breast cancer trials. *J. Clin. Oncol.* **2006**, *24*, 2028–2037. [CrossRef] [PubMed]
114. Anderson, S.J.; Wapnir, I.; Dignam, J.J.; Fisher, B.; Mamounas, E.P.; Jeong, J.H.; Geyer Jr, C.E.; Wickerham, D.L.; Costantino, J.P.; Wolmark, N. Prognosis after ipsilateral breast tumor recurrence and locoregional recurrences in patients treated by breast-conserving therapy in five National Surgical Adjuvant Breast and Bowel Project protocols of node-negative breast cancer. *J. Clin. Oncol.* **2009**, *27*, 2466–2473. [CrossRef]
115. Gennari, A.; Conte, P.; Rosso, R.; Orlandini, C.; Bruzzi, P. Survival of metastatic breast carcinoma patients over a 20-year period: A retrospective analysis based on individual patient data from six consecutive studies. *Cancer* **2005**, *104*, 1742–1750. [CrossRef]
116. Waldron, J. *Breast Screening Programme, England 2008-09*; NHS Digital: Leeds, UK, 2010.
117. CDC. Breast Cancer Screening Guidelines for Women. Available online: https://www.cdc.gov/cancer/breast/pdf/breastcancerscreeningguidelines.pdf (accessed on 1 April 2018).
118. Dos-Santos-Silva, I. Breast cancer control policies in Brazil: Where to go from here? *Cadernos De Saude Publica* **2018**, *34*. [CrossRef]
119. National Institute for Health and Care Excellence. *Familial Breast Cancer: Classification and Care of People at Risk of Familial Breast Cancer and Management of Breast Cancer and Related Risks in People with a Family History of Breast Cancer*; National Institute for Health and Care Excellence: London, UK, 2013.
120. Cuzick, J.; Sestak, I.; Bonanni, B.; Costantino, J.P.; Cummings, S.; DeCensi, A.; Dowsett, M.; Forbes, J.F.; Ford, L.; LaCroix, A.Z.; et al. Selective oestrogen receptor modulators in prevention of breast cancer: An updated meta-analysis of individual participant data. *Lancet* **2013**, *381*, 1827–1834. [CrossRef]
121. Townsend, N.; Bhatnagar, P.; Wilkins, E. *Cardiovascular Disease Statistics*; British Heart Foundation: London, UK, 2015.
122. CDC. Heart Disease. Available online: https://www.cdc.gov/nchs/fastats/heart-disease.htm (accessed on 17 March 2018).
123. Who Is at Risk for Coronary Heart Disease? Available online: https://www.nhlbi.nih.gov/health-topics/coronary-heart-disease#Risk-Factors (accessed on 17 March 2018).
124. American Heart Association. Cardiovascular Disease: A Costly Burden for America—Projections through 2035. Available online: http://www.heart.org/idc/groups/heart-public/@wcm/@adv/documents/downloadable/ucm_491543.pdf (accessed on 17 March 2018).
125. Population, total. Available online: https://data.worldbank.org/indicator/SP.POP.TOTL?view=chart (accessed on 7 November 2019).
126. Afana, M.; Brinjikji, W.; Cloft, H.; Salka, S. Hospitalization costs for acute myocardial infarction patients treated with percutaneous coronary intervention in the United States are substantially higher than Medicare payments. *Clin. Cardiol.* **2015**, *38*, 13–19. [CrossRef]
127. Office for National Statistics. Employee earnings in the UK: 2018. Available online: https://www.ons.gov.uk/employmentandlabourmarket/peopleinwork/earningsandworkinghours/bulletins/annualsurveyofhoursandearnings/2018 (accessed on 7 November 2019).
128. Bureau of Labor Statistics. Labor Force Statistics from the Current Population Survey. Available online: https://www.bls.gov/cps/earnings.htm#demographics (accessed on 7 November 2019).
129. Statistics Netherlands. Available online: www.cbs.nl (accessed on 7 November 2019).
130. World Economic Forum. The Global Gender Gap Report 2016. Available online: http://reports.weforum.org/global-gender-gap-report-2016/economies/#economy=CHN (accessed on 7 November 2019).
131. Brazilian Institute of Geography and Statistics. Estatísticas de Gênero - Indicadores sociais das mulheres no Brasil. Available online: https://www.ibge.gov.br/estatisticas-novoportal/multidominio/genero/20163-estatisticas-de-genero-indicadores-sociais-das-mulheres-no-brasil.html?=&t=o-que-e (accessed on 7 November 2019).
132. National Sample Survey Office. *Employment and Unemployment Survey, 68th Round, 2012-13, Government of India, Ministry of Statistics & Programme Implementation*; National Sample Survey Office (NSSO): New Delhi, India, 2013.
133. National Ovarian Cancer Coalition. Ovarian Cancer Recurrence: Discussion With an Expert. Available online: http://ovarian.org/component/content/article/33/385 (accessed on 7 November 2019).

134. National Institue for Health and Care Excellence (NICE). *Social Value Judgements: Principles for the Development of NICE Guidance*; National Institute for Health and Clinical Excellence: Cardiff, UK, 2008.
135. Ubel, P.A.; Hirth, R.A.; Chernew, M.E.; Fendrick, A.M. What is the price of life and why doesn't it increase at the rate of inflation? *Arch. Intern. Med.* **2003**, *163*, 1637–1641. [CrossRef]
136. *Richtlijn Voor Het Uitvoeren van Economische Evaluaties in de Gezondheidszorg*; Zorginstituut Nederland (National Health Care Institute, Netherlands): Diemen, The Netherlands, 2016. Available online: https://www.zorginstituutnederland.nl/publicaties/publicatie/2016/02/29/richtlijn-voor-het-uitvoeren-van-economische-evaluaties-in-de-gezondheidszorg (accessed on 21 March 2019).

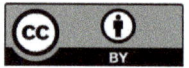

© 2020 by the authors. Licensee MDPI, Basel, Switzerland. This article is an open access article distributed under the terms and conditions of the Creative Commons Attribution (CC BY) license (http://creativecommons.org/licenses/by/4.0/).

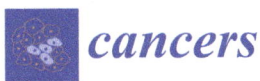

Article

Multi-Marker Longitudinal Algorithms Incorporating HE4 and CA125 in Ovarian Cancer Screening of Postmenopausal Women

Aleksandra Gentry-Maharaj [1,†], Oleg Blyuss [2,3,†], Andy Ryan [1], Matthew Burnell [1], Chloe Karpinskyj [1], Richard Gunu [4], Jatinderpal K. Kalsi [4], Anne Dawnay [5], Ines P. Marino [6], Ranjit Manchanda [1,7,8], Karen Lu [9], Wei-Lei Yang [9], John F. Timms [4], Mahesh Parmar [1], Steven J. Skates [10], Robert C. Bast, Jr. [9,‡], Ian J. Jacobs [4,11,‡], Alexey Zaikin [3,4,12,13,‡] and Usha Menon [1,‡,*]

1. MRC Clinical Trials Unit at UCL, Institute of Clinical Trials & Methodology, London WC1V 6LJ, UK; a.gentry-maharaj@ucl.ac.uk (A.G.-M.); a.ryan@ucl.ac.uk (A.R.); m.burnell@ucl.ac.uk (M.B.); c.karpinskyj@ucl.ac.uk (C.K.); r.manchanda@qmul.ac.uk (R.M.); m.parmar@ucl.ac.uk (M.P.)
2. School of Physics, Astronomy and Mathematics, University of Hertfordshire, Hatfield AL10 9AB, UK; o.blyuss@qmul.ac.uk
3. Department of Paediatrics and Paediatric Infectious Diseases, Sechenov First Moscow State Medical University, Moscow 119991, Russia; alexey.zaikin@ucl.ac.uk
4. Department of Women's Cancer, Institute for Women's Health, University College London, London WC1E 6BT, UK; r.gunu@ucl.ac.uk (R.G.); j.k.kalsi@ucl.ac.uk (J.K.K.); john.timms@ucl.ac.uk (J.F.T.); i.jacobs@unsw.edu.au (I.J.J.)
5. Clinical Biochemistry, Barts Health NHS Trust, London E1 8PR, UK; anne.dawnay@bartshealth.nhs.uk
6. Department of Biology and Geology, Physics and Inorganic Chemistry, Universidad Rey Juan Carlos, 28933 Madrid, Spain; ines.perez@urjc.es
7. Wolfson Institute of Preventive Medicine, Barts CRUK Cancer Centre, Queen Mary University of London, London EC1M 6BQ, UK
8. Department of Gynaecological Oncology, St Bartholomew's Hospital, Barts Health NHS Trust, London EC1A 7BE, UK
9. University of Texas M.D. Anderson Cancer Center, Houston, TX 77030, USA; khlu@mdanderson.org (K.L.); wlyang@mdanderson.org (W.-L.Y.); rbast@mdanderson.org (R.C.B.J.)
10. Massachusetts General Hospital and Harvard Medical School, Boston, MA 02114, USA; sskates@mgh.harvard.edu
11. University of New South Wales, Sydney 2052, Australia
12. Department of Applied Mathematics, Lobachevsky University of Nyzhniy Novgorod, Nizhniy Novgorod 603105, Russia
13. Department of Mathematics, University College London, London WC1H 0AY, UK
* Correspondence: u.menon@ucl.ac.uk; Tel.: +44-20-7670-4649
† These authors contributed equally to this paper.
‡ Joint last author.

Received: 8 June 2020; Accepted: 14 July 2020; Published: 17 July 2020

Abstract: Longitudinal CA125 algorithms are the current basis of ovarian cancer screening. We report on longitudinal algorithms incorporating multiple markers. In the multimodal arm of United Kingdom Collaborative Trial of Ovarian Cancer Screening (UKCTOCS), 50,640 postmenopausal women underwent annual screening using a serum CA125 longitudinal algorithm. Women (cases) with invasive tubo-ovarian cancer (WHO 2014) following outcome review with stored annual serum samples donated in the 5 years preceding diagnosis were matched 1:1 to controls (no invasive tubo-ovarian cancer) in terms of the number of annual samples and age at randomisation. Blinded samples were assayed for serum human epididymis protein 4 (HE4), CA72-4 and anti-TP53 autoantibodies. Multimarker method of mean trends (MMT) longitudinal algorithms were developed using the assay results and trial CA125 values on the training set and evaluated in the blinded validation set. The study set comprised of 1363 (2–5 per woman) serial samples from 179 cases and 181 controls. In the validation set, area under the curve (AUC) and sensitivity of longitudinal CA125-MMT algorithm were 0.911 (0.871–0.952) and 90.5% (82.5–98.6%). None of the longitudinal multi-marker algorithms (CA125-HE4, CA125-HE4-CA72-4, CA125-HE4-CA72-4-anti-TP53) performed better or improved on lead-time. Our population study suggests that longitudinal HE4, CA72-4, anti-TP53 autoantibodies adds little value to longitudinal serum CA125 as a first-line test in ovarian cancer screening of postmenopausal women.

Keywords: ovarian cancer; CA125; HE4; UKCTOCS; MMT; screening; postmenopausal women

1. Introduction

Ovarian cancer is the most fatal of all gynaecological malignancies [1]. Despite significant advances in treatment, the impact on mortality over the past three decades has been modest [2–5]. A key contributing factor is diagnosis at advanced stages when survival is poor (5-year survival rates for stage III/IV disease 35% versus 90% for stage I) [6]. Efforts over the past four decades have therefore focused on early detection. Advances in understanding the natural history has meanwhile clarified the need to focus on detecting invasive tubo-ovarian cancer (WHO 2014), especially Type II (high-grade serous) cancers as they account for most of the mortality.

Since its discovery in 1981, CA125 remains the best performing marker for ovarian cancer. It forms an integral part of differential diagnosis and has been studied extensively in the context of screening [7–10]. In screening, performance has been improved by the use of the Risk of Ovarian Cancer Algorithm (ROCA), which assesses serial changes in CA125 over time. As a first-line test for ovarian cancer screening, ROCA had a sensitivity of 85.8% in the United Kingdom Collaborative Trial of Ovarian Cancer Screening (UKCTOCS) during incidence screening [11]. Moreover, screening using the multimodal strategy (ROCA as the first-line test with transvaginal ultrasound as the second-line test) resulted for the first time in a stage shift in women diagnosed with invasive tubo-ovarian cancer compared with no screening, on an "intention to screen" analysis. The mortality benefit was however not definitive at the first analysis and further follow-up is underway [5]. Retrospective analysis using data from the trial suggests that other longitudinal CA125 algorithms such as parametric empirical Bayes (PEB) [12,13], parenclitic networks [14], deep learning [15] and method of mean trends (MMT) [16,17] are likely to perform similarly.

Over the years, data from small case–control studies [18,19] have suggested that markers like human epididymis protein 4 (HE4) and TP53 autoantibodies might complement CA125 in ovarian cancer screening. HE4 was the second best marker for invasive tubo-ovarian cancer after CA125 (sensitivity CA125 86%; HE4 73%) in a nested case–control study within the Prostate, Lung, Colorectal and Ovarian cancer screening (PLCO) trial using a single preclinical sample taken within 6 months of diagnosis [20]. Data from the Carotene and Retinol Efficacy Trial suggested that a panel including CA125, HE4 and mesothelin may provide a signal for ovarian cancer 3 years before diagnosis [21]. More recently, elevated anti-TP53 autoantibody levels were detected in 16% of cases not detected by ROCA in the UKCTOCS sample set, providing in these cases a lead time of 22 months [19]. Other studies have explored the performance of multi-marker (CA125, IGFBP2, LCAT, SHBG, GRP78 and calprotectin) [22] panels. All have used cut-offs for interpreting results. Longitudinal algorithms incorporating multiple markers have not been previously investigated.

We report on the performance of longitudinal multi-marker algorithms incorporating CA125, HE4, CA72-4 and anti-TP53 autoantibodies as a first-line test in ovarian cancer screening using the prospective specimen collection and the retrospective blinded evaluation (PRoBe) design [23] within the general population UKCTOCS trial.

2. Results

During a median follow-up of 11.1 (IQR 10.0–12.0) years, of the 46,237 women randomised to the multimodal screening (MMS) arm of UKCTOCS who had two or more annual screens, 238 were diagnosed with invasive tubo-ovarian cancer [24]. At the time of sample selection, 179 (75.2%) of the latter had adequate (>2 mL) serum in the biorepository. The final set comprised of 179 cases and 181 controls. Training and validation sets comprised of 181 women (90 invasive tubo-ovarian cancer cases, 91 controls; 676 annual samples) and 179 women (89 invasive tubo-ovarian cancer cases, 90 controls; 677 annual samples), respectively (Table 1), with 2–5 serial samples per woman.

Table 1. Details of cases (invasive tubo-ovarian cancer) and controls in training and validation sets.

Group	Overall		Annual Samples Available in Year Preceding Diagnosis	
	No. of Women	No. of Annual Samples	No. of Women	No. of Annual Samples
	Training Set			
Cases	90	317	68	68
Controls	91	359	113/167 *	608
	Validation Set			
Cases	89	332	74	74
Controls	90	355	105/173 *	613

* a case is included as a control until the screen is within a year of diagnosis for the purposes of this analysis—the first number is unique controls and the second number includes those who will become cases.

Of the cases, 68 and 74 were diagnosed within 1 year of sample in the training and validation set, respectively (Table 1). There was no difference in age between the cases and controls. Baseline and clinical characteristics of the women in the training and validation sets were well balanced (Table 2). There were 13 Type I, 74 Type II, and 3 Type uncertain tubo-ovarian cancers in the training set, and 11 Type I, 72 Type II, and 6 Type uncertain in the validation set. In the training set, four longitudinal multi-marker algorithms (CA125-HE4-MMT1, CA125-HE4-MMT2, CA125-HE4-CA72-4-MMT, CA125-HE4-CA72-4-anti-TP53-MMT) were derived and then applied to the validation set, which comprised of 670 annual samples from 179 women (Table 1).

For the detection of invasive tubo-ovarian cancers diagnosed within 1 year of last annual sample, at a fixed specificity of 87.6% (similar to ROCA as a first-line test in UKCTOCS), CA125, HE4 or CA72-4 alone had a sensitivity of 73%, 58.1%, and 37.8%, respectively (Table 3). Figure 1 shows the Receiver Operating Curve (ROC) for the performance of CA125-MMT versus the four newly developed models, CA125-HE4-MMT1, CA125-HE4-MMT2, CA125-HE4-CA72-4-MMT, CA125-HE4-CA72-4-anti-TP53-MMT, in the validation set. CA125-MMT provided a higher area under the curve (AUC) compared with any other model (0.911 versus 0.897–0.902) (Table 3). At a specificity of 87.6%, CA125-MMT outperformed all other multimarker models (sensitivity of 90.5% versus 81–86.5%) with CA125-HE4-MMT1 being the next best model.

Of the 74 invasive tubo-ovarian cancers in the validation set, 67 (90.5%) were detected by the CA125-MMT model, of whom 53 (79.1%) were Type II cancers (Table S1). Of the other models, the CA125-HE4-MMT1 detected 64 cancers with one additional woman with Type I cancer not detected by the CA125-MMT model.

In the lead time analysis, no multimarker algorithm outperformed CA125-MMT. The lead time from marker elevation/change point to diagnosis was on average 140–148 days (multimarker algorithms) compared with 152 days (CA125-MMT algorithm) (Table 4).

Table 2. Characteristics of cases and controls in training and validation sets.

Baseline Characteristics	Training Set	Validation Set
No. of women	181	179
Median age at recruitment (years)	63.54	63.68
BMI	26.46	25.99
OCP use	90 (49.7%)	88 (49.2%)
Median Duration of OCP use (years)	5 ($n = 89$)	5 ($n = 86$)
Hysterectomy	35 (19.3%)	34 (19.0%)
% White ethnicity	177 (97.8%)	174 (97.6%)
HRT use	25 (13.8%)	33 (18.4%)
Personal history of breast cancer	3 (1.66%)	7 (3.91%)
Morphology of Cases		
Invasive tubo-ovarian cancer	90	89
Histological Type of Invasive Tubo-Ovarian Cancer		
Type I	**13**	**11**
Endometrioid (low grade)	6	5
Serous (low grade)	1	2
Clear cell	6	4
Type II	**68**	**63**
High grade serous ovarian	57	62
Carcinoma, NOS	10	3
Endometrioid (high grade)	6	5
Carcinosarcoma	1	2
Type uncertain	**3**	**6**
Carcinoma, NOS	2	4
Serous (grade unknown)	1	2
Stage of Invasive Tubo-Ovarian Cancer		
I	21	20
II	12	10
III	47	53
IV	10	6

BMI, body mass index; OCP, oral contraceptive pill; HRT, hormone replacement therapy.

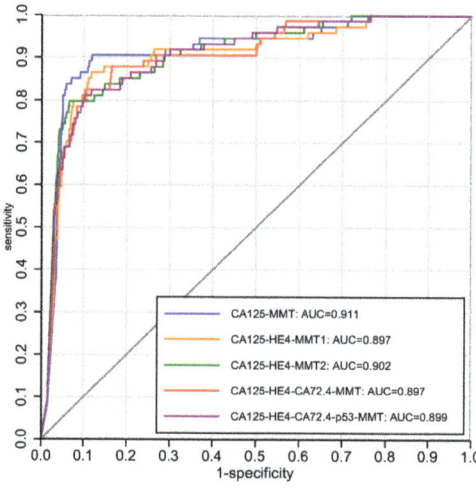

Figure 1. ROC curves with the AUC for each of the longitudinal algorithms.

Table 3. Sensitivity and area under the ROC curve (AUC) of algorithms for the detection of invasive tubo-ovarian cancer diagnosed within one year of sample in the validation set.

Algorithms	AUC (95%CI)	Sensitivity (95%CI) at 87.6% SPECIFICITY
CA125-MMT	91.1	90.5
	(87.1 to 95.2)	(82.5 to 98.6)
CA125-HE4-MMT1	89.7	86.5
	(85.6 to 93.8)	(77.7 to 95.2)
CA125-HE4-MMT2	90.2	81
	(86.4 to 94)	(71.8 to 90.4)
CA125-HE4-CA72-4-MMT	89.7	82.4
	(85.8 to 93.7)	(73.5 to 91.4)
CA125-HE4-CA72-4-anti-TP53-MMT	90	82.4
	(86.2 to 93.6)	(73.5 to 91.4)
CA125	86.5	73
	(81.1 to 91.9)	(61.1 to 84.8)
HE4	80.4	58.1
	(74.8 to 86)	(45.4 to 70.8)
CA72-4	71.7	37.8
	(65 to 78.5)	(22.9 to 49.8)

AUC, area under ROC curve; CI, confidence interval.

Table 4. Lead time of algorithms for the detection of invasive tubo-ovarian cancer in the validation set.

Algorithm	No. of Cases Detected by Algorithm	Mean Lead Time	SD
CA125-MMT	67	152	95
CA125-HE4-MMT1	64	148	95
CA125-HE4-MMT2	60	140	91
CA125-HE4-CA72-4-MMT	61	144	92
CA125-HE4-CA72-4-anti-TP53-MMT	61	144	92

The newer models offered no benefit in detecting poor prognostic cases (who died within 5 years of the last sample taken), with 12 of 67 (18.0%) women detected by the CA125-MMT model. The CA125-HE4-MMT2 model was able to detect 11 cases who died but at a cost of only detecting 60 cases. None of the other models were able to improve on this.

3. Discussion

3.1. Principal Findings

This is the first study to explore the added value of longitudinal multi-marker profiles to longitudinal CA125 for ovarian cancer screening. In this population-based case–control study, the addition of longitudinal HE4 or other markers such as CA72-4 and anti-TP53 did not improve on the performance of the longitudinal single marker CA125 algorithm in postmenopausal women [16]. There was also no improvement in lead time over longitudinal CA125. It would therefore be hard to justify the higher costs of including HE4 alongside CA125 in this population.

3.2. Results in Context

The current sensitivity of multimodal ovarian cancer screening is 87%. The MMS strategy consists of first-line screening using the longitudinal CA125 algorithm (ROCA) followed by repeat CA125 profiling and transvaginal ultrasound in women with intermediate or elevated test results. There has been longstanding interest in the possibility of increasing sensitivity by adding other markers that might help detect the 15% of the cases that are currently missed using the MMS strategy, which is probably due to the tumours not expressing CA125. HE4 has been the fore runner among potential markers ever since being highlighted in the study by Cramer and colleagues [20] using samples from the ovarian cancer screening arm of the PLCO trial. This study showed that out of 35 markers evaluated in a single sample taken 6 months prior to diagnosis in 118 women with ovarian cancer, HE4 (sensitivity 73%) was the second best marker to CA125 (sensitivity 86%). A previous exploratory study nested within the UKCTOCS cohort which was enriched for the missed cases also seemed to suggest that longitudinal HE4 and CA72-4 might improve sensitivity [25]. In the same UKCTOCS nested case–control study, p53 autoantibody profile was shown to complement CA125 in that it was able to detect 20.7% of those not detected by ROCA [19]. This was however not borne out in our rigorous study that used all available samples from the multimodal cohort. Our results using a cut-off as used in the PLCO analysis resulted in similar results (HE4 sensitivity 58.1% vs. 73% in PLCO; CA125 73% versus 86% in PLCO).

3.3. Clinical and Research Implications

There are now a number of longitudinal CA125 algorithms [16,26]. The advantage of the MMT methodologies presented here is that they incorporate longitudinal profiling of multiple biomarkers in a single algorithm. This sets the stage for future work incorporating novel markers as they gain recognition in ovarian cancer screening. Moreover, the longitudinal algorithms framework described here is applicable to other cancers and diseases where a serial profile of multiple markers is available.

3.4. Strengths and Limitations

The major strength is the decrease in bias through the use of a population-based nested case–control as per the PRoBE study design [23]. All samples were prospectively collected before outcome ascertainment. Linkage to electronic health records and independent outcome review of cases ensured complete and accurate data. The study has involved the largest dataset of serial samples up to 5 years prior to diagnosis of tubo-ovarian cancer in postmenopausal women from the general population that we are aware of. While the number of cases may seem small, the set consisted of 75% of all women who had two or more annual screens and were diagnosed with invasive tubo-ovarian cancer in the course of 343,156 screens. CA125, HE4 and CA72-4 assays were assayed by ELISA (enzyme-linked immunosorbent assay), the gold standard [27] in assaying markers. When applying the algorithm in the validation set, the statistician was blinded to the outcome. The algorithms described have a flexible modelling framework and hence can be used more widely. HE4 levels are known to increase with age in healthy people [28]. To address this in our design we have used age-matched controls. Moreover, as our models are based on trend indices rather than raw HE4 levels, the variation in age is unlikely to affect our results. While all women donated annual samples, it needs to be noted that the available serial repeat samples were influenced by the use of CA125 and ROCA in the trial. The results cannot be extrapolated to high-risk screening strategies where the frequency of screening is 6-monthly or less. In these high risk populations, ovarian cancer screening, if undertaken, usually starts at age 35 and in these premenopausal women HE4 may be helpful in ruling out endometriosis. We only used one control per case due to limited funds. Including a larger number of controls would have shed more light on the biological variation of HE4 in postmenopausal women.

4. Materials and Methods

4.1. Subjects

Between April 2001 and September 2005, 202,638 postmenopausal women aged 50–74 were recruited to UKCTOCS through 13 trial centres based in England, Wales and Northern Ireland (NI). The women were randomised to annual screening: (1) MMS using serum CA125 interpreted with the

ROCA followed by transvaginal ultrasound (TVS) as a second-line test ($n = 50{,}640$); (2) ultrasound (USS) screening using TVS alone ($n = 50{,}639$); or (3) no screening (control) group ($n = 101{,}359$) in a 1:1:2 ratio, as described previously [29,30]. In the MMS group, based on ROCA, women were triaged to (1) annual screening if normal; (2) repeat CA125 in 6 weeks if intermediate; (3) repeat CA125 and TVS if the risk was elevated. Women with abnormal ultrasound or persistent elevated risk (irrespective of scan findings) had clinical assessment by a trial clinician and additional investigations within the NHS. Women who had surgery or biopsy for suspected tubo-ovarian cancer after clinical assessment were considered trial-screen positive. Blood samples were taken at the trial centres in gel tubes (8 mL gel separation serum tubes; Greiner Bio-One 455071, Stonehouse, UK) and transported at room temperature overnight to the central UKCTOCS laboratory using the standard protocol [11,29,31]. The samples received within 56 h of venepuncture were processed by centrifuging at $1500\times g$ for 10 min. The serum was separated and assayed for CA125. The excess serum was pre-cooled at −80 °C and stored in 500 μL straws in liquid nitrogen at an off-site cryorepository until the sample was retrieved and thawed for the current analysis.

UKCTOCS was approved by the UK North West Multicentre Research Ethics Committees (North West MREC 00/8/34) on 21 June 2000 with site-specific approval from the local regional ethics committees and the Caldicott guardians (data controllers) of the primary care trusts. The current study was approved by the NRES (National Research Ethics Service) Committee North East-Tyne & Wear South (Ref: 15/NE/0025) on 20 January 2015.

All women were followed up through linkage via electronic health records for cancers and deaths as previously detailed [5,30] (NHS Digital, England and Wales; Northern Ireland Cancer Registry and NI Health and Social Care Business Services Organisation, NI). Women also completed two follow-up postal questionnaires; 3–5 years after randomisation, and in April 2014. As for the mortality analysis previously undertaken [5], cancer registrations received up to 5 April 2015 (England, Wales), and 9 April 2015 (NI) were used.

For all women with a possible diagnosis of ovarian cancer (one of 19 ICD-10 codes) [5], medical notes were requested and reviewed by a member of the independent Outcomes Review Committee (two pathologists and two gynaecological oncologists) who were masked to the randomisation group [5]. The Outcomes Review Committee [5] confirmed the final diagnosis—the primary cancer site (WHO 2014) [24]; the stage and morphology; and where possible, classified invasive tubo-ovarian cancer (WHO 2014 classification) [24] which included epithelial ovarian, fallopian tube and the primary peritoneal cancer as per WHO 2003 classification into Type I (low-grade serous, low-grade endometrioid, mucinous, clear cell) or Type II (high-grade serous, high-grade endometrioid, carcinosarcomas, undifferentiated) cancers or Type uncertain [32].

4.2. Sample Set and CA125, HE4, CA72-4 and Anti-TP53 Autoantibody Assays

The cases were all women in the MMS group diagnosed with invasive tubo-ovarian cancer [24] during follow-up, who had ≥2 serial samples taken within 5 years of diagnosis. Women with borderline epithelial and non-epithelial ovarian cancer were excluded. The controls were randomly chosen from the remaining women who did not have primary malignant neoplasm of the ovary. The cases were matched (1:1) to controls in terms of the number of annual samples available and age (±6 months) at randomisation.

The sample set for the study included all serial samples in the cases and controls where >2 mL serum was available in the cryorepository.

Once assayed for CA125 (Roche Diagnostics, Burgess Hill, UK), the excess serum was stored in liquid nitrogen in an off-site commercial cryorepository until it was retrieved for this study.

CA125 measurements (Roche, Burgess Hill, UK) completed as part of the UKCTOCS screening protocol were used along with anti-TP53 autoantibody values assayed during a previously reported study [19]. HE4 and CA72-4 (Roche Diagnostics, Burgess Hill) were assayed on all samples using the Roche Cobas analyser at the UCL Department of Women's Cancer Proteomics laboratory.

4.3. Method of Mean Trends (MMT) Algorithms Incorporating CA125, HE4, CA72-4 and Anti-TP53 Autoantibody

The MMT that evaluates the dynamics of longitudinal CA125 measurements has been described previously [16].

In brief, the serial pattern of a particular biomarker $Y_{i,j}$, $j = 1\ldots T$ of each woman "i" was mapped into a five-variable space. The new variables included the mean derivative weighted to the most recent measurement, the mean area under the time series (1), the coefficient of variation (2), the "centre of mass" of the time series (3) and the most recent measurement.

$$\left(\sum_{j=1}^{T-1} \frac{(Y_{i,j+1} - Y_{i,j})(t_{i,j+1} - t_{i,j})}{2}\right)/(T-1) \quad (1)$$

$$\sqrt{\frac{\sum_{j=1}^{T}(Y_{i,j} - \overline{Y}_i)^2}{T}}/\overline{Y}_i \quad (2)$$

$$\frac{\sum_{j=1}^{T} Y_{i,j} t_{i,j}}{\sum_{j=1}^{T} t_{i,j}} \quad (3)$$

The mean derivative was evaluated as $\sum_{j=1}^{T-1} w_{ij} \frac{Y_{i,j+1} - Y_{i,j}}{t_{i,j+1} - t_{i,j}}$ where weights w_j were computed for each interval between two consecutive measurements as $w_{ij} = \frac{1}{t_{i,T} - (t_{i,j+1} + t_{i,j})/2}$. Here, $t_{i,T}$ was the age of the patient at the time of the most recent sample, while $t_{i,j}$ was age of the patient when the j-th sample was taken.

To use this approach to incorporate multiple serial biomarkers, for each of the proteins, the aforementioned five variables were evaluated and combined together into a logistic regression with AIC (Akaike information criterion) used to select the predictors that explain the labels of the patients (control = 0, case = 1) in the most optimal way.

With the MMT approach, we generated four separate models for the prediction of the risk of ovarian cancer using the serial measurements of multiple biomarkers:

- CA125-HE4-MMT1, where variable selection was made only over HE4 indices added to the reported CA125-MMT model [16];
- CA125-HE4-MMT2, where five indices for both CA125 and HE4 were used with further variable selection;
- CA125-HE4-CA72-4-MMT, where five indices for CA125, HE4 and CA72-4 were used with further variable selection;
- CA125-HE4-CA72-4- anti-TP53-MMT, where five indices for CA125, HE4, CA72-4 and anti-TP53 were used with further variable selection.

The performance of these models was evaluated against the original CA125-MMT approach as well as the actual biomarkers levels.

4.4. Statistical Analysis

The cases and controls were randomly split into "training" and "validation" sets in a 1:1 ratio. Longitudinal CA125 MMT described previously [16], and four separate longitudinal multi-marker (CA125-HE4-MMT1, CA125-HE4-MMT2, CA125-HE4-CA72-4-MMT and CA125-HE4-CA72-4-anti-TP53-MMT) algorithms were built using all available serial samples from the cases and controls in the "training" set by OB. OB then applied them to the blinded "validation" set.

Statistical analysis was undertaken by MB to ensure blinding. The performance characteristics of the newly constructed algorithms as a first-line test were evaluated and compared with the CA125-MMT in terms of the following: (1) sensitivity at a fixed specificity of 87.6% similar to ROCA in UKCTOCS [11];

(2) average lead time for all cases detected (the date of detection is the date when risk given by algorithm is abnormal and for all further annual measurements it remains abnormal); (3) the area under the receiver operating characteristic (ROC) curve (AUC). Inference for the ROC curves was based on cluster-robust standard errors that accounted for the serially correlated nature of the samples [33]. At fixed specificity (87.6%), the performance characteristics of CA125 and HE4 cut-offs were compared with those of the newly derived algorithm.

Only annual samples were included in this analysis. The last blood sample was considered as true positive (if within 1 year from diagnosis) and all prior annual samples as true negatives. In the controls, all samples were included as true negatives.

To investigate whether any of the algorithms identified invasive tubo-ovarian cancer cases earlier than CA125-MMT, we performed lead time analysis, where the mean interval from detection to diagnosis was compared for all algorithms. For each algorithm, the average interval was calculated in days for only those cases that were detected as abnormal by the algorithm. Here, we assumed that an algorithm identified a cancer case at a particular measurement if both at this and at all subsequent measurements it classified the risk as abnormal. A further analysis explored how many of the cancers missed by ROCA during the trial (trial-screen negative cases) would have been detected by each of the algorithms.

5. Conclusions

In the context of screening, our study suggests that the additional value of HE4, CA72-4 and p53 autoantibodies to CA125 as a first line test in screening for ovarian cancer of postmenopausal women from the general population is limited. Further work on the value of these markers as a reflex test following elevated risk may show promise and strengthen the confidence in cancer diagnosis and thus shorten the period between the screening test and surgical intervention.

Supplementary Materials: The following are available online at http://www.mdpi.com/2072-6694/12/7/1931/s1, Table S1: Details of invasive epithelial cancers diagnosed within 1 year of sample detected/missed by algorithms in the validation set

Author Contributions: Conceptualisation, U.M., A.G.-M., O.B., A.Z., A.R., R.C.B.J.; literature search, U.M., A.G.-M.; support and development of CA72-4 and anti-TP53 autoantibody assays, K.L., W.-L.Y. and R.C.B.J.; preparation of the dataset, A.G.-M., A.R.; development of the MMT algorithm, O.B., A.Z.; trial conduct, C.K., R.G., J.K.K., A.D., R.M., M.P., S.J.S., I.J.J.; statistical analysis and preparation of figures and tables, O.B., I.P.M., M.B., J.F.T. All authors have read and agreed to the published version of the manuscript.

Funding: The analysis is part of PROMISE, which was funded through Cancer Research UK PRC Programme Grant A12677 and by The Eve Appeal. University College London investigators received support from the National Institute for Health Research University College London Hospitals Biomedical Research Centre and from MRC core funding (MR_UU_12023). UKCTOCS was core funded by the Medical Research Council (G9901012 and G0801228), Cancer Research UK (C1479/A2884), and the Department of Health with additional support from the Eve Appeal. J.F.T. received support from CRUK Early Detection Committee Project Award (C12077/A26223). S.J.S. received additional support from an NCI Early Detection Research Network grant (CA152990). R.C.B.J. was supported by funds from the Early Detection Research Network (5 U01 CA200462-02) and the MD Anderson Ovarian SPOREs (P50 CA83639 and P50 CA217685), National Cancer Institute, Department of Health and Human Services, the Cancer Prevention Research Institute of Texas (RP101382 and RP160145), Golfer's Against Cancer, the Mossy Foundation, the Roberson Endowment, National Foundation for Cancer Research, The K Yao Foundation, UT MD Anderson Women's Moon Shot and generous donations from Stuart and Gaye Lynn Zarrow. A.Z. acknowledges support by MRC grant MR/R02524X/1 and the grant of the Ministry of Education and Science of the Russian Federation Agreement No. 074-02-2018-330.

Acknowledgments: We are particularly grateful to the women throughout the UK who have participated in the trial. We thank all the staff involved in the trial for their hard work and dedication. We thank the Data Monitoring and Ethics Committee and the independent Trial Steering Committee members.

Conflicts of Interest: U.M. has stock ownership and has received research funding from Abcodia. I.J.J. reports personal fees from and stock ownership in Abcodia as the non-executive director and consultant. He reports personal fees from Women's Health Specialists as the director. He has a patent for the Risk of Ovarian Cancer algorithm and an institutional license to Abcodia with royalty agreement. He is a trustee (2012–14) and Emeritus Trustee (2015 to present) for The Eve Appeal. S.J.S. is a member of Scientific Advisory Boards for the LUNGevity Foundation and SISCAPA Assay Technologies. He is a consultant to Abcodia. Massachusetts General Hospital has co-licensed software for the Risk of Ovarian Cancer algorithm to Abcodia. All other authors declare no competing interests.

References

1. CRUK. Ten Most Common Causes of Cancer Death in Females. Available online: https://www.cancerresearchuk.org/health-professional/cancer-statistics/mortality/common-cancers-compared#heading-Two (accessed on 8 January 2019).
2. van Nagell, J.R., Jr.; Miller, R.W.; DeSimone, C.P.; Ueland, F.R.; Podzielinski, I.; Goodrich, S.T.; Elder, J.W.; Huang, B.; Kryscio, R.J.; Pavlik, E.J. Long-term survival of women with epithelial ovarian cancer detected by ultrasonographic screening. *Obs. Gynecol* **2011**, *118*, 1212–1221. [CrossRef] [PubMed]
3. Buys, S.S.; Partridge, E.; Black, A.; Johnson, C.C.; Lamerato, L.; Isaacs, C.; Reding, D.J.; Greenlee, R.T.; Yokochi, L.A.; Kessel, B.; et al. Effect of screening on ovarian cancer mortality: The Prostate, Lung, Colorectal and Ovarian (PLCO) Cancer Screening Randomized Controlled Trial. *JAMA J. Am. Med. Assoc.* **2011**, *305*, 2295–2303. [CrossRef] [PubMed]
4. Kobayashi, H.; Yamada, Y.; Sado, T.; Sakata, M.; Yoshida, S.; Kawaguchi, R.; Kanayama, S.; Shigetomi, H.; Haruta, S.; Tsuji, Y.; et al. A randomized study of screening for ovarian cancer: A multicenter study in Japan. *Int. J. Gynecol. Cancer Off. J. Int. Gynecol. Cancer Soc.* **2008**, *18*, 414–420. [CrossRef]
5. Jacobs, I.J.; Menon, U.; Ryan, A.; Gentry-Maharaj, A.; Burnell, M.; Kalsi, J.K.; Amso, N.N.; Apostolidou, S.; Benjamin, E.; Cruickshank, D.; et al. Ovarian cancer screening and mortality in the UK Collaborative Trial of Ovarian Cancer Screening (UKCTOCS): A randomised controlled trial. *Lancet (Lond. Engl.)* **2016**, *387*, 945–956. [CrossRef]
6. CRUK. Ovarian Cancer Survival by Stage at Diagnosis. Available online: http://www.cancerresearchuk.org/health-professional/cancer-statistics/statistics-by-cancer-type/ovarian-cancer/survival#heading-Three (accessed on 12 December 2018).
7. Lu, K.H.; Skates, S.; Hernandez, M.A.; Bedi, D.; Bevers, T.; Leeds, L.; Moore, R.; Granai, C.; Harris, S.; Newland, W.; et al. A 2-stage ovarian cancer screening strategy using the Risk of Ovarian Cancer Algorithm (ROCA) identifies early-stage incident cancers and demonstrates high positive predictive value. *Cancer* **2013**, *119*, 3454–3461. [CrossRef] [PubMed]
8. Menon, U.; Skates, S.J.; Lewis, S.; Rosenthal, A.N.; Rufford, B.; Sibley, K.; Macdonald, N.; Dawnay, A.; Jeyarajah, A.; Bast, R.C., Jr.; et al. Prospective study using the risk of ovarian cancer algorithm to screen for ovarian cancer. *J. Clin. Oncol. Off. J. Am. Soc. Clin. Oncol.* **2005**, *23*, 7919–7926. [CrossRef] [PubMed]
9. Skates, S.J.; Horick, N.; Yu, Y.; Xu, F.J.; Berchuck, A.; Havrilesky, L.J.; de Bruijn, H.W.; van der Zee, A.G.; Woolas, R.P.; Jacobs, I.J.; et al. Preoperative sensitivity and specificity for early-stage ovarian cancer when combining cancer antigen CA-125II, CA 15-3, CA 72-4, and macrophage colony-stimulating factor using mixtures of multivariate normal distributions. *J. Clin. Oncol. Off. J. Am. Soc. Clin. Oncol.* **2004**, *22*, 4059–4066. [CrossRef]
10. Skates, S.J.; Pauler, D.K.; Jacobs, I.J. Screening Based on the Risk of Cancer Calculation From Bayesian Hierarchical Changepoint and Mixture Models of Longitudinal Markers. *J. Am. Stat. Assoc.* **2001**, *96*, 429–439. [CrossRef]
11. Menon, U.; Ryan, A.; Kalsi, J.; Gentry-Maharaj, A.; Dawnay, A.; Habib, M.; Apostolidou, S.; Singh, N.; Benjamin, E.; Burnell, M.; et al. Risk Algorithm Using Serial Biomarker Measurements Doubles the Number of Screen-Detected Cancers Compared With a Single-Threshold Rule in the United Kingdom Collaborative Trial of Ovarian Cancer Screening. *J. Clin. Oncol. Off. J. Am. Soc. Clin. Oncol.* **2015**, *33*, 2062–2071. [CrossRef]
12. Drescher, C.W.; Shah, C.; Thorpe, J.; O'Briant, K.; Anderson, G.L.; Berg, C.D.; Urban, N.; McIntosh, M.W. Longitudinal screening algorithm that incorporates change over time in CA125 levels identifies ovarian cancer earlier than a single-threshold rule. *J. Clin. Oncol. Off. J. Am. Soc. Clin. Oncol.* **2013**, *31*, 387–392. [CrossRef]
13. McIntosh, M.W.; Urban, N. A parametric empirical Bayes method for cancer screening using longitudinal observations of a biomarker. *Biostatistics* **2003**, *4*, 27–40. [CrossRef]
14. Whitwell, H.J.; Blyuss, O.; Menon, U.; Timms, J.F.; Zaikin, A. Parenclitic networks for predicting ovarian cancer. *Oncotarget* **2018**, *9*, 22717–22726. [CrossRef] [PubMed]

15. Vázquez, M.A.; Mariño, I.P.; Blyuss, O.; Ryan, A.; Gentry-Maharaj, A.; Kalsi, J.; Manchanda, R.; Jacobs, I.; Menon, U.; Zaikin, A. A quantitative performance study of two automatic methods for the diagnosis of ovarian cancer. *Biomed. Signal Process. Control* **2018**, *46*, 86–93. [CrossRef] [PubMed]
16. Blyuss, O.; Burnell, M.; Ryan, A.; Gentry-Maharaj, A.; Marino, I.P.; Kalsi, J.; Manchanda, R.; Timms, J.F.; Parmar, M.; Skates, S.J.; et al. Comparison of Longitudinal CA125 Algorithms as a First-Line Screen for Ovarian Cancer in the General Population. *Clin. Cancer Res. Off. J. Am. Assoc. Cancer Res.* **2018**, *24*, 4726–4733. [CrossRef]
17. Whitwell, H.J.; Worthington, J.; Blyuss, O.; Gentry-Maharaj, A.; Ryan, A.; Gunu, R.; Kalsi, J.; Menon, U.; Jacobs, I.; Zaikin, A.; et al. Improved early detection of ovarian cancer using longitudinal multimarker models. *Br. J. Cancer* **2020**, *122*, 847–856. [CrossRef] [PubMed]
18. Simmons, A.R.; Fourkala, E.O.; Gentry-Maharaj, A.; Ryan, A.; Sutton, M.N.; Baggerly, K.; Zheng, H.; Lu, K.H.; Jacobs, I.; Skates, S.; et al. Complementary Longitudinal Serum Biomarkers to CA125 for Early Detection of Ovarian Cancer. *Cancer Prev. Res.* **2019**, *12*, 391–400. [CrossRef] [PubMed]
19. Yang, W.L.; Gentry-Maharaj, A.; Simmons, A.; Ryan, A.; Fourkala, E.O.; Lu, Z.; Baggerly, K.A.; Zhao, Y.; Lu, K.H.; Bowtell, D.; et al. Elevation of TP53 Autoantibody Before CA125 in Preclinical Invasive Epithelial Ovarian Cancer. *Clin. Cancer Res. Off. J. Am. Assoc. Cancer Res.* **2017**, *23*, 5912–5922. [CrossRef]
20. Cramer, D.W.; Bast, R.C., Jr.; Berg, C.D.; Diamandis, E.P.; Godwin, A.K.; Hartge, P.; Lokshin, A.E.; Lu, K.H.; McIntosh, M.W.; Mor, G.; et al. Ovarian cancer biomarker performance in prostate, lung, colorectal, and ovarian cancer screening trial specimens. *Cancer Prev. Res.* **2011**, *4*, 365–374. [CrossRef]
21. Anderson, G.L.; McIntosh, M.; Wu, L.; Barnett, M.; Goodman, G.; Thorpe, J.D.; Bergan, L.; Thornquist, M.D.; Scholler, N.; Kim, N.; et al. Assessing lead time of selected ovarian cancer biomarkers: A nested case-control study. *J. Natl. Cancer Inst.* **2010**, *102*, 26–38. [CrossRef]
22. Russell, M.R.; Graham, C.; D'Amato, A.; Gentry-Maharaj, A.; Ryan, A.; Kalsi, J.K.; Ainley, C.; Whetton, A.D.; Menon, U.; Jacobs, I.; et al. A combined biomarker panel shows improved sensitivity for the early detection of ovarian cancer allowing the identification of the most aggressive type II tumours. *Br. J. Cancer* **2017**, *117*, 666–674. [CrossRef]
23. Pepe, M.S.; Feng, Z.; Janes, H.; Bossuyt, P.M.; Potter, J.D. Pivotal evaluation of the accuracy of a biomarker used for classification or prediction: Standards for study design. *J. Natl. Cancer Inst.* **2008**, *100*, 1432–1438. [CrossRef]
24. Kurman, R.J.; Carcangiu, M.L.; Herrington, S.; Young, R.H. *WHO Classification of Tumours of Female Reproductive Organs (IARC WHO Classification of Tumours)*, 4th ed.; IARC: Lyon, France, 2014; Volume 6.
25. Simmons, A.; Fourkala, E.O.; Gentry-Maharaj, A.; Ryan, A.; Baggerly, K.A.; Zheng, H.; Lu, K.H.; Jacobs, I.; Skates, S.J.; Menon, U.; et al. Validation of longitudinal performance of a multi-marker panel for the early detection of ovarian cancer. *Cancer Prev. Res.* **2019**, in press.
26. Mariño, I.P.; Blyuss, O.; Ryan, A.; Gentry-Maharaj, A.; Timms, J.F.; Dawnay, A.; Kalsi, J.; Jacobs, I.; Menon, U.; Zaikin, A. Change-point of multiple biomarkers in women with ovarian cancer. *Biomed. Signal Process. Control* **2017**, *33*, 169–177. [CrossRef]
27. Thiha, A.; Ibrahim, F. A Colorimetric Enzyme-Linked Immunosorbent Assay (ELISA) Detection Platform for a Point-of-Care Dengue Detection System on a Lab-on-Compact-Disc. *Sensors* **2015**, *15*, 11431–11441. [CrossRef] [PubMed]
28. Moore, R.G.; Miller, M.C.; Eklund, E.E.; Lu, K.H.; Bast, R.C., Jr.; Lambert-Messerlian, G. Serum levels of the ovarian cancer biomarker HE4 are decreased in pregnancy and increase with age. *Am. J. Obstet. Gynecol.* **2012**, *206*, 349.e1–349.e7. [CrossRef]
29. Menon, U.; Gentry-Maharaj, A.; Hallett, R.; Ryan, A.; Burnell, M.; Sharma, A.; Lewis, S.; Davies, S.; Philpott, S.; Lopes, A.; et al. Sensitivity and specificity of multimodal and ultrasound screening for ovarian cancer, and stage distribution of detected cancers: Results of the prevalence screen of the UK Collaborative Trial of Ovarian Cancer Screening (UKCTOCS). *Lancet Oncol.* **2009**, *10*, 327–340. [CrossRef]
30. Menon, U.; Gentry-Maharaj, A.; Ryan, A.; Sharma, A.; Burnell, M.; Hallett, R.; Lewis, S.; Lopez, A.; Godfrey, K.; Oram, D.; et al. Recruitment to multicentre trials–lessons from UKCTOCS: Descriptive study. *BMJ* **2008**, *337*, a2079. [CrossRef] [PubMed]
31. Blyuss, O.; Gentry-Maharaj, A.; Fourkala, E.-O.; Ryan, A.; Zaikin, A.; Menon, U.; Jacobs, I.; Timms, J.F. Serial Patterns of Ovarian Cancer Biomarkers in a Prediagnosis Longitudinal Dataset. *BioMed Res. Int.* **2015**, *2015*, 681416. [CrossRef] [PubMed]

32. Kurman, R.J.; Shih Ie, M. The origin and pathogenesis of epithelial ovarian cancer: A proposed unifying theory. *Am. J. Surg. Pathol.* **2010**, *34*, 433–443. [CrossRef] [PubMed]
33. Rogers, W. Regression standard errors in clustered samples. *Stata Tech. Bull.* **1993**, *13*, 19–23.

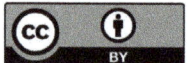
© 2020 by the authors. Licensee MDPI, Basel, Switzerland. This article is an open access article distributed under the terms and conditions of the Creative Commons Attribution (CC BY) license (http://creativecommons.org/licenses/by/4.0/).

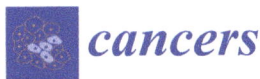

Review

Rare Germline Genetic Variants and the Risks of Epithelial Ovarian Cancer

Marina Pavanello [1,2,†], Isaac HY Chan [1,†], Amir Ariff [1,2], Paul DP Pharoah [3], Simon A. Gayther [4,5] and Susan J. Ramus [1,2,*]

1. School of Women's and Children's Health, Faculty of Medicine, University of New South Wales, Sydney 2052, Australia; m.pavanello@student.unsw.edu.au (M.P.); isaac.chan@unsw.edu.au (I.H.C.); amir.ariff@unsw.edu.au (A.A.)
2. Adult Cancer Program, Lowy Cancer Research Centre, University of New South Wales, Sydney 2052, Australia
3. Strangeways Research Laboratory, University of Cambridge, Cambridge CB1 8RN, UK; pp10001@medschl.cam.ac.uk
4. Center for Cancer Prevention and Translational Genomics, Cedars Sinai Medical Center, Los Angeles, CA 90048, USA; simon.gayther@cshs.org
5. Applied Genomics, Computation and Translational Core, Cedars Sinai Medical Center, Los Angeles, CA 90048, USA
* Correspondence: s.ramus@unsw.edu.au
† These authors have contributed equally to this work.

Received: 16 September 2020; Accepted: 14 October 2020; Published: 19 October 2020

Simple Summary: Several genes have been confirmed as risk genes for epithelial ovarian cancer (EOC). There are five main types of EOC, with different molecular changes and clinical characteristics, suggesting they should be considered different diseases. This review summarises the contribution of rare inherited mutations to EOC susceptibility, focussing on the frequency in each EOC type. Susceptibility genes can have a major clinical impact, reducing ovarian cancer incidence by screening of family members to detect women at higher risk than the general population. They can also lead to the development of new targeted treatments.

Abstract: A family history of ovarian or breast cancer is the strongest risk factor for epithelial ovarian cancer (EOC). Germline deleterious variants in the *BRCA1* and *BRCA2* genes confer EOC risks by age 80, of 44% and 17% respectively. The mismatch repair genes, particularly *MSH2* and *MSH6*, are also EOC susceptibility genes. Several other DNA repair genes, *BRIP1*, *RAD51C*, *RAD51D*, and *PALB2*, have been identified as moderate risk EOC genes. EOC has five main histotypes; high-grade serous (HGS), low-grade serous (LGS), clear cell (CCC), endometrioid (END), and mucinous (MUC). This review examines the current understanding of the contribution of rare genetic variants to EOC, focussing on providing frequency data for each histotype. We provide an overview of frequency and risk for pathogenic variants in the known susceptibility genes as well as other proposed genes. We also describe the progress to-date to understand the role of missense variants and the different breast and ovarian cancer risks for each gene. Identification of susceptibility genes have clinical impact by reducing disease-associated mortality through improving risk prediction, with the possibility of prevention strategies, and developing new targeted treatments and these clinical implications are also discussed.

Keywords: ovarian cancer risk; rare germline variants; susceptibility genes

1. Introduction

Epithelial ovarian cancer (EOC) is the seventh most common cancer in women worldwide, with over 295,000 incident cases each year, and is the leading cause of mortality relating to gynaecological malignancies, with 184,000 deaths each year [1]. Typically, EOCs are stratified into five main histological subtypes: High grade serous, which account for up to 70% of all EOC cases, endometrioid (~10%), clear cell (~10%), mucinous (~3%), and low-grade serous carcinomas (<5%) [2]. The five different histotypes have different risk factors and molecular characteristics. The inherited genetics of each histotype is also likely to be different.

The prognosis of ovarian cancer is poor, with a five-year survival rate of just 47% [3]. Ovarian cancer is difficult to diagnose early in its disease course, and 80% of cases are diagnosed after extensive metastasis at stage III or IV, which carry a five-year survival rate of 41% and 20% respectively [3]. However, outcomes are good if ovarian cancer is detected early, with an 89% five-year survival in stage I cancers [3]. Screening for ovarian cancer is of limited utility and no studies investigating ovarian cancer screening have shown a significant impact of screening on mortality [4,5]. As a result, population-based screening for ovarian cancer is not recommended in the guidelines of any major society. As the prognosis of EOC is related to its stage at diagnosis, the ability to use genetic information to predict EOC risk and intervene before disease development would reduce overall mortality and morbidity in ovarian cancer [6].

A family history of EOC confers an increase in relative risk (RR) of ovarian cancer of 2.96. The known EOC risk genes explain less than half of the excess familial risk for EOC, suggesting that there are still undiscovered ovarian cancer predisposing genes to be found [7,8]. The known ovarian cancer predisposing genes are from two different DNA repair pathways. The homologous recombination (HR) DNA repair pathway and the mismatch repair (MMR) DNA repair pathway. The majority of the genes are part of the HR DNA repair pathway. *BRCA1* and *BRCA2* have been confirmed as highly penetrant predisposition genes for EOC [9]. Several other genes—*BRIP1*, *RAD51C*, *RAD51D*, and *PALB2*, recently described as moderate risk genes, are also part of this pathway [10–12]. The mismatch repair genes *MLH1*, *MSH2*, *MSH6*, and *PSM2* are also confirmed moderate risk EOC susceptibility genes [13]. The frequency of disease-associated variants in these genes is different for the different EOC histotypes. Thirty-seven common variants have been identified for ovarian cancer, using genome-wide association studies (GWAS) [14,15]. The ability to derive accurate risk estimates for ovarian cancer from genetic information in asymptomatic women has significant implications for ovarian cancer management.

This review aims to summarise the progress to date in efforts to understand the contribution of rare genetic variants to ovarian cancer and histotype specific differences, as well as the clinical implications of these discoveries. In the first part of this review, we describe germline protein truncating variants (insertion/deletions or nonsense) in confirmed EOC susceptibility genes, followed by an overview of the role of missense variants in these genes. Lastly, we described germline protein truncating variants in other proposed genes that have not been validated as EOC susceptibility genes.

2. Protein Truncating Variants in Confirmed Susceptibility Genes

2.1. BRCA1 and BRCA2

These two major breast/ovarian cancer susceptibility genes encode proteins that work in DNA replication pathways to avoid double-strand DNA damage. Deleterious protein truncating variants include small insertions and deletions and single base changes, as well as large genomic alterations, which account for approximately 10% of *BRCA1* variants [16]. Several deleterious missense variants have also been described.

The prevalence and penetrance of deleterious variants in *BRCA1* and *BRCA2* has been extensively studied in ovarian cancer patients. The case ascertainment, either from families with a history of breast or ovarian cancer or from the general ovarian cancer population, has a major impact on the results. The presence of founder mutations in the population also affects the prevalence and has important implications for clinical testing. The presence of founder mutations can allow for cheap and rapid testing and the potential for population screening. In the Ashkenazi Jewish population, there are three *BRCA* founder mutations (185delAG and 5382insC in *BRCA1* and 6174delT in *BRCA2*) that accounts for almost all mutations present in this population [17]. In the Icelandic population, there is a single founder mutation, 999del5, in the *BRCA2* gene. Most of the breast and ovarian cancer cases in Icelandic families have this *BRCA2* founder mutation, while mutations in *BRCA1* are very rare [18]. Founder mutations in the *BRCA* genes have also been reported in many other populations, including Russians [19,20], Polish [21], Norwegian [22], Finnish [23], Japanese [24], and Chinese [25]. While some mutations are restricted to isolated regions or certain populations, others are common across different countries, such as *BRCA1* 5382insC mutation that is common in many European populations [17].

Early studies of cases selected for a family history of breast or ovarian cancer found that 24–76% had deleterious variants in *BRCA1* and 1–17% had deleterious variants in *BRCA2* [17]. Recent studies using clinical testing laboratory data have reported the prevalence of *BRCA1/2* pathogenic variants in 5020 and 7489 cases from the USA [26,27], 4409 cases from France [28], and 3230 cases from a meta-analysis of 48 multi-gene panel testing-based studies [29]. In these studies, the frequency of germline pathogenic variants in *BRCA1* in ovarian cancer cases were 5.1%, 3.6%, 3.7%, and 8.6%, respectively, and 3.9%, 3.3%, 4.0%, and 4.5% in *BRCA2* [26–29].

Testing of unselected ovarian cancer cases in non-Ashkenazi Jewish populations shows that the frequency of deleterious *BRCA1* and *BRCA2* variants ranged from 3–10% and 0.6–6%, respectively [17]. Recent population-based studies from Table 1 found that 3.8–11.1% of cases have *BRCA1* deleterious variants and 4.3–6.4% had *BRCA2* deleterious variants.

In a large prospective study of *BRCA* carriers ascertained through family clinics, the cumulative risk, by age 80, of ovarian cancer in women with pathogenic variants in *BRCA1* and *BRCA2* was estimated to be 44% (95% confidence interval (CI), 36–53%) and 17% (95% CI, 11–25%), respectively [9]. The histotypes of ovarian cancer diagnosed in the study were not described [9]. Breast cancer was also assessed and the cumulative risk at the age of 80 years was estimated to be 72% (95% CI, 65–79%) for *BRCA1* carriers and 69% (95% CI, 61–77%) for *BRCA2* [9]. Variants in these *BRCA* genes are also associated with increased risk of pancreatic cancer [30] and high-grade prostate cancer [31].

Four studies, with cases unselected for age or family history, provided information on histotype (Table 1). Due to the small numbers of the much rarer histotypes (END, CCC, LGS, and MUC), the frequencies of germline pathogenic variants varied significantly. In an effort to estimate the frequency in these rarer histotypes, we have combined the results across studies. This showed that the frequency of deleterious variants in *BRCA1* were approximately 7.8% in HGS, 3% in END, 3.6% in CCC, 3.7% in LGS, and <1% in MUC [32–35]. In *BRCA2*, deleterious variants were seen in approximately 5.9% of HGS cases, 2.9% of END, 0.9% of CCC, 2.0% of LGS, and <1% of MUC [33–35] (Table 1). According to these data, both genes have a higher frequency of variants in the HGS histotype compared to the non-HGS histotypes, and a much lower frequency in mucinous cases. Available cumulative risks from these retrospective studies are comparable to the prospective study previously mentioned [9] (Table 1).

Ovarian cancer patients with deleterious variants in *BRCA1* and *BRCA2* are characterized by genomic instability within their tumours. They have a better response to platinum-based chemotherapies, resulting in improved five-year overall survival. Five-year overall survival for non-carriers was reported to be 36% (95% CI 34–38) compared to 44% (95% CI 40–48) for *BRCA1*-carriers and 52% (95% CI 46–58) for *BRCA2*-carriers [36]. However, this survival advantage was not present when follow-up was extended to 10 years [37,38].

Identifying pathogenic variants associated with increased risk of ovarian cancer has major clinical implications. Due to the magnitude of ovarian cancer risk associated with variants in *BRCA1* and *BRCA2*, risk-reducing salpingo-oophorectomy (RRSO) is currently recommended as a prevention strategy for *BRCA1* carriers by age 35 to 40 years, once the woman's childbearing is complete, and for *BRCA2* carriers by age 40 to 45 [39].

Table 1. Frequency of germline pathogenic variants in BRCA1/2 in epithelial ovarian cancer (EOC) histotypes, in cases from population studies.

Gene	Study	Cases Carriers/Total (Frequency)							Controls Carriers/Total (Frequency)		OR (95% CI)	Cumulative Risk (95% CI) [a]
		HGS	END	CCC	LGS	MUC	Mixed/Unk [b]	All EOC	Matched	Publicly Available		
BRCA1	Walsh et al., 2011 [34]	31/242 ** (12.8%)	2/23 (8.7%)	1/17 (5.9%)	**	-	6/78 (7.7%)	40/360 (11.1%)	-	-	NC	NC
	Alsop et al., 2012 [†] [32]	74/709 ** (10.4%)	7/119 (5.9%)	4/63 (6.3%)	**	-	3/110 (2.7%)	88/1001 (8.79%)	-	-	NC	NC
	Song et al., 2014 [^] [33]	58/1105 * (5.2%)	3/322 (0.9%)	3/192 (1.6%)	6/172 (3.5%)	1/157 (0.6%)	13/274 (4.7%)	84/2222 (3.78%)	1/1528 (0.07%)	-	60 [#] (10–2100)	61% (15–99%)
	Norquist et al., 2016 [35]	155/1498 (10.3%)	4/77 (5.2%)	4/58 (6.9%)	3/70 (4.3%)	0/16 (0%)	16/196 (8.2%)	142/1915 (7.41%)	-	114/36276 (0.31%)	48.9 (24–100)	NC
	Total	278/3554 (7.82%)	16/541 (2.95%)	12/330 (3.63%)	9/242 (3.72%)	1/173 (0.58%)	38/658 (5.77%)	354/5498 (6.43%)	1/1528 (0.07%)	-	-	-
BRCA2	Walsh et al., 2011 [34]	18/242 ** (7.4%)	0/23 (0%)	0/17 (0%)	**	-	5/78 (6.4%)	23/360 (6.38%)	-	-	NC	NC
	Alsop et al., 2012 [†] [32]	44/709 ** (6.2%)	3/119 (2.5%)	0/63 (0%)	**	-	6/110 (5.4%)	53/1001 (5.29%)	-	-	NC	NC
	Song et al., 2014 [^] [33]	64/1105 * (5.8%)	10/322 (3.1%)	3/192 (1.6%)	4/172 (2.3%)	1/157 (0.6%)	12/274 (4.4%)	94/2222 (4.23%)	4/1528 (0.26%)	-	17 [#] (6.3–63)	24% (10–62%)
	Norquist et al., 2016 [35]	85/1498 (5.7%)	3/77 (3.9%)	0/58 (0%)	1/70 (1.4%)	0/16 (0%)	9/196 (4.6%)	98/1915 (5.11%)	-	149/36276 (0.41%)	14 (8.2–23.8)	NC
	Total	211/3554 (5.93%)	16/541 (2.95%)	3/330 (0.91%)	5/242 (2.0%)	1/173 (0.57%)	32/658 (4.86%)	268/5498 (4.87%)	4/1528 (0.26%)	-	-	-

-: Not available, NC: Not calculated due to no controls or not described, ** Frequency of serous combined, * Frequency of HGS and serous undifferentiated, [#] Odds ratio (OR) for the matched controls analysis, [a] Risks based on all cases combined, [b] Mixed/Unknown includes some other histotypes, [†] Mucinous ovarian cancer cases were excluded, [^] Not screened for large genomic alterations. Bold: highlight info.

Furthermore, understanding the role of *BRCA1/2* variants in ovarian cancer has allowed for the development of targeted therapies, namely PARP (poly[adenosine diphosphate–ribose] polymerase) inhibitors, which improve progression-free survival in selected women with ovarian cancer. Approximately 50% of HGS cases present defects in DNA repair mechanisms due to pathogenic variants in the homologous recombination deficiency (HRD) genes, such as *BRCA1/2*, or due to functional inactivation through methylation [40]. PARPi have shown highly efficacious activity particularly in women with platinum-sensitive disease carrying *BRCA1/2* variants, or women with other homologous recombination deficiencies [41–43]. Improved activity has also been seen in women with recurrent disease regardless of their *BRCA* status [44]. As *BRCA1/2* status affects clinical management of affected women, current guidelines recommend *BRCA1/2* testing in all non-mucinous ovarian cancer cases [39].

2.2. BRIP1

The protein encoded by *BRIP1* is part of the Fanconi anaemia group (FANCJ) and is involved in the repair of DNA double-strand breaks by homologous recombination. *BRIP1* was described as a candidate risk gene by Walsh et al. that identified germline loss-of-function variants in 1% of ovarian cancer cases not selected for age or family history [34]. Pathogenic germline variants in *BRIP1* are the most common mutation found in ovarian cancer after *BRCA1/2* with a frequency of approximately 1% of the EOC cases [11].

The contribution of germline protein truncating variants in *BRIP1* have not yet been assessed in prospective studies. Ramus et al. described a relative risk associated with protein truncating variants in *BRIP1* of 11.2 (95% CI 3.2–34.1), with an estimated cumulative risk of 5.8% (95% CI 3.6–9.1%) by the age of 80 years [11] (Table 3). The association between protein truncating variants in *BRIP1* and risk of ovarian cancer has been confirmed in other analyses (associated risks ranged from 2.6 to 6.4 [27–29,35,45]) (Tables 2 and 3). The frequency of protein truncating variants in population-based studies, separated by ovarian cancer histotypes are given in Table 3, and the frequency in the other retrospective studies, mostly family studies or with women referred to clinical testing, are given in Table 2. Some of the studies in Table 2 have included predicted deleterious missense changes that cannot be separated from the totals, and these are indicated.

Three studies have reported the frequency of protein truncating variants in *BRIP1* by ovarian cancer histotype. Combining these data show that approximately 1.2% of HGS and END cases and 0.8% of LGS cases had protein truncating variants in *BRIP1* [11,34,35] (Table 3). No variants were observed in CCC and MUC, but the total number of cases examined were low. Additional studies are needed to further assess the contribution of germline protein truncating variants in *BRIP1* in the ovarian cancer histotypes.

Available data for *BRIP1* consistently have shown an increased risk of ovarian cancer, with cumulative risk estimated to be approximately 6% by age of 80, and the National Comprehensive Cancer Network, USA, now recommends RRSO for women, starting from ages 45 to 50 [39].

2.3. RAD51C and RAD51D

RAD51C and *RAD51D* are homologous recombination genes, which encode proteins that interact with *BRCA1/2* and participate in the DNA repair process. Ovarian cancer risk attributed to protein truncating variants in *RAD51C* and *RAD51D* was first described by Meindl et al. in 2010 and Loveday et al. in 2011 [46,47].

Song et al. and Norquist et al. provided the frequency of protein truncating variants in the *RAD51C/D* genes in population-based studies by ovarian cancer histotypes [35,48] (Table 3). Combining their data, approximately 0.4–0.5% of HGS, END and CCC cases and 0.2% of LGS had protein truncating variants in *RAD51C*. For *RAD51D*, 0.5% of HGS cases and 0.9% of END cases had protein truncating variants. These variants were not detected in CCC, LGS, and MUC cases, although so far, the number of cases of these histotypes in the datasets are low. The frequency of deleterious variants in family-based studies that combined all EOC cases are given in Table 2. The estimated risk associated with *RAD51C/D* described in the two population-studies were OR 5.2 (95% CI 1.1–24) and 3.4 (95% CI 1.5–7.6) for *RAD51C* and 12.0 (95% CI 1.5–90) and 10.9 (95% CI 4.6–26) for *RAD51D* (Table 3) [35,48]. Three additional case-control studies which included only individuals referred to clinical testing estimated a risk of OR 4.9 (95%CI 3.0–8.0), OR 14.6 (95% CI 5.3 –29.5), and SRR 5.12 (95% CI 3.7–6.9) for *RAD51C*. For *RAD51D*, associated risks were OR 4.78 (95% CI 2.1–10.7), OR 11.8 (95% CI 1.1–40), and SRR 6.34 (95% CI 3.1–11.3) (Table 2) [26–28].

More recently, Yang et al. performed a study of 125 families with pathogenic variants in *RAD51C* and 60 families with pathogenic variants in *RAD51D* and confirmed an increased risk of ovarian cancer associated with pathogenic variants in both genes (*RAD51C*, RR 7.55, 95% CI 5.6–10.2 and *RAD51D*, RR 7.6, 95% CI 5.6–10.3) [10]. The cumulative risk of having ovarian cancer by age 80 was estimated to be 11% (95% CI 6–21%) for *RAD51C* and 13% (95% CI 7–23%) for *RAD51D* based on their segregation analysis [10] (Table 2). *RAD51C/D* were also shown to be associated with breast cancer with cumulative risk of 21% (95% CI 15–29%) and 20% (95% CI 14–28%) for these genes by the age of 80 years, respectively [10].

There is no consensus about the EOC risk threshold for surgical prevention, although the acceptability of RRSO for women with a lifetime risk greater than 10% is well-established. It has been recently suggested that this threshold should be lower and was demonstrated that prophylactic surgery is cost-effective for women at lifetime risk of 5% [49–51]. Considering the current cumulative risk estimates for *RAD51C* and *RAD51D*, women carrying pathogenic variants in these genes could be offered preventive surgery starting from ages 45 to 50, once childbearing is complete.

2.4. PALB2

PALB2 is a confirmed breast cancer susceptibility gene with a cumulative risk estimated to be 44% by 80 years [52], and therefore clinical testing for germline pathogenic variants in this gene is part of breast cancer standard of care. *PALB2* is needed to recruit *BRCA2* in the HR DNA repair pathway [53].

Initial analysis of 3227 EOC cases and 3444 matched-controls suggested that larger numbers of samples were required to determine if *PALB2* was an ovarian cancer susceptibility gene (p 0.08) [11]. Evidence of risk association was observed in case-control analysis of 1915 EOC cases compared to publicly available controls with the OR estimated to be 4.4 (95% CI 2.1–9.1) [35]. Recently, *PALB2* has been confirmed as a risk gene by targeted sequencing in 5123 HGS cases and 5202 controls, WES data from 829 cases and 913 controls, and genotyping data from an independent set of ~14,000 EOC cases and 29,000 controls [54]. The odds ratio was estimated to be 3.01 (95% CI 1.59–5.68) [54] (Table 3).

Histotype data are only available from the first two studies, and combined show that approximately 0.4% of HGS cases had protein truncating variants in *PALB2* (Table 3). A lower frequency was found for LGS (0.2%) and no variants were found in END and MUC. In contrast CCC cases had a frequency of 2.4%. The total number of non-HGS cases examined to date, particularly for CCC, is very low, thus larger numbers are needed to establish the true frequency of *PALB2* pathogenic variants in the rarer histotypes.

An increased risk of ovarian cancer has recently been confirmed in a study of 976 individuals with protein truncating variants in *PALB2* from 524 families, where complex segregation analysis adjusted for ascertainment was performed. The relative risk was estimated to be 2.91 (95% CI 1.4–6.0) [12] (Table 2). Cumulative risks were estimated to be approximately 5% (95% CI 2–10%) by the age of 80 years in the family-based study [12] and 3.2% (95% CI 1.8–5.7%) by the same age in the case-control study previously described [54]. Discussions in the clinical community on whether or not these women should be eligible for prophylactic surgery are still ongoing.

Yang et al. also showed that protein truncating variants in *PALB2* were associated with increased risk of female and male breast cancer (RR 7.18 95% CI 5.8–8.8 and 7.34 95% CI 1.2–42.8, respectively) and pancreatic cancer (RR 2.37 95% CI 1.2–4.5) [12].

Table 2. Frequency of germline pathogenic variants in *BRIP1*, *RAD51C*, *RAD51D*, and *PALB2*, in EOC cases from family history studies.

Gene	Study	Type of Study	Cases Carriers/Total (Frequency) All EOC	Controls (Carriers/Total Frequency) Matched	Controls (Carriers/Total Frequency) Publicly Available	Risk (95% CI)	Cumulative Risk (95% CI)
BRIP1	Lilyquist et al., 2017 ¶ [27]	Clinical testing lab	58/6294 (0.92%)	-	ExAC	SRR: 4.99 (3.8-6.4)	NC
	Kurian et al., 2017 ¶ [26]	Clinical testing lab	36/5020 (0.71%)	161/64,649 (0.24%)	-	OR: 2.62 (1.7-3.9)	NC
	Castera et al., 2018 ¶ [28]	Genetic counselling	21/4408 (0.48%)	-	72/36,276 [a] (0.20%)	OR: 3.77 (0.7-9.4)	NC
	Suszynska et al., 2020 [45]	Meta-analysis ^	200/22,494 (0.89%)	-	209/115,375 [b] (0.18%)	OR: 4.94 (4.0-6.0)	NC
	Meindl et al., 2010 [46]	Family study	6/480 families	-	-	NC	NC
	Lilyquist et al., 2017 ¶ [27]	Clinical testing lab	44/6294 (0.7%)	-	ExAC	SRR: 5.12 (3.7-6.9)	NC
RAD51C	Kurian et al., 2017 ¶ [26]	Clinical testing lab	32/5020 (0.6%)	72/64,649	-	OR: 4.98 (3.0-8.0)	NC
	Castera et al., 2018 ¶ [28]	Genetic counselling	23/4309 (0.5%)	-	43/36,276 [a] (0.12%)	OR: 14.6 (5.3-29.5)	NC
	Suszynska et al., 2019 [29]	Meta-analysis ^^	21/3791 (0.6%)	-	-	OR: 4.3 (2.5-7.5)	NC
	Yang et al., 2020 [10]	*RAD51C* families #	125 families	-	-	RR: 7.55 (5.6-10.2)	11% (15-29%)
	Suszynska et al., 2020 [45]	Meta-analysis ^	149/23,802 (0.62%)	-	130/115,475 [b] (0.11%)	OR: 5.59 (4.4-7.0)	NC
	Loveday et al., 2011 [47]	Family study	8/911 families	1/1060 (0.09%)	-	RR: 6.30 (2.8-13.8)	NC
RAD51D	Lilyquist et al., 2017 ¶ [27]	Clinical testing lab	11/5743 (0.2%)	-	ExAC	SRR: 6.34 (3.1-11.3)	NC
	Kurian et al., 2017 ¶ [26]	Clinical testing lab	9/5020 (0.2%)	40/64,649 (0.06%)	-	OR: 4.78 (2.1-10.7)	NC
	Castera et al., 2018 ¶ [28]	Genetic counselling	9/4011 (0.2%)	-	18/36,276 [a] (0.05%)	OR: 11.8 (1.1-40)	NC
	Suszynska et al., 2019 [29]	Meta-analysis ^^	19/3258 (0.6%)	-	-	OR: 11.6 (5.9-23)	NC
	Yang et al., 2020 [10]	*RAD51D* families #	60 families	-	-	RR: 7.6 (5.6-10.3)	13% (7-23%)
	Suszynska et al., 2020 [45]	Meta-analysis ^	94/22,787 (0.45%)	-	72/120,688 [b] (0.06%)	OR: 6.9 (5.1-9.4)	NC
PALB2	Yang et al., 2020 [12]	*PALB2* families #	524 families	-	-	RR: 2.91 (1.4-6.0)	5% (2-10%)

Abbreviations: RR —Relative risk; OR—odds ratio; SRR—Standardized risk ratio; PVs—Pathogenic variants; -: Not available, NC: Not calculated, [a] ExAC NFE non-TCGA, [b] gnomAD NFE non-TCGA, ¶ deleterious missense changes included, ^ [45] Overlapped with 6 studies included in this review; ^^ [29] Overlapped with 1 study included in this review; # Segregation analysis. Bold: highlight info.

Table 3. Frequency of germline protein truncating variants in *BRIP1*, *RAD51C*, *RAD51D*, and *PALB2* in EOC histotypes, in cases from population studies.

Gene	Study	Cases Carriers/Total (Frequency)							Controls Carriers/Total (Frequency)		Risk (95% CI)	Cumulative Risk (95% CI) [a]
		HGS	END	CCC	LGS	MUC	Mixed/Unk [b]	All EOC	Matched	Publicly Available		
BRIP1	Walsh et al., 2011 [34]	2/242 ** (0.8%)	1/23 (4.3%)	0/17 (0%)	**	-	1/78 (1.3%)	4/360 (1.1%)	-	-	NC	NC
	Ramus et al., 2015 [11]	26/2535 * (1.0%)	0/65 (0%)	0/25 (0%)	4/416 (0.9%)	0/26 (0%)	0/160 (0%)	30/3227 (0.92%)	3/3444 (0.09)	-	RR: 11.2 # (3.2–34.1)	5.8% (3.6–9.1%)
	Norquist et al., 2016 [35]	22/1498 (1.5%)	1/77 (1.3%)	0/58 (0%)	0/70 (0%)	0/16 (0%)	3/196 (1.5%)	26/1915 (1.36%)	-	60/36276 [c] (0.17%)	OR: 6.4 (3.8–10.6)	NC
	Total	50/4275 (1.17%)	2/165 (1.21%)	0/100 (0%)	4/486 (0.82%)	0/42 (0%)	4/434 (0.9%)	60/5502 (1.1%)	3/3444 (0.09%)	-	-	-
RAD51C	Song et al., 2015 [48] [†]	10/1806 * (0.6%)	1/383 (0.3%)	1/225 (0.4%)	1/405 (0.2%)	0/166 (0%)	1/444 (0.2%)	14/3429 (0.40%)	2/2772 (0.07%)	-	OR: 5.2 # (1.1–24)	5.2% [¶] (1.1–22%)
	Norquist et al., 2016 [35] [†]	7/1498 (0.5%)	1/77 (1.3%)	0/58 (0%)	0/70 (0%)	0/16 (0%)	3/196 (1.5%)	11/1915 (0.57%)	-	39/36276 [c] (0.11%)	OR: 3.4 (1.5–7.6)	NC
	Total	17/3304 (0.51%)	2/460 (0.43%)	1/283 (0.35%)	1/475 (0.21%)	0/182 (0%)	4/640 (0.62%)	25/5344 (0.47%)	2/2772 (0.07%)	-	-	-
RAD51D	Song et al., 2015 [48]	9/1806 * (0.5%)	3/383 (0.8%)	0/225 (0%)	0/405 (0%)	0/166 (0%)	0/444 (0%)	12/3429 (0.35%)	1/2772 (0.04%)	-	OR: 12 # (1.5–90)	12% [¶] (1.5–60%)
	Norquist et al., 2016 [35]	7/1498 (0.5%)	1/77 (1.3%)	0/58 (0%)	0/70 (0%)	0/16 (0%)	3/196 (1.5%)	11/1915 (0.57%)	-	14/36276 [c] (0.04%)	OR: 10.9 (4.6–26.0)	NC
	Total	16/3304 (0.48%)	4/460 (0.87%)	0/283 (0%)	0/475 (0%)	0/182 (0%)	3/640 (0.47%)	23/5344 (0.43%)	1/2772 (0.04%)	-	-	-
PALB2	Ramus et al., 2015 [11]	6/2535 * (0.24%)	0/65 (0%)	1/25 (4%)	1/416 (0.24%)	0/26 (0%)	1/160 (0.62%)	9/3227 (0.28%)	3/3444 (0.09%)	-	NC	NC
	Norquist et al., 2016 [35]	9/1498 (0.60%)	0/77 (0%)	1/58 (1.7%)	0/70 (0%)	0/16 (0%)	2/196 (1.0%)	12/1915 (0.62%)	-	39/36276 [c] (0.10%)	OR: 4.4 (2.1–9.1)	NC
	Song et al., 2019 [54]	18/5123 (0.35%)	-	-	-	-	-	18/5123 (0.35%)	6/5202 (0.12%)	-	OR: 3.01 # (1.6–5.7)	3.2% (1.8–5.7%)
	Total [^]	15/4033 (0.37%)	0/142 (0%)	2/83 (2.4%)	1/486 (0.2%)	0/42 (0%)	3/356 (0.84%)	21/5142 (0.41%)	3/3444 (0.09%)	-	-	-

Abbreviations: RR—Relative risk; OR—odds ratio; SRR—Standardized risk ratio; -: Not available, NC: Not calculated due to no controls or not described, ** Frequency of serous combined, * Frequency of HGS and serous undifferentiated, # OR for the matched controls analysis, [†] Studies included one known deleterious missense variant [55], [a] Risks based on all cases combined, [b] Mixed/Unknown includes some other histotypes, [c] ExAC NFE-nonTCGA, [¶] Cumulative risks by age 70. Song et al., 2019 [54], study as extensive overlap with Ramus et al., 2015 [11]. Bold: highlight info.

2.5. Mismatch Repair (MMR) Genes

Germline protein truncating and known deleterious missense variants in four MMR genes are associated with Lynch syndrome, which is an inherited disorder that increases the risk of many types of cancers including colon, endometrial, ovarian, pancreatic, small-bowel, and ureteric. In ovarian cancer cases from Lynch syndrome families, deleterious variants in the MMR genes were mostly seen in END and CCC cases and were more prevalent in the *MSH2* and *MSH6* genes [56]. This histotype-specific characteristic has been confirmed by population-based cohorts of EOC [33,34].

Germline deleterious MMR gene variants in ovarian cancer cases appear to be very rare, which may partly be because they are associated with the rare histotypes of disease [33]. Three studies have described MMR gene mutation frequencies by ovarian cancer histotypes [33–35] (Table 4).

We have combined the data across studies to provide an estimate of the frequency in these rarer histotypes (Table 4). Deleterious variants in these genes were more frequent in END and CCC cases than HGS. No variants were reported in MUC or LGS cases, although some studies combined HGS and LGS cases. Variants were more frequently found in *MSH6* than the other genes, with CCC and END cases both having greater than 1% frequency.

Five other case-control studies have investigated MMR frequencies between 2000 and 7500 EOC cases, four of which included data from commercial laboratories where clinical grade testing was performed in women with hereditary cancer risk [26–28,57], while another was a meta-analysis [29]. These studies have estimated the OR for mutation carriers of these genes. For *MLH1* carriers the OR was 3 (95% CI, 1.47–6.59) [26], for *MSH2* carriers, OR data from different studies ranged from 2 to 14 [26–29], and for *MSH6* carriers, ranged from 2 to 9 [26–29,57]. For the MMR genes combined, the OR was estimated to be 2.3 (95% CI, 0.83–8.2) with a cumulative risk of ovarian cancer by age 80 years of 3.7% (95% CI, 1.4–13%) in cases from a population-based study [33].

A Lynch syndrome prospective study had estimated the cumulative risk of ovarian cancer as a unique disease to be 10% (95% CI 4.8–15.4%) for *MLH1* carriers by the age of 75 years, 17% (95% CI 5.7–28.0%) for *MSH2* carriers, and 13% (95% CI 0.1–31.2%) for *MSH6* carriers [13]. The risk in the different EOC histotypes was not reported [13], although it is known that they are mostly seen in END and CCC cases.

The cumulative risk of endometrial cancer by the age of 75 years was estimated to be 43% (95% CI 33.1–52.3%), 57% (95% CI 41.8–71.6%), and 46% (95% CI 27.3–65.0%) for *MLH1*, *MSH2*, and *MSH6* carriers, respectively [13]. Due to the increased risk of both ovarian and endometrial cancer in women with Lynch syndrome, discussion about RRSO with hysterectomy is recommended. MMR carriers from these Lynch syndrome families were also reported to have an increased risk of colorectal, upper gastrointestinal, urinary tract, prostate, and brain cancers [13].

3. Missense Variants in Confirmed Susceptibility Genes

Protein truncating variants have been classified as deleterious, however a relatively large number of missense variants, including some rare predicted pathogenic missense variants have also been identified in these genes. Determining if any of these missense variants are also pathogenic is important for patient management and risk prediction in families.

3.1. BRCA1/2 and MMR Genes

Over many years, due to efforts of commercial labs, independent research groups, and large consortia, many missense variants of unknown significance (VUS) or unclassified variants (UV) have been reclassified as either pathogenic or benign. However, there are still many variants that remain unclassified. Large-scale consortia efforts, such as the Evidence-based Network for the Interpretation of Germline Mutant Alleles (ENIGMA) are in the process of investigating and classifying these variants in the *BRCA1/2* genes and the interpretation of the results of genetic testing for reporting and counselling [58].

Table 4. Frequency of germline pathogenic variants in the mismatch repair (MMR) genes in EOC histotypes, in cases from population studies.

Gene	Study	Cases Carriers/Total (Frequency)							Controls Carriers/Total (Frequency)
		HGS	END	CCC	LGS	MUC	Mixed/Unk [a]	All EOC	Matched
MLH1	Song et al., 2014 [33]	0/1105 * (0%)	0/322 (0%)	1/192 (0.52%)	0/172 (0%)	0/157 (0%)	0/274 (0%)	1/2222 (0.04%)	2/1528 (0.13%)
	Norquist et al., 2016 [35]	0/1498 (0%)	0/77 (0%)	0/58 (0%)	0/70 (0%)	0/16 (0%)	1/196 [b] (0.51%)	1/1915 (0.05%)	-
	Total	0/2603 (0%)	0/399 (0%)	1/250 (0.40%)	0/242 (0%)	0/173 (0%)	1/470 (0.21%)	2/4137 (0.04%)	2/1528 (0.13%)
MSH2	Song et al., 2014 [33]	1/1105 * (0.09%)	0/322 (0%)	1/192 (0.52%)	0/172 (0%)	0/157 (0%)	0/274 (0%)	2/2222 (0.09%)	0/1528 (0%)
	Total	1/1105 (0.09%)	0/322 (0%)	1/192 (0.52%)	0/172 (0%)	0/157 (0%)	0/274 (0%)	2/2222 (0.09%)	0/1528 (0%)
MSH6	Walsh et al., 2011 [34]	0/242 ** (0%)	2/23 (8.7%)	0/17 (0%)	**	-	0/78 (0%)	2/360 (0.55%)	-
	Song et al., 2014 [33]	4/1105 * (0.36%)	2/322 (0.62%)	3/192 (1.56%)	0/172 (0%)	0/157 (0%)	0/274 (0%)	9/2222 (0.40%)	1/1528 (0.06%)
	Norquist et al., 2016 [35]	1/1498 (0.06%)	2/77 (2.59%)	0/58 (0%)	0/70 (0%)	0/16 (0%)	0/196 (0%)	3/1915 (0.15%)	-
	Total	5/2845 (0.17%)	6/422 (1.42%)	3/267 (1.12%)	0/242 (0%)	0/173 (0%)	0/548 (0%)	14/4497 (0.31%)	1/1528 (0.06%)
PMS2	Song et al., 2014 [33]	0/1105 * (0%)	1/322 (0.31%)	0/192 (0%)	0/172 (0%)	0/157 (0.6%)	0/274 (0%)	1/2222 (0.04%)	0/1528 (0%)
	Norquist et al., 2016 [35]	4/1498 (0.3%)	0/77 (0%)	0/58 (0%)	0/70 (0%)	0/16 (0%)	0/196 (0%)	4/1915 (0.20%)	-
	Total	4/2603 (0.15%)	1/399 (0.25%)	0/250 (0%)	0/242 (0%)	0/173 (0%)	0/470 (0%)	5/4137 (0.12%)	0/1528 (0%)
All 4 genes	Total [$]	10/2845 (0.35%)	7/422 (1.65%)	5/267 (1.87%)	0/242 (0%)	0/173 (0%)	1/548 (0.18%)	23/4497 (0.51%)	3/1528 (0.19%)

-: Not available, ** serous combined, * HGS and serous undifferentiated, [a] Mixed/Unknown includes some other histotypes, [b] MLH1 variant found in carcinosarcoma, [$] Totals did not include overlapped studies. Bold: highlight info.

To date, the National Institutes of Health (NIH) repository, ClinVar, has reported approximately 7000 pathogenic or likely pathogenic variants and 7400 VUS in *BRCA1/2* genes (mostly missense changes, but also in-frame deletions and insertions, and intronic and exonic variants that may affect splicing efficiency) [59]. The same clinical challenge occurs in patients with variants in the MMR genes, approximately 30% of all variants are classified as VUS [60].

Individual studies may include analysis of missense variants using bioinformatic tools such as SIFT [61], PolyPhen-2 [62], and Provean [63] to predict the functional effect of variants. Association between predicted deleterious rare missense variants and ovarian cancer risk can be assessed using burden tests, such as the rare admixture maximum likelihood test (RAML), that accounts for differences in risk of each associated variant [64]. Song et al. have performed this type of analysis in 131 predicted deleterious missense variants in *BRCA1/2* and the MMR genes (*MLH1*, *MSH2*, *MSH6*, and *PMS2*) and found little evidence for ovarian cancer risk association between these variants in any of the six genes [33].

3.2. BRIP1, RAD51C/D and PALB2

Missense variants in the moderate-risk genes recently confirmed as susceptibility genes in ovarian cancer need further investigation to determine if any are likely to be pathogenic. Some studies have included predicted deleterious missense variants in estimating mutation frequencies.

Ramus et al. used SIFT, PolyPhen-2, and Provean scores to predict if uncommon (minor allele frequency (MAF) < 1%) and rare (MAF < 0.1%) missense variants were potentially deleterious and identified 35 for *BRIP1* and 26 in *PALB2*. They performed the RAML burden test and found an increased risk association for uncommon and rare missense variants in *BRIP1*, but not for *PALB2* [11,54].

In *RAD51C/D*, Song et al. performed the RAML test for 28 rare predicted deleterious missense variants (12 in *RAD51C* and 16 in *RAD51D*) [48]. Evidence for an association of rare predicted deleterious missense variants with an increased risk of ovarian cancer was observed in both genes [48] (Table 5).

The data from the RAML burden test suggest that some of the predicted deleterious missense variants in *BRIP1*, *RAD51C*, and *RAD51D* likely increase disease risk, but it does not indicate how many or which ones. There is no evidence for specific missense variants.

Table 5. Predicted deleterious missense variants in known moderate risk genes for EOC.

Genes	Study	Cases Del Missense/Total (Frequency)	Predicted Deleterious	Evidence of Risk from RAML
BRIP1	Ramus et al., 2015 [11]	35/3227 [a] (1.1%)	SIFT, PolyPhen-2 and Provean	Yes (All EOC, but stronger in HGS)
	Suszynska et al., 2020 [45]	2 */22494	Described in ClinVar	-
RAD51C	Song et al., 2015 [11]	12/3429 [b] (0.32%)	SIFT, PolyPhen-2 and Provean	Yes (All EOC, but stronger in HGS)
	Lilyquist et al., 2017 [27]	2 $/6294	Described in ClinVar	-
	Norquist et al., 2016 [35]	1 #/1915 [c]	Functional assay [65]	-
	Suszynska et al., 2020 [45]	3 ˆ/22,494	Described in ClinVar	-
RAD51D	Song et al., 2015 [11]	16/3429 (0.46%)	SIFT, PolyPhen-2 and Provean	Yes (Only in HGS)
	Suszynska et al., 2020 [45]	1 ¶/22,494	Described in ClinVar	-
PALB2	Ramus et al., 2015 [11]	26/3227 (0.80%)	SIFT, PolyPhen-2 and Provean	No
	Song et al., 2019 [54]	40/5123 [a] (0.78%)	SIFT, PolyPhen-2 and Provean	No

-: Not available. [a] All variants reported in HGS. [b] One variant found in LGS – (histotype not available for the other variants). [c] Variant found in a serous carcinoma. ClinVar reported variants: * p.Gln169 = and p.Ala349Pro; $ p.C135Y and p.L138F; # p.Q143R; ˆ p.Cys135Tyr, p.Cys135Ser and p.Leu138Phe; ¶ p.Ser207Leu.

4. Deleterious Variants in Other Proposed Susceptibility Genes

4.1. FANCM

FANCM is part of the Fanconi anemia group together with *BRCA2*, *BRIP1* and *PALB2* (also known as *FANCD1*, *FANCJ*, and *FANCN*). A case-control study was performed by Dicks et al. where *FANCM* targeted sequencing was performed in 3107 HGS cases, 1491 cases of other histotypes, and 3368 unaffected matched controls [66]. A significantly higher frequency of protein truncating variants was found in the HGS cases compared to the controls (p 0.008) and no evidence of association was observed with other histotypes (p 0.82) [66]. The relative risk for HGS was estimated to be 2.5 (95% CI 1.3–5) with lifetime average risk of 3.8% (80% CI 2.2–4.5%) [66]. Lifetime risk was increased when known ovarian cancer risk factors such as common risk alleles and lifestyle factors were taken into account (4.6% (80% CI 3.1–7.0%) and 5.2% (80% CI 3.4–7.8%), respectively) [66]. Additionally, the RAML test was performed for 243 uncommon predicted deleterious missense variants (effect given by at least two of the three function prediction programs Polyphen-2, Provean, and SIFT), but there was no difference in the frequency of these variants in cases compared to controls [66].

Although this study had shown evidence of association between germline protein truncating variants in *FANCM* and moderate increase in risk of HGS ovarian cancer, larger and prospective studies are still needed to confirm this.

4.2. ATM

ATM is a candidate ovarian cancer susceptibility gene due to its role in breast [67] and pancreatic cancer [68]. Germline heterozygous pathogenic *ATM* variants are associated with fivefold higher risk of breast cancer by the age of 50 years [67] and some rare variants have been shown to have penetrance as high as the *BRCA2* gene [69].

In ovarian cancer, case-control studies mainly enriched for a family history of breast or ovarian cancer, have suggested that pathogenic or likely pathogenic variants in *ATM* might be associated with moderate increased risk (OR 1.69, 95% CI 1.2–2.4 [26]; Standardized risk ratio (SRR) 2.25, 95% CI 1.7–3 [27]; OR 1.97, 95% CI 1.3–3 [29]; OR 2.4, 95% CI 1.2–4.7 [35]; OR 2.85, 95% CI 1.3–6.3 [57]), however the cumulative lifetime risk has been estimated to be lower than 3%.

4.3. BARD1 and NBN

The *BARD1* and *NBN* genes were included in breast/ovarian cancer genetic panel tests, due to their breast cancer risk, despite the ovarian cancer risk for deleterious variants in these genes being unknown. The *BARD1* encoded protein interacts closely with the *BRCA1* protein due to sharing the N-terminal RING finger and the BRCA1 C-terminal domains. Interaction between these genes affects double-strand break repair and apoptosis suggesting that this protein may play an important role in *BRCA1* tumour suppression [70]. Consequently, *BARD1* was considered a potential candidate susceptibility gene for ovarian cancer. However, Ramus et al. found no significant differences in *BARD1* deleterious variants frequency in a cohort of ~3200 ovarian cancer cases compared with ~3400 matched-controls (p 0.39) [11]. Several additional case-control studies confirmed that no evidence of association was observed between ovarian cancer risk and pathogenic variants in *BARD1* (OR 0.59, 95% CI 0.21–1.68 [26]; SSR 1.28, 95% CI 0.55–2.51 [27]; OR 1.4, 95% CI 0.7–2.9 [29]). A moderate increase in breast cancer risk has been suggested but more evidence is needed to validate these findings [70,71].

The *NBN* encoded protein interacts with *MRE11A* and *RAD50* encoded proteins as a large complex, which interacts with the protein produced by the *ATM* gene. These combined proteins have an important role in identifying broken strands of DNA and repairing it. Due to its essential function in the DNA repair pathway and because this gene is commercially available in gene testing panels for ovarian cancer, case-controls studies have examined if they are susceptibility genes. However, most studies have not found a higher frequency of pathogenic variants in *NBN*, *MRE11A*, or *RAD50* in cases compared to controls (*NBN*: *p* 0.61 [11] and 0.09 [35]; *MRE11A*: *p* 1.0 [35]; *RAD50*: *p* 0.63 [35]) and therefore no evidence of association with risk was observed in any of these 3 genes.

4.4. CHECK2

Germline pathogenic variants in *CHECK2* (a cell cycle checkpoint regulator) are associated with an increased risk of breast cancer [72] and *CHECK2* was proposed to be a candidate gene for ovarian cancer risk on that basis. A prospective study had shown that in estrogen receptor–positive breast cancer, CHEK2*1100delC heterozygosity was associated with increased risk of early death, breast cancer–specific death, and risk of a second breast cancer [72]. However, numerous retrospective case-control studies did not find an association between pathogenic variants in *CHECK2* and an increased risk of ovarian cancer [26,27,35].

4.5. Other Genes

TP53 was suggested as a potential candidate susceptibility gene for ovarian cancer from a case only study [34] and from a whole-exome sequencing analysis where protein truncating variants were identified at a greater frequency in ovarian cancer cases compared to publicly available controls (OR 18.5; 95% CI, 2.6–808.1) [34,57]. This gene has not been validated in other targeted sequencing and WES studies [26,35].

Other candidate genes selected for targeted sequencing validation in cases and controls have shown weak evidence of association with ovarian cancer risk for protein truncating variants in *POLK*, *SLX4* (also known as *FANCP*), and *FBXO10*, but further studies are required to confirm this [54]. Several Fanconi Anaemia genes (*FANCA, FANCB, FANCC, FANCD2, FANCE, FANCG, FANCI,* and *FANCL*) have been tested in these case-control studies but a risk association has not been detected [54]. A large number of other genes have been examined and not been shown to be ovarian cancer risk genes [48,57,66].

5. Discussion

We have presented a comprehensive review of the contribution of rare genetic variants to ovarian cancer, with a focus on the relationship between genetic variation and ovarian cancer histotypes, using data mostly only presented as supplementary in the original papers.

For *BRCA1/2*, deleterious germline variants are more common in HGS (8% for *BRCA1* and 6% for *BRCA2*), but there is a significant frequency of variants in END (3% for both genes), CCC (3% for *BRCA1* and 1% for *BRCA2*), and LGS (3% for *BRCA1* and 2% for *BRCA2*) patients. Consequently, the current guidelines recommend *BRCA1/2* testing in all non-mucinous ovarian cancer cases. For the MMR genes, the frequency of deleterious germline variants is higher in END and CCC patients, with variants in *MSH6* being more common than variants in *MLH1, MSH2,* and *PMS2* (greater than 1% in *MSH6* and approximately or less than 0.5% in *MLH1/MSH2/PMS2*). For *BRIP1*, the frequency of protein truncating variants seems to be similar for HGS and END (approximately 1.2%), but slightly lower for LGS cases (0.8%). For *RAD51C*, a slightly higher frequency of variants in the HGS cases is observed (0.5%), and frequencies range from 0.2 to 0.4% in END, CCC, and LGS. No variants in MUC were found. In contrast, a higher frequency of protein truncating variants in END cases is seen for *RAD51D* (0.9%), compared to the HGS cases (0.5%). No variants were detected in CCC, LGS, or MUC. A higher frequency of protein truncating variants in CCC is seen in *PALB2*, compared to 0.4% in HGS and 0.2% in LGS. However, larger numbers of the non-HGS cases are needed to confirm these frequencies especially in the moderate risk genes that have been recently confirmed as susceptibility genes for ovarian cancer.

The role of individual missense variants in the known ovarian cancer genes is not yet known. Work by the ENIGMA consortium is underway to identify deleterious missense variants in *BRCA1* and *BRCA2*, and ongoing efforts will be required for other genes [58].

The frequency of large genomic alternations (insertions, deletions, and rearrangements) have been examined in *BRCA1/2* and the MMR genes [17,73]. These types of changes make up 8–40% of *BRCA1* mutations, depending on the population [17]. We do not yet know how frequent they are in the *BRIP1*,

RAD51C, *RAD51D*, and *PALB2* genes, and this could affect prevalence estimates. These types of changes cannot be detected with the methods currently used for targeted sequencing in clinical panel testing.

As outcomes in ovarian cancer are linked to its stage at diagnosis, the ability to identify women at risk earlier or before diagnosis has important clinical implications. The use of multigene panel testing has allowed women to be tested for multiple genetic variants associated with increased cancer risk, enabling personalised risk estimates to be developed [74,75]. While screening for ovarian cancer has not been shown to reduce mortality, RRSO can be offered to women at a sufficiently high risk of developing ovarian cancer [4,5].

There has been some debate as to what level of lifetime cancer risk justifies prophylactic surgical intervention. Traditionally, a threshold of greater than 10% lifetime ovarian cancer risk was used, allowing for RRSO in women carrying *BRCA1*, *BRCA2*, or mismatch repair gene mutations, which confer lifetime ovarian cancer risk well in excess of 10% [76]. The more recent discovery of moderate penetrance genes has prompted formal studies into risk thresholds for invention, and recent analyses have suggested that offering RRSO to women with a lifetime risk as low as 4–5% can be cost-effective [50]. On that basis, women carrying variants in *BRIP1*, *RAD51C*, and *RAD51D* may also be offered RRSO [77,78].

The best approach to managing patients with genetic variants that do not sufficiently increase ovarian cancer risk to justify RRSO but increase risk to higher than that of the general population is not yet known. While it is plausible that targeting these women for screening may allow for detection of cancers at an earlier stage, this has not been studied. Studies investigating the impact of ovarian cancer screening using ultrasonographic and biochemical methods in both the general population, and high-risk groups (greater than 10% risk on the basis of family history or presence of genetic variants) have been associated with stage-shift, but have not been shown to significantly reduce mortality [5,79].

Genetic testing is fraught with ethical, legal, and psychosocial implications for patients, and the rate of advancement in our understanding of cancer genetics often outstrips our ability to use information in the clinic [80,81]. It is important to note that genetic susceptibility to EOC cancer does not exist in isolation, and variants conferring increased ovarian cancer risk also often increase the risk of developing other cancers—most notably breast cancer in *BRCA1* and *BRCA2*, and colon cancer in Lynch syndrome. Furthermore, breast and ovarian cancer genes are often combined into a single panel test, potentially uncovering variants in genes for which pathogenicity is disputed. As an example, *PALB2* is associated with a lifetime breast cancer risk of 53%, but also lifetime risks of 5% and 2–3% for ovarian and pancreatic malignancies, respectively [12]. While a 53% lifetime breast cancer risk is clearly clinically actionable, the risk of ovarian and pancreatic cancers associated with *PALB2* exists in an area of clinical uncertainty. The opposite is seen for deleterious variants in *BRIP1*, with an increased risk of ovarian cancer but no increase in breast cancer risk. For these reasons, all women undergoing genetic testing for familial susceptibility to ovarian cancer should receive appropriate pre- and post-test counselling, and follow-up with relevant clinical services. Genetic information should be applied cautiously in the clinic, after careful evaluation of the available literature, as some genes included on so called "ovarian cancer" panel tests have now been shown not to increase ovarian cancer risk [82,83] (Table 6). The risks of ovarian and breast cancer for genes in the double-strand DNA break repair pathway are shown in Figure 1.

Current testing guidelines do not recommend population-based genetic testing for ovarian cancer, however population-based testing approaches may be effective in groups with a small number of common founder mutations such as the three *BRCA1/2* variants in Ashkenazi Jews [86,87]. With the decreasing costs of sequencing methods, these approaches may also become cost effective in other populations. Population-based genetic testing has many issues, including cultural and psychosocial, that need to be investigated [87]. The majority of the genetic studies in ovarian cancer have been performed in white populations, and work on other ethnic groups is ongoing [88].

Table 6. Summary of the frequency of deleterious variants by EOC histotype for each homologous recombination (HR) gene and the MMR genes, and a comparison of risk and clinical management for ovarian and breast cancer patients.

Genes	Frequency (%)						Risk Est. ^		Risk Level		Clinical Management $	
	HGS	END	CCC	LGS	MUC	EOC	BC	EOC	BC	EOC	BC
BRCA1	7.8	2.9	3.6	3.7	<1	60	72% *	Very high	Very high	RRSO age 35 to 45 PARPi	RRM age 25 to 40
BRCA2	5.9	2.9	<1	2	<1	17	69% *	High	Very high		
MMR	<1	1.6	1.9	0	0	2.3	-	Mod	None	RRSO with hysterectomy for LS	No increased risk
BRIP1	1.2	1.2	0	<1	0	11.2	-	Mod	None	RRSO age 45 to 50 no consensus	Insufficient evidence
RAD51C	<1	<1	<1	<1	0	5.2	1.9	Mod	None		
RAD51D	<1	<1	0	0	0	12	1.8	Mod	None		
PALB2	<1	0	2.4	<1	0	3.0	7.2	Low	Mod	Insufficient evidence	Annual mammography/breast MRI age 30 no consensus
TP53	Insufficient data					Insuf	Insuf	Low	Mod	Insufficient evidence	Insufficient evidence
CHEK2	No increased risk					-	3.0	None	Low	No increased risk	Annual mammography/breast MRI age 40 no consensus
ATM	No increased risk					-	2.8	None	Low		
NBN	No increased risk					-	2.7	None	Low		
RAD50	No increased risk					-	Insuf	None	Low	No increased risk	Insufficient evidence
MRE11A	No increased risk					-	Insuf	None	Low		

Abbreviations: BC—breast cancer; RRM—Risk-reducing mastectomy; LS—Lynch Syndrome; MRI—Magnetic Resonance Imaging; Insuf—Insufficient. ^ From Tables 1, 3 and 4. EOC BRCA1/2 from ref [33], MMR from ref [33], BRIP1 from ref [11], RAD51C/D from ref [9], PALB2 from ref [48]. BC BRCA1/2 from ref [54]. BC BRCA1/2 from ref [10], PALB2 from ref [12], CHEK2/ATM/NBN from ref [84]. $ BRCA1/2 from ref [13], BRIP1/RAD51C/D from ref [49], MMR from refs [39,85], PALB2/CHEK2/ATM/NBN from refs [77,84]. * Cumulative risk data by the age of 80.

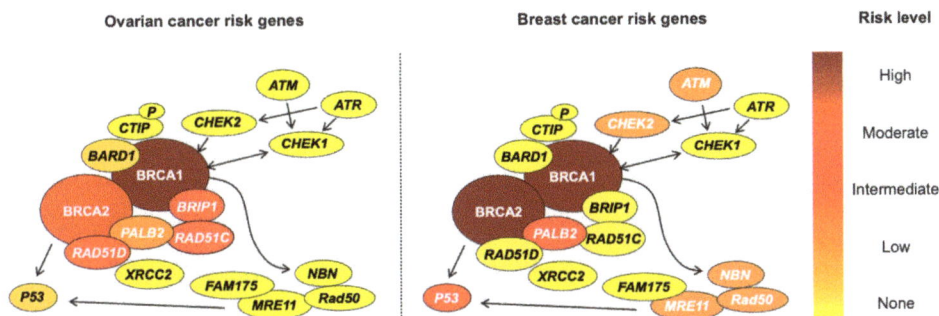

Figure 1. Susceptibility genes present in the double-strand DNA break repair pathway for ovarian and breast cancer and its different correspondent risks levels in each disease.

Identifying ovarian cancer genes has translated to novel therapeutic options for patients. PARP inhibitors, which target double-stranded DNA repair in cells with deficient homologous recombination, including cells with dysfunctional BRCA DNA repair pathways, have been shown to improve progression free survival (PFS) in serous and endometrioid ovarian cancers [89–92]. The impact of PARP inhibitors on PFS is most dramatic in patients with mutations in *BRCA1* and *BRCA2*, but can also benefit women without BRCA mutations if they are found to have deficiencies in homologous recombination, such as variants in the DNA repair genes discussed above [92]. However, improvements in PFS do not necessarily translate to improved overall survival, and the impact of PARP inhibitors on the overall survival endpoint has not yet been reported [92].

To date, ovarian cancer has largely been treated as a single entity. However, as outlined above, the five main histotypes of epithelial ovarian cancer appear to be characterised by distinct genetic mutations. The tumours also have different molecular profiles, and patients have different treatment responses [93]. Therefore, it has become increasingly clear that ovarian cancer represents not just a single disease but encompasses a number of distinct cancers. Most of our understanding of ovarian cancer genes relates to high-grade serous tumours, as they represent the majority of ovarian cancers. Identifying genetic variants contributing to non-serous ovarian cancers has posed an ongoing challenge for researchers, as finding rare variants for rare cancers requires studies with sample sizes that are not yet feasible.

Despite significant advancements in our understanding of the genetic epidemiology of ovarian cancer, the known ovarian cancer risk variants explain less than half of the excess familial risk for ovarian cancer [8]. Efforts to identify novel genetic variants associated with ovarian cancer are ongoing. The discovery of new genetic variants should be accompanied by efforts to accurately quantify the exact magnitude of increased risk associated with that variant. Case-control studies, the most commonly used study design in gene discovery, are only able to generate relative risks, from which absolute risks are extrapolated.

Prospective population-based studies, which have been used to provide gold-standard estimates of lifetime cancer risk in *BRCA1*, *BRCA2*, and the mismatch repair genes, would provide more accurate risk estimates for moderate penetrance ovarian cancer genes, but are costly, and require long-term investment. Segregation analysis from large international consortia has been used to calculate ovarian cancer risks in *RAD51C*, *RAD51D*, and *PALB2*, and could be applied to other moderate risk ovarian cancer genes [10,12].

Genetic association studies, by their design, are unable to establish a causal relationship between germline variant status and cancer phenotype. The discovery of novel ovarian cancer risk genes should be followed-up by further efforts to characterise the functional mechanisms by which they contribute to cancer development and identify potential therapeutic targets.

6. Conclusions

Ovarian cancer is the most lethal gynaecological malignancy, and an improved understanding of the contribution of rare genetic variants to the development of ovarian cancer allows for better clinical management of at-risk women. Based on the best available evidence, variants in BRCA1, BRCA2, BRIP1, RAD51C, RAD51D, and the mismatch repair genes confer ovarian cancer risks that warrant the consideration of risk-reducing surgery. The best approach for managing women with deleterious variants in ovarian cancer genes that do not warrant prophylactic surgery requires further investigation.

Funding: M.P. is funded by UNSW Sydney, the Yarrow Family and the Australian Government Research Training Program Scholarship. This work was funded by Cancer Australia, priority-driven Collaborative Cancer Research Scheme (1147276). The content is solely the responsibility of the individual authors and does not reflect the views of Cancer Australia.

Conflicts of Interest: The authors declare no conflict of interest.

References

1. Bray, F.; Ferlay, J.; Soerjomataram, I.; Siegel, R.L.; Torre, L.A.; Jemal, A. Global cancer statistics 2018: GLOBOCAN estimates of incidence and mortality worldwide for 36 cancers in 185 countries. *CA Cancer J. Clin.* **2018**, *68*, 394–424. [CrossRef]
2. Prat, J. Ovarian carcinomas: Five distinct diseases with different origins, genetic alterations, and clinicopathological features. *Virchows Arch.* **2012**, *460*, 237–249. [CrossRef]
3. Torre, L.A.; Trabert, B.; DeSantis, C.E.; Miller, K.D.; Samimi, G.; Runowicz, C.D.; Gaudet, M.M.; Jemal, A.; Siegel, R.L. Ovarian cancer statistics, 2018. *CA Cancer J. Clin.* **2018**, *68*, 284–296. [CrossRef]
4. Buys, S.S.; Partridge, E.; Black, A.; Johnson, C.C.; Lamerato, L.; Isaacs, C.; Reding, D.J.; Greenlee, R.T.; Yokochi, L.A.; Kessel, B.; et al. Effect of screening on ovarian cancer mortality: The Prostate, Lung, Colorectal and Ovarian (PLCO) Cancer Screening Randomized Controlled Trial. *JAMA* **2011**, *305*, 2295–2303. [CrossRef]
5. Jacobs, I.J.; Menon, U.; Ryan, A.; Gentry-Maharaj, A.; Burnell, M.; Kalsi, J.K.; Amso, N.N.; Apostolidou, S.; Benjamin, E.; Cruickshank, D.; et al. Ovarian cancer screening and mortality in the UK Collaborative Trial of Ovarian Cancer Screening (UKCTOCS): A randomised controlled trial. *Lancet* **2016**, *387*, 945–956. [CrossRef]
6. Jayson, G.C.; Kohn, E.C.; Kitchener, H.C.; Ledermann, J.A. Ovarian cancer. *Lancet* **2014**, *384*, 1376–1388. [CrossRef]
7. Thomas, D.M.; James, P.A.; Ballinger, M.L. Clinical implications of genomics for cancer risk genetics. *Lancet Oncol.* **2015**, *16*, e303–e308. [CrossRef]
8. Jervis, S.; Song, H.; Lee, A.; Dicks, E.; Tyrer, J.; Harrington, P.; Easton, D.F.; Jacobs, I.J.; Pharoah, P.P.; Antoniou, A.C. Ovarian cancer familial relative risks by tumour subtypes and by known ovarian cancer genetic susceptibility variants. *J. Med. Genet.* **2014**, *51*, 108–113. [CrossRef]
9. Kuchenbaecker, K.B.; Hopper, J.L.; Barnes, D.R.; Phillips, K.A.; Mooij, T.M.; Roos-Blom, M.J.; Jervis, S.; van Leeuwen, F.E.; Milne, R.L.; Andrieu, N.; et al. Risks of Breast, Ovarian, and Contralateral Breast Cancer for BRCA1 and BRCA2 Mutation Carriers. *JAMA* **2017**, *317*, 2402–2416. [CrossRef]
10. Yang, X.; Song, H.; Leslie, G.; Engel, C.; Hahnen, E.; Auber, B.; Horváth, J.; Kast, K.; Niederacher, D.; Turnbull, C.; et al. Ovarian and Breast Cancer Risks Associated With Pathogenic Variants in RAD51C and RAD51D. *J. Natl. Cancer Inst.* **2020**, *112*. [CrossRef]
11. Ramus, S.J.; Song, H.; Dicks, E.; Tyrer, J.P.; Rosenthal, A.N.; Intermaggio, M.P.; Fraser, L.; Gentry-Maharaj, A.; Hayward, J.; Philpott, S.; et al. Germline Mutations in the BRIP1, BARD1, PALB2, and NBN Genes in Women With Ovarian Cancer. *J. Natl. Cancer Inst.* **2015**, *107*. [CrossRef]
12. Yang, X.; Leslie, G.; Doroszuk, A.; Schneider, S.; Allen, J.; Decker, B.; Dunning, A.M.; Redman, J.; Scarth, J.; Plaskocinska, I.; et al. Cancer Risks Associated with Germline PALB2 Pathogenic Variants: An International Study of 524 Families. *J. Clin. Oncol.* **2020**, *38*, 674–685. [CrossRef]
13. Møller, P.; Seppälä, T.T.; Bernstein, I.; Holinski-Feder, E.; Sala, P.; Gareth Evans, D.; Lindblom, A.; Macrae, F.; Blanco, I.; Sijmons, R.H.; et al. Cancer risk and survival in path_MMR carriers by gene and gender up to 75 years of age: A report from the Prospective Lynch Syndrome Database. *Gut* **2018**, *67*, 1306–1316. [CrossRef]

14. Kar, S.P.; Berchuck, A.; Gayther, S.A.; Goode, E.L.; Moysich, K.B.; Pearce, C.L.; Ramus, S.J.; Schildkraut, J.M.; Sellers, T.A.; Pharoah, P.D.P. Common Genetic Variation and Susceptibility to Ovarian Cancer: Current Insights and Future Directions. *Cancer Epidemiol. Biomark. Prev.* **2018**, *27*, 395. [CrossRef]
15. Phelan, C.M.; Kuchenbaecker, K.B.; Tyrer, J.P.; Kar, S.P.; Lawrenson, K.; Winham, S.J.; Dennis, J.; Pirie, A.; Riggan, M.J.; Chornokur, G.; et al. Identification of 12 new susceptibility loci for different histotypes of epithelial ovarian cancer. *Nat. Genet.* **2017**, *49*, 680–691. [CrossRef]
16. Ramus, S.J.; Harrington, P.A.; Pye, C.; DiCioccio, R.A.; Cox, M.J.; Garlinghouse-Jones, K.; Oakley-Girvan, I.; Jacobs, I.J.; Hardy, R.M.; Whittemore, A.S.; et al. Contribution of BRCA1 and BRCA2 mutations to inherited ovarian cancer. *Hum. Mutat.* **2007**, *28*, 1207–1215. [CrossRef]
17. Ramus, S.J.; Gayther, S.A. The Contribution of BRCA1 and BRCA2 to Ovarian Cancer. *Mol. Oncol.* **2009**, *3*, 138–150. [CrossRef]
18. Johannesdottir, G.; Gudmundsson, J.; Bergthorsson, J.T.; Arason, A.; Agnarsson, B.A.; Eiriksdottir, G.; Johannsson, O.T.; Borg, A.; Ingvarsson, S.; Easton, D.F.; et al. High Prevalence of the 999del5 Mutation in Icelandic Breast and Ovarian Cancer Patients. *Cancer Res.* **1996**, *56*, 3663–3665.
19. Gayther, S.A.; Harrington, P.; Russell, P.; Kharkevich, G.; Garkavtseva, R.F.; Ponder, B.A. Frequently occurring germ-line mutations of the BRCA1 gene in ovarian cancer families from Russia. *Am. J. Hum. Genet.* **1997**, *60*, 1239–1242.
20. Sokolenko, A.P.; Rozanov, M.E.; Mitiushkina, N.V.; Sherina, N.Y.; Iyevleva, A.G.; Chekmariova, E.V.; Buslov, K.G.; Shilov, E.S.; Togo, A.V.; Bit-Sava, E.M.; et al. Founder mutations in early-onset, familial and bilateral breast cancer patients from Russia. *Fam. Cancer* **2007**, *6*, 281–286. [CrossRef] [PubMed]
21. Menkiszak, J.; Gronwald, J.; Górski, B.; Jakubowska, A.; Huzarski, T.; Byrski, T.; Foszczyńska-Kłoda, M.; Haus, O.; Janiszewska, H.; Perkowska, M.; et al. Hereditary ovarian cancer in Poland. *Int. J. Cancer* **2003**, *106*, 942–945. [CrossRef]
22. Heimdal, K.; Maehle, L.; Apold, J.; Pedersen, J.C.; Møller, P. The Norwegian founder mutations in BRCA1: High penetrance confirmed in an incident cancer series and differences observed in the risk of ovarian cancer. *Eur. J. Cancer* **2003**, *39*, 2205–2213. [CrossRef]
23. Sarantaus, L.; Huusko, P.; Eerola, H.; Launonen, V.; Vehmanen, P.; Rapakko, K.; Gillanders, E.; Syrjäkoski, K.; Kainu, T.; Vahteristo, P.; et al. Multiple founder effects and geographical clustering of BRCA1 and BRCA2 families in Finland. *Eur. J. Hum. Genet.* **2000**, *8*, 757–763. [CrossRef]
24. Sekine, M.; Nagata, H.; Tsuji, S.; Hirai, Y.; Fujimoto, S.; Hatae, M.; Kobayashi, I.; Fujii, T.; Nagata, I.; Ushijima, K.; et al. Mutational analysis of BRCA1 and BRCA2 and clinicopathologic analysis of ovarian cancer in 82 ovarian cancer families: Two common founder mutations of BRCA1 in Japanese population. *Clin. Cancer Res.* **2001**, *7*, 3144–3150.
25. Khoo, U.S.; Chan, K.Y.; Cheung, A.N.; Xue, W.C.; Shen, D.H.; Fung, K.Y.; Ngan, H.Y.; Choy, K.W.; Pang, C.P.; Poon, C.S.; et al. Recurrent BRCA1 and BRCA2 germline mutations in ovarian cancer: A founder mutation of BRCA1 identified in the Chinese population. *Hum. Mutat.* **2002**, *19*, 307–308. [CrossRef]
26. Kurian, A.W.; Hughes, E.; Handorf, E.A.; Gutin, A.; Allen, B.; Hartman, A.-R.; Hall, M.J. Breast and Ovarian Cancer Penetrance Estimates Derived from Germline Multiple-Gene Sequencing Results in Women. *JCO Precis. Oncol.* **2017**, *1*, 1–12. [CrossRef]
27. Lilyquist, J.; LaDuca, H.; Polley, E.; Davis, B.T.; Shimelis, H.; Hu, C.; Hart, S.N.; Dolinsky, J.S.; Couch, F.J.; Goldgar, D.E. Frequency of mutations in a large series of clinically ascertained ovarian cancer cases tested on multi-gene panels compared to reference controls. *Gynecol. Oncol.* **2017**, *147*, 375–380. [CrossRef]
28. Castéra, L.; Harter, V.; Muller, E.; Krieger, S.; Goardon, N.; Ricou, A.; Rousselin, A.; Paimparay, G.; Legros, A.; Bruet, O.; et al. Landscape of pathogenic variations in a panel of 34 genes and cancer risk estimation from 5131 HBOC families. *Genet. Med.* **2018**, *20*, 1677–1686. [CrossRef]
29. Suszynska, M.; Klonowska, K.; Jasinska, A.J.; Kozlowski, P. Large-scale meta-analysis of mutations identified in panels of breast/ovarian cancer-related genes—Providing evidence of cancer predisposition genes. *Gynecol. Oncol.* **2019**, *153*, 452–462. [CrossRef]
30. Iqbal, J.; Ragone, A.; Lubinski, J.; Lynch, H.T.; Moller, P.; Ghadirian, P.; Foulkes, W.D.; Armel, S.; Eisen, A.; Neuhausen, S.L.; et al. The incidence of pancreatic cancer in BRCA1 and BRCA2 mutation carriers. *Br. J. Cancer* **2012**, *107*, 2005–2009. [CrossRef]

31. Pritchard, C.C.; Mateo, J.; Walsh, M.F.; De Sarkar, N.; Abida, W.; Beltran, H.; Garofalo, A.; Gulati, R.; Carreira, S.; Eeles, R.; et al. Inherited DNA-Repair Gene Mutations in Men with Metastatic Prostate Cancer. *N. Engl. J. Med.* **2016**, *375*, 443–453. [CrossRef]
32. Alsop, K.; Fereday, S.; Meldrum, C.; deFazio, A.; Emmanuel, C.; George, J.; Dobrovic, A.; Birrer, M.J.; Webb, P.M.; Stewart, C.; et al. BRCA mutation frequency and patterns of treatment response in BRCA mutation-positive women with ovarian cancer: A report from the Australian Ovarian Cancer Study Group. *J. Clin. Oncol.* **2012**, *30*, 2654–2663. [CrossRef]
33. Song, H.; Cicek, M.S.; Dicks, E.; Harrington, P.; Ramus, S.J.; Cunningham, J.M.; Fridley, B.L.; Tyrer, J.P.; Alsop, J.; Jimenez-Linan, M.; et al. The contribution of deleterious germline mutations in BRCA1, BRCA2 and the mismatch repair genes to ovarian cancer in the population. *Hum. Mol. Genet.* **2014**, *23*, 4703–4709. [CrossRef]
34. Walsh, T.; Casadei, S.; Lee, M.K.; Pennil, C.C.; Nord, A.S.; Thornton, A.M.; Roeb, W.; Agnew, K.J.; Stray, S.M.; Wickramanayake, A.; et al. Mutations in 12 genes for inherited ovarian, fallopian tube, and peritoneal carcinoma identified by massively parallel sequencing. *Proc. Natl. Acad. Sci. USA* **2011**, *108*, 18032–18037. [CrossRef]
35. Norquist, B.M.; Harrell, M.I.; Brady, M.F.; Walsh, T.; Lee, M.K.; Gulsuner, S.; Bernards, S.S.; Casadei, S.; Yi, Q.; Burger, R.A.; et al. Inherited Mutations in Women with Ovarian Carcinoma. *JAMA Oncol.* **2016**, *2*, 482–490. [CrossRef]
36. Bolton, K.L.; Chenevix-Trench, G.; Goh, C.; Sadetzki, S.; Ramus, S.J.; Karlan, B.Y.; Lambrechts, D.; Despierre, E.; Barrowdale, D.; McGuffog, L.; et al. Association between BRCA1 and BRCA2 Mutations and Survival in Women with Invasive Epithelial Ovarian Cancer. *JAMA* **2012**, *307*, 382–390. [CrossRef]
37. Kotsopoulos, J.; Rosen, B.; Fan, I.; Moody, J.; McLaughlin, J.R.; Risch, H.; May, T.; Sun, P.; Narod, S.A. Ten-year survival after epithelial ovarian cancer is not associated with BRCA mutation status. *Gynecol. Oncol.* **2016**, *140*, 42–47. [CrossRef]
38. McLaughlin, J.R.; Rosen, B.; Moody, J.; Pal, T.; Fan, I.; Shaw, P.A.; Risch, H.A.; Sellers, T.A.; Sun, P.; Narod, S.A. Long-Term Ovarian Cancer Survival Associated with Mutation in BRCA1 or BRCA2. *J. Natl. Cancer Inst.* **2013**, *105*, 141–148. [CrossRef]
39. National Comprehensive Cancer Network. Genetics Screening (Version 2.2019). Available online: https://www.nccn.org/professionals/physician_gls/pdf/genetics_screening.pdf (accessed on 11 June 2020).
40. Cancer Genome Atlas Research Network. Integrated genomic analyses of ovarian carcinoma. *Nature* **2011**, *474*, 609–615. [CrossRef]
41. Kaufman, B.; Shapira-Frommer, R.; Schmutzler, R.K.; Audeh, M.W.; Friedlander, M.; Balmaña, J.; Mitchell, G.; Fried, G.; Stemmer, S.M.; Hubert, A.; et al. Olaparib monotherapy in patients with advanced cancer and a germline BRCA1/2 mutation. *J. Clin. Oncol.* **2015**, *33*, 244–250. [CrossRef]
42. Swisher, E.M.; Lin, K.K.; Oza, A.M.; Scott, C.L.; Giordano, H.; Sun, J.; Konecny, G.E.; Coleman, R.L.; Tinker, A.V.; O'Malley, D.M.; et al. Rucaparib in relapsed, platinum-sensitive high-grade ovarian carcinoma (ARIEL2 Part 1): An international, multicentre, open-label, phase 2 trial. *Lancet Oncol.* **2017**, *18*, 75–87. [CrossRef]
43. Oza, A.M.; Tinker, A.V.; Oaknin, A.; Shapira-Frommer, R.; McNeish, I.A.; Swisher, E.M.; Ray-Coquard, I.; Bell-McGuinn, K.; Coleman, R.L.; O'Malley, D.M.; et al. Antitumor activity and safety of the PARP inhibitor rucaparib in patients with high-grade ovarian carcinoma and a germline or somatic BRCA1 or BRCA2 mutation: Integrated analysis of data from Study 10 and ARIEL2. *Gynecol. Oncol.* **2017**, *147*, 267–275. [CrossRef]
44. Gelmon, K.A.; Tischkowitz, M.; Mackay, H.; Swenerton, K.; Robidoux, A.; Tonkin, K.; Hirte, H.; Huntsman, D.; Clemons, M.; Gilks, B.; et al. Olaparib in patients with recurrent high-grade serous or poorly differentiated ovarian carcinoma or triple-negative breast cancer: A phase 2, multicentre, open-label, non-randomised study. *Lancet Oncol.* **2011**, *12*, 852–861. [CrossRef]
45. Suszynska, M.; Ratajska, M.; Kozlowski, P. BRIP1, RAD51C, and RAD51D mutations are associated with high susceptibility to ovarian cancer: Mutation prevalence and precise risk estimates based on a pooled analysis of ~30,000 cases. *J. Ovarian Res.* **2020**, *13*, 50. [CrossRef]
46. Meindl, A.; Hellebrand, H.; Wiek, C.; Erven, V.; Wappenschmidt, B.; Niederacher, D.; Freund, M.; Lichtner, P.; Hartmann, L.; Schaal, H.; et al. Germline mutations in breast and ovarian cancer pedigrees establish RAD51C as a human cancer susceptibility gene. *Nat. Genet.* **2010**, *42*, 410–414. [CrossRef]

47. Loveday, C.; Turnbull, C.; Ramsay, E.; Hughes, D.; Ruark, E.; Frankum, J.R.; Bowden, G.; Kalmyrzaev, B.; Warren-Perry, M.; Snape, K.; et al. Germline mutations in RAD51D confer susceptibility to ovarian cancer. *Nat. Genet.* **2011**, *43*, 879–882. [CrossRef]
48. Song, H.; Dicks, E.; Ramus, S.J.; Tyrer, J.P.; Intermaggio, M.P.; Hayward, J.; Edlund, C.K.; Conti, D.; Harrington, P.; Fraser, L.; et al. Contribution of Germline Mutations in the RAD51B, RAD51C, and RAD51D Genes to Ovarian Cancer in the Population. *J. Clin. Oncol.* **2015**, *33*, 2901–2907. [CrossRef]
49. Manchanda, R.; Legood, R.; Antoniou, A.; Pearce, L.; Menon, U. Commentary on changing the risk threshold for surgical prevention of ovarian cancer. *BJOG An. Int. J. Obstet. Gynaecol.* **2018**, *125*, 541–544. [CrossRef]
50. Manchanda, R.; Legood, R.; Antoniou, A.C.; Gordeev, V.S.; Menon, U. Specifying the ovarian cancer risk threshold of 'premenopausal risk-reducing salpingo-oophorectomy' for ovarian cancer prevention: A cost-effectiveness analysis. *J. Med. Genet.* **2016**, *53*, 591–599. [CrossRef]
51. Manchanda, R.; Legood, R.; Pearce, L.; Menon, U. Defining the risk threshold for risk reducing salpingo-oophorectomy for ovarian cancer prevention in low risk postmenopausal women. *Gynecol. Oncol.* **2015**, *139*, 487–494. [CrossRef]
52. Antoniou, A.C.; Casadei, S.; Heikkinen, T.; Barrowdale, D.; Pylkas, K.; Roberts, J.; Lee, A.; Subramanian, D.; De Leeneer, K.; Fostira, F.; et al. Breast-cancer risk in families with mutations in PALB2. *N. Engl. J. Med.* **2014**, *371*, 497–506. [CrossRef]
53. Ducy, M.; Sesma-Sanz, L.; Guitton-Sert, L.; Lashgari, A.; Gao, Y.; Brahiti, N.; Rodrigue, A.; Margaillan, G.; Caron, M.C.; Côté, J.; et al. The Tumor Suppressor PALB2: Inside out. *Trends Biochem. Sci.* **2019**, *44*, 226–240. [CrossRef]
54. Song, H.; Ramus, S.; Dicks, E.; Tyrer, J.; Intermaggio, M.; Chenevix-Trench, G.; Bowtell, D.; Traficante, N.; Brenton, J.; Goranova, T.; et al. Population based targeted sequencing of 54 candidate genes identifies PALB2 as a susceptibility gene for high grade serous ovarian cancer. *J Med Genet.* **2020**. [CrossRef]
55. Osorio, A.; Endt, D.; Fernández, F.; Eirich, K.; de la Hoya, M.; Schmutzler, R.; Caldés, T.; Meindl, A.; Schindler, D.; Benitez, J. Predominance of pathogenic missense variants in the RAD51C gene occurring in breast and ovarian cancer families. *Hum. Mol. Genet.* **2012**, *21*, 2889–2898. [CrossRef]
56. Ketabi, Z.; Bartuma, K.; Bernstein, I.; Malander, S.; Grönberg, H.; Björck, E.; Holck, S.; Nilbert, M. Ovarian cancer linked to Lynch syndrome typically presents as early-onset, non-serous epithelial tumors. *Gynecol. Oncol.* **2011**, *121*, 462–465. [CrossRef]
57. Lu, H.M.; Li, S.; Black, M.H.; Lee, S.; Hoiness, R.; Wu, S.; Mu, W.; Huether, R.; Chen, J.; Sridhar, S.; et al. Association of Breast and Ovarian Cancers with Predisposition Genes Identified by Large-Scale Sequencing. *JAMA Oncol.* **2019**, *5*, 51–57. [CrossRef]
58. Spurdle, A.B.; Healey, S.; Devereau, A.; Hogervorst, F.B.; Monteiro, A.N.; Nathanson, K.L.; Radice, P.; Stoppa-Lyonnet, D.; Tavtigian, S.; Wappenschmidt, B.; et al. ENIGMA—Evidence-based network for the interpretation of germline mutant alleles: An international initiative to evaluate risk and clinical significance associated with sequence variation in BRCA1 and BRCA2 genes. *Hum. Mutat* **2012**, *33*, 2–7. [CrossRef]
59. Li, H.; LaDuca, H.; Pesaran, T.; Chao, E.C.; Dolinsky, J.S.; Parsons, M.; Spurdle, A.B.; Polley, E.C.; Shimelis, H.; Hart, S.N.; et al. Classification of variants of uncertain significance in BRCA1 and BRCA2 using personal and family history of cancer from individuals in a large hereditary cancer multigene panel testing cohort. *Genet. Med.* **2020**, *22*, 701–708. [CrossRef]
60. Thompson, B.A.; Spurdle, A.B.; Plazzer, J.P.; Greenblatt, M.S.; Akagi, K.; Al-Mulla, F.; Bapat, B.; Bernstein, I.; Capellá, G.; den Dunnen, J.T.; et al. Application of a 5-tiered scheme for standardized classification of 2,360 unique mismatch repair gene variants in the InSiGHT locus-specific database. *Nat. Genet.* **2014**, *46*, 107–115. [CrossRef]
61. Ng, P.C.; Henikoff, S. SIFT: Predicting amino acid changes that affect protein function. *Nucleic Acids Res.* **2003**, *31*, 3812–3814. [CrossRef]
62. Adzhubei, I.; Jordan, D.M.; Sunyaev, S.R. Predicting functional effect of human missense mutations using PolyPhen-2. *Curr. Protoc. Hum. Genet.* **2013**, *76*, 7–20. [CrossRef]
63. Choi, Y.; Chan, A.P. PROVEAN web server: A tool to predict the functional effect of amino acid substitutions and indels. *Bioinformatics* **2015**, *31*, 2745–2747. [CrossRef]
64. Tyrer, J.P.; Guo, Q.; Easton, D.F.; Pharoah, P.D. The admixture maximum likelihood test to test for association between rare variants and disease phenotypes. *BMC Bioinform.* **2013**, *14*, 177. [CrossRef]

65. Bouwman, P.; van der Gulden, H.; van der Heijden, I.; Drost, R.; Klijn, C.N.; Prasetyanti, P.; Pieterse, M.; Wientjens, E.; Seibler, J.; Hogervorst, F.B.; et al. A high-throughput functional complementation assay for classification of BRCA1 missense variants. *Cancer Discov.* **2013**, *3*, 1142–1155. [CrossRef]
66. Dicks, E.; Song, H.; Ramus, S.J.; Oudenhove, E.V.; Tyrer, J.P.; Intermaggio, M.P.; Kar, S.; Harrington, P.; Bowtell, D.D.; Group, A.S.; et al. Germline whole exome sequencing and large-scale replication identifies FANCM as a likely high grade serous ovarian cancer susceptibility gene. *Oncotarget* **2017**, *8*, 50930–50940. [CrossRef]
67. Thompson, D.; Duedal, S.; Kirner, J.; McGuffog, L.; Last, J.; Reiman, A.; Byrd, P.; Taylor, M.; Easton, D.F. Cancer Risks and Mortality in Heterozygous ATM Mutation Carriers. *JNCI J. Natl. Cancer Inst.* **2005**, *97*, 813–822. [CrossRef]
68. Roberts, N.J.; Jiao, Y.; Yu, J.; Kopelovich, L.; Petersen, G.M.; Bondy, M.L.; Gallinger, S.; Schwartz, A.G.; Syngal, S.; Cote, M.L.; et al. ATM mutations in patients with hereditary pancreatic cancer. *Cancer Discov.* **2012**, *2*, 41–46. [CrossRef]
69. Goldgar, D.E.; Healey, S.; Dowty, J.G.; Da Silva, L.; Chen, X.; Spurdle, A.B.; Terry, M.B.; Daly, M.J.; Buys, S.M.; Southey, M.C.; et al. Rare variants in the ATM gene and risk of breast cancer. *Breast Cancer Res.* **2011**, *13*, R73. [CrossRef]
70. Weber-Lassalle, N.; Borde, J.; Weber-Lassalle, K.; Horváth, J.; Niederacher, D.; Arnold, N.; Kaulfuß, S.; Ernst, C.; Paul, V.G.; Honisch, E.; et al. Germline loss-of-function variants in the BARD1 gene are associated with early-onset familial breast cancer but not ovarian cancer. *Breast Cancer Res.* **2019**, *21*, 55. [CrossRef]
71. Couch, F.J.; Shimelis, H.; Hu, C.; Hart, S.N.; Polley, E.C.; Na, J.; Hallberg, E.; Moore, R.; Thomas, A.; Lilyquist, J.; et al. Associations between Cancer Predisposition Testing Panel Genes and Breast Cancer. *JAMA Oncol.* **2017**, *3*, 1190–1196. [CrossRef]
72. Weischer, M.; Nordestgaard, B.G.; Pharoah, P.; Bolla, M.K.; Nevanlinna, H.; Van't Veer, L.J.; Garcia-Closas, M.; Hopper, J.L.; Hall, P.; Andrulis, I.L.; et al. CHEK2*1100delC heterozygosity in women with breast cancer associated with early death, breast cancer-specific death, and increased risk of a second breast cancer. *J. Clin. Oncol. Off. J. Am. Soc. Clin. Oncol.* **2012**, *30*, 4308–4316. [CrossRef]
73. Gylling, A.; Ridanpää, M.; Vierimaa, O.; Aittomäki, K.; Avela, K.; Kääriäinen, H.; Laivuori, H.; Pöyhönen, M.; Sallinen, S.-L.; Wallgren-Pettersson, C.; et al. Large genomic rearrangements and germline epimutations in Lynch syndrome. *Int. J. Cancer* **2009**, *124*, 2333–2340. [CrossRef]
74. Easton, D.F.; Pharoah, P.D.; Antoniou, A.C.; Tischkowitz, M.; Tavtigian, S.V.; Nathanson, K.L.; Devilee, P.; Meindl, A.; Couch, F.J.; Southey, M.; et al. Gene-panel sequencing and the prediction of breast-cancer risk. *N. Engl. J. Med.* **2015**, *372*, 2243–2257. [CrossRef] [PubMed]
75. Prapa, M.; Solomons, J.; Tischkowitz, M. The use of panel testing in familial breast and ovarian cancer. *Clin. Med.* **2017**, *17*, 568–572. [CrossRef]
76. Menon, U.; Karpinskyj, C.; Gentry-Maharaj, A. Ovarian Cancer Prevention and Screening. *Obstet Gynecol.* **2018**, *131*, 909–927. [CrossRef]
77. Domchek, S.M.; Robson, M.E. Update on Genetic Testing in Gynecologic Cancer. *J. Clin. Oncol.* **2019**, *37*, 2501–2509. [CrossRef]
78. Manchanda, R.; Menon, U. Setting the Threshold for Surgical Prevention in Women at Increased Risk of Ovarian Cancer. *Int. J. Gynecol. Cancer* **2018**, *28*, 34–42. [CrossRef]
79. Rosenthal, A.N.; Fraser, L.S.M.; Philpott, S.; Manchanda, R.; Burnell, M.; Badman, P.; Hadwin, R.; Rizzuto, I.; Benjamin, E.; Singh, N.; et al. Evidence of Stage Shift in Women Diagnosed with Ovarian Cancer during Phase II of the United Kingdom Familial Ovarian Cancer Screening Study. *J. Clin. Oncol.* **2017**, *35*, 1411–1420. [CrossRef] [PubMed]
80. Clayton, E.W. Ethical, legal, and social implications of genomic medicine. *N. Engl. J. Med.* **2003**, *349*, 562–569. [CrossRef]
81. Mersch, J.; Brown, N.; Pirzadeh-Miller, S.; Mundt, E.; Cox, H.C.; Brown, K.; Aston, M.; Esterling, L.; Manley, S.; Ross, T. Prevalence of Variant Reclassification Following Hereditary Cancer Genetic Testing. *JAMA* **2018**, *320*, 1266–1274. [CrossRef]
82. LaDuca, H.; Stuenkel, A.J.; Dolinsky, J.S.; Keiles, S.; Tandy, S.; Pesaran, T.; Chen, E.; Gau, C.-L.; Palmaer, E.; Shoaepour, K.; et al. Utilization of multigene panels in hereditary cancer predisposition testing: Analysis of more than 2,000 patients. *Genet. Med. Off. J. Am. Coll. Med Genet.* **2014**, *16*, 830–837. [CrossRef] [PubMed]

83. Tandy-Connor, S.; Guiltinan, J.; Krempely, K.; LaDuca, H.; Reineke, P.; Gutierrez, S.; Gray, P.; Tippin Davis, B. False-positive results released by direct-to-consumer genetic tests highlight the importance of clinical confirmation testing for appropriate patient care. *Genet. Med.* **2018**, *20*, 1515–1521. [CrossRef] [PubMed]
84. Tung, N.; Domchek, S.M.; Stadler, Z.; Nathanson, K.L.; Couch, F.; Garber, J.E.; Offit, K.; Robson, M.E. Counselling framework for moderate-penetrance cancer-susceptibility mutations. *Nat. Rev. Clin. Oncol.* **2016**, *13*, 581–588. [CrossRef] [PubMed]
85. Giuliano, A.E.; Boolbol, S.; Degnim, A.; Kuerer, H.; Leitch, A.M.; Morrow, M. Society of Surgical Oncology: Position statement on prophylactic mastectomy. Approved by the Society of Surgical Oncology Executive Council, March 2007. *Ann. Surg Oncol.* **2007**, *14*, 2425–2427. [CrossRef] [PubMed]
86. Gabai-Kapara, E.; Lahad, A.; Kaufman, B.; Friedman, E.; Segev, S.; Renbaum, P.; Beeri, R.; Gal, M.; Grinshpun-Cohen, J.; Djemal, K.; et al. Population-based screening for breast and ovarian cancer risk due to *BRCA1* and *BRCA2*. *Proc. Natl. Acad. Sci. USA* **2014**, *111*, 14205–14210. [CrossRef] [PubMed]
87. Manchanda, R.; Loggenberg, K.; Sanderson, S.; Burnell, M.; Wardle, J.; Gessler, S.; Side, L.; Balogun, N.; Desai, R.; Kumar, A.; et al. Population Testing for Cancer Predisposing BRCA1/BRCA2 Mutations in the Ashkenazi-Jewish Community: A Randomized Controlled Trial. *JNCI J. Natl. Cancer Inst.* **2014**, *107*. [CrossRef] [PubMed]
88. Chen, K.; Ma, H.; Li, L.; Zang, R.; Wang, C.; Song, F.; Shi, T.; Yu, D.; Yang, M.; Xue, W.; et al. Genome-wide association study identifies new susceptibility loci for epithelial ovarian cancer in Han Chinese women. *Nat. Commun.* **2014**, *5*, 4682. [CrossRef]
89. Coleman, R.L.; Fleming, G.F.; Brady, M.F.; Swisher, E.M.; Steffensen, K.D.; Friedlander, M.; Okamoto, A.; Moore, K.N.; Efrat Ben-Baruch, N.; Werner, T.L.; et al. Veliparib with First-Line Chemotherapy and as Maintenance Therapy in Ovarian Cancer. *N. Engl. J. Med.* **2019**, *381*, 2403–2415. [CrossRef]
90. Ray-Coquard, I.; Pautier, P.; Pignata, S.; Pérol, D.; González-Martín, A.; Berger, R.; Fujiwara, K.; Vergote, I.; Colombo, N.; Mäenpää, J.; et al. Olaparib plus Bevacizumab as First-Line Maintenance in Ovarian Cancer. *N. Engl. J. Med.* **2019**, *381*, 2416–2428. [CrossRef]
91. González-Martín, A.; Pothuri, B.; Vergote, I.; DePont Christensen, R.; Graybill, W.; Mirza, M.R.; McCormick, C.; Lorusso, D.; Hoskins, P.; Freyer, G.; et al. Niraparib in Patients with Newly Diagnosed Advanced Ovarian Cancer. *N. Engl. J. Med.* **2019**, *381*, 2391–2402. [CrossRef]
92. Longo, D.L. Personalized Medicine for Primary Treatment of Serous Ovarian Cancer. *N. Engl. J. Med.* **2019**, *381*, 2471–2474. [CrossRef] [PubMed]
93. Lheureux, S.; Gourley, C.; Vergote, I.; Oza, A.M. Epithelial ovarian cancer. *Lancet* **2019**, *393*, 1240–1253. [CrossRef]

Publisher's Note: MDPI stays neutral with regard to jurisdictional claims in published maps and institutional affiliations.

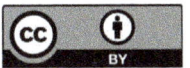

© 2020 by the authors. Licensee MDPI, Basel, Switzerland. This article is an open access article distributed under the terms and conditions of the Creative Commons Attribution (CC BY) license (http://creativecommons.org/licenses/by/4.0/).

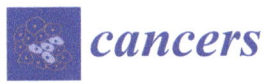

Article

Women's Intentions to Engage in Risk-Reducing Behaviours after Receiving Personal Ovarian Cancer Risk Information: An Experimental Survey Study

Ailish Gallagher [1], Jo Waller [2], Ranjit Manchanda [3,4], Ian Jacobs [5] and Saskia Sanderson [1,6,*]

[1] Research Department of Behavioural Science and Health, University College London, Gower Street, London WC1E 6BT, UK; Ailish.gallagher@gstt.nhs.uk
[2] Cancer Prevention Group, School of Cancer & Pharmaceutical Sciences, King's College London, Guy's Hospital, Great Maze Pond, London SE1 9RT, UK; jo.waller@kcl.ac.uk
[3] Wolfson Institute of Preventive Medicine, Barts Cancer Institute, Queen Mary University of London, Charterhouse Square, London EC1M 6BQ, UK; r.manchanda@qmul.ac.uk
[4] Department of Gynaecological Oncology, Barts Health NHS Trust, London EC1A 7BE, UK
[5] Department of Women's Health, University of New South Wales, Australia, Level 1, Chancellery Building, Sydney 2052, Australia; i.jacobs@unsw.edu.au
[6] Early Disease Detection Research Project UK (EDDRP UK), 2 Redman Place, London E20 1JQ, UK
* Correspondence: saskia.sanderson@ucl.ac.uk

Received: 5 October 2020; Accepted: 24 November 2020; Published: 27 November 2020

Simple Summary: Risk stratification using genetic testing to identify women at increased risk of ovarian cancer may increase the number of patients to whom risk-reducing surgery (e.g., salpingo-oophorectomy) may be offered. However, little is known about public acceptability of such approaches. Our online experimental survey aimed to explore whether women aged 45–75 in the general population are willing to undergo ovarian cancer risk assessment, including genetic testing, and whether women's potential acceptance of risk-reducing surgery differs depending on their estimated risk. We looked at whether psychological and cognitive factors mediated women's decision-making. The majority of participants would be interested in having genetic testing. In response to our hypothetical scenarios, a substantial proportion of participants were open to the idea of surgery to reduce risk of ovarian cancer, even if their absolute lifetime risk is only increased from 2% to 5 or 10%.

Abstract: Risk stratification using genetic and/or other types of information could identify women at increased ovarian cancer risk. The aim of this study was to examine women's potential reactions to ovarian cancer risk stratification. A total of 1017 women aged 45–75 years took part in an online experimental survey. Women were randomly assigned to one of three experimental conditions describing hypothetical personal results from ovarian cancer risk stratification, and asked to imagine they had received one of three results: (a) 5% lifetime risk due to single nucleotide polymorphisms (SNPs) and lifestyle factors; (b) 10% lifetime risk due to SNPs and lifestyle factors; (c) 10% lifetime risk due to a single rare mutation in a gene. Results: 83% of women indicated interest in having ovarian cancer risk assessment. After receiving their hypothetical risk estimates, 29% of women stated they would have risk-reducing surgery. Choosing risk-reducing surgery over other behavioural responses was associated with having higher surgery self-efficacy and perceived response-efficacy, but not with perceptions of disease threat, i.e., perceived risk or severity, or with experimental condition. A substantial proportion of women age 45–75 years may be open to the idea of surgery to reduce risk of ovarian cancer, even if their absolute lifetime risk is only increased to as little as 5 or 10%.

Keywords: risk stratification; genomics; questionnaires; attitudes

1. Introduction

Ovarian cancer is the sixth most common cancer among women in the UK. The general population lifetime risk of developing ovarian cancer is approximately 2%, and incidence is predicted to rise by 26% in the UK, 14% in Europe, and by 55% worldwide over the next two decades [1]. The risk of ovarian cancer rises with age, increasing significantly in women over 45 years [2]. DNA variants in a number of cancer susceptibility genes are known to be associated with ovarian cancer: women with a high penetrance genetic variant, such as a *BRCA1* or *BRCA2* mutation, are considered to be at high risk for developing breast and ovarian cancer [3–5]. Historically, genetic testing for ovarian cancer risk has been clinically indicated only for women with a strong family history of breast and/or ovarian cancer. However, using a family history based approach misses over half the cancer susceptibility gene (CSG) carriers at risk [6,7], and is associated with restricted access and limited utilization of genetic testing [8]. Additionally, the majority of cases of ovarian cancer do not occur in affected families [9]. There is increasing interest in the idea of adopting a risk-stratified approach to ovarian cancer prevention by offering genetic testing to all women regardless of family history [10–12].

In addition to rare variants of high penetrance, genome-wide association studies have to date identified a number of common single nucleotide polymorphisms (SNPs) associated with slightly increased risk of ovarian cancer [13]. SNP-based information and certain lifestyle factors each increase ovarian cancer risk by a small amount individually, but this becomes clinically significant when the information is combined, e.g., from 2% to between 5% and 10% lifetime risk [9,14,15]. Surgical prevention has been shown to be cost-effective at the 4–5% ovarian cancer risk threshold [16,17]. Newer risk models and recently validated intermediate risk genes can identify individuals at these risk thresholds. Risk stratification using multigene testing to identify women at increased risk of ovarian cancer is potentially more cost- and time-effective than single gene testing and increases the number of patients to whom risk-reducing surgery (e.g., salpingo-oophorectomy) may be offered [18]. While clinical practice has gradually begun to change [19], data on public acceptability of such approaches are limited.

An initial quantitative study assessing attitudes towards population-based genetic testing for ovarian cancer risk in a general population sample found high levels of support for risk-stratified ovarian cancer screening based on prior genetic risk assessment [20]. There is good evidence to suggest that population-wide genetic testing for ovarian cancer is acceptable, feasible and cost-effective amongst Ashkenazi Jewish populations [6,7,21–23]. Preliminary data from the general population also indicate that population-based personalised ovarian cancer risk stratification is feasible, acceptable, has high satisfaction, reduces cancer worry/risk perception, and does not negatively impact psychological health or quality of life [12].

Bilateral risk-reducing salpingo-oophorectomy (surgical removal of the ovaries and fallopian tubes, hereafter referred to as "risk-reducing salpingo-oophorectomy" or "RRSO") is currently recommended as the main and most effective preventative strategy for ovarian cancer in women at increased risk of ovarian cancer such as *BRCA* mutation carriers. RRSO can reduce ovarian cancer risk by 85–90% [24]. Traditionally the most common group of women undergoing surgical prevention have been *BRCA* carriers, who have a 17–44% lifetime risk of ovarian cancer [5,25]. In the UK, women with an estimated lifetime ovarian cancer risk of greater than 10%, who have completed their families, have traditionally been offered risk-reducing surgery [15]. Undertaking surgery on the basis of family history alone in the absence of a known mutation (at lower than *BRCA* levels of risk) has thus been clinical practice in the UK and other countries for many years [25,26]. Recently, the 10% threshold was relaxed to 4–5% [14,15]. A number of new ovarian cancer risk genes have been identified, such as *RAD51C* (lifetime risk 11%) [27], *RAD51D* (lifetime risk 13%), *PALB2* (lifetime risk 5%) [28], and *BRIP1* (lifetime risk 5.8%) [29], testing for which is part of routine clinical practice. RRSO is now offered and being undertaken for these CSGs too. Thus a number of clinical teams now offer RRSO to women in the "intermediate" risk category (5–10%) as well as those in the "high" risk category (over 10%) [15]. Additionally, more complex models using SNP profiles, in combination with other epidemiological and genetic risk factors, are being validated, which will provide absolute lifetime risk estimates in these ranges in the not too distant future [12].

National screening programmes for ovarian cancer are unavailable. In a large randomised control trial designed to establish the effect of early detection by ovarian screening in the general low-risk population, no conclusive significant impact on mortality from ovarian cancer was found [30], and definitive mortality data are awaited in 2021. Surveillance for those identified as high-risk (or in some cases moderate-to-high-risk) for ovarian cancer currently consists of serial 3–4 monthly serum CA125 (Cancer Antigen 125 protein; a tumour marker) measurement (and annual transvaginal ultrasound) aiming to detect pre-symptomatic cancer in the earlier stages and/or low volume disease where treatment is more effective [31]. This 4 monthly longitudinal CA125 biomarker driven surveillance strategy, using the risk of the ovarian cancer (ROCA) algorithm, may be beneficial in women at high risk of ovarian cancer [31]. We have shown that this is associated with a significant stage shift, which can be a surrogate for improved survival [31]. Identifying those at increased risk using a population wide risk-stratified approach may result in more timely risk reduction options and could have a significant impact on disease burden: modelling suggests that 13% of the female UK population have greater than 4% lifetime risk and 9% have greater than 5% lifetime risk [15]. Manchanda et al. (2018) suggest that, based on National Institute for Health and Care Excellence (NICE) cost-effectiveness guidelines, risk-reducing surgery may be cost effective for postmenopausal women over the age of 50, with a lifetime ovarian cancer risk of ≥5%. Wider implementation of targeted surgical prevention for women at greater than 4–5% lifetime risk threshold provides a huge opportunity for cost-effective targeted primary prevention.

Offering risk stratification to women in the general population, including communicating personal ovarian cancer risk information and offering risk-reducing surgery, has the potential to be a feasible way to reduce ovarian cancer mortality and reduce the population burden of the disease. However, risk stratification will only lead to improved ovarian cancer prevention and early diagnosis if women whose results indicate increased risk take action to reduce their risk. Women with a family history of breast and ovarian cancer have been found to opt for risk reduction surgery, e.g., among *BRCA1* and *BRCA2* mutation carriers, the majority underwent risk-reducing surgery (salpingo-oophorectomy) after their risk was communicated to them [25,32]. However, although quite a lot is known about how genetic risk information impacts psychological wellbeing and behaviours among women from families affected with ovarian (and/or breast) cancer, less is known about how women in the wider non-Jewish population might react to being informed they have an increased genetic risk of ovarian cancer [33–37]. Further research is needed to determine how women in the general population might respond if presented with ovarian cancer risk information indicating they are at high risk based on genetic as well as other risk factors.

Based on research prior to 2016, the evidence does not support the hypothesis that communicating CSG-based risk estimates motivates lifestyle behaviour changes [33,38]. CSG-based risk information also has not been associated with negative psychological outcomes [7,33,38,39]. More recently, a nested study within the Predicting Risk of Cancer at Screening (PROCAS) study was conducted comparing the psychological impact of providing women with personalised breast cancer risk estimates based on: (a) the Tyrer–Cuzick (T–C) risk algorithm including breast density, or (b) T–C including breast density plus SNPs, versus (c) comparison women awaiting results. This study found little evidence of either psychological harm or of differences between women provided with risk estimates based on SNPs versus others. However, women categorised as high-risk were excluded from the study, so no conclusions could be drawn regarding high-risk results specifically. It remains to be seen whether the source of the risk may have impacted psychological factors or if it had an effect on acceptance of the risk information in this study [40]. In another recent study that examined the impact of returning secondary findings (including *BRCA1/2*) from genomic sequencing to unselected populations, few adverse psychological effects were found [41].

As an initial step to providing some empirical data on the question of how women in the general population might respond to personal ovarian cancer risk information indicating increased risk (as against moderate risk [40]), we conducted an experimental survey study with women in the general population, using the Extended Parallel Process Model (EPPM) [42] as our theoretical framework, and to inform our selection of variables and measures. The EPPM is a social cognition model of information processing and behaviour: it posits that how individuals react to threatening information is informed by (a) their perceptions of the threat (perceived risk or susceptibility, and perceived severity), and (b) their perceptions of the recommended action to reduce the threat (self-efficacy, i.e., their confidence in their ability to carry out the recommended behaviour, and perceived response efficacy, i.e., their confidence that the recommended behaviour will effectively reduce the threat to their health).

Our specific aims were to: (1) explore whether women in the general population are willing to undergo ovarian cancer risk assessment which includes genetic testing; (2) examine whether women's potential acceptance of risk-reducing surgery differs depending on whether their estimated risk is 5% or 10%; (3) examine whether women's potential acceptance of risk-reducing surgery differs depending on whether their estimated risk is based on a single rare genetic variant of high penetrance or a more complex combination of genetic and non-genetic factors. We also explored whether threat and efficacy cognitions mediated any observed between-group differences, and examined the associations between these cognitions (threat, efficacy) and acceptance of risk-reducing surgery in the sample overall.

2. Results

2.1. Sample Characteristics

Table 1 provides an overview of the participant characteristics. Age ranged from 45 to 75 years with a mean of 57.50 (SD = 8.13). The majority were White (95.6%) with 3.8% from other ethnic backgrounds. Educational attainment was fairly evenly split between General Certificate of Secondary Education (GCSE) or equivalent (34.6%), A levels or equivalent (23.8%), and undergraduate degree or equivalent (24.1%). The majority (85.2%) of women were either perimenopausal (beginning menopause) or post-menopausal. See Figure 1 for the Consolidated Standards of Reporting Trials (CONSORT) flow diagram of participants throughout the study.

Table 1. Sample characteristics and interest in genetic testing overall and in each randomised experimental group (total n = 1017).

Variables	Group 1: 5% SNPs and Lifestyle (n = 340)	Group 2: 10% SNPs and Lifestyle (n = 343)	Group 3: 10% Rare Genetic Variant (n = 334)
Demographics		n (%)	
Age Mean (SD)	57.43 (8.32)	57.37 (7.78)	58.08 (8.19)
Age group			
45–50	89 (26.2)	82 (23.9)	73 (21.9)
51–55	71 (20.9)	66 (19.2)	67 (20.1)
56–60	59 (17.4)	70 (20.4)	65 (19.5)
61–65	53 (15.6)	70 (20.4)	61 (18.3)
66–70	42 (12.4)	34 (9.9)	38 (11.4)
71–75	26 (7.6)	21 (6.1)	30 (9.0)
Ethnicity			
White (Any background)	327 (96.2)	324 (94.5)	321 (96.1)
Other ethnic group	11 (3.2)	17 (5.0)	11 (3.3)
Educational Attainment			
No Formal Qualification	26 (7.6)	23 (6.7)	17 (5.1)
GCSE or equivalent	115 (33.8)	126 (36.7)	111 (33.2)
A-Levels or equivalent	75 (22.1)	80 (23.3)	87 (26.0)
Undergraduate degree/equivalent	89 (26.2)	77 (22.4)	79 (23.7)
Postgraduate degree/equivalent	31 (9.1)	30 (8.7)	31 (9.3)
Other	4 (1.2)	7 (2.0)	9 (2.7)

Table 1. Cont.

Variables	Group 1: 5% SNPs and Lifestyle ($n = 340$)	Group 2: 10% SNPs and Lifestyle ($n = 343$)	Group 3: 10% Rare Genetic Variant ($n = 334$)
Relationship Status			
Married/Cohabiting/In a relationship	245 (72.1)	232 (67.6)	233 (69.8)
Single/Separated/divorced/widowed	93 (27.4)	111 (32.4)	99 (29.6)
Health Characteristics			
Menopause status			
Premenopausal	41 (12.1)	37 (10.8)	43 (12.9)
During/post menopause	283 (83.2)	298 (86.9)	285 (85.3)
Personal History of Cancer			
Yes	17 (5.0)	16 (4.7)	17 (5.1)
No/Not sure	323 (95.0)	327 (95.3)	317 (94.9)
Family History of Cancer			
Yes	214 (62.4%)	206 (59.7%)	201 (58.8%)
No/Not sure	129 (37.6%)	139 (40.3%)	141 (41.2%)
Cervical Screening			
Regular	192 (72.7)	214 (76.7)	179 (67.8)
Irregular	72 (27.3)	65 (23.3)	85 (32.2)
Not eligible	58 (17.1)	44 (12.8)	62 (18.6)
Breast Screening			
Regular	196 (81.0)	201 (79.4)	196 (79.7)
Irregular	46 (19.0)	52 (20.6)	50 (20.3)
Not eligible	72 (21.2)	59 (17.2)	61 (18.3)
Interest in ovarian cancer risk assessment			
Yes Definitely	139 (40.9)	122 (35.6)	125 (37.4)
Yes Probably	151 (44.4)	156 (45.5)	153 (45.8)
No Probably not	36 (10.6)	46 (13.4)	46 (13.8)
No definitely not	14 (4.1)	19 (5.5)	10 (3.0)

SNPs: single nucleotide polymorphisms; SD: standard deviation; GCSE: General Certificate of Secondary Education.

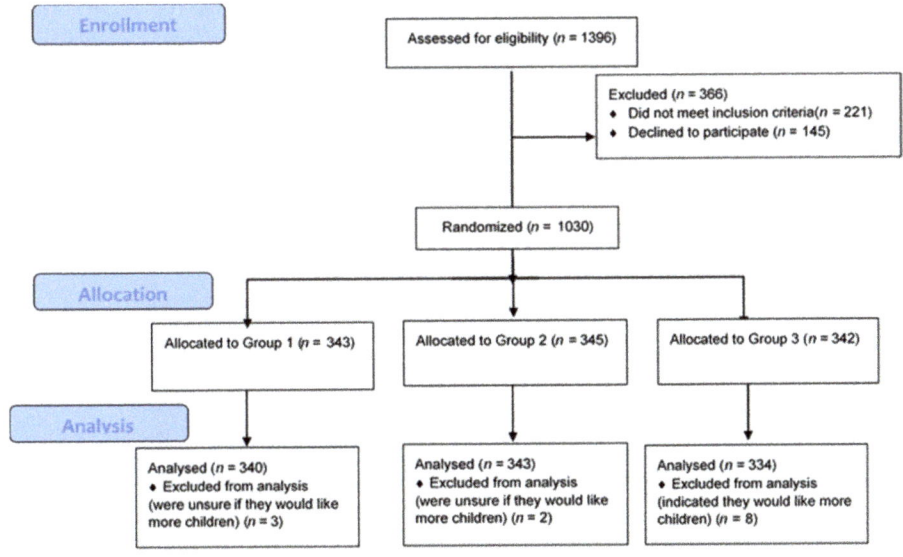

Figure 1. CONSORT 2010 Flow Diagram.

2.2. Interest in Ovarian Cancer Risk Assessment

Overall, 83.2% of women indicated they would "yes definitely" (38.0%) or "yes probably" (45.2%) have an ovarian cancer risk assessment if it was offered to them by their general practitioner (GP) on the National Health Service (NHS) (see Table 1 and Figure 2).

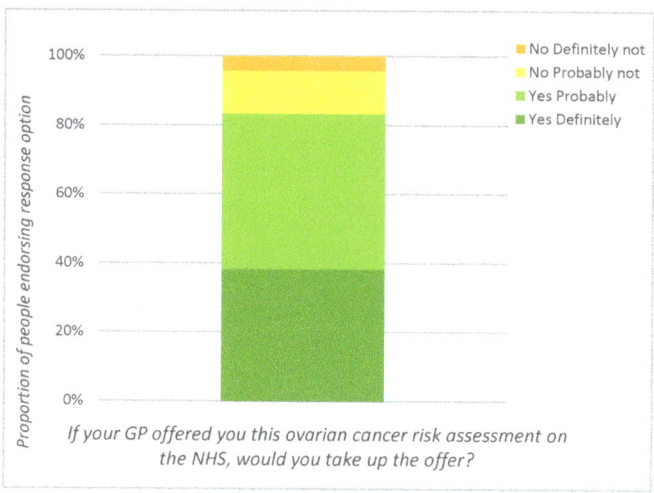

Figure 2. Interest in ovarian cancer risk assessment.

2.3. Behavioural Response to Personalised Ovarian Cancer Risk Information

After receiving their hypothetical risk result, 28.5% of women said they would opt for risk-reducing surgery, 33.9% for increased surveillance (transvaginal ultrasound), and 20.9% would make lifestyle changes (e.g., quitting smoking, maintaining a healthy weight; see Figure 3 and Table S1).

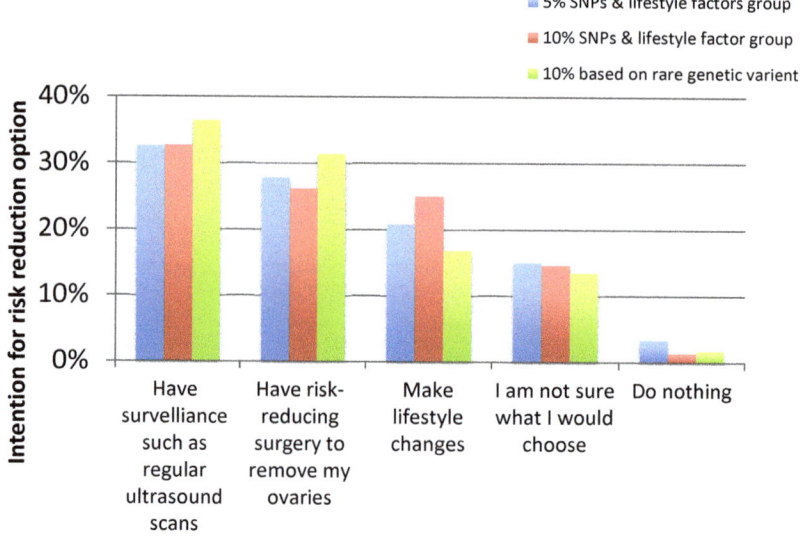

Figure 3. Behavioural intentions after exposure to hypothetical risk scenario compared between groups.

2.4. Differences by Experimental Condition

Women's intentions to have risk-reducing surgery did not differ significantly between the 5% and 10% multifactorial SNPs + lifestyle groups (27.9% vs. 26.2%, respectively) ($\chi^2(1) = 0.314$, $p = 0.61$). Women who received a 10% risk result based on a rare genetic variant were no more likely to opt for RRSO over other risk-reducing options than women who received a 10% risk result based on multifactorial SNPs + lifestyle factors (31.4% vs. 26.2%, respectively) ($\chi^2(1) = 2.512$, $p = 0.13$).

2.5. EPPM Variables

The mean (M) and standard deviation (SD) of the EPPM variables were: perceived risk (M = 3.51, SD = 0.82), perceived severity (M = 4.52, SD = 0.58), perceived response-efficacy (M = 4.03, SD = 0.78), perceived self-efficacy (M = 2.98, SD = 1.34). Means by exposure group are shown in the Supplementary Materials (Table S2).

2.6. Intention to Have Risk-Reducing Surgery (RRSO) versus Other Risk-Management Options

A binary logistic regression was conducted to investigate what factors were associated with hypothetical intention to have risk-reducing surgery vs. other behavioural options. Independent variables included in the model were age, ethnicity, educational attainment, previous breast and cervical screening participation, experimental group and EPPM variables (perceived risk, perceived severity, self-efficacy, perceived response-efficacy). In unadjusted analyses, women reporting higher perceived risk of ovarian cancer and higher perceived severity of ovarian cancer (i.e., the perceived threat variables), and higher surgery self-efficacy and perceived response-efficacy (i.e., variables relating to perceptions of the risk-reducing behaviour) were more likely than other women to opt for risk-reducing surgery. In the multivariable model, perceived response-efficacy (odds ratio (OR) = 2.22; 95% confidence interval (CI): 1.64–3.00) and self-efficacy (OR = 1.90; 95% CI: 1.63–2.22) remained significantly associated, whereas the perceived threat variables were no longer significantly associated, with choosing risk-reducing surgery over other behavioural options. None of the measured socio-demographic or health-related factors were significantly associated with intention to have surgery (see Table 2).

Table 2. Logistic regression predicting likelihood of intending to have risk-reducing surgery vs. other behavioural response ($n = 1017$).

Variable	Intention to Have Risk-Reducing Surgery	Odds Ratios (95% CI)	
Demographic Factors	n (%)	Unadjusted	Adjusted
Age			
45–50	74 (30.3)	Ref	Ref
51–55	65 (31.9)	1.07 (0.72–1.61)	0.94 (0.51–1.74)
56–60	60 (30.9)	1.03 (0.68–1.55)	1.00 (0.53–1.87)
61–65	49 (26.6)	0.83 (0.55–1.28)	0.62 (0.32–1.19)
66–70	27 (23.7)	0.71 (0.43–1.19)	0.48 (0.14–1.65)
71–75	15 (19.5)	0.56 (0.30–1.04)	0.29 (0.06–1.50)
Ethnicity			
White (Any background)	278 (28.6)	Ref	Ref
Other ethnic group	11 (28.2)	0.98 (0.48–2.00)	1.16 (0.38–3.50)
Educational Attainment			
No formal qualifications	16 (24.2)	Ref	
GCSE/O Levels	111 (31.5)	1.44 (0.79–2.64)	
A-Levels or Equivalent	68 (28.1)	1.22 (0.68–2.29)	
Undergraduate degree	59 (24.1)	0.99 (0.53–1.87)	
Postgraduate degree	28 (30.4)	1.37 (0.67–2.80)	
Other	8 (40.0)	2.08 (0.72–6.00)	

Table 2. Cont.

Variable	Intention to Have Risk-Reducing Surgery	Odds Ratios (95% CI)	
		Unadjusted	Adjusted
Demographic Factors	n (%)		
Relationship Status			
Not married/in a relationship	82 (27.1)	Ref	
Married/in a relationship	207 (29.2)	1.11 (0.82–1.50)	
Health history			
Cervical Screening Attendance (n = 807)			
Regular	200 (34.2)	Ref	Ref
Irregular	49 (22.1)	0.59 (0.41–0.85) *	0.67 (0.41–1.11)
Breast Screening Attendance (n = 741)			
Regular	205 (34.6)	Ref	Ref
Irregular	35 (23.6)	0.53 (0.36–0.80) *	0.67 (0.38–1.17)
Menopause status			
Pre-menopause	35 (28.9)	Ref	Ref
Peri/Post-menopause	243 (28.1)	0.96 (0.63–1.46)	
Extended Parallel Processing Model Variables			
Perceived Risk		1.43 (1.19–1.71) **	1.14 (0.90–1.45)
Perceived Severity		1.42 (1.11–1.82) *	1.08 (0.74–1.57)
Self-Efficacy		2.19 (1.94–2.47) **	1.90 (1.63–2.22) **
Perceived Response Efficacy		3.15 (2.50–3.96) **	2.22 (1.64–3.00) **
Experimental condition			
5% SNPs & Lifestyle	95 (32.8)	Ref	Ref
10% SNPS & Lifestyle	90 (31.0)	0.92 (0.66–1.29)	1.08 (0.67–1.73)
10% rare genetic variant	105 (36.2)	1.18 (0.85–1.65)	1.87 (1.17–3.00) **

** Predictor significant at the 0.01 level (2-tailed), * Predictor significant at the 0.05 level (2-tailed), CI = Confidence Interval. Ref = reference category.

3. Discussion

A high proportion (83%) of women in this sample indicated they would be interested in having an ovarian cancer risk assessment if offered by their GP on the NHS. This is consistent with previous research by Meisel et al. (2016), who found that 88% of a general population sample of women in the UK would be interested in genetic testing for ovarian cancer risk if it were offered by the NHS, and included information about breast cancer risk, echoing previous support from qualitative research for the availability of genetic testing and risk-stratified screening [43]. It is also consistent with uptake of genetic testing in our population-based studies [12,21].

We also found that a substantial proportion of British women over the age of 45 years might be open to the idea of having RRSO, even if their absolute lifetime risk were increased from a general population risk of 2% to as little as 5% or 10%. In addition, we also demonstrated in multivariable analyses that perceptions of risk-reducing surgery (self-efficacy and perceived response-efficacy) were independently associated with choosing surgery over other options, whereas the perceived threat of ovarian cancer (perceived risk and perceived severity) was not.

Although over a quarter (29%) of women opted for RRSO, slightly more women opted for surveillance (34%). The observed preference for surveillance may be due to the invasiveness of surgery, and could also potentially be due to the generally positive attitude towards cancer screening in the UK [44]. Lack of detailed information on the efficacy of each risk management option due to the hypothetical nature of this study may have resulted in participants deciding on the less invasive option, i.e., surveillance. Research suggests perceptions about risk-reducing surgery and surveillance are potentially modifiable: Mai et al. (2017) identified misperceptions about ovarian cancer risk and benefits of screening as important factors influencing decisions about risk-reducing surgery versus surveillance [45]. The concept of common genetic variants of low penetrance single nucleotide polymorphisms (SNPs) may be unfamiliar to the majority of individuals in the general public. For example, in a study by French et al. (2018), there was considerable variation in understanding of test results. The role of SNPs in cancer risk may be less familiar to individuals than more widely publicised rare genetic variants such as those in the *BRCA* genes [40]. Additionally, lifestyle factors may be perceived as being under greater personal control and, therefore, less serious than rare genetic variants.

Our study findings suggest that individuals interpreted the two levels of risk (5% vs. 10%) similarly, with the difference in communicated risk having a non-significant impact on participants' intentions to have RRSO. This supports previous research exploring the effect of risk information on behaviour, suggesting there is not a simple linear relationship between increments in risk and risk perception [39,40].

In addition to the lack of impact on perceived risk of ovarian cancer, we similarly found that different presentations of risk in the hypothetical scenarios (5% SNPs + lifestyle vs. 10% SNPs + lifestyle risk; 10% rare genetic variant vs. 10% SNPs + lifestyle) did not lead to differences in any other cognitive factors considered in the EPPM framework (i.e., perceived severity of ovarian cancer, perceived response-efficacy of risk-reducing surgery, self-efficacy to undertake risk-reducing surgery).

In contrast, we found that, in the sample overall, opting for risk-reducing surgery was associated with higher self-efficacy and higher perceived response-efficacy of risk-reducing surgery. According to the Extended Parallel Processing Model [46], higher perceptions of self-efficacy and/or response-efficacy relating to the recommended behaviour are associated with greater likelihood that systematic processing of threatening (risk) information will occur. Conversely, when perceptions of efficacy are low, people are more likely to avoid threatening risk information. Together, our findings suggest that if women perceive or believe that RRSO is being recommended to them clinically, this may have a greater impact on their decision-making than the details of their risk result (i.e., whether their risk is 5% or 10%, and whether that risk is based on a single rare genetic variant or a more complex combination of SNPs and lifestyle factors). The observation that psychological variables had a greater impact on intentions than the absolute risk numbers suggest that this might be important to consider in any potential future national rollouts. Offering psychological support for those who need it as part of the RRSO discussion and decision-making process is part of routine clinical practice in many centres today. Our study highlights the importance of incorporating this into future national guidelines.

In previous research using hypothetical scenarios, there has been some evidence to suggest that genetic information leads to more deterministic responses than non-genetic information [33,38,47–49]. Our study did not include a non-genetic condition and so does not speak to this aspect of how people respond to personal genetic versus non-genetic information.

The present study had several limitations. The cross-sectional design of the study did not allow for causation to be inferred. However, exploratory experimental studies such as this one can be valuable in informing hypotheses before moving on to study designs designed to trial real risk assessments. The use of hypothetical scenarios was both a strength and a limitation. This study attempted to model a "real life" scenario in which genetic risk information was provided to the general population. However, many of the contextual details and additional resources that accompany risk information are not available in hypothetical scenarios, which may limit the ecological validity of the study. This study was concerned with behavioural intention, as ovarian cancer population surveillance or population-wide genetic testing is not currently clinically available, so actual behaviour could not be measured. The presence of a potential intention behaviour gap is well established for other clinical interventions and cannot be excluded here.

The measures used in this study are adapted from previous research; however, they were almost all single-item measures, which may not be sensitive enough to adequately represent the underlying construct being measured due to the lack of psychometric information (e.g., test-retest reliability, discriminant or convergent validity). Prior knowledge may have an influence on how individuals appraise threatening health information [50]: this study did not measure previous ovarian cancer and genetic risk knowledge or previous genetic testing, which may have had an impact on behavioural intention (however this may be unlikely given this type of genetic testing is not widely available in the UK). In addition, we did not assess understanding of the information provided, and it is possible that some concepts (e.g., SNPs) may not have been well understood.

The sample was predominately White British and, therefore, may not be generalisable to other ethnic groups, given decisions about risk-reducing surgery and psychological effects may differ cross-culturally. In addition, the restricted age-range of the sample limits the generalisability of the findings (e.g., to younger women age 35 years and over who may also be offered risk-reducing surgery if they are at high risk). However, most women from the general population who are at increased risk of ovarian cancer will fall in the intermediate risk (5–10% lifetime risk) category [9]. RRSO at intermediate ovarian cancer risk levels (including for moderate penetrance CSGs) is recommended to be undertaken over the age of 45–50 years [15]. The sample was self-selected and may have had greater interest in the topic than the wider general population; the generalizability of the findings is therefore uncertain. Finally, as with any experimental study, we are unable to rule out the possibility of demand characteristics, i.e., participants responding in a way they think is expected according to their perceptions of the aim of the study. Despite the limitations, this study provides insights on the effects of experimentally manipulating genetic risk information for ovarian cancer on outcomes, comparing different sources and levels of risk on risk management behavioural intentions and psychological variables in the general population.

The information provided before being exposed to the hypothetical risk scenario on ovarian cancer, risk factors, and the efficacy of risk management was necessarily basic and brief, which may be an additional limitation. However, previous research did not find any difference in behavioural outcomes between use of gist and extended versions of decision aids in relation to ovarian cancer risk management [51]. Future research might usefully provide more detailed information containing details about the efficacy of a particular risk management behaviour to encourage "danger control" cognitive processing. This may aid in changing risk management preferences.

Future research might also benefit from including measures of other psychological and cognitive factors as potential predictors of risk management, e.g., causal beliefs. In addition, further research is needed on communicating risk information incorporating genetics to people in the general population outside of traditional clinical genetics department settings. Furthermore, a control group where participants are given a general population-based risk estimate would be useful for future research, as we were unable to compare between the general population risk and increased risk in this study.

The mean age of participants in this study was 57 years, with the majority of participants having completed having children and/or being past childbearing age, with most participants reporting they had begun menopause or were post-menopausal. Future research should explore the psychological and cognitive effects of ovarian cancer risk information being offered to younger women. In addition, there were relatively few women in the oldest age group (71–75 years) in this study, and so it is possible the apparent trend of increasing age being less associated with interest in surgery was due to the study being underpowered. This could also be a topic of investigation in future research.

Risk-reducing surgery, specifically RRSO, is at present the most effective risk management option available to women at increased risk of ovarian cancer. Our findings suggest there are a number of cognitive factors that influence intention to have ovarian cancer risk-reducing clinical interventions, beyond perceptions of risk. Future research should explore other possible factors that may have an impact on decision-making about risk management strategies. It is imperative to identify whether and/or how genetic risk information about common complex diseases will be translated into public health benefit: this is arguably especially urgent for diseases, such as ovarian cancer, which are characterised by being notoriously difficult to detect early and by having a high prevalence of late-stage diagnosis. Combined testing for multiple genetic factors together with lifestyle and other risk factors may lead to the ability to stratify the population for ovarian cancer risk for targeted prevention thus potentially saving lives.

Population testing provides a new paradigm for ovarian cancer prevention and can prevent thousands more cancers than the current clinical approach [52]. Jewish population studies support population testing for CSGs [53]. Our pilot study shows that population testing for lifetime risk of ovarian cancer is feasible, acceptable and has high satisfaction in general population women [12].

However, there is now need for large implementation studies, with long term outcomes, to provide real world evidence and develop context-specific models for implementing this approach for women in the general population. This will valuably inform future policy decisions regarding population-wide risk stratified approaches for risk-adapted ovarian cancer screening and prevention.

4. Materials and Methods

4.1. Overview

Participants ($n = 1017$) were women aged 45–75 years recruited via online survey company Survey Sampling International (SSI) in July 2017. An email containing a web link was sent to SSI panellists who fit the study criteria with respect to gender and age, inviting them to take part. The email did not contain information about the topic of the study. Those responding were directed to a short screening questionnaire. Eligible participants were then presented with a consent form. Incentive points, which can be exchanged for shopping vouchers, were awarded to SSI panellists for their time (equivalent to ~£0.50 for this 10 min study).

All participants were given information about ovarian cancer, including that on average around 2% of women will develop ovarian cancer in their lifetime; asked to imagine that they had had an ovarian cancer risk assessment via the NHS; and asked to imagine they had received a result indicating they were at increased risk of ovarian cancer (see Appendix A).

Women were randomly assigned to one of three experimental conditions using a software algorithm (See Figure 1). They were asked to imagine they had undergone an ovarian cancer risk assessment and had received this personalised risk estimate from their GP: (a) 5% ovarian cancer risk due to common genetic variants and lifestyle factors; (b) 10% ovarian cancer risk due to common genetic variants and lifestyle factors; or (c) 10% ovarian cancer risk due to a single rare variant in a cancer susceptibility gene such as *BRCA2* (see Appendix B).

The study was approved by the University College London ethics committee (Project ID Number: 10251/001).

4.2. Inclusion Criteria

Eligible participants were women aged 45–75 years, with no previous history of breast or ovarian cancer diagnosis. Women who indicated they were unsure of, or had not completed childbearing, were excluded from analyses ($n = 13$).

4.3. Measures

All measures are shown in Appendix C.

4.3.1. Interest in Ovarian Cancer Risk Assessment

Interest was assessed before exposure to the hypothetical test results, with the item, "If your GP offered you this ovarian cancer risk assessment on the NHS, would you take up the offer?" (adapted from [20]. Response options were "no, definitely not"; "no probably not"; "yes, probably" and "yes, definitely". The information women read before answering the question explained that the risk assessment would involve providing lifestyle information as well as a blood sample for genetic testing (see Appendix A).

4.3.2. Perceived Risk of Ovarian Cancer

Perceived risk was measured using a single item, "If I had just received this personal ovarian cancer risk result, I would feel that my risk of developing ovarian cancer was" adapted from [54]. Responses for these questions were recorded on a 5-point Likert scale with response options ranging from "much lower than other women of my age" to "much higher than women of my age". A higher score on the 5-point scale indicated greater perceived risk.

4.3.3. Perceived Severity of Ovarian Cancer

Perceived severity was measured using two questions adapted from [55]: "Developing ovarian cancer would have major consequences on my life" and "ovarian cancer is a serious condition" with five response options ranging from "strongly agree" to "strongly disagree". A higher score on the (possible scores 1–5) scale indicated greater perceived severity.

4.3.4. Self-Efficacy for Risk-Reducing Surgery

One item, adapted from [56], assessed participants' confidence in their ability to have risk-reducing surgery. Individuals were asked "How confident are you that you would go through with risk-reducing surgery if you were motivated to do so". The response options ranged from "not at all confident" to "extremely confident". A higher score on the scale indicated greater perceived self-efficacy.

4.3.5. Perceived Response-Efficacy of Risk-Reducing Surgery

For perceived response-efficacy of risk-reducing surgery, participants were asked to indicate how effective they felt risk-reducing surgery would be in lowering their ovarian cancer risk using a single item adapted from [56]: "Having surgery to remove your ovaries and fallopian tubes is an effective way to lower your risk of ovarian cancer". The response options were "strongly agree" to "strongly disagree". Items were reverse coded: a higher score on the (possible scores 1–5) scale indicated greater perceived response-efficacy.

4.3.6. Behavioural Intention

To assess women's potential behavioural reactions to their risk results, they were asked: "If I had just received this personal ovarian cancer risk result, I would choose to...". The response options were: "have risk-reducing surgery to remove my ovaries"; "have surveillance such as regular ultrasound scans"; "make lifestyle changes"; "do nothing"; and "I am not sure what I would do".

4.3.7. Demographic and Health Characteristic Measures

Information on demographics was collected from all participants including: age, ethnicity, educational attainment, relationship status, health characteristics, family history of cancer, personal history of cancer, menopause status, and breast and cervical screening attendance. Ethnicity (White vs. other ethnic group), menopause status (pre-menopausal vs. peri/post-menopause) and breast and cervical screening attendance (regular vs. irregular or not yet eligible) were dichotomised.

4.4. Data Analyses

A power calculation based on the primary binary outcome, intention to have risk-reducing surgery, taking into account group comparisons of three groups, suggested a sample size of 782 was required (medium effect size, power of 90%, alpha of 0.05). All statistical analyses of the data were carried out using SPSS 24. Analyses of variance (ANOVAs) and chi-square tests were conducted to explore between-group differences. Logistic regression was used to explore predictors of willingness to have risk-reducing surgery (vs. other behavioural responses to the risk information). Unadjusted and adjusted models were examined to explore the predictive effect of the experimental group and psychological variables on intention to have surgery and address possible demographic and health-related covariates.

5. Conclusions

The findings of this study contribute to a growing body of risk stratification research exploring the potential usefulness and clinical utility of population-wide risk assessment incorporating genetic testing alongside other risk factors. The need for risk stratification is perhaps particularly urgent for diseases, such as ovarian cancer, where survival outcomes are poor and population-wide screening for the disease is not currently recommended. We provide initial evidence, suggesting that a substantial proportion of women aged 45 years and over are open to the idea of risk stratification and having surgery to reduce their risk of ovarian cancer in response to increased risk results, even if their absolute lifetime risk is only increased by a few percentage points in absolute terms. Our findings do not speak to other barriers that might prevent women's behavioural intentions or preferences being translated into actions—barriers such as lack of timely access to healthcare services.

Supplementary Materials: The following are available online at http://www.mdpi.com/2072-6694/12/12/3543/s1, Table S1: Data for Figure 3, Table S2: Mean EPPM variables by experimental group.

Author Contributions: Conceptualization, S.S. and J.W.; methodology, J.W., A.G., S.S., R.M.; formal analysis, A.G., J.W., S.S.; resources, I.J., R.M., J.W.; data curation, A.G., S.S., J.W.; writing—original draft preparation, A.G.; writing—review and editing, J.W., S.S., I.J., R.M.; visualization, A.G., J.W., S.S.; supervision, J.W., S.S., I.J., R.M.; project administration, A.G.; funding acquisition, J.W. All authors have read and agreed to the published version of the manuscript.

Funding: The fieldwork for this study was funded by Cancer Research UK as part of a programme grant awarded to Professor Jane Wardle.

Acknowledgments: We are grateful to the women who took part in the study.

Conflicts of Interest: Ian Jacobs is a Director and shareholder in Abcodia, Ltd., a company focused on biomarkers for early detection of cancer. He is a co-inventor of the Risk of Ovarian Cancer Algorithm, which has been licensed to Abcodia by Massachusetts General Hospital, and has a right to a royalty stream. The other authors declare no conflict of interest. The funders had no role in the design of the study; in the collection, analyses, or interpretation of data; in the writing of the manuscript, or in the decision to publish the results.

Appendix A

Ovarian cancer and risk information

Section 1: Hypothetical scenario

> Please imagine that you have gone to your GP, and they have offered you a new approach to assessing your risk of developing ovarian cancer in the future. When your GP offered this to you, they gave you some written information to help you decide whether or not you want to have the risk assessment done. This information is below. Please read the information, and then answer the question that follows.

Assessing ovarian cancer risk

> Ovarian cancer is the sixth most common cancer among women in the UK: 2% of women will be diagnosed with ovarian cancer during their lifetime. Ovarian cancer is caused by many genetic and non-genetic factors. Currently, ovarian cancer is often detected at a late stage because symptoms are hard to spot. This means that it is often very hard to treat effectively.
> A new ovarian cancer risk assessment has been developed. This risk assessment combines lots of different types of information about you to estimate how likely you are to develop ovarian cancer in your lifetime. The types of information included in the risk assessment include lifestyle factors, rare genetic variants, and common genetic variants.
> Lifestyle factors: Lifestyle factors that may increase a woman's risk of ovarian cancer include tobacco smoking and being overweight.
> Common genetic variants: Single nucleotide polymorphisms, frequently called SNPs (pronounced "snips"), are the most common type of genetic variation among people. SNPs occur normally throughout a person's DNA. Most SNPs have no effect on health, but some are important to a person's health. Some SNPs can influence a woman's risk of developing ovarian cancer. Individually, each one of these SNPs only influences ovarian cancer risk by a tiny amount, but if a woman has a large number of these SNPs then her risk of ovarian cancer may be increased.
> Rare genetic variants: Some ovarian cancers are caused by a rare variant in a person's DNA. These rare variants can have quite a strong effect on a woman's risk of developing ovarian cancer. For example, variants in the *BRCA2* gene can increase a woman's lifetime risk of ovarian cancer up to between 10% and 20%.
> If you want to have this ovarian cancer risk assessment carried out, you will need to provide your GP with the information they request, including about your lifestyle. You will also need to have a blood test, so that the scientists can see whether you have any of the genetic variants that increase your risk.

Appendix B

Generic Risk Scenarios

> Next, regardless of how you answered in the previous question, please imagine that you have had the ovarian cancer risk assessment done, and your GP has now given you the result from the assessment. Please read your hypothetical result below.

Your personal ovarian cancer risk assessment: results [Group 1 only]

> Your result indicates that your lifetime risk of developing ovarian cancer is 5%. This is higher than the average risk for women, which is 2%.
> Your risk of ovarian cancer is higher than average because you have been found to have at least one lifestyle factor and several common genetic variants which are known to put women at increased risk of developing ovarian cancer.

OR

Your personal ovarian cancer risk assessment: results [Group 2 only]

> Your result indicates that your lifetime risk of developing ovarian cancer is 10%. This is higher than the average risk for women, which is 2%.
> Your risk of ovarian cancer is higher than average because you have been found to have at least one lifestyle factor and several common genetic variants which are known to put women at increased risk of developing ovarian cancer.

OR

Your personal ovarian cancer risk assessment: results [Group 3 only]

> Your result indicates that your lifetime risk of developing ovarian cancer is 10%. This is higher than the average risk for women, which is 2%.
> Your risk of ovarian cancer is higher than average because you have been found to have a rare genetic variant which is known to put women at increased risk of developing ovarian cancer.

AND

[All groups]

> There are several options for women who are at higher than average risk of ovarian cancer.
> Risk-reducing surgery involves removing the ovaries and fallopian tubes to prevent ovarian cancer from developing. However, removing the ovaries has downsides. For example, it causes a woman who has not yet been through her menopause to start her menopause (a natural process that usually happens in a woman's early 50 s).
> Surveillance includes having a regular (e.g., annual) ultrasound of your ovaries to see if a tumour is present. This ultrasound is usually an internal (transvaginal) ultrasound. Effective screening has not been established.
> Lifestyle changes include maintaining a healthy weight and quitting smoking. These types of lifestyle changes may reduce a woman's risk of developing ovarian cancer.

Appendix C

Questionnaire

> Please carefully imagine what you would think and how you would feel if you had received this personal result from the ovarian cancer risk assessment. Now please answer the following questions.

Intention for Genetic Screening

Q1. If your GP offered you this ovarian cancer risk assessment on the NHS, would you take up the offer?

- No definitely not
- No probably not
- Yes probably
- Yes definitely

Q2. How likely do you think you are to develop ovarian cancer in your lifetime?

(a)   ... Not at all likely
(b)   ... Not very likely
(c)   ... Quite likely
(d)   ... Extremely likely

Behavioural outcome

Q3. If I had just received this personal ovarian cancer risk result, I would choose to ...

(a)   ... have risk-reducing surgery to remove my ovaries.
(b)   ... have surveillance such as regular ultrasound scans.
(c)   ... make lifestyle changes.
(d)   ... do nothing.
(e)   ... I am not sure what I would choose.

   (Please select one option only)

Perceived risk

Q4. If I had just received this personal ovarian cancer risk result, I would feel that my risk of developing ovarian cancer was ...

(a)   ... much lower than other women of my age
(b)   ... lower than other women of my age
(c)   ... the same as other women of my age
(d)   ... higher than other women of my age
(e)   ... much higher than other women of my age

Perceived Response efficacy

> How much do you agree or disagree with the following statement based on how you would feel if you had received this personal ovarian cancer risk result from the ovarian cancer risk assessment.

Q7. There is little that can be done to prevent ovarian cancer.

(a)   ... Strongly agree
(b)   ... Agree
(c)   ... Neither agree or disagree
(d)   ... Disagree
(e)   ... Strongly disagree

Q8. Having surgery to remove your ovaries and fallopian tubes is an effective way to lower your risk of ovarian cancer.

(a)   ... Strongly agree
(b)   ... Agree
(c)   ... Neither agree or disagree
(d)   ... Disagree
(e)   ... Strongly disagree

Perceived Response efficacy

Q9. Regular screening through transvaginal ultrasound is an effective way to lower your risk of ovarian cancer.

(a)   … Strongly agree
(b)   … Agree
(c)   … Neither agree or disagree
(d)   … Disagree
(e)   … Strongly disagree

Perceived severity

Q10. Developing ovarian cancer would have major consequences on my life

(a)   … Strongly agree
(b)   … Agree
(c)   … Neither agree or disagree
(d)   … Disagree
(e)   … Strongly disagree

Perceived severity

Q11. Ovarian cancer is a serious condition.

(a)   … Strongly agree
(b)   … Agree
(c)   … Neither agree or disagree
(d)   … Disagree
(e)   … Strongly disagree

Self-efficacy

Q12. How confident are you that you could go through with having risk-reducing surgery if you were motivated to do so?

(a)   … not at all confident
(b)   … somewhat confident
(c)   … fairly confident
(d)   … very confident
(e)   … extremely confident

Q13. Have you ever been diagnosed with cancer? (Please select one)

Yes
No
Not sure

Q14. If yes, what type of cancer is it/was it?
… … … … … … … … … … … … … … … … …

Q15. Do you have a family history of cancer?
Have any first-degree family member (parents, brothers, sisters, children) or second-degree (aunts, uncles, nieces, nephews, grandparents, grandchildren) been diagnosed with cancer.

Yes

No
Not sure

Q15a. If yes, what type(s) of cancer?
… … … … … … … … … … … … … … … … … ..

Q16. What is your current menstrual status? (Please select one)

Premenopausal (before menopause; having regular periods)
Perimenopause (menopause transition—changes in periods, but have not gone 12 months in a row without a period)
Postmenopausal (After menopause; periods have stopped for at least 12 months)
Don't know

Q17. If you have indicated that you have not had a period in the previous 12 months, what age were you at your last period?

Q18. If you are still having periods, how often do they occur? (Please respond in days)

Q19. Is there a recent change in how often you have periods?

Yes/No

Q20. Was your menopause:

Spontaneous ("natural")
Surgical (removal of both ovaries)
Due to chemotherapy or radiation therapy
Other
n/a—haven't yet reached menopause
(If indicated they are still having periods don't ask this question)

Q21. Women aged 25–49 years are invited for cervical screening (also called a smear or Pap test) every 3 years, and women aged 50–64 are invited every 5 years. Which of these statements best describes you?

I'm up to date with cervical screening
I'm overdue for cervical screening
I've never been for cervical screening
I'm 65 or over so I'm not invited any more

Q22. Women aged 50–70 years are invited for breast screening (also called a mammogram or mammography) every 3 years. Which of these statements best describes you?

I'm up to date with breast screening
I'm overdue for breast screening
I've never been for breast screening
I'm under 50 or over 70 so I'm not eligible for breast screening.

Q23. How old are you?
_____

Q24. How would you describe your ethnic background? (Please select one)

White British
White non-British

Black
Asian
Mixed
Other
Do not wish to answer

Q25. What is the highest level of education you have achieved? (Please select one)

No formal qualifications
GCSEs/O levels or equivalent
A-Levels or equivalent
Undergraduate degree or equivalent
Postgraduate degree or equivalent
Other (please state)

Q26. What is your relationship status? (Please select one)

Single
In a relationship
Living with a partner
Married
Separated/divorced/widowed

Q27. How many children do you have? (Please select one)

0
1
2
3
4
5 or more

Q28. Do you plan to have any (more) children in the future? (Please select one)

Yes
No
Not sure

END OF SURVEY

References

1. Cancer Research UK, Ovarian Cancer Statistics. 2016. Available online: https://www.cancerresearchuk.org/health-professional/cancer-statistics/statistics-by-cancer-type/ovarian-cancer (accessed on 25 June 2017).
2. Hunn, J.; Rodriguez, G.C. Ovarian Cancer: Etiology, risk factors, and epidemiology. *Clin. Obstet. Gynecol.* **2012**, *55*, 3–23. [CrossRef] [PubMed]
3. Levy-Lahad, E.; Gabai-Kapara, E.; Kaufman, B.; Catane, R.; Segev, S.; Renbaum, P.; Beller, U.; King, M.; Lahad, A. Identification of BRCA1/BRCA2 carriers by screening in the healthy population and its implications. *J. Clin. Oncol.* **2011**, *29*, 1513. [CrossRef]
4. King, M.-C.; Levy-Lahad, E.; Lahad, A. Population-Based Screening for BRCA1 and BRCA2. *JAMA* **2014**, *312*, 1091–1092. [CrossRef] [PubMed]
5. Kuchenbaecker, K.B.; Hopper, J.L.; Barnes, D.R.; Phillips, K.-A.; Mooij, T.M.; Roos-Blom, M.-J.; Jervis, S.E.; Van Leeuwen, F.; Milne, R.L.; Andrieu, N.; et al. Risks of Breast, Ovarian, and Contralateral Breast Cancer for BRCA1 and BRCA2 Mutation Carriers. *JAMA* **2017**, *317*, 2402–2416. [CrossRef] [PubMed]

6. Manchanda, R.; Burnell, M.; Gaba, F.; Desai, R.; Wardle, J.; Gessler, S.; Side, L.; Sanderson, S.; Loggenberg, K.; Brady, A.F.; et al. Randomised trial of population-based BRCA testing in Ashkenazi Jews: Long-term outcomes. *BJOG: Int. J. Obstet. Gynaecol.* **2019**, *127*, 364–375. [CrossRef] [PubMed]
7. Manchanda, R.; Loggenberg, K.; Sanderson, S.; Burnell, M.; Wardle, J.; Gessler, S.; Side, L.; Balogun, N.; Desai, R.; Kumar, A.; et al. Population testing for cancer predisposing BRCA1/BRCA2 mutations in the Ashkenazi-Jewish community: A randomized controlled trial. *J. Natl. Cancer Inst.* **2014**, *107*, 379. [CrossRef]
8. Manchanda, R.; Blyuss, O.; Gaba, F.; Gordeev, V.S.; Jacobs, C.; Burnell, M.; Gan, C.; Taylor, R.; Turnbull, C.; Legood, R.; et al. Current detection rates and time-to-detection of all identifiable BRCA carriers in the Greater London population. *J. Med. Genet.* **2018**, *55*, 538–545. [CrossRef]
9. Jervis, S.; Song, H.; Lee, A.; Dicks, E.; Harrington, P.; Baynes, C.; Manchanda, R.; Easton, D.F.; Jacobs, I.; Pharoah, P.P.D.; et al. A risk prediction algorithm for ovarian cancer incorporating BRCA1, BRCA2, common alleles and other familial effects. *J. Med. Genet.* **2015**, *52*, 465–475. [CrossRef]
10. Manchanda, R.; Gaba, F. Population Based Testing for Primary Prevention: A Systematic Review. *Cancers* **2018**, *10*, 424. [CrossRef]
11. Evans, O.; Gaba, F.; Manchanda, R. Population-based genetic testing for Women's cancer prevention. *Best Pr. Res. Clin. Obstet. Gynaecol.* **2020**, *65*, 139–153. [CrossRef]
12. Gaba, F.; Blyuss, O.; Liu, X.; Goyal, S.; Lahoti, N.; Chandrasekaran, D.; Kurzer, M.; Kalsi, J.K.; Sanderson, S.C.; Lanceley, A.; et al. Population Study of Ovarian Cancer Risk Prediction for Targeted Screening and Prevention. *Cancers* **2020**, *12*, 1241. [CrossRef] [PubMed]
13. Rahman, B.; Side, L.; Gibbon, S.; Meisel, S.F.; Fraser, L.; Gessler, S.; Wardle, J.; Lanceley, A. Moving towards population-based genetic risk prediction for ovarian cancer. *BJOG: Int. J. Obstet. Gynaecol.* **2017**, *124*, 855–858. [CrossRef]
14. Manchanda, R.; Legood, R.; Antoniou, A.; Pearce, L.; Menon, U. Commentary on changing the risk threshold for surgical prevention of ovarian cancer. *BJOG: Int. J. Obstet. Gynaecol.* **2017**, *125*, 541–544. [CrossRef] [PubMed]
15. Manchanda, R.; Menon, U. Setting the Threshold for Surgical Prevention in Women at Increased Risk of Ovarian Cancer. *Int. J. Gynecol. Cancer* **2018**, *28*, 34–42. [CrossRef] [PubMed]
16. Manchanda, R.; Legood, R.; Antoniou, A.C.; Gordeev, V.S.; Menon, U. Specifying the ovarian cancer risk threshold of 'premenopausal risk-reducing salpingo-oophorectomy' for ovarian cancer prevention: A cost-effectiveness analysis. *J. Med. Genet.* **2016**, *53*, 591–599. [CrossRef] [PubMed]
17. Manchanda, R.; Legood, R.; Pearce, L.; Menon, U. Defining the risk threshold for risk reducing salpingo-oophorectomy for ovarian cancer prevention in low risk postmenopausal women. *Gynecol. Oncol.* **2015**, *139*, 487–494. [CrossRef] [PubMed]
18. Manchanda, R.; Patel, S.; Gordeev, V.S.; Antoniou, A.C.; Smith, S.; Lee, A.; Hopper, J.L.; MacInnis, R.J.; Turnbull, C.G.N.; Ramus, S.J.; et al. Cost-effectiveness of Population-Based BRCA1, BRCA2, RAD51C, RAD51D, BRIP1, PALB2 Mutation Testing in Unselected General Population Women. *J. Natl. Cancer Inst.* **2018**, *110*, 714–725. [CrossRef]
19. Chandrasekaran, D.; Manchanda, R. Germline and somatic genetic testing in ovarian cancer patients. *BJOG: Int. J. Obstet. Gynaecol.* **2018**, *125*, 1460. [CrossRef]
20. Meisel, S.F.; for the PROMISE-2016 Study Team; Rahman, B.; Side, L.; Fraser, L.; Gessler, S.; Lanceley, A.; Wardle, J. Genetic testing and personalized ovarian cancer screening: A survey of public attitudes. *BMC Women's Health* **2016**, *16*, 46. [CrossRef]
21. Manchanda, R.; Burnell, M.; Loggenberg, K.; Desai, R.; Wardle, J.; Sanderson, S.C.; Gessler, S.; Side, L.; Balogun, N.; Kumar, A.; et al. Cluster-randomised non-inferiority trial comparing DVD-assisted and traditional genetic counselling in systematic population testing for BRCA1/2 mutations. *J. Med. Genet.* **2016**, *53*, 472–480. [CrossRef]
22. Manchanda, R.; Legood, R.; Burnell, M.; McGuire, A.; Raikou, M.; Loggenberg, K.; Wardle, J.; Sanderson, S.; Gessler, S.; Side, L.; et al. Cost-effectiveness of Population Screening for BRCA Mutations in Ashkenazi Jewish Women Compared with Family History-Based Testing. *J. Natl. Cancer Inst.* **2015**, *107*, 380. [CrossRef] [PubMed]
23. Manchanda, R.; Patel, S.; Antoniou, A.C.; Levy-Lahad, E.; Turnbull, C.; Evans, D.G.; Hopper, J.L.; MacInnis, R.J.; Menon, U.; Jacobs, I.; et al. Cost-effectiveness of population based BRCA testing with varying Ashkenazi Jewish ancestry. *Am. J. Obstet. Gynecol.* **2017**, *217*, 578.e1–578.e12. [CrossRef] [PubMed]

24. Rebbeck, T.R.; Lynch, H.T.; Neuhausen, S.L.; Narod, S.A.; Veer, L.V.; Garber, J.E.; Evans, G.; Isaacs, C.; Daly, M.B.; Matloff, E.; et al. Prophylactic Oophorectomy in Carriers of BRCA1 or BRCA2 Mutations. *N. Engl. J. Med.* **2002**, *346*, 1616–1622. [CrossRef] [PubMed]
25. Manchanda, R.; Burnell, M.; Abdelraheim, A.; Johnson, M.; Sharma, A.; Benjamin, E.; Brunell, C.; Saridogan, E.; Gessler, S.; Oram, D.; et al. Factors influencing uptake and timing of risk reducing salpingo-oophorectomy in women at risk of familial ovarian cancer: A competing risk time to event analysis. *BJOG: Int. J. Obstet. Gynaecol.* **2012**, *119*, 527–536. [CrossRef]
26. Manchanda, R.; Abdelraheim, A.; Johnson, M.; Rosenthal, A.N.; Benjamin, E.; Brunell, C.; Burnell, M.; Side, L.; Gessler, S.; Saridogan, E.; et al. Outcome of risk-reducing salpingo-oophorectomy in BRCA carriers and women of unknown mutation status. *BJOG: Int. J. Obstet. Gynaecol.* **2011**, *118*, 814–824. [CrossRef]
27. Yang, X.; Song, H.; Leslie, G.; Engel, C.; Hahnen, E.; Auber, B.; Horváth, J.; Kast, K.; Niederacher, D.; Turnbull, C.; et al. Ovarian and Breast Cancer Risks Associated with Pathogenic Variants in RAD51C and RAD51D. *J. Natl. Cancer Inst.* **2020**. [CrossRef]
28. Yang, X.; Leslie, G.; Doroszuk, A.; Schneider, S.; Allen, J.; Decker, B.; Dunning, A.M.; Redman, J.; Scarth, J.; Plaskocinska, I.; et al. Cancer Risks Associated with Germline PALB2 Pathogenic Variants: An International Study of 524 Families. *J. Clin. Oncol.* **2020**, *38*, 674–685. [CrossRef]
29. Ramus, S.J.; Song, H.; Dicks, E.; Tyrer, J.P.; Rosenthal, A.N.; Intermaggio, M.P.; Fraser, L.; Gentry-Maharaj, A.; Hayward, J.; Philpott, S.; et al. Germline Mutations in the BRIP1, BARD1, PALB2, and NBN Genes in Women with Ovarian Cancer. *J. Natl. Cancer Inst.* **2015**, *107*. [CrossRef]
30. Jacobs, I.; Menon, U.; Ryan, A.; Gentry-Maharaj, A.; Burnell, M.; Kalsi, J.K.; Amso, N.N.; Apostolidou, S.; Benjamin, E.; Cruickshank, D.; et al. Ovarian cancer screening and mortality in the UK Collaborative Trial of Ovarian Cancer Screening (UKCTOCS): A randomised controlled trial. *Lancet* **2016**, *387*, 945–956. [CrossRef]
31. Rosenthal, A.N.; Fraser, L.S.; Philpott, S.; Manchanda, R.; Burnell, M.; Badman, P.; Hadwin, R.; Rizzuto, I.; Benjamin, E.C.; Singh, N.; et al. Evidence of Stage Shift in Women Diagnosed with Ovarian Cancer during Phase II of the United Kingdom Familial Ovarian Cancer Screening Study. *J. Clin. Oncol.* **2017**, *35*, 1411–1420. [CrossRef]
32. Kauff, N.D.; Domchek, S.M.; Friebel, T.M.; Robson, M.E.; Lee, J.; Garber, J.E.; Isaacs, C.; Evans, D.G.; Lynch, H.; Eeles, R.A.; et al. Risk-Reducing Salpingo-Oophorectomy for the Prevention of BRCA1- and BRCA2-Associated Breast and Gynecologic Cancer: A Multicenter, Prospective Study. *J. Clin. Oncol.* **2008**, *26*, 1331–1337. [CrossRef] [PubMed]
33. Hollands, G.J.; French, D.P.; Griffin, S.J.; Prevost, A.T.; Sutton, S.; King, S.; Marteau, T.M. The impact of communicating genetic risks of disease on risk-reducing health behaviour: Systematic review with meta-analysis. *BMJ* **2016**, *352*, i1102. [CrossRef] [PubMed]
34. Hallowell, N.; kConFab Psychosocial Group on Behalf of the kConFab Investigators; Baylock, B.; Heiniger, L.; Butow, P.N.; Patel, D.; Meiser, B.; Saunders, C.M.; Price, M.A. Looking different, feeling different: Women's reactions to risk-reducing breast and ovarian surgery. *Fam. Cancer* **2011**, *11*, 215–224. [CrossRef] [PubMed]
35. Meiser, B.; Butow, P.; Friedlander, M.; Barratt, A.; Schnieden, V.; Watson, M.; Brown, J.; Tucker, K. Psychological impact of genetic testing in women from high-risk breast cancer families. *Eur. J. Cancer* **2002**, *38*, 2025–2031. [CrossRef]
36. Pruthi, S.; Gostout, B.S.; Lindor, N.M. Identification and Management of Women with BRCA Mutations or Hereditary Predisposition for Breast and Ovarian Cancer. *Mayo Clinic Proc.* **2010**, *85*, 1111–1120. [CrossRef]
37. Rebbeck, T.R.; Kauff, N.D.; Domchek, S.M. Meta-analysis of Risk Reduction Estimates Associated with Risk-Reducing Salpingo-oophorectomy in BRCA1 or BRCA2 Mutation Carriers. *J. Natl. Cancer Inst.* **2009**, *101*, 80–87. [CrossRef]
38. Marteau, T.M.; French, D.P.; Griffin, S.J.; Prevost, T.; Sutton, S.; Watkinson, C.; Attwood, S.; Hollands, G.J. Effects of communicating DNA-based disease risk estimates on risk-reducing behaviours. *Cochrane Database Syst. Rev.* **2010**, CD007275. [CrossRef]
39. Cameron, L.D.; Sherman, K.; Marteau, T.M.; Brown, P.M. Impact of genetic risk information and type of disease on perceived risk, anticipated affect, and expected consequences of genetic tests. *Health Psychol.* **2009**, *28*, 307–316. [CrossRef]

40. French, D.P.; Southworth, J.; Howell, A.; Harvie, M.; Stavrinos, P.; Watterson, D.; Sampson, S.; Evans, D.G.; Donnelly, L.S. Psychological impact of providing women with personalised 10-year breast cancer risk estimates. *Br. J. Cancer* **2018**, *118*, 1648–1657. [CrossRef]
41. Hart, M.R.; Biesecker, B.B.; Blout, C.L.; Christensen, K.D.; Amendola, L.M.; Bergstrom, K.L.; Biswas, S.; Bowling, K.M.; Brothers, K.B.; Conlin, L.K.; et al. Secondary findings from clinical genomic sequencing: Prevalence, patient perspectives, family history assessment, and health-care costs from a multisite study. *Genet. Med.* **2019**, *21*, 1100–1110. [CrossRef]
42. Witte, K.; Allen, M. A Meta-Analysis of Fear Appeals: Implications for Effective Public Health Campaigns. *Heal. Educ. Behav.* **2000**, *27*, 591–615. [CrossRef] [PubMed]
43. Meisel, S.F.; Side, L.; Fraser, L.; Gessler, S.; Wardle, J.; Lanceley, A. Population-Based, Risk-Stratified Genetic Testing for Ovarian Cancer Risk: A Focus Group Study. *Public Health Genom.* **2013**, *16*, 184–191. [CrossRef] [PubMed]
44. Waller, J.L.; Osborne, K.; Wardle, J.F.C. Enthusiasm for cancer screening in Great Britain: A general population survey. *Br. J. Cancer* **2015**, *112*, 562–566. [CrossRef] [PubMed]
45. Mai, P.L.; Piedmonte, M.; Han, P.K.J.; Moser, R.P.; Walker, J.L.; Rodriguez, G.C.; Boggess, J.; Rutherford, T.J.; Zivanovic, O.; Cohn, D.E.; et al. Factors associated with deciding between risk-reducing salpingo-oophorectomy and ovarian cancer screening among high-risk women enrolled in GOG-0199: An NRG Oncology/Gynecologic Oncology Group study. *Gynecol. Oncol.* **2017**, *145*, 122–129. [CrossRef] [PubMed]
46. Witte, K. Putting the fear back into fear appeals: The extended parallel process model. *Commun. Monogr.* **1992**, *59*, 329–349. [CrossRef]
47. Claassen, L.; Henneman, L.; De Vet, R.; Knol, D.; Marteau, T.M.; Timmermans, D. Fatalistic responses to different types of genetic risk information: Exploring the role of Self-Malleability. *Psychol. Health* **2010**, *25*, 183–196. [CrossRef] [PubMed]
48. Marteau, T.M. Genetic risk and behavioural change. *BMJ* **2001**, *322*, 1056–1059. [CrossRef]
49. Marteau, T.M.; Weinman, J. Self-regulation and the behavioural response to DNA risk information: A theoretical analysis and framework for future research. *Soc. Sci. Med.* **2006**, *62*, 1360–1368. [CrossRef]
50. Evans, R.E.; Beeken, R.J.; Steptoe, A.; Wardle, J. Cancer information and anxiety: Applying the Extended Parallel Process Model. *J. Health Psychol.* **2012**, *17*, 579–589. [CrossRef]
51. Meisel, S.F.; Freeman, M.; Waller, J.; Fraser, L.; Gessler, S.; Jacobs, I.; Kalsi, J.K.; Manchanda, R.; Rahman, B.; Side, L.; et al. Impact of a decision aid about stratified ovarian cancer risk-management on women's knowledge and intentions: A randomised online experimental survey study. *BMC Public Health* **2017**, *17*, 882. [CrossRef]
52. Evans, O.; Manchanda, R. Population-based Genetic Testing for Precision Prevention. *Cancer Prev. Res.* **2020**, *13*, 643–648. [CrossRef] [PubMed]
53. Manchanda, R.; Lieberman, S.; Gaba, F.; Lahad, A.; Levy-Lahad, E. Population Screening for Inherited Predisposition to Breast and Ovarian Cancer. *Annu. Rev. Genom. Hum. Genet.* **2020**, *21*, 373–412. [CrossRef] [PubMed]
54. Gurmankin, A.D.; Shea, J.; Williams, S.V.; Quistberg, D.A.; Armstrong, K. Measuring Perceptions of Breast Cancer Risk. *Cancer Epidemiol. Biomarkers Prev.* **2006**, *15*, 1893–1898. [CrossRef] [PubMed]
55. Peipins, L.A.; Mccarty, F.; Hawkins, N.A.; Rodriguez, J.L.; Scholl, L.E.; Leadbetter, S. Cognitive and affective influences on perceived risk of ovarian cancer. *Psycho-Oncology* **2015**, *24*, 279–286. [CrossRef] [PubMed]
56. Rawl, S.; Champion, V.; Menon, U.; Loehrer, P.J.; Vance, G.H.; Skinner, C.S. Validation of Scales to Measure Benefits of and Barriers to Colorectal Cancer Screening. *J. Psychosoc. Oncol.* **2001**, *19*, 47–63. [CrossRef]

Publisher's Note: MDPI stays neutral with regard to jurisdictional claims in published maps and institutional affiliations.

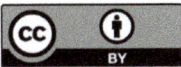

© 2020 by the authors. Licensee MDPI, Basel, Switzerland. This article is an open access article distributed under the terms and conditions of the Creative Commons Attribution (CC BY) license (http://creativecommons.org/licenses/by/4.0/).

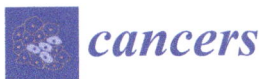

Review

Identifying Ovarian Cancer in Symptomatic Women: A Systematic Review of Clinical Tools

Garth Funston [1,*], Victoria Hardy [1], Gary Abel [2], Emma J. Crosbie [3,4], Jon Emery [1,5], Willie Hamilton [2] and Fiona M. Walter [1,5]

1. The Primary Care Unit, Department of Public Health and Primary Care, University of Cambridge, Cambridge CB1 8RN, UK; veh29@medschl.cam.ac.uk (V.H.); jon.emery@unimelb.edu.au (J.E.); fmw22@medschl.cam.ac.uk (F.M.W.)
2. University of Exeter Medical School, University of Exeter, Exeter EX1 1TX, UK; G.A.Abel@exeter.ac.uk (G.A.); W.Hamilton@exeter.ac.uk (W.H.)
3. Gynaecological Oncology Research Group, Division of Cancer Sciences, University of Manchester, Manchester M13 9WL, UK; emma.crosbie@manchester.ac.uk
4. Department of Obstetrics and Gynaecology, Manchester University NHS Foundation Trust, Manchester Academic Health Sciences Centre, Manchester M13 9WL, UK
5. Centre for Cancer Research and Department of General Practice, University of Melbourne, Melbourne, VIC 3000, Australia
* Correspondence: gf272@medschl.cam.ac.uk

Received: 12 November 2020; Accepted: 4 December 2020; Published: 8 December 2020

Simple Summary: Most women with ovarian cancer are diagnosed after they develop symptoms—identifying symptomatic women earlier has the potential to improve outcomes. Tools, ranging from simple symptom checklists to diagnostic prediction models that incorporate tests and risk factors, have been developed to help identify women at increased risk of undiagnosed ovarian cancer. In this review, we systematically identified studies evaluating these tools and then compared the reported diagnostic performance of tools. All included studies had some quality concerns and most tools had only been evaluated in a single study. However, four tools were evaluated in multiple studies and showed moderate diagnostic performance, with relatively little difference in performance between tools. While encouraging, further large and well-conducted studies are needed to ensure these tools are acceptable to patients and clinicians, are cost-effective and facilitate the early diagnosis of ovarian cancer.

Abstract: In the absence of effective ovarian cancer screening programs, most women are diagnosed following the onset of symptoms. Symptom-based tools, including symptom checklists and risk prediction models, have been developed to aid detection. The aim of this systematic review was to identify and compare the diagnostic performance of these tools. We searched MEDLINE, EMBASE and Cochrane CENTRAL, without language restriction, for relevant studies published between 1 January 2000 and 3 March 2020. We identified 1625 unique records and included 16 studies, evaluating 21 distinct tools in a range of settings. Fourteen tools included only symptoms; seven also included risk factors or blood tests. Four tools were externally validated—the Goff Symptom Index (sensitivity: 56.9–83.3%; specificity: 48.3–98.9%), a modified Goff Symptom Index (sensitivity: 71.6%; specificity: 88.5%), the Society of Gynaecologic Oncologists consensus criteria (sensitivity: 65.3–71.5%; specificity: 82.9–93.9%) and the QCancer Ovarian model (10% risk threshold—sensitivity: 64.1%; specificity: 90.1%). Study heterogeneity precluded meta-analysis. Given the moderate accuracy of several tools on external validation, they could be of use in helping to select women for ovarian cancer investigations. However, further research is needed to assess the impact of these tools on the timely detection of ovarian cancer and on patient survival.

Keywords: ovarian cancer; symptoms; early detection; risk assessment; diagnostic prediction model; triage tool; ovarian cancer symptoms

1. Introduction

Ovarian cancer is the eighth most common cancer to affect women worldwide, accounting for over 384,000 deaths in 2018 [1]. Outcomes are strongly linked to stage at diagnosis, with five-year survivals of 90% and 4% for UK women diagnosed at stages I and IV, respectively [2]. Given this, large ovarian cancer screening trials have been conducted, but these have so far failed to demonstrate a significant reduction in long-term mortality [3,4]. In the absence of effective screening programs, the majority of ovarian cancers are diagnosed following symptomatic presentation [5,6], and a focus has been placed on the early detection of symptomatic disease [7].

While once regarded as a 'silent killer', many studies have demonstrated that a range of symptoms are more common in women with ovarian cancer than in control subjects and that symptoms occur at all stages of the disease [8]. Clinical guidelines in countries around the world recommend that patients presenting with symptoms of possible ovarian cancer undergo investigation, although debate remains over which symptoms are indicative of disease and should be included in guidelines [7]. To facilitate the early detection of symptomatic cancer, researchers have developed a number of symptom-based checklists for use either when patients first present in the clinical setting or in 'symptom-triggered screening' programs, in which symptoms are proactively solicited [9–11]. More sophisticated tools, which can take the form of diagnostic prediction models [12], have also been developed to incorporate test results and ovarian cancer risk factors alongside symptoms, in a bid to improve tool performance. Several of these tools have been incorporated into clinical computer systems, which, then, automatically alert the clinician to consider ovarian cancer investigations when relevant symptoms are present or when the risk of undiagnosed cancer reaches a certain level. However, the relative limitations and merits of the various available tools remain unclear. In this systematic review, we aimed to identify and compare the diagnostic performances of symptom-predicated tools for the detection of ovarian cancer.

2. Methods

2.1. Eligibility Criteria and Searches

This review was conducted and is reported in accordance with the Preferred Reporting Items for Systematic Reviews and Meta-Analysis (PRISMA) guidelines (Table S1); a study protocol was registered with PROSPERO [CRD42020149879]. We searched MEDLINE, EMBASE and Cochrane CENTRAL for keywords relating to ovarian cancer, symptoms and prediction/diagnostic tools to identify papers published between 1 January 2000 and 3 March 2020 (Text S1). The start date was chosen to predate the publication of key ovarian cancer symptom papers [13,14]. No language restrictions or restrictions on methodological design were applied. No restrictions were placed on study setting, so studies conducted in the general population or in primary, secondary, or tertiary care were all eligible for inclusion. Reference lists of included papers were screened to identify any additional relevant papers.

Studies were included if they (a) described the development and or evaluation of a multivariable tool designed to identify patients with undiagnosed ovarian cancer and (b) provided the sensitivity and specificity of the tool or gave sufficient data to allow these metrics to be calculated. For the purposes of this review, we defined a multivariable tool as a combination of three or more variables used to detect or predict the risk of undiagnosed ovarian cancer. This broad definition encompasses traditional multivariable diagnostic prediction models and clinical prediction rules [12,15]. We considered variable 'checklists', in which any one variable in the list needed to be present for a positive result, to be a form of multivariable tool. As the focus of this review was on symptom-based tools, the tool under investigation had to include at least one symptom for a study to be eligible. No other restrictions were placed on the type of variable that could be included in a tool. Studies on tools intended to estimate future risk of developing ovarian cancer rather than the current risk of having an undiagnosed ovarian cancer were excluded, as were studies on tools that solely provide an indication of the risk of relapse or recurrence. We excluded studies in which all participants had a pelvic mass—as this represents a highly selected high-risk population—and studies undertaken solely in paediatric (<18 years) populations. Non-primary research studies were also excluded.

2.2. Study Selection

The online Rayyan software was used to facilitate abstract screening and study selection [16]. Following removal of duplicates, two reviewers (G.F. and V.H.) independently screened titles and abstracts against eligibility criteria. Potentially eligible papers identified at the screening stage were obtained and the full texts were independently examined against eligibility criteria by two reviewers (G.F. and V.H.). Any disagreements were resolved by consensus.

2.3. Data Extraction and Synthesis

Data extraction was performed by one reviewer (G.F.) and checked against full-text papers by a second reviewer (V.H.) to ensure accuracy. Using a predeveloped template, information was extracted on study characteristics (year of publication and location), study design (methodology, population, data source and outcome definition), tools (variables and tool development methods), and tool performance metrics (sensitivity, specificity and other diagnostic metrics). Where a study evaluated multiple tools, data relating to each tool were extracted separately.

Sensitivity and specificity were used to compare tool accuracy. For diagnostic prediction models, area under the receiver operator characteristic curve (AUC) was used to compare discrimination (the ability of a tool to identify those with a condition from those without a condition) and calibration (agreement between estimated and observed outcomes). Due to the marked heterogeneity of included studies in terms of the study designs, populations, variable definitions, outcome definitions and use of different tool thresholds, and the failure of multiple studies to report numbers of patients with true positive/true negative/false positive/false negative results, we were unable to perform any meta-analyses. Instead, performance characteristics were summarised in tabular form and using a narrative synthesis approach. When synthesising data, we paid particular attention to several study and tool characteristics. First, the source of participant recruitment. For example, whether controls were recruited from the general population or after entry into healthcare, as symptoms may be more common in clinical controls than population controls, which could influence measures of tool sensitivity and specificity [17]. Second, whether the measures of tool accuracy were obtained directly from the patient sample in which the tool was developed (apparent performance), by applying internal validation methods, such as splitting the sample into development and validation sets or using cross-validation techniques (internal validation), or from a separate analysis in a distinct population (external validation) [12]. Tools usually exhibit poorer diagnostic performance in external validation studies than when evaluated in the original development sample, and external validation of tools is recommended before they are used in clinical practice [12]. Third, we considered whether tools consisted solely of symptoms or symptoms in addition to other variables, as this is likely to impact the clinical utility of the tool.

2.4. Risk of Bias Assessment

The Quality Assessment of Diagnostic Accuracy Studies 2 (QUADAS-2) tool was used to assess the risk of bias and applicability of the included studies [18]. QUADAS-2 includes signalling questions (intended to identify areas of potential bias or concern over study applicability) covering four domains: (1) patient selection, (2) index test(s), (3) reference standard and (4) flow and timing. Each domain was rated as having "high", "low" or "unclear" (where insufficient information is provided) risk of bias. Domains 1–3 were also rated for applicability as "high", "low" or "unclear" concern. Two reviewers (G.F. and V.H.) independently assessed each study using QUADAS-2. Ratings were compared and disagreements were resolved by consensus.

3. Results

3.1. Study Selection

In total, 2331 records were identified from database searches, of which 708 were duplicates. Two additional records were identified from examination of reference lists. A total of 1625 titles and abstracts were screened, and 35 full-text papers were examined. Sixteen studies met the eligibility criteria and were included (Figure 1).

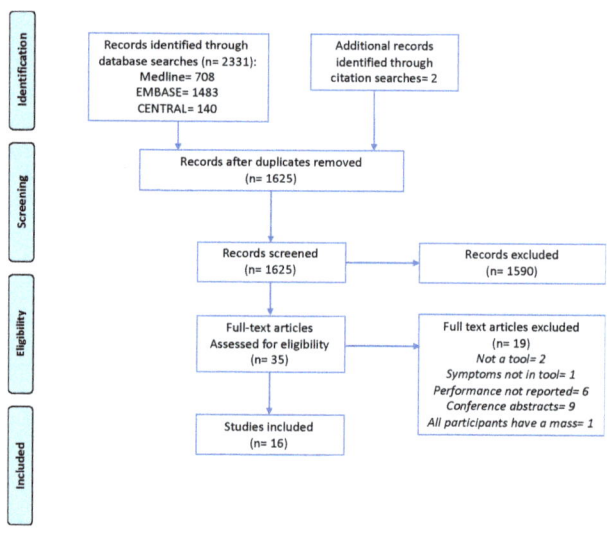

Figure 1. Preferred Reporting Items for Systematic Reviews and Meta-Analysis (PRISMA) flow diagram illustrating the study selection process.

3.2. Study Characteristics

The characteristics of the included studies are summarised in Table 1 and additional exclusion criteria are detailed in Supplementary Material Table S2. Three studies were population-based [19–21], five studies were based in a primary care setting [14,22–25], four studies were entirely hospital-based [26–29] and four studies were hospital-based but also recruited controls from screening studies [30–33]. All population- and hospital-based studies were of case-control design. Two of the studies that recruited from the hospital setting included a proportion of controls with benign ovarian pathology [26,28]. Three of the five primary care studies were of cohort design [22–24], and the remaining two were of case-control design [14,25]. The studies used a variety of data sources for variables, including pre-existing routinely collected primary care data ($n = 6$), information from surveys or patient interviews ($n = 11$) and blood samples ($n = 4$). Study sizes varied markedly, with 75–1,908,467 participants and 24–1885 women with ovarian cancer per study. While all studies used ovarian cancer as an outcome, how this was defined differed, with some only including invasive epithelial cancer or specifically stating that they excluded borderline tumours [19–21,26–29], and others apparently including both invasive and borderline epithelial tumours or all ovarian cancers [14,22–25,30–33]. One study included ovarian cancer alongside other common cancers in a composite outcome, but tool performance characteristics for each cancer were given separately [23]. Seven studies developed entirely new tools [14,19,22,23,25,30,33], six modified existing tools [26–29,31,32] and eight externally validated existing tools [20,21,24,26–29,33].

Table 1. Study characteristics.

Author, Date, Country	Design		Objective			Primary Outcome	Candidate Variable Data Sources	Participants	Study Sample
	Case Control	Cohort	Develop New Tool	Modify Existing Tool	Externally Validate Existing Tool				
Population based									
Lurie, 2009, USA	•					Primary invasive ovarian carcinoma	In-person patient interviews using a structured survey	Cases: Women aged 19-88 years histologically-confirmed primary invasive ovarian carcinoma (1993–2007) Controls: Aged ≥ 18 years, Hawaii resident ≥ 1 year, randomly selected from statutory state survey Frequency-matched to cases (1:1) by age, ethnicity, interview time	Cases: 432 Controls: 491
Rossing, 2010, USA	•				•	Primary invasive epithelial OC [a]	In-person interviews	Cases: Residents in western Washington State, aged 35–74 years, diagnosed with a primary invasive epithelial ovarian tumour (January 2002–December 2005) Controls: Selected by random digit dialling with stratified sampling in 5-year age categories, 1-year calendar intervals and two (urban vs. suburban or rural) county strata	Cases: 594 Controls: 1313
Jordan, 2010, Australia	•				•	Invasive epithelial OC	Patient survey	Cases: Aged 20–79 years with suspected OC, subsequently diagnosed with invasive epithelial OC (January 2002–June 2005) Controls: Frequency-matched based on age (5-year groups) and state of residence identified from electoral roll [34]	Cases: 1215 Controls: 1456
Primary care population									
Hamilton, 2009, England	•		•			Primary OC, including borderline	Researcher-coded GP records	Cases: Aged ≥ 40 years with primary OC diagnosed between 2000 and 2007 Controls: Matched on age, sex and GP practice	Cases: 212 Controls: 1060
Hippisley-Cox, 2012, England and Wales		•	•			OC (NOS)	QResearch database [35]	Aged 30–84 years, registered with GP practices between 1 January 2000 and 30 September 2010	Development (2/3)—1,158,723 women with 976 OCs Validation (1/3)—608,862 women with 538 OCs

Table 1. Cont.

Author, Date, Country	Design		Objective			Primary Outcome	Candidate Variable Data Sources	Participants	Study Sample
	Case Control	Cohort	Develop New Tool	Modify Existing Tool	Externally Validate Existing Tool				
Hippisley-Cox, 2013, England and Wales		•	•			OC (NOS) and 10 other cancers	QResearch database [35]	Aged 25–89 years, registered with GP practices between 1 January 2000 and 1 April 2012	Development (2/3)—1,240,864 women with 1279 OCs Validation (1/3)—667,603 women with 606 OCs
Grewal, 2013, England	•		•			Primary OC, including borderline	Researcher-coded GP records	Cases: Aged ≥ 40 years with primary OC diagnosed between 2000 and 2007 Controls: Matched on age, sex and GP practice	Cases: 212 Controls: 1060
Collins, 2013, UK		•			•	OC (NOS)	THIN database [36]	Women aged 30–84 years registered with GP practices between 1 January 2000 and 30 June 2008	1,054,818 women with 735 cancers
Hospital + screening populations									
Goff, 2007, USA	•		•			OC, including borderline	Patient survey	Cases: Women with a pelvic mass recruited in secondary care prior to OC diagnosis Controls: (a) Healthy 'high-risk' [b] women enrolled in a screening study [37], (b) women who presented for pelvic/abdominal US	Development Cases: 74 Controls: 243 Validation Cases: 75 Controls: 245
Andersen, 2008, USA	•			•		OC (NOS)	Patient survey, blood sample	Cases: Women with a pelvic mass, recruited prior to OC diagnosis Controls: Healthy 'high risk' [b] women enrolled in a screening study [37]	Cases: 75 Controls: 254
Andersen, 2010, USA	•			•		OC (NOS)	Patient survey, blood sample	Cases: Women with a pelvic mass recruited in secondary care prior to OC diagnosis Controls: Healthy 'high risk' [b] women enrolled in a screening study [37], frequency matched to cases on age (</>50 years)	Cases: 74 Controls: 137
Lim, 2012, UK	•		•		•	OC, including borderline	(a) Survey, (b) telephone interview, (c) GP notes	Cases: Women aged 50–79 years with primary OC recruited prior to diagnosis (February 2006–February 2008) Controls: Screening trial participants [38], frequency matched on year of birth and agreement to a telephone interview	Cases: 194 [c] Controls: 268 [c]

Table 1. Cont.

Author, Date, Country	Design		Objective			Primary Outcome	Candidate Variable Data Sources	Participants	Study Sample
	Case Control	Cohort	Develop New Tool	Modify Existing Tool	Externally Validate Existing Tool				
Hospital based population									
Kim, 2009, Korea	•			•	•	Epithelial OC (NOS)	Patient survey, blood sample	Cases: OC diagnosis Controls: Women with benign ovarian cysts recruited prior to surgery and those undergoing routine pap smear	Cases: 116 Controls: 209 (Benign: 74, Pap smear: 135)
Macuks, 2011, Latvia	•			•	•	Epithelial OC (NOS)	Patient survey, blood sample	Cases: Women with epithelial OC recruited prior to surgery/diagnosis Controls: Age-matched 'healthy women' attending a gynaecology outpatient clinic [d]	Cases: 24 Controls: 31 [d]
Shetty, 2015, India	•			•	•	OC, excluding borderline	Patient survey	Cases: Women admitted to hospital for investigation and subsequently diagnosed with OC Controls: (a) Women with benign ovarian pathology; (b) those undergoing a 'gynaecological check-up'	Cases: 74 Controls: 218 (benign: 144, gynaecological check-up: 74)
Jain, 2018, India	•			•	•	OC, excluding borderline	Patient survey, blood sample	Cases: Women undergoing surgery for a pelvic mass, subsequently diagnosed with ovarian cancer Controls: First-degree healthy relatives of cases	Cases: 45 Controls: 90

[a] Data collected on borderline tumours but not included in their tool performance evaluation. [b] Women with high-risk family histories consistent with a possible BRCA1/2 mutation in their families, participating in the Ovarian Cancer Early Detection Study (OCEDS) [37]. [c] Numbers varied by study component: questionnaire (191 cases, 268 controls), telephone interview (111 cases, 125 controls) and GP notes (171 cases, 227 controls). [d] Controls with benign gynaecological disease were also included in study but are excluded from the review, as performance was examined separately to healthy controls and no overall specificity measure was given. Study design and Objectives denoted by "•". Abbreviations: OC = Ovarian cancer; NOS = Not otherwise specified; GP = General practice; US = Ultrasound.

3.3. Risk of Bias

The main potential sources of bias were identified in the "patient selection" and the "index test" domains (Figure 2). As the case-control design can lead to overestimation of test performance [18], 13 studies were flagged as being at high risk of bias for patient selection. Key potential sources of bias identified for studies in the "index test" domain included failing to pre-define the tool threshold and retrospectively administering the tool after the outcome had been determined, e.g., questioning participants after the ovarian cancer diagnosis had been made. The risk of bias was generally judged as low for the "reference standard" and "flow and timing" domains. However, all primary care studies were flagged as being at high risk of bias in the "reference standard" domain as they relied on general practitioner (GP) records to identify ovarian cancer diagnoses, supplemented in two studies by death registration data [22,23] rather than hospital or cancer registry histological diagnoses. Concern over the applicability of studies was judged as low, save for the "reference standard" domain of one study which used a composite cancer outcome [23].

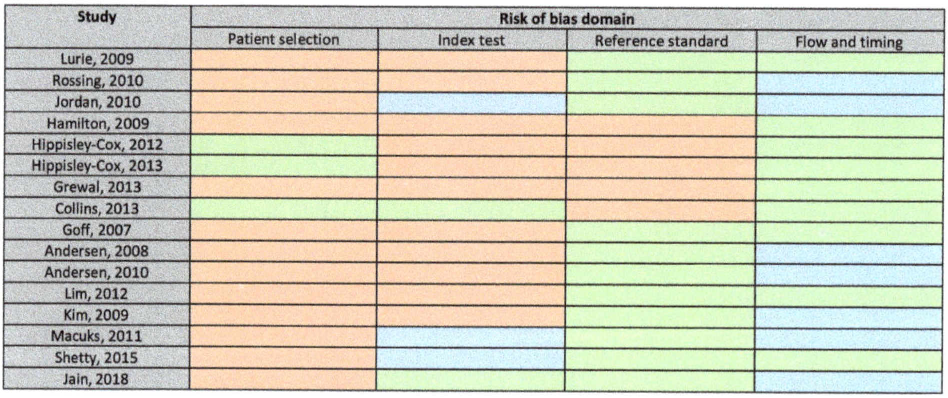

Study	Risk of bias domain			
	Patient selection	Index test	Reference standard	Flow and timing
Lurie, 2009	high	high	low	low
Rossing, 2010	high	high	low	unclear
Jordan, 2010	high	unclear	low	low
Hamilton, 2009	high	high	low	low
Hippisley-Cox, 2012	low	low	high	low
Hippisley-Cox, 2013	low	low	high	low
Grewal, 2013	low	high	low	low
Collins, 2013	low	high	low	low
Goff, 2007	high	high	low	low
Andersen, 2008	high	high	low	low
Andersen, 2010	high	high	low	unclear
Lim, 2012	high	high	low	low
Kim, 2009	high	high	low	unclear
Macuks, 2011	high	unclear	low	low
Shetty, 2015	high	unclear	low	low
Jain, 2018	high	high	low	low

Figure 2. QUADAS-2 Risk of Bias Assessment. Green = "low", orange = "high", blue = "unclear" risk of bias.

4. Tool Variables

The studies evaluated a total of 21 distinct tools, of which five were diagnostic prediction models developed using appropriate statistical methods from which variable weights were derived [12]. We grouped variables included in the tools into four categories: (1) patient demographics, (2) personal and family medical history, (3) symptoms and (4) test results (Table 2). By definition, all tools included symptoms, with 14 including only symptoms. Four tools incorporated demographics, two incorporated personal and family medical history and six incorporated test results. Five symptoms (abdominal pain, pelvic pain, distension, bloating and appetite loss) were included in more than half ($\geq$11) of the tools and a further six symptoms (feeling full quickly, difficulty eating, postmenopausal bleeding, urinary frequency, palpable abdominal mass/lump and rectal bleeding) were included in at least a quarter ($\geq$6) of the tools. Six tools were based on an existing tool—the Goff Symptom Index (SI)—which was modified to include additional symptom or test result variables. Specifications of each tool, including how variables were defined, are included in the Supplementary Material Table S3.

Table 2. Variables included in the final tools.

Tool (Study, Year)	Demographics		Personal/Family History		Symptoms (Symptom checklists)													Test Results		
	Age	Other	PMH	FH	Abdo. Pain	Pelvic Pain	Increase Abdo. Size/Distens.	Bloat.	Appetite Loss	Feeling Full	Difficulty Eating	Weight Loss	Postmen. Bleeding	Rectal Bleeding	Palpable Abdo. Mass/lump	Urinary Freq.	Other	Hb	CA125	HE4
Goff SI (Goff, 2007)					•	•	•	•												
Modified Goff SI 1 (Kim, 2009)					•	•	•	•		•	•						Urinary urgency			
Lurie 7-SI (Lurie, 2009)					•	•	•		•						•	•	Bowel symptoms, difficulty emptying bladder, dysuria, fatigue, abnormal vaginal bleed.			
Lurie 5-SI (Lurie, 2009)					•	•	•								•	•	Difficulty emptying bladder, dysuria, abnormal vaginal bleed.			
Lurie 4-SI (Lurie, 2009)						•	•								•		Abnormal vaginal bleed.			
Lurie 3-SI (Lurie, 2009)						•									•		Abnormal vaginal bleed.			
Hamilton SI (Hamilton, 2009)					•	•	•	•	•				•	•						
SGO consensus criteria * (Rossing, 2010)					•	•		•		•						•	Urinary urgency			
Lim SI 1 (Lim, 2012)					•	•	•	•	•		•	•			•	•				
Lim SI 2 (Lim, 2012)					•	•		•	•						•	•	Vaginal discharge			
Hippisley-Cox SI (Hippisley-Cox, 2012)					•		•		•			•	•	•						

Table 2. Cont.

Tool (Study, Year)	Demographics		Personal/Family History		Symptoms														Test Results		
	Age	Other	PMH	FH	Abdo. Pain	Pelvic Pain	Increase Abdo. Size/Distens.	Bloat.	Appetite Loss	Feeling Full	Difficulty Eating	Weight Loss	Postmen. Bleeding	Rectal Bleeding	Palpable Abdo. Mass/lump	Urinary Freq.	Urinary urgency	Other	Hb	CA125	HE4
Modified Goff SI 2 (Shetty, 2015)					•	•	•	•	•	•	•	•				•					
Augmented symptom checklists																					
Goff SI + CA125 (Andersen, 2008)					•	•	•	•	•	•	•	•								•	
Goff SI + HE4 (Andersen, 2010)					•	•	•	•	•	•	•	•									•
Goff SI + HE4 + CA125 (Andersen, 2010)					•	•	•	•	•	•	•	•								•	•
Goff SI + CA125 + menopause (Macuks, 2011)		Menopause			•	•	•	•	•	•	•	•								•	
Prediction models																					
QCancer Ovarian (Hippisley-Cox, 2012)	•		OC		•		•		•			•	•	•					•		
QCancer Female (Hippisley-Cox, 2013)	•	Townsend score, smoking, alcohol, BMI	T2DM, COPD, endomet. hyperplasia or polyp, chronic pancreatitis	OC, GI cancer, breast cancer	•				•			•	•	•				Difficulty swallowing, heartburn/indigestion, blood in urine, blood in vomit, blood when cough, irregular menstrual bleeding, vaginal bleeding after sex, breast lump, breast skin tethering or nipple discharge, breast pain, lump in neck, night sweats, venous thromboembolism, CIBH, constipation, cough, unexplained bruising	•		

Table 2. Cont.

Tool (Study, Year)	Demographics		Personal/Family History		Symptoms												Test Results		
	Age	Other	PMH	FH	Abdo. Pain	Pelvic Pain	Increase Abdo. Size/Distens.	Bloat.	Appetite Loss	Feeling Full	Difficulty Eating	Weight Loss	Postmen. Bleeding	Rectal Bleeding	Palpable Abdo. Mass/lump	Urinary Freq.	Other	Hb	CA125	HE4
OC Score A (Grewal, 2013)					•		•	•	•				•	•		•				
OC Score B (Grewal, 2013)					•		•	•	•				•	•		•				
OC Score C (Grewal, 2013)	•						•	•	•				•	•		•				

* Consensus statement released by the Society of Gynaecologic Oncologists (SGO), the Gynaecologic Cancer Foundation and the American Cancer Society. The presence of a variable within a model is denoted by "•". The terms used to describe a given symptom varied subtly between studies—full details of each tool, including symptom terminology and duration and frequency criteria, are included in Supplementary Material Table S3. Abbreviations: PMH = past medical history; FH = family history; Abdo. = abdominal; Distens. = distension; Bloat. = bloating; Postmen. = postmenopausal; bleed. = bleeding; Freq. = frequency; Hb = haemoglobin; CA125 = cancer antigen 125; HE4 = human epididymis protein 4; SI = symptom index; OC = ovarian cancer; BMI = body mass index; endomet. = endometrial; T2DM = type 2 diabetes mellites; COPD = chronic obstructive pulmonary disease; GI = gastrointestinal; CIBH = change in bowel habit.

4.1. Evaluation of Tool Performance

The diagnostic performance of the included tools is summarised in Table 3. Measures of diagnostic performance for the majority of the tools were obtained directly from the patient sample with which the tool was developed (apparent performance) or by applying internal validation methods, such as splitting the sample into development and validation sets (internal validation), with only four tools—the Society of Gynaecologic Oncology (SGO) consensus criteria, Goff SI, QCancer Ovarian, Modified Goff SI 1—undergoing independent validation with an external dataset. Although the Goff SI in combination with CA125 was evaluated in several studies, the CA125 thresholds used varied markedly, so no studies were considered to have externally validated the same combination. There was overlap in evaluation of tools between healthcare settings, but no tool evaluated in primary care was evaluated in another setting or vice versa.

The most widely studied tool was the Goff SI, which was evaluated in nine studies [20,21,26,27,29–33], but two of these used data from subsets of women in the original tool development study [31,32]. Apparent deviations from the original Goff SI in how variables were defined were noted in several studies (Table S4). The Goff SI was the only tool to be externally validated in groups of women recruited from more than one setting.

4.2. Tool Diagnostic Accuracy

4.2.1. Hospital Setting

All but two tools evaluated in hospital populations incorporated the Goff SI. Two of these underwent external evaluation—the original Goff SI and a modified version incorporating additional symptoms (Modified Goff SI 1). The Goff SI, which was externally validated in six studies, demonstrated sensitivities which ranged from 56.9% to 83.3% (an outlier result) and specificities from 48.3% (an outlier result) to 98.9%. A modified version of the Goff SI (Modified Goff SI 1) demonstrated a sensitivity of 71.6% and a specificity of 88.5% in a single external validation study.

Augmenting symptom checklists with baseline risk factors and test results generally led to a reduction in sensitivity and an increase in specificity, or vice versa, depending on the threshold used. For example, the addition of the serum ovarian cancer biomarker CA125 to the Goff SI by Anderson et al. (2008) led to a reduction in tool sensitivity—if both variables were required to be abnormal for a positive tool result—or in tool specificity—if only one was required to be abnormal for a positive tool result [31].

4.2.2. Population Setting

In women recruited from the population setting, two symptom checklists were externally validated side by side—the Goff SI and the SGO consensus criteria. While the sensitivities and specificities of the tools differed between the studies, within each study, they were similar, with an in-study maximum difference in sensitivity of 3.4% and specificity of 2.4% between the tools.

4.2.3. Primary Care

A single tool (QCancer Ovarian), which took the form of a prediction model and combined symptom variables with demographics, family history and routine blood test results, underwent external validation in a primary care setting. When the threshold for abnormality was set to include the 5% of women at the highest predicted risk, QCancer Ovarian had a sensitivity of 43.8% and a specificity of 95%, while when the threshold was set to include women at the 10% highest risk, the sensitivity increased to 64.1% but the specificity fell to 90.1%. Several scores, developed by Grewal et al., demonstrated higher sensitivities and specificities than QCancer Ovarian at the 5% risk threshold (OC Score B $\geq$ 4) and 10% risk threshold (OC Score C $\geq$ 4), but diagnostic accuracy measures were derived from the same dataset used in score development.

Table 3. Tool diagnostic accuracy.

Tool	Study	Recruitment				Source of Accuracy Estimate			Sensitivity (95% CI)	Specificity (95% CI)	PPV	AUC (95% CI)
		Population Level	1° Care	Hospital + Screening	Hospital	Apparent Performance	Internal Validation	External Validation				
Symptom checklists												
Goff SI	Goff, 2007			•		•			≥50 yrs: 66.7 <50 yrs: 86.7	≥50 yrs: 90 <50 yrs: 86.7	-	-
	Andersen, 2008 [a]			•		•			64 (52.1-74.8)	88.2 (83.6-91.9)	-	-
	Kim, 2009				•				56.9	87.6	-	-
	Rossing, 2010	•						•	67.5 (65.4-69.6)	94.9 (93.9-95.8)	0.77-1.12 [b]	-
	Jordan, 2010	•						•	68.1 (65.5-70.7)	85.3	0.09 [c] (≥55 yrs: 0.21-0.31 <55 yrs: 0.04) [d]	-
	Andersen, 2010 [a]			•			•		63.5 (51.5-74.4)	88.3 (81.7-93.2)	-	-
	Macuks, 2011				•		•		83.3	48.3	-	-
	Jain, 2018				•		•		77.8	87.8	-	-
	Lim, 2012			•				•	61.4-75.7 [e]	89.6-98.9 [e]	-	-
Modified Goff SI 1	Kim, 2009				•	•			65.5	84.7	-	-
	Shetty, 2015				•			•	71.6	88.5	-	-
7-symptom Index	Lurie, 2009	•				•			85	40	-	-
5-symptom Index	Lurie, 2009	•				•			80	63	-	-
4-symptom Index	Lurie, 2009	•				•			74	77	-	-
3-symptom Index	Lurie, 2009	•				•			54	93	-	-
Hamilton SI	Hamilton, 2009		•						85	85	-	-
SGO consensus criteria	Rossing, 2010	•						•	65.3 (63.1-67.4)	93.9 (92.8-95)	0.63-0.92 [b]	-
	Jordan, 2010	•							71.5 (69-74.1)	82.9 (81-84.8)	0.08 [c] (≥55 yrs: 0.18-0.27 <55 yrs: 0.05) [d]	-
Lim SI 1	Lim, 2012			•			•		69.6-91 [e]	76-91 [e]	-	-

Table 3. Cont.

Tool	Study	Recruitment				Source of Accuracy Estimate			Sensitivity (95% CI)	Specificity (95% CI)	PPV	AUC (95% CI)
		Population Level	1° Care	Hospital + Screening	Hospital	Apparent Performance	Internal Validation	External Validation				
Lim SI 2	Lim, 2012			•				•	67.3–91 [e]	82.4–94 [e]	-	-
Hippisley-Cox SI	Hippisley-Cox, 2012		•					•	71.9	82.9	0.5	-
Modified Goff SI 2	Shetty, 2015				•	•			77	88.5	-	-
Augmented symptom checklists												
Goff SI or CA125 [f]	Andersen, 2008			•		•			89.3 (80.1–95.3)	83.5 (78.3–87.8)	-	-
Goff SI or CA125 (>35 U/mL)	Jain, 2018				•	•			97.8	68.9	-	-
Goff SI & CA125 (>21 U/mL)	Macuks, 2011				•	•			79.1	100	-	-
Goff SI & CA125 (>35 U/mL)	Macuks, 2011				•	•			70.8	100	-	-
Goff SI & CA125 (>65 U/mL)	Macuks, 2011				•	•			70.8	100	-	-
Goff SI or CA125 [f]	Andersen, 2010			•		•			91.9 (83.2–97)	83.2 (75.9–89)	-	-
Goff SI or HE4 [f]	Andersen, 2010			•		•			91.9 (83.2–97)	84.7 (77.5–90.3)	-	-
Any 1 of 3 (Goff SI or CA125 or HE4) [f]	Andersen, 2010			•		•			94.6 (86.7–98.5)	79.6 (71.8–86)	-	-
Any 2 of 3 (Goff SI or CA125 or HE4) [f]	Andersen, 2010			•		•			83.8 (73.4–91.3)	98.5 (94.8–99.8)	-	-
Goff SI & 1 or more of CA125 or HE4 [f]	Andersen, 2010			•		•			58.1 (46.1–69.5)	98.5 (94.8–99.8)	-	-
Goff SI & CA125 (>25 U/mL) & menopause	Macuks, 2011				•	•			50	100	-	-
Goff SI & CA125 (>35 U/mL) & menopause	Macuks, 2011				•	•			45.8	100	-	-
Goff SI & CA125 (>65 U/mL) & menopause	Macuks, 2011				•	•			45.8	100	-	-
Prediction models												

Table 3. Cont.

Tool	Study	Recruitment				Source of Accuracy Estimate			Sensitivity (95% CI)	Specificity (95% CI)	PPV	AUC (95% CI)
		Population Level	1° Care	Hospital + Screening	Hospital	Apparent Performance	Internal Validation	External Validation				
QCancer Ovarian (Top 10% risk)	Hippisley-Cox, 2012		•				•		63.2	90.8	0.8	0.84 (0.83–0.86)
	Collins, 2013		•					•	64.1	90.1	0.5	0.86 (0.84–0.87)
QCancer Ovarian (Top 5% risk)	Hippisley-Cox, 2012		•				•		42.2	95.6	1.1	-
	Collins, 2013		•					•	43.8	95	0.6	-
QCancer Ovarian (Top 1% risk)	Hippisley-Cox, 2012		•				•		13.9	99.3	2.1	-
QCancer Ovarian (Top 0.5% risk)	Hippisley-Cox, 2012		•				•		11	99.6	3.2	-
QCancer Ovarian (Top 0.1% risk)	Hippisley-Cox, 2012		•				•		3.9	99.9	5.5	-
QCancer Female (Top 10% risk)	Hippisley-Cox, 2013		•				•		61.6	90	0.6	0.84 (0.82–0.86)
OC Score A (Score ≥ 3)	Grewal, 2013		•			•			58.5	97.3	-	0.89
OC Score A (Score ≥ 4)	Grewal, 2013		•			•			57.6	97.3	-	
OC Score B (Score ≥ 3)	Grewal, 2013		•			•			75	90.1	-	0.89
OC Score B (Score ≥ 4)	Grewal, 2013		•			•			58.9	97.3	-	
OC Score C (Score ≥ 3)	Grewal, 2013		•			•			85.4	85.1	-	0.88
OC Score C (Score ≥ 4)	Grewal, 2013		•			•			72.6	91.3	-	

[a] Study used a subset of patients from Goff, 2007. [b] Calculated using external data from screening studies. [39,40]. [c] Calculated using external Australian population-level data. [d] Calculated using external data from US and UK screening studies and Australian population-level data. [41,42]. [e] Sensitivity and specificity varied by data collection method (questionnaire, telephone interview, GP notes). [f] Biomarker level (CA125, HE4) dichotomised at 95th percentile in control group—levels above that deemed abnormal. The Recruitment setting and the source of accuracy estimate are denoted by "•". Abbreviations: OC = ovarian cancer; CI = confidence interval; AUC = area under the receiver operator characteristic curve; PPV = positive predictive values; yrs = years.

Discrimination was reported for five tools (Table 3), all of which had similar AUCs within the 'good' range (0.84–0.89), with QCancer Ovarian exhibiting an AUC of 0.86 on external validation. Tool calibration was assessed for QCancer tools by graphically comparing the predicted cancer risk at two years with the observed risk by predicted risk deciles [22–24]. Authors reported good calibration on internal validation. On external validation, QCancer Ovarian had reasonable calibration but overpredicted risk, particularly in older women [24].

4.2.4. Positive Predictive Values

The three cohort studies conducted in primary care reported positive predictive values (PPV) for QCancer tools at a range of thresholds (Table 3). The PPVs at any given risk threshold were similar—for example, values ranged from 0.5 to 0.8% when the threshold was set to identify the 10% of women at highest risk. Two case control studies (Rossing et al. and Jordan et al.) used external disease prevalence figures from screening studies and available population-level statistics to estimate the PPVs of the Goff SI and SGO consensus criteria—if they were to be used in general populations. The tools had similar estimated PPVs within each study, but PPVs were higher in Rossing et al. (0.63–1.12%) than in Jordan et al. (<55 years: 0.04–0.05%, ≥55 years: 0.18–0.31%).

5. Discussion

To our knowledge, this is the first systematic review to compare the diagnostic performance of existing symptom-based tools for ovarian cancer detection. We identified 21 symptom-based tools designed to help identify women with undiagnosed ovarian cancer. These tools comprised simple symptom checklists, checklists which included both symptoms and tests and more complex diagnostic prediction models which incorporated symptoms, test results and baseline risk factors. While the diagnostic performances of most tools were evaluated solely within the study development datasets, four tools were independently externally validated, with one being validated in multiple population settings. Externally validated tools demonstrated similar moderate diagnostic performances. Our findings should inform future studies evaluating the clinical impact of validated symptom-based tools when implemented in clinical practice.

5.1. Study Strengths and Limitations

The main strengths of this study were its systematic approach, broad search strategy and liberal eligibility criteria, which enabled us to identify and compare the performances of a wide variety of tools. However, the identified studies were extremely heterogeneous in their designs, populations, variable definitions, outcome definitions and thresholds, which ultimately precluded any meaningful meta-analyses. For example, although the Goff SI was evaluated in nine studies, there was overlap between the participants in three studies, control groups ranged from apparently healthy general population participants to hospital gynaecology patients (with or without benign pathology), ovarian cancer definitions differed and deviations in the parameters of the SI itself, in terms of symptom duration and frequency criteria, were noted in several studies. While meta-analysis was not deemed appropriate, our results demonstrate how the Goff SI performs under different conditions. An additional limitation was that all included studies were at high risk of bias in at least one QUADAS-2 domain, which limits the conclusions that can be drawn.

5.2. Comparison of Tools

Although all tools were symptom-based and designed to help identify women with ovarian cancer, they varied markedly in the symptoms they included. This mirrors discrepancies in the literature and within national guidelines as to which symptoms are associated with the disease and probably reflects differences in study methodologies and study populations [7]. Despite this, the symptoms with the highest positive likelihood ratios for ovarian cancer in a recent systematic review (distension, bloating, abdominal or pelvic pain) were incorporated into the majority of tools [8]. The more cancer-associated symptoms that are included in a checklist, the higher the sensitivity of the tool is likely to be, but at the cost of reducing specificity, as demonstrated by several of the included studies [19,26,33]. This was cited by Goff et al. as a rationale for not including urinary symptoms in the Goff SI [30]. Ultimately, variation in which additional symptoms a tool includes may have limited impact on tool performance; on external validation, two studies reported similar diagnostic accuracy metrics for the Goff SI and the SGO criteria (which differed on several symptoms), and on internal validation, Lim et al. concluded that changing several of the symptoms made relatively little difference to tool diagnostic accuracy [33].

In multiple studies, symptom checklists were augmented by ovarian cancer biomarkers with the aim of improving tool diagnostic accuracy. This approach naturally led to a reduction in tool specificity (where either symptoms or an abnormal test resulted in a positive tool) or sensitivity (where symptoms and an abnormal test were needed for a positive tool). If ovarian cancer biomarkers are to be included alongside symptoms within tools, this loss of performance could be avoided by incorporating them within prediction models, as per the inclusion of anaemia in QCancer Ovarian. As the prediction model threshold can be set at a desired risk level, biomarkers, such as CA125 and HE4, could be incorporated without harming tool performance. However, this would require women to have specialist ovarian cancer markers performed in order for the tool to be used, which significantly limits clinical utility. A more practical approach would be to incorporate tools within a two-step pathway in which symptom-based tools (which do not include specialist test variables) are used to help select higher-risk women for specialist ovarian cancer tests.

Variation in the reported sensitivity and specificity of the most widely evaluated tool, the Goff SI, was noted between studies. This variation is likely to be due, in part, to the marked differences in study design, populations and outcome definitions which precluded meta-analysis across these studies. Despite these differences, in 5 of the 6 external validation studies (including two large population-based studies), the Goff SI had a sensitivity in excess of 60%, and in all but the smallest study, which included only 24 ovarian cancers and 31 controls, its specificity exceeded 85%. The sensitivities and specificities of the two other externally validated symptom checklists—the SGO consensus criteria and the modified Goff SI 1—were similar, as were those of the only externally validated diagnostic prediction model—QCancer Ovarian (applying a 10% risk threshold). Given the similarity in performance of the various existing validated tools, future research efforts may be better directed at evaluating the impact of using available tools in practice rather than developing further tools consisting of different symptom combinations.

5.3. Clinical Relevance

Two distinct uses for tools were identified by the authors of the included studies: (1) assessment of women presenting symptomatically in the standard clinical setting to identify those at higher risk of undiagnosed cancer and to inform decision making and further investigation, and (2) proactive 'symptom-triggered screening' programs in which women are actively screened using the tool, with further testing for ovarian cancer occurring if the tool is positive. Several of the tools identified in this review are already available for use within the standard clinical setting in the form of electronic clinical decision support tools (eCDSTs). QCancer tools are integrated within some UK general practice IT systems and alert the clinician if the risk of ovarian cancer in an individual reaches a certain level, prompting them to consider ovarian cancer as a possible diagnosis. eCDSTs have been shown to improve practitioner performance and patient care, but there are multiple barriers to their implementation and they do not always lead to improved outcomes [43,44]. Therefore, even if eCDSTs are deemed to have acceptable diagnostic accuracy, their cost-effectiveness, acceptability to patients and clinicians and their impact on timely ovarian cancer detection and survival need to be evaluated. Currently, a large, clustered, randomised control trial is seeking to help to address this by investigating the clinical impact of implementing a suite of electronic cancer risk assessment tools (including an electronic version of the Hamilton ovarian SI) in UK general practice [45]. Studies have also sought to evaluate the impact of using tools as part of 'symptom-triggered screening' programs, but none have taken the form of randomised control trials—the gold standard approach—and so findings should be interpreted with caution. In one study, 5000 women were approached in primary care clinics and screened for symptoms using the Goff SI, with further investigations performed if the Goff SI was positive [11]. However, conclusions were limited as only two ovarian cancers were identified in the study window. The Diagnosing Ovarian and Endometrial Cancer Early (DOvEE) trial also employs a proactive symptom-triggered testing approach, supported by media campaigns, in which women can self-refer and are screened for range of symptoms prior to study inclusion. Although the final DOvEE results are yet to be published, a pilot study reported that participants had lower tumour burden and more resectable disease than women diagnosed via the standard clinical pathway [9].

When considering the clinical utility of a tool, it is important to assess the proportion of women who are 'tool-positive' who ultimately have ovarian cancer, i.e., the PPV. Primary care cohort studies indicated that between 1 in 200 and 1 in 100 women who were QCancer tool-positive (5% or 10% risk) had the disease. Although these figures may appear low, evidence indicates that patients would opt for cancer testing at PPVs of 1% [46]. Further, having a positive tool result in the clinical setting does not necessarily mean that further investigation will automatically occur, as there may be a clear alternative cause for the symptoms—the tool is simply intended as a diagnostic aid to highlight the risk of ovarian cancer to the clinician. In addition, the most common follow-up tests—CA125 and transvaginal ultrasound—are relatively non-invasive, and CA125 is known to perform well when used in a symptomatic primary care population [47], although invasive investigations/surgery may ultimately be needed to determine whether ovarian cancer is present. In proactive symptom-triggered screening programs, the tool is more than just a diagnostic aid—it is the initial screening step which will dictate whether further ovarian cancer tests take place. The two population studies reporting PPVs relied on external ovarian cancer prevalence figures, but their PPV estimates were similar to that reported in the pilot DOvEE study (0.76% in women ≥ 50 years) [9]. Further research is needed to help determine whether, given this PPV, follow-up testing in proactive symptom-triggered testing programs is acceptable to women and improves outcomes. The definitive diagnosis of ovarian cancer often involves invasive procedures/surgery, which has contributed to patient morbidity in key ovarian cancer screening trials [3,39]. Although initial findings indicate that proactive symptom triggered testing approaches lead to minimal unnecessary surgery [9,11], large trials are needed to confirm that the implementation of symptom-based tools in clinical practice does not lead to significant excess morbidity.

6. Conclusions

Over 20 symptom-based tools have been developed in different populations to help assess women for ovarian cancer, but the majority have not been validated. Four symptom-based tools—the Goff SI, a modified version of the Goff symptom Index, SGO consensus criteria and QCancer Ovarian—have undergone independent external validation and exhibit similar sensitivities and specificities. These tools could have an important role to play in the detection of ovarian cancer, but further large well-conducted studies are needed to assess their cost-effectiveness, their acceptability, their effect on the timeliness of ovarian cancer diagnosis and their impact on clinical outcomes, including patient survival.

Supplementary Materials: The following are available online at http://www.mdpi.com/2072-6694/12/12/3686/s1, Table S1: PRISMA Checklist. Text S1: MEDLINE search strategy. Table S2: Specific study exclusions. Table S3: Tool specifications. Table S4: Deviations from the original Goff SI in validation studies.

Author Contributions: Conceptualization, G.F.; methodology, G.F., F.M.W. and W.H.; formal analysis, G.F. and V.H.; data curation, G.F. and V.H.; writing—original draft preparation, G.F.; writing—review and editing, G.F., V.H., G.A., E.J.C., W.H., F.M.W. and J.E.; supervision, F.M.W., G.A., E.J.C. and W.H.; funding acquisition, F.M.W. and W.H. All authors have read and agreed to the published version of the manuscript.

Funding: This research arises from the CanTest Collaborative, which is funded by Cancer Research UK [C8640/A23385], of which G.F. is Clinical Research Fellow, V.H. is a PhD student, G.A. is the Senior Statistician, J.E. is Associate Director, and W.H. and F.M.W. are Directors. E.J.C. is supported through the NIHR Manchester Biomedical Research Centre (IS-BRC-1215-20007). The funders of this study had no role in the study design, data collection, data analysis, data interpretation, or writing of the report.

Conflicts of Interest: Two studies included in this review were conducted by W.H. W.H. played no role in study selection or quality assessment. All other authors declare no conflicts of interest. The funders had no role in the design of the study; in the collection, analyses, or interpretation of data; in the writing of the manuscript, or in the decision to publish the results.

References

1. Bray, F.; Ferlay, J.; Soerjomataram, I.; Siegel, R.L.; Torre, L.A.; Jemal, A. Global cancer statistics 2018: GLOBOCAN estimates of incidence and mortality worldwide for 36 cancers in 185 countries. *CA Cancer J. Clin.* **2018**, *68*, 394–424. [CrossRef] [PubMed]
2. Cancer Research UK. Ovarian Cancer Survival Statistics. Available online: http://www.cancerresearchuk.org/health-professional/cancer-statistics/statistics-by-cancer-type/ovarian-cancer/survival#heading-Three (accessed on 20 May 2020).
3. Jacobs, I.J.; Menon, U.; Ryan, A.; Gentry-Maharaj, A.; Burnell, M.; Kalsi, J.K.; Amso, N.N.; Apostolidou, S.; Benjamin, E.; Cruickshank, D.; et al. Ovarian cancer screening and mortality in the UK Collaborative Trial of Ovarian Cancer Screening (UKCTOCS): A randomised controlled trial. *Lancet* **2016**, *387*, 945–956. [CrossRef]
4. Pinsky, P.F.; Yu, K.; Kramer, B.S.; Black, A.; Buys, S.S.; Partridge, E.; Gohagan, J.; Berg, C.D.; Prorok, P.C. Extended mortality results for ovarian cancer screening in the PLCO trial with median 15 years follow-up. *Gynecol. Oncol.* **2016**, *143*, 270–275. [CrossRef] [PubMed]
5. Barrett, J.; Sharp, D.J.; Stapley, S.; Stabb, C.; Hamilton, W. Pathways to the diagnosis of ovarian cancer in the UK: A cohort study in primary care. *BJOG* **2010**, *117*, 610–614. [CrossRef]
6. National Cancer Intellegence Network. Routes to Diagnosis 2006–2016 by year, V2.1a. Available online: http://www.ncin.org.uk/publications/routes_to_diagnosis (accessed on 21 May 2020).
7. Funston, G.; Melle, V.M.; Ladegaard Baun, M.-L.; Jensen, H.; Helpser, C.; Emery, J.; Crosbie, E.; Thompson, M.; Hamilton, W.; Walter, F.M. Variation in the initial assessment and investigation for ovarian cancer in symptomatic women: A systematic review of international guidelines. *BMC Cancer* **2019**, *19*, 1028. [CrossRef]
8. Ebell, M.H.; Culp, M.B.; Radke, T.J. A Systematic Review of Symptoms for the Diagnosis of Ovarian Cancer. *Am. J. Prev. Med.* **2016**, *50*, 384–394. [CrossRef]
9. Gilbert, L.; Basso, O.; Sampalis, J.; Karp, I.; Martins, C.; Feng, J.; Piedimonte, S.; Quintal, L.; Ramanakumar, A.V.; Takefman, J.; et al. Assessment of symptomatic women for early diagnosis of ovarian cancer: Results from the prospective DOvE pilot project. *Lancet Oncol.* **2012**, *13*, 285–291. [CrossRef]
10. Goff, B.A.; Lowe, K.A.; Kane, J.C.; Robertson, M.D.; Gaul, M.A.; Andersen, M.R. Symptom triggered screening for ovarian cancer: A pilot study of feasibility and acceptability. *Gynecol. Oncol.* **2012**, *124*, 230–235. [CrossRef]
11. Andersen, M.R.; Lowe, K.A.; Goff, B.A. Value of Symptom-Triggered Diagnostic Evaluation for Ovarian Cancer. *Obstet. Gynecol.* **2014**, *123*, 73–79. [CrossRef]
12. Moons, K.G.M.; Altman, D.G.; Reitsma, J.B.; Ioannidis, J.P.A.; Macaskill, P.; Steyerberg, E.W.; Vickers, A.J.; Ransohoff, D.F.; Collins, G.S. Transparent reporting of a multivariable prediction model for individual prognosis or diagnosis (TRIPOD): Explanation and elaboration. *Ann. Intern. Med.* **2015**, *162*, W1–W73. [CrossRef]
13. Goff, B.A.; Mandel, L.S.; Melancon, C.H.; Muntz, H.G. Frequency of symptoms of ovarian cancer in women presenting to primary care clinics. *JAMA* **2004**, *291*, 2705–2712. [CrossRef] [PubMed]
14. Hamilton, W.; Peters, T.J.; Bankhead, C.; Sharp, D. Risk of ovarian cancer in women with symptoms in primary care: Population based case-control study. *BMJ* **2009**, *339*, b2998. [CrossRef] [PubMed]
15. Laupacis, A.; Sekar, N.; Stiell, I.G. Clinical prediction rules: A review and suggested modifications of methodological standards. *J. Am. Med. Assoc.* **1997**, *277*, 488–494. [CrossRef]
16. Ouzzani, M.; Hammady, H.; Fedorowicz, Z.; Elmagarmid, A. Rayyan-a web and mobile app for systematic reviews. *Syst. Rev.* **2016**, *5*, 210. [CrossRef]
17. Usher-Smith, J.A.; Sharp, S.J.; Griffin, S.J. The spectrum effect in tests for risk prediction, screening, and diagnosis. *BMJ* **2016**, *353*, i3139. [CrossRef]
18. Whiting, P.F.; Rutjes, A.W.S.; Westwood, M.E.; Mallett, S.; Deeks, J.J.; Reitsma, J.B.; Leeflang, M.M.G.; Sterne, J.A.C.; Bossuyt, P.M.M. Quadas-2: A revised tool for the quality assessment of diagnostic accuracy studies. *Ann. Intern. Med.* **2011**, *155*, 529–536. [CrossRef]

19. Lurie, G.; Thompson, P.J.; McDuffie, K.E.; Carney, M.E.; Goodman, M.T. Prediagnostic symptoms of ovarian carcinoma: A case-control study. *Gynecol. Oncol.* **2009**, *114*, 231–236. [CrossRef]
20. Rossing, M.A.; Wicklund, K.G.; Cushing-Haugen, K.L.; Weiss, N.S. Predictive value of symptoms for early detection of ovarian cancer. *J. Natl. Cancer Inst.* **2010**, *102*, 222–229. [CrossRef]
21. Jordan, S.J.; Coory, M.D.; Webb, P.M. Re: Predictive Value of Symptoms for Early Detection of Ovarian Cancer. *JNCI J. Natl. Cancer Inst.* **2010**, *102*, 1599–1601. [CrossRef]
22. Hippisley-Cox, J.; Coupland, C. Identifying women with suspected ovarian cancer in primary care: Derivation and validation of algorithm. *BMJ* **2012**, *344*, d8009. [CrossRef]
23. Hippisley-Cox, J.; Coupland, C. Symptoms and risk factors to identify women with suspected cancer in primary care: Derivation and validation of an algorithm. *Br. J. Gen. Pract.* **2013**, *63*, e11–e21. [CrossRef]
24. Collins, G.S.; Altman, D.G. Identifying women with undetected ovarian cancer: Independent and external validation of QCancer® (Ovarian) prediction model. *Eur. J. Cancer Care (Engl.)* **2013**, *22*, 423–429. [CrossRef]
25. Grewal, K.; Hamilton, W.; Sharp, D. Ovarian cancer prediction: Development of a scoring system for primary care. *BJOG An Int. J. Obstet. Gynaecol.* **2013**, *120*, 1016–1019. [CrossRef]
26. Kim, M.-K.; Kim, K.; Kim, S.M.; Kim, J.W.; Park, N.-H.; Song, Y.-S.; Kang, S.-B. A hospital-based case-control study of identifying ovarian cancer using symptom index. *J. Gynecol. Oncol.* **2009**, *20*, 238–242. [CrossRef]
27. Macuks, R.; Baidekalna, I.; Donina, S. Diagnostic test for ovarian cancer composed of ovarian cancer symptom index, menopausal status and ovarian cancer antigen CA125. *Eur. J. Gynaecol. Oncol.* **2011**, *32*, 286–288.
28. Shetty, J.; Priyadarshini, P.; Pandey, D.; Manjunath, A.P. Modified Goff Symptom Index: Simple triage tool for ovarian malignancy. *Sultan Qaboos Univ. Med. J.* **2015**, *15*, e370–e375. [CrossRef]
29. Jain, S.; Danodia, K.; Suneja, A.; Mehndiratta, M.; Chawla, S. Symptom index for detection of ovarian malignancy in indian women: A hospital-based study. *J. Indian Acad. Clin. Med.* **2018**, *19*, 27–32.
30. Goff, B.A.; Mandel, L.S.; Drescher, C.W.; Urban, N.; Gough, S.; Schurman, K.M.; Patras, J.; Mahony, B.S.; Robyn Andersen, M. Development of an ovarian cancer symptom index: Possibilities for earlier detection. *Cancer* **2007**, *109*, 221–227. [CrossRef]
31. Andersen, M.R.; Goff, B.A.; Lowe, K.A.; Scholler, N.; Bergan, L.; Dresher, C.W.; Paley, P.; Urban, N. Combining a symptoms index with CA 125 to improve detection of ovarian cancer. *Cancer* **2008**, *113*, 484–489. [CrossRef]
32. Andersen, M.R.; Goff, B.A.; Lowe, K.A.; Scholler, N.; Bergan, L.; Drescher, C.W.; Paley, P.; Urban, N. Use of a Symptom Index, CA125, and HE4 to predict ovarian cancer. *Gynecol. Oncol.* **2010**, *116*, 378–383. [CrossRef] [PubMed]
33. Lim, A.W.W.; Mesher, D.; Gentry-Maharaj, A.; Balogun, N.; Jacobs, I.; Menon, U.; Sasieni, P. Predictive value of symptoms for ovarian cancer: Comparison of symptoms reported by questionnaire, interview, and general practitioner notes. *J. Natl. Cancer Inst.* **2012**, *104*, 114–124. [CrossRef] [PubMed]
34. Merritt, M.A.; Green, A.C.; Nagle, C.M.; Webb, P.M.; Bowtell, D.; Chenevix-Trench, G.; Green, A.; Webb, P.; DeFazio, A.; Gertig, D.; et al. Talcum powder, chronic pelvic inflammation and NSAIDs in relation to risk of epithelial ovarian cancer. *Int. J. Cancer* **2008**, *122*, 170–176. [CrossRef] [PubMed]
35. QResearch The QResearch Database. Available online: https://www.qresearch.org (accessed on 8 January 2019).
36. THIN® The Health Improvement Network. Available online: https://www.the-health-improvement-network.com/en/ (accessed on 9 November 2020).
37. Lowe, K.A.; Shah, C.; Wallace, E.; Anderson, G.; Paley, P.; McIntosh, M.; Andersen, M.R.; Scholler, N.; Bergan, L.; Thorpe, J.; et al. Effects of personal characteristics on serum CA125, mesothelin, and HE4 levels in healthy postmenopausal women at high-risk for ovarian cancer. *Cancer Epidemiol. Biomark. Prev.* **2008**, *17*, 2480–2487. [CrossRef]
38. Menon, U.; Gentry-Maharaj, A.; Hallett, R.; Ryan, A.; Burnell, M.; Sharma, A.; Lewis, S.; Davies, S.; Philpott, S.; Lopes, A.; et al. Sensitivity and specificity of multimodal and ultrasound screening for ovarian cancer, and stage distribution of detected cancers: Results of the prevalence screen of the UK Collaborative Trial of Ovarian Cancer Screening (UKCTOCS). *Lancet Oncol.* **2009**, *10*, 327–340. [CrossRef]
39. Buys, S.S.; Partridge, E.; Greene, M.H.; Prorok, P.C.; Reding, D.; Riley, T.L.; Hartge, P.; Fagerstrom, R.M.; Ragard, L.R.; Chia, D.; et al. Ovarian cancer screening in the Prostate, Lung, Colorectal and Ovarian (PLCO) cancer screening trial: Findings from the initial screen of a randomized trial. *Am. J. Obstet. Gynecol.* **2005**, *193*, 1630–1639. [CrossRef]

40. Jacobs, I.; Prys Davies, A.; Bridges, J.; Stabile, I.; Fay, T.; Lower, A.; Grudzinskas, J.G.; Oram, D. Prevalence screening for ovarian cancer in postmenopausal women by CA 125 measurement and ultrasonography. *Br. Med. J.* **1993**, *306*, 1030–1034. [CrossRef]
41. *Cancer Incidence Projections Australia 2002 to 2011*; Australian Institute of Health and Welfare; Australasian Association of Cancer Registries; National Cancer Strategies Group: Canberra, Australia, 2005.
42. *Australian Demographic Statistics*; Australian Bureau of Statistics D: Canberra, Australia, 2007.
43. Chima, S.; Milley, K.; Reece, J.C.; Milton, S.; McIntosh, J.G.; Emery, J.D. Decision support tools to improve cancer diagnostic decision making in primary care: A systematic review. *Br. J. Gen. Pract.* **2019**, *69*, e809–e818. [CrossRef]
44. Chiang, P.C.; Glance, D.; Walker, J.; Walter, F.M.; Emery, J.D. Implementing a qcancer risk tool into general practice consultations: An exploratory study using simulated consultations with Australian general practitioners. *Br. J. Cancer* **2015**, *112*, S77–S83. [CrossRef]
45. Hamilton, W. Electronic Risk Assessment for Cancer for Patients in General Practice (ISRCTN22560297). Available online: http://www.isrctn.com/ISRCTN22560297 (accessed on 30 October 2020).
46. Banks, J.; Hollinghurst, S.; Bigwood, L.; Peters, T.J.; Walter, F.M.; Hamilton, W. Preferences for cancer investigation: A vignette-based study of primary-care attendees. *Lancet Oncol.* **2014**, *15*, 232–240. [CrossRef]
47. Funston, G.; Hamilton, W.; Abel, G.; Crosbie, E.J.; Rous, B.; Walter, F.M. The diagnostic performance of CA125 for the detection of ovarian and non-ovarian cancer in primary care: A population-based cohort study. *PLoS Med.* **2020**, *17*, e1003295. [CrossRef]

Publisher's Note: MDPI stays neutral with regard to jurisdictional claims in published maps and institutional affiliations.

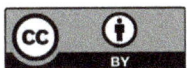

© 2020 by the authors. Licensee MDPI, Basel, Switzerland. This article is an open access article distributed under the terms and conditions of the Creative Commons Attribution (CC BY) license (http://creativecommons.org/licenses/by/4.0/).

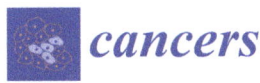

Article

Long-Term Evaluation of Women Referred to a Breast Cancer Family History Clinic (Manchester UK 1987–2020)

Anthony Howell [1,2,3,*], Ashu Gandhi [1,2,3], Sacha Howell [1,2,3], Mary Wilson [1], Anthony Maxwell [1,4,*], Susan Astley [1,2,4], Michelle Harvie [1], Mary Pegington [1,3], Lester Barr [1], Andrew Baildam [1,5], Elaine Harkness [1,4], Penelope Hopwood [1,6], Julie Wisely [1,7], Andrea Wilding [1], Rosemary Greenhalgh [1], Jenny Affen [1], Andrew Maurice [1], Sally Cole [1], Julia Wiseman [1], Fiona Lalloo [1,8], David P. French [9] and D. Gareth Evans [1,2,4,8,10,11]

1. Nightingale Breast Screening Centre & Prevent Breast Cancer Unit Wythenshawe Hospital, Manchester University NHS Foundation Trust, Manchester M23 9LT, UK; ashu.gandhi@mft.nhs.uk (A.G.); sacha.howell@manchester.ac.uk (S.H.); mary.wilson@mft.nhs.uk (M.W.); Sue.astley@manchester.ac.uk (S.A.); michelle.harvie@manchester.ac.uk (M.H.); Mary.pegington@manchester.ac.uk (M.P.); lester.barr@mft.nhs.uk (L.B.); aetab2@btinternet.com (A.B.); elaine.harkness@manchester.ac.uk (E.H.); penny.hopwood@icr.ac.uk (P.H.); julie.wisely@mft.nhs.uk (J.W.); Andrea.Wilding@MFT.NHS.UK (A.W.); rosemary.greenhalgh@mft.nhs.uk (R.G.); jenny.affen@mft.nhs.uk (J.A.); Andrew.maurice@nhs.net (A.M.); Sally.cole@mft.nhs.uk (S.C.); julia.wiseman@mft.nhs.uk (J.W.); fiona.lalloo@mft.nhs.uk (F.L.); Gareth.Evans@mft.nhs.uk (D.G.E.)
2. Manchester Breast Centre, The Christie Hospital, Manchester M23 9LT, UK
3. Division of Cancer Sciences, Medicine and Health, University of Manchester, Manchester Academic Health Science Centre, Manchester M23 9LT, UK
4. Division of Informatics, Imaging & Data Sciences, School of Health Sciences, Faculty of Biology, Medicine and Health, University of Manchester, Manchester M13 9PT, UK
5. Department of Surgery, King Edward VII's Hospital, London W1G6AA, UK
6. Clinical Trials and Statistics Unit, The Institute of Cancer Research, London SM25PT, UK
7. Department of Psychology, University Hospital of South Manchester NHS Trust, Wythenshawe, Manchester M23 9LT, UK
8. Manchester Centre for Genomic Medicine, Manchester University Hospitals NHS Foundation Trust, Manchester M23 9LT, UK
9. Division of Psychology and Mental Health, School of Health Sciences, Manchester Centre of Health Psychology, University of Manchester, Manchester M23 9LT, UK; david.french@manchester.ac.uk
10. NW Genomic Laboratory Hub, Manchester Centre for Genomic Medicine, Manchester University Hospitals NHS Foundation Trust, Manchester M13 9WL, UK
11. Faculty of Biology, Division of Evolution and Genomic Sciences, School of Biological Sciences, Medicine and Health, University of Manchester, Manchester Academic Health Science Centre, Manchester M23 9LT, UK
* Correspondence: anthony.howell@manchester.ac.uk (A.H.); anthony.maxwell@manchester.ac.uk (A.M.)

Received: 22 November 2020; Accepted: 5 December 2020; Published: 9 December 2020

Simple Summary: This study reports the management of women at high risk for breast cancer over a 33 years period. The aim was to summarize the numbers seen and to report the results of our studies on gene testing, the outcomes of screening and the success of preventive methods including lifestyle change, chemoprevention and risk-reducing mastectomy. We also discuss how the clinical Family History Service may be improved in the future.

Abstract: Clinics for women concerned about their family history of breast cancer are widely established. A Family History Clinic was set-up in Manchester, UK, in 1987 in a Breast Unit serving a population of 1.8 million. In this review, we report the outcome of risk assessment, screening and prevention strategies in the clinic and propose future approaches. Between 1987–2020,

14,311 women were referred, of whom 6.4% were from known gene families, 38.2% were at high risk (≥30% lifetime risk), 37.7% at moderate risk (17–29%), and 17.7% at an average/population risk who were discharged. A total of 4168 (29.1%) women were eligible for genetic testing and 736 carried pathogenic variants, predominantly in *BRCA1* and *BRCA2* but also other genes (5.1% of direct referrals). All women at high or moderate risk were offered annual mammographic screening between ages 30 and 40 years old: 646 cancers were detected in women at high and moderate risk (5.5%) with a detection rate of 5 per 1000 screens. Incident breast cancers were largely of good prognosis and resulted in a predicted survival advantage. All high/moderate-risk women were offered lifestyle prevention advice and 14–27% entered various lifestyle studies. From 1992–2003, women were offered entry into IBIS-I (tamoxifen) and IBIS-II (anastrozole) trials (12.5% of invitees joined). The NICE guidelines ratified the use of tamoxifen and raloxifene (2013) and subsequently anastrozole (2017) for prevention; 10.8% women took up the offer of such treatment between 2013–2020. Since 1994, 7164 eligible women at ≥25% lifetime risk of breast cancer were offered a discussion of risk-reducing breast surgery and 451 (6.2%) had surgery. New approaches in all aspects of the service are needed to build on these results.

Keywords: family history; breast cancer; risk; genes; screening; prevention

1. Introduction

In the 1980s, the rising incidence of breast cancer (BC) and the introduction in the UK of the NHS National Health Service Breast Screening Programme (NHSBSP) led women with a family history of the disease to seek advice concerning management of their personal risk. In response to concerns expressed by primary care physicians and colleagues within our breast oncology service, we established a referral Family History Clinic (FHC) in Manchester, UK, in 1987 with a cancer genetics service (CGS) initiated in 1990 (DGRE, FL). The clinic serves a catchment population of 1.8 million, (just over half the population of Greater Manchester), although women at high-risk may be specifically referred to the centre from a population of approximately 5 million in North West England.

The aims of the FHC were to introduce a service for the estimation and management of BC risk for women with familial risk and to evaluate the short- and long-term effectiveness of the clinic. At presentation, an individual's risk was explained, annual breast screening initiated and advice given concerning diet and lifestyle factors which might affect risk. Later, chemoprevention (1992 as part of the IBIS I clinical trial), genetic testing (1994) and risk-reducing surgery (1994) were introduced. In 1994, we published local guidelines for the management of women with a family history of BC [1]. These were followed by national guidelines for the UK [2,3] and the USA [4,5].

Management was undertaken by a multi-disciplinary team. Following referral, each woman was sent a questionnaire to assess family history and breast factors and, if eligible, offered a clinic appointment. Women were initially seen by geneticists (DGRE, FL) or medical oncologists (AH, SJH). Breast examination was undertaken and advice given by specially trained nurses (RG, JW, AW) and annual mammography and MRIs performed by radiologists within the Breast Unit (represented by MW and AM). Risk-reducing surgery was performed by a team of surgeons (represented by AB, AG and LB). Quality of life aspects of risk communication, mutation testing and risk-reducing mastectomy (RRM) were an integrated part of the FHC clinical and research agenda provided by psycho-oncologists and a health psychologist (PH, JW, DF).

The aims of this paper were to present the results of each aspect of the service and to suggest potential future improvements. The results include the numbers of referrals, estimation of their BC risks and results of genetic testing, screening and uptake to lifestyle prevention, chemoprevention and risk-reducing surgery interventions. The main quality of life outcomes are also reported. The second half of this paper then suggests improvements to the service based on our own studies and those of others.

2. Results

2.1. Referrals to the Clinic

Over the period from September 1987 to September 2020, 14,311 women were referred to the clinic. Referrals were from primary care (GPs, 55.9%), from secondary care (mainly breast surgeons, 15.1%) and from the local Clinical Genetics Service for further follow up after risk assessment (20.9%). Women were also referred from a research study (notably, 3.1% from PROCAS—Prediction Risk Of Cancer At Screening, [6]) or from "other" sources such as relatives at risk attending with a proband (5.0%). The age at entry ranged from 16–81 years (median 39.9; interquartile range (IQR) 33.9–46.9, with 83% of women (11,878/14,311) below age 50 (Table 1). The number of referrals by year is shown in Figure 1 and ranged between approximately 300–700 per year following the initial 3 years lead in the period after the clinic was established.

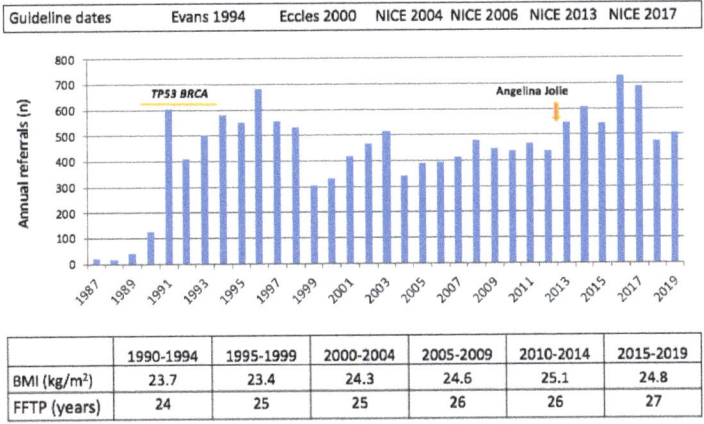

	1990-1994	1995-1999	2000-2004	2005-2009	2010-2014	2015-2019
BMI (kg/m^2)	23.7	23.4	24.3	24.6	25.1	24.8
FFTP (years)	24	25	25	26	26	27

Figure 1. Annual referrals to the Manchester FHC between 1987 and 2020. Increases in referral were seen during the period when the first breast cancer genes, *TP53* and *BRCA1/2*, were identified and also related to the publicity surrounding Angelina Jolie when she indicated that she was a *BRCA1* PV carrier. The increase in median body mass index (BMI) and median age at first full-term pregnancy (FFTP) over this period are shown. Over the period of 33 years, lifetime risk of BC in the population increased from 1 in 12 to 1 in 8, an increase presumed to be associated with change in modifiable risk factors. These trends were apparent in the FHC. For example, the median age of first full-term pregnancy increased from 24 years to 27 years ($p < 0.001$), and median BMI at clinic entry increased from 23.7 to 24.8 kg/m^2 ($p < 0.001$).

Table 1. Number of referrals to the Family History Clinic (FHC) according to the source of referral, NICE guideline [3] risk category and BCA1/2 status.

Group	Number	% of All Referrals	Known Gene in Family	%	High Risk	%	Moderate	%	Average	%	BRCA +v at Last Follow Up	%	Number
GP	8004	55.9%	165	2.1%	2646	33.1%	3542	44.3%	1651	20.6%	222	2.77%	8004
Surgery	2157	15.1%	38	1.8%	751	34.9%	831	38.6%	537	24.9%	55	2.55%	2157
Genetics	2868	20.0%	662	23.5%	1445	51.5%	594	21.2%	168	6.0%	406	14.16%	2868
PROCAS	448	3.1%	2	0.4%	311	69.4%	124	27.7%	11	2.5%	0	0.00%	448
Other	833	5.8%	54	6.5%	307	36.9%	299	35.9%	173	20.8%	53	6.36%	833
Totals	14,311		921	6.4%	5460	38.2%	5390	37.7%	2540	17.7%	736	5.14%	

GP, general practitioner; PROCAS, Prediction Risk Of Cancer At Screening.

2.2. Estimated Lifetime BC Risk

Risk was estimated initially by a modification of the Claus method with the addition of hormonal and lifestyle factors, such as age of first pregnancy and BMI, and by the Tyrer–Cuzick and BOADICEA models from 2004 [7–9]. We demonstrated that the modified Claus and the Tyrer–Cuzick models gave similar distributions of risk accurately, but the Gail model underpredicted risk [10,11].

Risk was reported as moderate (17–29% lifetime risk) and high (30%+) according to our original clinic guidelines (Evans 1994) and thereafter using the NICE Guidelines risk categories (2004) [1,3]. Overall, 44.6% of women were at high-risk (including 6.4% either with a pathogenic variant (PV) or a known PV in a close family member), 37.7% at moderate risk and 17.7% at average risk (Table 1). Following assessment of the referral questionnaire, women at average risk were referred back to primary care. It was clear that more higher risk women were referred to the Clinical Genetics Service reflecting a referral pathway from primary care to the Clinical Genetics Service for the highest risk women. (Table 1). After excluding referrals at average risk, 43.7% (n = 3397) of women directly referred to the clinic from primary and secondary care were estimated to be at high-risk and 56.7% (n = 4373) were at moderate risk.

2.3. Risk Perception and Cancer Worry

Risk was uniformly given as a proportion (e.g., 1 in 4 or 1 in 5). Our early studies reported that women had a relatively inaccurate perception of personal and population risk at presentation which improved when reassessed after risk counselling [12,13]. In another study, we demonstrated that the proportion of women with accurate personal risk perceptions significantly improved after risk counselling from 12% pre-counselling to 67% 3 months post-counselling (p < 0.001), which was maintained for 1 year [14]. Reassuringly, this improvement in accuracy of women's risk appraisal was not associated with increased anxiety. A subsequent analysis of questionnaire data from 500 FHC attendees over time indicated that BC risk counselling reduced self-reported cancer worry in women who initially overestimated their risk, with no significant change in levels for other risk perception groups, even if the risk was greater than they had estimated pre-counselling [15,16].

2.4. Genetic Testing

Genetic testing in the clinic began in 1991 just after the discovery of *TP53* and then the *BRCA1* (1994) and *BRCA2* (1995) genes [17–19]. Initially, testing was by single-strand confirmation polymorphism (SSCP) and protein truncation testing (PTT) [20], then, from 2001, Sanger sequencing all coding exons [20], and from 2013, next generation sequencing [21]. All samples, including retrospectively, were tested for large deletions and duplications by multiple ligation-dependent probe amplification (MLPA). All mutations detected by PTT or SSCP were confirmed by sequencing. From 2004, the probability of a *BRCA1* or *BRCA2* PV in the family was estimated using the Tyrer–Cuzick model [8] the BOADICEA model [9] or the Manchester Score [20,21]. The NICE Guidelines (2004) [3] initially indicated that the proband required the probability of a PV in BRCA1/2 of ≥20% for genetic testing in England and Wales [3]. In 2013, this was reduced to a ≥10% likelihood [22]. At present, gene testing in the UK is restricted to the *BRCA1*, *BRCA2*, and *PALB2* genes (National Genomic Test Directory (2020)) [23].

Of the 14,311 referrals to the FHC, *BRCA1* and *BRCA2* testing was completed for 4168 individuals (29.1%) or their affected family member. A total of 736 women (5.1% of the whole FHC cohort and 17.6% of those tested) were identified as *BRCA* PV carriers (*BRCA1* = 364, *BRCA2* = 372). However, only 2.5% of unaffected direct referrals to the FHC without a known gene in the family subsequently tested positive. No systematic approach to testing for PVs in other genes was undertaken. However, 35 potential BC and other risk genes were tested on a research basis in a subpopulation of 808 women unaffected by breast cancer representative of the risk distribution of direct referrals to the FHC [24]. Of the 808 tests there were 29 (3.6%) with PVs in other potentially actionable genes (*ATM* = 11, *CHEK2* = 11,

PALB2 = 7). These data indicate that approximately 6.1% of women directly referred to the FHC carry a PV in one of the actionable BC-associated genes.

2.5. Mammographic Screening

Annual mammography and clinical breast examination were offered from the inception of the clinic. Women were screened between the ages of 35 and 50 years (moderate risk) or 35 to 60 years (high risk), plus from 5 years younger than the earliest family diagnosis of BC. These screening periods were in accordance with an initial in-house protocol [25] and later, NICE guidelines [3,22]. Women with *BRCA1* and *BRCA2* PVs and others of equivalent high risk were screened by annual MRI between age 30 and 50 and annual mammography from age 30 to 70 according to NICE Guidelines [3,22].

Between 1987 and 2020, there were 129,119 women years of follow up; 646 BCs occurred prospectively, giving an annual incidence rate of 5.0 per 1000 which was approximately 1.7 times higher than the general population's annual rate of 3 per 1000 women aged 50–75 in the NHSBSP. Three hundred and ninety-four breast cancers occurred whilst on the screening programme or within 18 months of a screen. The majority of invasive cancers were lymph node negative (72.9%), small (≤20 mm, 73.2%) and stage 1 (61.4%). Cancers in women with *BRCA1* and *BRCA2* PVs were smaller overall with 75.0% and 85.4% being ≤20 mm, respectively, reflecting the benefits of MRI screening [26]. Breast cancer-specific survival at 10 years was 91.3% (87.4–94.0), compared with the current 10 year survival from BC in England, from 2013–2017, of 75.9% (74.9–77.0). Overall, 30.5% (92/322) of invasive cancers were oestrogen receptor negative (ER−) and 11/51 (21.5%) of carcinoma in situ (not assessed 21) were ER−.

2.6. Lifestyle Prevention

Excess weight, weight gain, sedentary lifestyle and high alcohol intake were established risk factors for BC before initiation to the FHC, and so verbal and standard written lifestyle advice was given to all women referred to the clinic. Lifestyle risk factors were common amongst high-risk women in the FHC with a similar prevalence of unhealthy lifestyles to women in the general population (57% are overweight/obese, 30% report <150 min moderate intensity physical activity/week and 45% have alcohol intakes of >14 units per week) [27]. Adult weight gain is a well-documented risk factor for BC (6% increased risk per 5 kg gain) [28]. We and others have reported that maintained weight loss of 5% or more before or after menopause in an unselected population cohort is associated with reductions of 39% and 23%, respectively, in the risk of post-menopausal BC [29]. Thus, women were advised to avoid weight gain if at a healthy weight and reduce weight by at least 5% if overweight/obese. Current guidelines include advising at least 150 min of moderate exercise per week and no more than 14 units of alcohol per week.

Since 2001 we conducted a series of randomised studies to determine the optimal methods for introducing and supporting weight control and other lifestyle changes amongst women in the FHC. These indicated that intermittent energy restriction (2 days of 50–60% energy restriction and 5 days of normal healthy eating/week) was associated with greater reductions in weight and insulin resistance than continuous energy restriction [30,31]. We also demonstrated that remotely supported (i.e., web and phone) weight loss/lifestyle behaviour change programmes are feasible and particularly effective amongst higher risk women producing ≥5% weight loss in approximately 60% of women at 12 months [32]. Uptake to these weight loss trials amongst moderate and high-risk women was between 14% and 27%.

2.7. Chemoprevention

Chemoprevention was not available at the inception of the FHC. However, women were randomised to tamoxifen or placebo in the IBIS-I trial (ISRCTN91879928). Between 1992 and 2001 and to anastrozole or placebo in the IBIS-II trial (SRCTN31488319). Between 2003 and 2012 [33,34]. Of the 7865 women invited to join these trials, 1003 women (12.8%) agreed (Table 2). These and other studies resulted in tamoxifen use being advised by NICE in the 2013 guidelines and anastrozole in the 2017 guidelines [22]. From 2013, 5121 women were invited to take either drug as part of management. To date, 282 have chosen chemoprevention and a further 284 in clinical trials so that overall 10.8% of eligible women have accepted treatment since 2013 (Table 2).

2.8. Risk-Reducing Mastectomy

Risk-reducing mastectomies were being performed, particularly in the USA, at the time of inception of the clinic. In 1994, we decided to offer this service in the FHC. Since then, 7164 women with a lifetime BC risk ≥25%, including *BRCA1/2* PV carriers, were offered a discussion concerning RRM according to a published protocol [35]. Of a total cohort of 7195 women at a ≥25% lifetime risk of BC, 451 (6.2%) without a current or previous breast cancer diagnosis elected to undergo RRM. Uptake of RRM was 49.3% in 479 *BRCA1/2* PV carriers and 5.2% in 6685 in non-carriers (9.4% for 1261 women at a ≥40% lifetime risk (non-BRCA), 4.9% in 3561 women at 30–39% risk and 3.0% in 1783 women at 25–29% lifetime risk).

In Cox regression analyses, factors which independently predicted risk-reducing mastectomy uptake included either the death of a sister with BC <50 years or mother <60 years, having children, having a breast biopsy or younger age at assessment (<30 years).

Of the 451 women who underwent RRM, four developed post-surgery BCs (all in *BRCA1/2* PV carriers) compared to 94 expected over a period of follow up of 7894 years, giving a risk reduction of 95.8%.

Twenty women (5.7%) had no reconstruction, whereas 352 (78%) had implant-based reconstruction (nipple sparing in 31% of these) and 63 (14%) flap-based reconstruction. The number of planned surgical procedures per patient was 2.41 ± 1.11 SD [36].

Two studies assessing psychological distress in our FHC patients undergoing risk-reducing mastectomy have been published [37,38]. Between 1995 and 1999, quality of life was assessed in 52 of 76 (79%) women undergoing surgery one-year post-operatively. At this point, 1 in 6 women had high scores for mental health problems on the General Health Questionnaire but for most, psychological distress appeared to be comparable with women at high risk who did not have surgery. Body image changes on the Body Image Scale were generally minor in degree with the most frequently reported changes reported in sexual attractiveness (55% responders), feeling less physically attractive (53%) and self-consciousness about appearance (53%). For the majority of women there was no evidence of significant mental health or body image problems in the first 3 years following RRM. Careful pre-operative preparation and long-term monitoring was advocated. In a second study, 79 women who chose to have surgery were compared with 64 women who declined surgery [38]. The main findings were that risk-reducing mastectomy reduced psychological morbidity and anxiety and did not have a significant detrimental impact on women's body image or sexual functioning.

Table 2. Number of women (A) randomised into the IBIS I or IBIS II trial 1992 and 2012; (B) number of women prescribed chemoprevention (CP) from 2013 either outside or as part of in-house trials.

	A				B					
Group	Number Seen	Randomised to IBIS I/II Trial	Number Invited to Trial	% Joined Trial	Seen Since 2013	Prescribed Chemoprevention	%	Joined Chemoprevention Trial	%	Either Trial or CP
Known gene in family	921	11	554	1.99%	364	2	0.55%	2	0.55%	4	1.10%
High	5488	465	3178	14.63%	2604	162	6.22%	168	6.45%	323	12.40%
Moderate	5370	431	3200	13.47%	2221	118	5.31%	113	5.09%	226	10.18%
Average	2532	112	1188	9.43%	609	0		0		0	
Total	14,311	1019	8120	12.55%	5798	282	4.86%	283	4.88%	553	9.54%

3. Discussion

We summarised the developments that occurred since the inception of the clinic including updated models for risk and gene testing estimation (i.e., Tyrer-Cuzick v8 2017 [39], BOADICEA-V2019 [40], the Manchester Score [20,21] consistent use of mammography and MRI (NICE 2013 [22], a more po-active approach to lifestyle change [32], chemoprevention [41] and RRM [42]. We now suggest potential improvements to the service in each of the areas considered above based on our own studies and those of others.

3.1. Referrals

The numbers of referrals have remained relatively stable over the years and are still mainly instituted by women concerned about their family history and primary and secondary care clinicians who refer according the NICE familial breast FHC guidelines [3]. Our own and the reports of others indicate that approximately 10% of women in the UK have a first degree relative with BC; however, we estimate that <20% of these are referred [43]. It is interesting that referrals to FHCs and Clinical Genetics Services increased over two-fold after Angelina Jolie made her *BRCA1* PV carrier status and breast and ovarian surgery public [44,45]. This suggests that lack of awareness of the services may be an issue. Lack of uptake may also be related to a complex referral system which requires a visit to primary care for referral and the completion of extensive questionnaires. The latter is illustrated in our study of risk estimation in women undergoing breast screening. Thirty-seven percent of women invited completed a two-page questionnaire concerning their risk factors [6]. The cohort included 13% of women with a first-degree relative with breast cancer. Of 673 women found to be at high risk and invited for counselling and treatment at the FHC, 500 (74.3%) attended [46]. These data indicate a greater interest in risk management if the system is streamlined, suggesting that progress may best be made by more effort to align risk estimation with screening programmes. Referral would then be less dependent on health care professionals and would make it a more routine and streamlined service.

3.2. Risk Estimation

We demonstrated that the modified Claus model used in the clinic before 2004 gave similar results to the Tyrer–Cuzick model, suggesting consistent risk estimation for the duration of the clinic to date [10,11]. However, several studies indicate that the accuracy of risk estimation increases with the number of risk factors that are incorporated into the models used [47–50]. Recently, mammographic density (MD) and polygenic risk scores (PRS) based on single nucleotide polymorphism (SNP) results) have been added to risk models such as Tyrer–Cuzick (v8) and BOADICEA V [39,40]. In patients under follow up at the FHC, we assessed the effect on risk of incorporating the first 18 BC risk-associated SNPs discovered into the Tyrer–Cuzick model [51,52]. Adding SNP18 resulted in a change to the original given risk using Tyrer–Cuzick (version 6) in half the population of women: 25% had an increase in risk and 27% had a decrease in risk, indicating the potential importance of additional risk factors [53].

In the screening population we demonstrated that when both mammographic density and a PRS score were added to the Tyrer–Cuzick (v8), the proportion of women at elevated risk (>5% 10 years risk) increased from 12% to 18%. Ten percent of women changed from average to high risk and 4% from high to average [54,55]. These studies illustrate that using standard models may give erroneous risks and adding more risk factors may result in more appropriate management. However, more work is required to routinely apply optimal risk models in the clinic and deal with change in risk estimation over time.

3.3. Genes

Of the women directly referred to the FHC in which there was no currently known PVs, 2.5% were *BRCA1/2* PV carriers and 3.6% were found to have PVs in other genes after multigene panel testing [24]. This low pickup rate reflects that over 50% of referrals were at moderate risk and many of those at higher risk had undergone testing in themselves or their family (Table 1). At the FHC, much time was used to calculate the probability that the proband or her family are likely to carry a breast cancer gene PV. At present our Clinical Genetics Service forwards primary care referrals for women unlikely to carry a PV immediately to the FHC; conversely, we refer relatives of known PV carriers to the Clinical Genetics Service. A simple method where primary and secondary care physicians could estimate PV risk and refer appropriately would be invaluable. A more widespread use of the simple Manchester Score needs to be evaluated in this regard [20,21]. Currently, the NHS guidelines to the UK genetics departments allow estimation of *BRCA1/2* and *PALB2* (as well as syndromic genes where indicated such as *PTEN* in Cowden disease) [23]. The recent report illustrating the nine genes (*BRCA1, BRCA2, PALB2, CHEK2, ATM, CDH1, STK11, PTEN, TP53*) in which PVs more than doubles the risk of BC and three genes at the two-fold threshold (*RAD51C, RAD51D, BARD1*) might allow better selection for appropriate gene testing and a reduction in the need for multigene testing which, in the UK, is in the commercial sector [24].

3.4. Breast Screening

Mammographic screening in this at-risk population detects more cancers annually (5/1000 screened) than in the national programme (3/1000) as expected. It also results in the detection of smaller, better risk cancers. Three studies in the UK, one in our clinic and two in association with other clinics in the UK indicated that screening at-risk women results in a survival advantage compared (in non-randomised trials) with age matched populations [56–58]. The latest study was designed to assess the value of screening both moderate- and high-risk women from age 35–39 and confirmed a survival advantage even in the moderate-risk group [58].

Countries where national screening programmes begin at age 40 will already be screening in the high-risk groups. A review of the value of screening from age 40 in the general population concluded it was of equivocal value [59]. In the UK, screening is every 3 years for all from the age of 50, but a recent study now suggests a survival advantage in the general population when screening begins annually at the age of 40. This may lead to a change in UK policy [60]. The results of two randomised trials of risk adapted screening will inform a potential change in policy since they both screen women from age 40 onwards (WISDOM [61] MyPebs UNICANCER 2018 [62]). Further, a programme of work carried out in Manchester is considering how best to implement risk adapted screening to optimise the ratio of benefits and harms, including how to include ethnically minority women and to minimise harms of screening for women at low risk [63].

In countries where screening begins at 50 (e.g., the UK), consideration should be given to offering all women a one-off mammogram at age 40, together with risk estimation to determine future screening frequency. Mammographic density could be assessed automatically using artificial intelligence methods [64,65] and SNPs used only to determine precise risk where needed. The trials of risk and density-adapted screening and determination of the value of supplemental imaging techniques, such as whole breast ultrasound, contrast-enhanced mammography and abbreviated MRI, would further refine the management advice offered to women with high MD. Currently, at the FHC, women are offered an MRI if they carry a PV of a high-risk gene or if they have a 10 year risk of ≥8% aged 30 or ≥12% aged 40, based on the finding in trials that MRIs detect smaller tumours and may offer a survival advantage [66–70]. However, neither MRIs nor ultrasounds are routinely available (or proven) for a large group of women at increased risk outside those in very high-risk groups.

3.5. Lifestyle Advice

Women at high risk who have a high BMI [71], low physical activity levels, high alcohol intake [72] and smoke [73] have proportionately higher BC risks than similar women at population risk [71–73]. These potentially modifiable risk factors have also been associated in women at high risk due to the fact of family history or high PRS [72,73]. Thus, there is a rationale for focussing on lifestyle change in this higher risk group, and it is probable that the more avenues to promote change that are pursued, the greater the likelihood of success [74].

Women at high risk present a challenge for achieving lifestyle behaviour change. Firstly, some women can view their BC risk as unchangeable because of their family history [75]. This is consistent with a large body of literature that indicates education around disease risk does not alter behaviour by itself and that people require an appropriate level of support to achieve and sustain lifestyle behavioural change [76]. Lifestyle behaviour change programmes need to address the often complex psychological issues amongst women who have a high burden of cancer diagnoses and bereavements in their family. For many women, the majority of excess weight is acquired between the age of 18 and 35 years [76], indicating that lifestyle programmes should begin at younger ages. Interviews with young, high-risk women (under 35 years) in our FHC indicate that those women require a supportive weight control lifestyle programme that is remotely accessible, provides a point of contact within the high-risk service and promotes general wellbeing as well as cancer risk reduction [76]. There is a need for wider testing of low-cost programmes for lifestyle prevention which can reach and engage the maximum number of women across the network of UK FHCs.

3.6. Chemoprevention

The reduction of risk of BC by 30–50% by the use of SERMs and AIs such as tamoxifen, raloxifene and anastrozole are well known [77]. More recently, long-term follow up of the IBIS I and IBIS II trials indicate that risk reduction continues long after the usual five-year prescription period [41,78]. A recent analysis by NICE indicates that the use of anastrozole, in particular, is cost saving to the NHS in women at moderate to high risk of BC. However, whilst reduction of risk is of benefit, none of the trials to date have shown a survival benefit. This has led to the suggestion that premarin should be used for women at least 5 years post-menopausal and without a uterus, since in this group the Women's Health Initiative trial use was associated with a survival advantage [79].

Our report of recent uptake of chemoprevention being relatively low at 10% is consistent with many but not all studies [80,81]. Part of the reason for the low uptake concerns the side effects, although our own and other studies show that the observed frequency of side effects are comparable to controls [33,34,81–84]. We found four themes associated with low uptake: the perceived impact of side effects, the impact of others' experience on beliefs about tamoxifen, tamoxifen as a "cancer drug" and the daily reminder of cancer risk [80]. These reasons are understandable and consistent with other studies. Future developments require better communication of the pros and cons of therapy and alternative approaches including low dose or topical tamoxifen [85]. New agents such as antiprogestins [86], and denosumab [87] are currently being trialled in the FHC and elsewhere.

3.7. Risk-Reducing Surgery

Historically, our unit performed approximately 10–12 operations per year. With recent increases in publicity surrounding RRM [44], this has increased approximately three-fold in our own and other units [45]. The seminal paper by Hartmann [88] indicated BC a risk reduction of 92%, similar to our observed reduction of 95.8%. Over the years, our surgical approaches have evolved to reflect refinements in surgical technique and improved technology. Initially, mastectomy inevitably involved sacrifice of the nipple areolar complex, and immediate reconstructions relied exclusively on submuscular implant placement or use of the transverse rectus abdominus flap. In recent years, with the increasing appreciation of patient reported outcome measures in women undergoing risk reducing surgery [89], surgeons have sought more aesthetically focussed reconstruction options whilst not compromising risk-reduction principles. This has allowed the safe introduction of skin sparing and nipple sparing mastectomy [90] and autologous reconstruction with deep inferior epigastric perforator flaps [91] or single-stage prepectoral implant-based reconstruction [92]. The use of acellular dermal matrices has revolutionised implant-based reconstruction, allowing structural support of implants within a reconstruction to mimic natural breast ptosis [93]. Further improvements may come from the use of lipomodelling to improve aesthetics and thus patient satisfaction [94].

In *BRCA* PV carriers, RRM results in an improvement in survival, especially in women with *BRCA1* PVs, a result also found by others [95,96]. There may also be an improvement in women with *BRCA2* PVs with longer follow up [97]. Our previous studies indicated good acceptance and psychological health after RRM [37,38] More recent overviews have emphasised the enormous importance of excellent pre-surgical explanation, the presence of a psychologist in the multidisciplinary team and improved surgical techniques have been emphasised (Braude 2017) [98].

3.8. Summary

Here, we summarised the updated results from the Manchester FHC which spans the period from the inception of such clinics in the UK up to the present. A large proportion of these clinics in the UK are associated with Breast Units and work in conjunction with local Clinical Genetics Services.

The question remains regarding how their services may be improved (Table 3). At present, relatively small numbers of women are referred, partly because of the emphasis on family history for referral. Inclusion in FHCs of women at increased risk due to the presence of non-familial risk factors awaits the widespread introduction of MD and SNPs to risk prediction models. The introduction of new risk factors, such as MD and SNPs, is particularly important, as there is evidence that without them women are currently being given erroneous risk estimates that may result in imprecise treatment stratification. Clinical Genetics Services would be helped by more precise prediction of PVs. Consideration might be given to abandoning large panel tests and focussing on the nine genes in which the PVs are associated with a two-fold or more risk of BC [24].

Table 3. Summary of "current practice" and issues to be addressed for each of the interventions discussed.

Intervention	Current Practice	Issues to Be Addressed
Referral	Referrals from primary & secondary care established	Only 20% of women with FH referred Very few with 'other' risk factors
Risk estimation	Evolved to include more risk factors eg. mammographic density & SNPs	Using all factors approximately 20% of population at moderate & high risk
Gene testing	BRCA1/2 & PALB2 available in NHS 10% threshold for PV used (NICE)	New data suggest panel of 9 genes be should be used
Screening	Annual mammography & MRI established	Breast density & SNPs being tested in trials of risk & density adapted screening
Lifestyle change	Observational studies suggest introduction would be valuable	Mechanisms for general application being tested
Chemoprevention	Longer term risk and benefits established	Application suboptimal—consider assessment at home and primary care
Risk reducing surgery	Offer at appropriate risk levels established	Continue improvements in psychological and surgical techniques

We are currently testing the feasibility of introducing identification and referral of higher risk women as part of routine screening, i.e., research with a focus on implementation as part of routine care in a NHSBSP could bring about a "step change" if implemented [6]. There is already some evidence that communicating breast cancer risk estimates as part of routine screening does not produce the harms that have been anticipated [99]. For instance, communicating risk estimates in this setting did not produce adverse emotional effects or effects on screening uptake [100].

It appears that it is timely to consider introduction of the service into primary care as is seen in the USA [101]. A challenge to implementation is that the risk estimation and treatment algorithms have become more complex and efforts to introduce the two models we have focussed on here have led to legitimate difficulties amongst busy primary care physicians [102,103]. Even the mainstream estimation of cardiovascular risk on practice computer systems is apparently only applied to half of those in need and only half of these who need it are treated (Q-RISK; Hippisley-Cox 2017) [104] suggesting difficulties with the primary care approach.

A possible approach, pioneered in Melbourne, is to develop a simplified version of the Tyrer–Cuzick model, called iPrevent, and to make it widely available to all women. The model is user friendly and provides suggested treatment pathways in addition to an individual's risk. If made widely available this could lead to patient-initiated referral for initial screening and SNP estimation to define definitive management [105]. Other measures may be to establish one-off breast density assessment for all women at a certain age (e.g., 40 years, as suggested above) to estimate BC risk and introduce further screening and preventive measures for those found to be at high risk [99,106].

4. Conclusions

We reported the activity in a clinic designed for referral of women concerned about their family history of breast cancer. The long period of the clinic illustrates the changes in risk estimation and management over the years. The time span also allows for multiple studies on the effectiveness of management, for example, the effectiveness of breast screening. It also allows for the study of and introduction of preventive approaches such as use of tamoxifen and anastrozole.

A major aim of the clinic is to reduce the incidence of and deaths from breast cancer. These will be reduced by screening, lifestyle change and chemoprevention. Improvements in their effectiveness depends upon more widespread introduction not only into the current at-risk population but also into the large proportion of women unknowingly at high risk

Author Contributions: Conceptualisation, A.H. and D.G.E.; Data curation, D.G.E.; Formal analysis, E.H. and D.G.E.; Investigation, A.G., S.H., M.W., A.M. (Anthony Maxwell), S.A., M.H., M.P., L.B., A.B., E.H., P.H., J.W. (Julie Wisely), A.W., R.G., J.A., A.M. (Andrew Maurice), S.C., J.W. (Julia Wiseman), F.L., D.P.F. and D.G.E.; Project administration, A.H. and D.G.E.; Writing—original draft, A.H., A.G., S.H., M.W., A.W., S.A., M.H., M.P., L.B., E.H., P.H., J.W. (Julie Wisely), F.L., D.P.F. and D.G.E.; Writing—review and editing, A.H., A.G., S.H., M.W., A.M. (Anthony Maxwell), S.A., M.H., M.P., L.B., A.B., E.H., P.H., J.W. (Julie Wisely), A.W., R.G., J.A., A.M. (Andrew Maurice), J.W., (Julia Wiseman), F.L. and D.G.E. All authors have read and agreed to the published version of the manuscript.

Funding: This paper received no external funding.

Acknowledgments: D.G.E., E.F.H., S.J.H., D.P.F. and A.H. are supported by the National Institute for Health Research (NIHR) BRC Manchester (Grant Reference Number: 1215-200074). This work was also supported by Prevent Breast Cancer and Breast Cancer Now. We thank all the women referred to the clinic, the many unnamed individuals who have helped run the clinic over the years and the many investigators who have assisted with our clinical studies. We also thank Lorna McWilliam for comments on the manuscript.

Conflicts of Interest: The authors declare no conflict of interest.

References

1. Evans, D.G.; Fentiman, I.S.; McPherson, K.; Asbury, D.; Ponder, B.A.; Howell, A. Fortnightly review: Familial breast cancer. *BMJ* **1994**, *15*, 183–187. [CrossRef]
2. Eccles, D.M.; Evans, D.G.R.; Mackay, J. Guidelines for a genetic risk based approach to advising women with a family history of breast cancer. *J. Med. Genet.* **2000**, *37*, 203–209. [CrossRef]
3. McIntosh, A.; Shaw, C.; Evans, G.; Turnbull, N.; Bahar, N.; Barclay, M.; Easton, D.; Emery, J.; Gray, J.; Halpin, J.; et al. (2004 updated 2006 and 2013) Clinical Guidelines and Evidence Review for The Classification and Care of Women at Risk of Familial Breast Cancer, London: National Collaborating Centre for Primary Care/University of Sheffield. NICE Guideline CG164. Available online: https://www.nice.org.uk/Guidance/CG164 (accessed on 15 November 2020).
4. Hoskins, K.F.; Stopfer, J.E.; Calzone, K.A.; Merajver, S.D.; Rebbeck, T.R.; Garber, J.E.; Weber, B.L. Assessment and counseling for women with a family history of breast cancer. A guide for clinicians. *JAMA* **1995**, *15*, 577–585. [CrossRef]

5. Merajver, S.D.; Milliron, K. Breast cancer risk assessment: A guide for clinicians using the NCCN Breast Cancer Risk Reduction Guidelines. *J. Natl. Comp. Cancer Netw.* **2003**, *1*, 297–301. [CrossRef]
6. Evans, D.G.; Astley, S.; Stavrinos, P.; Harkness, E.; Donnelly, L.S.; Dawe, S.; Jacob, I.; Harvie, M.; Cuzick, J.; Brentnall, A.; et al. Improvement in Risk Prediction, Early Detection and Prevention of Breast Cancer in the NHS Breast Screening Programme and Family History Clinics: A Dual Cohort Study. *Southampt. (UK) NIHR J. Libr.* **2016**. [CrossRef]
7. Claus, E.B.; Risch, N.; Thompson, W.D. Genetic analysis of breast cancer in the cancer and steroid hormone study. *Am. J. Hum. Genet.* **1991**, *48*, 232–242.
8. Tyrer, J.; Duffy, S.W.; Cuzick, J. A breast cancer prediction model incorporating familial and personal risk factors. *Stat. Med.* **2004**, *23*, 1111–1130. [CrossRef]
9. Antoniou, A.C.; Pharoah, P.P.; Smith, P.; Easton, D.F. The BOADICEA model of genetic susceptibility to breast and ovarian cancer. *Br. J. Cancer* **2004**, *18*, 1580–1590. [CrossRef]
10. Amir, E.; Evans, D.G.; Shenton, A.; Lalloo, F.; Moran, A.; Boggis, C.; Wilson, M.; Howell, A. Evaluation of Breast Cancer Risk Assessment Packages in the Family History Evaluation and Screening Programme. *J. Med. Genet.* **2003**, *40*, 807–814. [CrossRef]
11. Evans, D.G.; Ingham, S.; Dawe, S.; Roberts, L.; Lalloo, F.; Brentnall, A.R.; Stavrinos, P.; Howell, A. Breast cancer risk assessment in 8,824 women attending a family history evaluation and screening programme. *FAM Cancer* **2014**, *13*, 189–196. [CrossRef]
12. Evans, D.G.R.; Burnell, L.; Hopwood, P.; Howell, A. Perception of risk in women with a family history of breast cancer. *Br. J. Cancer* **1993**, *67*, 612–614. [CrossRef] [PubMed]
13. Evans, D.G.R.; Blair, V.; Greenhalgh, R.; Hopwood, P.; Howell, A. The impact of genetic counselling on risk perception in women with a family history of breast cancer. *Br. J Cancer* **1994**, *70*, 934–938. [CrossRef] [PubMed]
14. Hopwood, P.; Keeling, F.; Long, A.; Pool, C.; Evans, G.; Howell, A. Psychological support needs for women at high genetic risk of breast cancer: Some preliminary indicators. *Psycho-Oncology* **1998**, *7*, 402–412. [CrossRef]
15. Hopwood, P.; Shenton, A.; Lalloo, F.; Evans, D.G.; Howell, A. Risk perception and cancer worry: An exploratory study of the impact of genetic risk counselling in women with a family history of breast cancer. *J. Med. Genet.* **2001**, *38*, 139. [CrossRef] [PubMed]
16. Hopwood, P.; Howell, A.; Lalloo, F.; Evans, G. Do women understand the odds? Risk perceptions and recall of risk information in women with a family history of breast cancer. *Community Genet.* **2003**, *6*, 214–223. [CrossRef]
17. Malkin, D.; Li, F.P.; Strong, L.C.; Fraumeni, J.F., Jr.; Nelson, C.E.; Kim, D.H.; Kassel, J.; Gryka, M.A.; Bischoff, F.Z.; Tainsky, M.A.; et al. Germ line p53 mutations in a familial syndrome of breast cancer, sarcomas, and other neoplasms. *Science* **1990**, *30*, 1233–1238. [CrossRef] [PubMed]
18. Miki, Y.; Swensen, J.; Shattuck-Eidens, D.; Futreal, P.A.; Harshman, K.; Tavtigian, S.; Liu, Q.; Cochran, C.; Bennett, L.M.; Ding, W.; et al. A strong candidate for the breast and ovarian cancer susceptibility gene BRCA1. *Science* **1994**, *266*, 66–71. [CrossRef]
19. Wooster, R.; Bignell, G.; Lancaster, J.; Swift, S.; Seal, S.; Mangion, J.; Collins, N.; Gregory, S.; Gumbs, C.; Micklem, G. Identification of the breast cancer susceptibility gene BRCA2. *Nature* **1995**, *378*, 789–792. [CrossRef]
20. Evans, D.G.; Eccles, D.M.; Rahman, N.; Young, K.; Bulman, M.; Amir, E.; Shenton, A.; Howell, A.; Lalloo, F. A new scoring system for the chances of identifying a BRCA1/2 mutation outperforms existing models including BRCAPRO. *J. Med. Genet.* **2004**, *41*, 474–480. [CrossRef]
21. Evans, D.G.; Harkness, E.F.; Plaskocinska, I.; Wallace, A.J.; Clancy, T.; Woodward, E.R.; Howell, A.; Tischkowitz, M.; Lalloo, F. Pathology update to the Manchester Scoring System based on testing in over 4000 families. *J. Med. Genet.* **2017**, *54*, 674–681. [CrossRef]
22. Familial Breast Cancer: Classification, care and Managing Breast Cancer and Related Risks in People with a Family History of Breast Cancer Clinical Guideline Published: 25 June 2013. Available online: www.nice.org.uk/guidance/cg164 (accessed on 12 October 2020).
23. NHS England. National Genomic Test Directory 2020. Available online: https://www.england.nhs.uk/publication/national-genomic-test-directories/ (accessed on 12 October 2020).

24. Dorling, L.; Carvalho, S.; Allen, J.; González-Neira, A.; Luccarini, C.; Wahlström, C.; Pooley, K.A.; Parsons, M.T.; Fortuno, C. Breast cancer risk genes: Association analysis of rare coding variants in 34 genes in 60,466 cases and 53,461 controls. *N. Engl. J. Med.* **2020**, *383*. in press.
25. Lalloo, F.; Boggis, C.R.; Evans, D.G.; Shenton, A.; Threlfall, A.G.; Howell, A. Screening by mammography, women with a family history of breast cancer. *Eur. J. Cancer* **1998**, *34*, 937–940. [CrossRef]
26. Leach, M.O.; Boggis, C.R.; Dixon, A.K.; Easton, D.F.; Eeles, R.A.; Evans, D.G.; Gilbert, F.J.; Griebsch, I.; Hoff, R.J.; Kessar, P.; et al. MARIBS study group. Screening with magnetic resonance imaging and mammography of a UK population at high familial risk of breast cancer: A prospective multicentre cohort study (MARIBS). *Lancet* **2005**, *365*, 1769–1778. [CrossRef] [PubMed]
27. Pegington, M.; Evans, D.G.; Howell, A.; Donnelly, L.S.; Wiseman, J.; Cuzick, J.M.; Harvie, M.N. Lifestyle behaviours and health measures of women at increased risk of breast cancer taking chemoprevention. *Eur. J. Cancer Prev.* **2019**, *28*, 500–506. [CrossRef] [PubMed]
28. World Cancer Research Fund. Diet, Nutrition, Physical Activity and Breast Cancer 2018. Available online: https://www.wcrf.org/sites/default/files/Breast-cancer-report.pdf (accessed on 12 October 2020).
29. Harvie, M.; Howell, A.; Vierkant, R.A.; Kumar, N.; Cerhan, J.R.; Kelemen, L.E.; Folsom, A.R.; Sellers, T.A. Association of gain and loss of weight before and after menopause with risk of postmenopausal breast cancer in the Iowa women's health study. *Cancer Epidemiol. Biomark. Prev.* **2005**, *14*, 656–661. [CrossRef]
30. Harvie, M.N.; Pegington, M.; Mattson, M.P.; Frystyk, J.; Dillon, B.; Evans, G.; Cuzick, J.; Jebb, S.A.; Martin, B.; Cutler, R.G.; et al. The effects of intermittent or continuous energy restriction on weight loss and metabolic disease risk markers: A randomized trial in young overweight women. *Int. J. Obes. (Lond.)* **2011**, *35*, 714–727. [CrossRef]
31. Harvie, M.; Wright, C.; Pegington, M.; McMullan, D.; Mitchell, E.; Martin, B.; Cutler, R.G.; Evans, G.; Whiteside, S.; Maudsley, S.; et al. The effect of intermittent energy and carbohydrate restriction v. daily energy restriction on weight loss and metabolic disease risk markers in overweight women. *Br. J. Nutr.* **2013**, *110*, 1534–1547. [CrossRef]
32. Harvie, M.; French, D.P.; Pegington, M.; Evans, D.G.R. Howell. Family History Lifestyle Study. *ISRCTN Regist.* **2020**, serial online.
33. Cuzick, J.; Forbes, J.; Edwards, R.; Baum, M.; Cawthorn, S.; Coates, A.; Hamed, A.; Howell, A.; Powles, T. IBIS investigators. First results from the International Breast Cancer Intervention Study (IBIS-I): A randomised prevention trial. *Lancet* **2002**, *360*, 817–824. [CrossRef]
34. Cuzick, J.; Sestak, I.; Forbes, J.F.; Dowsett, M.; Knox, J.; Cawthorn, S.; Saunders, C.; Roche, N.; Mansel, R.E.; von Minckwitz, G.; et al. Anastrozole for prevention of breast cancer in high-risk postmenopausal women (IBIS-II): An international, double-blind, randomised placebo-controlled trial. *Lancet* **2014**, *383*, 1041–1048. [CrossRef]
35. Lalloo, F.; Baildam ABrain, A.; Hopwood, P.; Evans, D.G.; Howell, A. A protocol for preventative mastectomy in women with an increased lifetime risk of breast cancer. *Eur. J. Surg. Oncol.* **2000**, *26*, 711–713. [CrossRef]
36. Gandhi, A.; Duxbury, P.; Murphy, J.; Foden, P.; Lalloo, F.; Clancy, T.; Wisely, J.; Howell, A.; Evans, D.G. Patient Reported Outcome Measures in a Cohort of Patients at High Risk of Breast Cancer Treated by Bilateral Risk Reducing Mastectomy and Breast Reconstruction. *Plast. Reconstr. Surg.*. in press.
37. Hopwood, P.; Lee, A.; Shenton, A.; Baildam, A.; Brain, A.; Lalloo, F.; Evans, G.; Howell, A. Clinical follow-up after bilateral risk reducing ('prophylactic') mastectomy: Mental health and body image outcomes. *Psychooncology* **2000**, *9*, 462–472. [CrossRef]
38. Hatcher, M.B.; Fallowfield, L.; A'Hern, R. The psychosocial impact of bilateral prophylactic mastectomy: Prospective study using questionnaires and semistructured interviews. *BMJ* **2001**, *322*, 76. [CrossRef] [PubMed]
39. Tyrer-Cuzick (IBIS) Risk Evaluation Tool. Available online: riskevaluator@ems-trials.org (accessed on 20 October 2020).
40. Lee, A.; Mavaddat, N.; Wilcox, A.N.; Cunningham, A.P.; Carver, T.; Hartley, S.; Babb de Villiers, C.; Izquierdo, A.; Simard, J.; Schmidt, M.K.; et al. Version 2.BOADICEA: A comprehensive breast cancer risk prediction model incorporating genetic and nongenetic risk factors. *Genet. Med.* **2019**, *21*, 1708–1718. [CrossRef] [PubMed]

41. Cuzick, J.; Sestak, I.; Forbes, J.F.; Dowsett, M.; Cawthorn, S.; Mansel, R.E.; Loibl, S.; Bonanni, B.; Evans, D.G.; Howell, A.; et al. Use of anastrozole for breast cancer prevention (IBIS-II): Long-term results of a randomised controlled trial. *Lancet* **2020**, *395*, 117–122. [CrossRef]
42. Evans, D.G.; Lalloo, F.; Ashcroft, L.; Shenton, A.; Clancy, T.; Baildam, A.D.; Brain, A.; Hopwood, P.; Howell, A. Uptake of risk-reducing surgery in unaffected women at high risk of breast and ovarian cancer is risk, age, and time dependent. *Cancer Epidemiol. Biomark. Prev.* **2009**, *18*, 2318–2324. [CrossRef]
43. Evans, D.G.; Brentnall, A.R.; Harvie, M.; Dawe, S.; Sergeant, J.C.; Stavrinos, P.; Astley, S.; Wilson, M.; Ainsworth, J.; Cuzick, J.; et al. Breast cancer risk in young women in the national breast screening programme: Implications for applying NICE guidelines for additional screening and chemoprevention. *Cancer Prev. Res. (Phila.)* **2014**, *7*, 993–1001. [CrossRef]
44. Evans, D.G.; Barwell, J.; Eccles, D.M.; Collins, A.; Izatt, L.; Jacobs, C.; Donaldson, A.; Brady, A.F.; Cuthbert, A.; Harrison, R.; et al. The Angelina Jolie effect: How high celebrity profile can have a major impact on provision of cancer related services. *Breast Cancer Res.* **2014**, *16*, 442. [CrossRef]
45. Evans, D.G.; Wisely, J.; Clancy, T.; Lalloo, F.; Wilson, M.; Johnson, R.; Duncan, J.; Barr, L.; Gandhi, A.; Howell, A. Longer term effects of the Angelina Jolie effect: Increased risk-reducing mastectomy rates in BRCA carriers and other high-risk women. *Breast Cancer Res.* **2015**, *17*, 143. [CrossRef]
46. Evans, D.G.; Donnelly, L.S.; Harkness, E.F.; Astley, S.M.; Stavrinos, P.; Dawe, S.; Watterson, D.; Fox, L.; Sergeant, J.C.; Ingham, S.; et al. Breast cancer risk feedback to women in the UK NHS breast screening population. *Br. J. Cancer* **2016**, *114*, 1045–1052. [CrossRef] [PubMed]
47. Vachon, C.M.; Pankratz, V.S.; Scott, C.G.; Haeberle, L.; Ziv, E.; Jensen, M.R.; Brandt, K.R.; Whaley, D.H.; Olson, J.E.; Heusinger, K.; et al. The contributions of breast density and common genetic variation to breast cancer risk. *J. Natl. Cancer Inst.* **2015**, *107*, dju397. [CrossRef] [PubMed]
48. Zhang, X.; Rice, M.; Tworoger, S.S.; Rosner, B.A.; Eliassen, A.H.; Tamimi, R.M.; Joshi, A.D.; Lindstrom, S.; Qian, J. Addition of a polygenic risk score, mammographic density, and endogenous hormones to existing breast cancer risk prediction models: A nested case-control study. *PLoS Med.* **2018**, *15*, e1002644. [CrossRef] [PubMed]
49. Terry, M.B.; Liao, Y.; Whittemore, A.S.; Leoce, N.; Buchsbaum, R.; Zeinomar, N.; Dite, G.S.; Chung, W.K.; Knight, J.A.; Southey, M.C.; et al. 10-year performance of four models of breast cancer risk: A validation study. *Lancet Oncol.* **2019**, *20*, 504–517. [CrossRef]
50. Pal, C.P.; Wilcox, A.N.; Brook, M.N.; Zhang, Y.; Ahearn, T.; Orr, N.; Coulson, P.; Schoemaker, M.J.; Jones, M.E.; Gail, M.H.; et al. Comparative Validation of Breast Cancer Risk Prediction Models and Projections for Future Risk Stratification. *J. Natl. Cancer Inst.* **2020**, *112*, 278–285. [CrossRef]
51. Easton, D.F.; Pooley, K.A.; Dunning, A.M.; Pharoah, P.D.; Thompson, D.; Ballinger, D.G.; Struewing, J.P.; Morrison, J.; Field, H.; Luben, R.; et al. Genome-wide association study identifies novel breast cancer susceptibility loci. *Nature* **2007**, *447*, 1087–1093. [CrossRef]
52. Turnbull, C.; Ahmed, S.; Morrison, J.; Pernet, D.; Renwick, A.; Maranian, M.; Seal, S.; Ghoussaini, M.; Hines, S.; Healey, C.S.; et al. Genome-wide association study identifies five new breast cancer susceptibility loci. *Nat. Genet.* **2010**, *42*, 504–507. [CrossRef]
53. Evans, D.G.; Brentnall, A.; Byers, H.; Harkness, E.; Stavrinos, P.; Howell, A.; FH-risk study Group; Newman, W.G.; Cuzick, J. The impact of a panel of 18 SNPs on breast cancer risk in women attending a UK familial screening clinic: A case-control study. *J. Med. Genet.* **2017**, *54*, 111–113. [CrossRef]
54. Van Veen, E.M.; Brentnall, A.R.; Byers, H.; Harkness, E.F.; Astley, S.M.; Sampson, S.; Howell, A.; Newman, W.G.; Cuzick, J.; Evans, D.G.R. Use of Single-Nucleotide Polymorphisms and Mammographic Density Plus Classic Risk Factors for Breast Cancer Risk Prediction. *JAMA Oncol.* **2018**, *4*, 476–482. [CrossRef]
55. Brentnall, A.R.; van Veen, E.M.; Harkness, E.F.; Rafiq, S.; Byers, H.; Astley, S.M.; Sampson, S.; Howell, A.; Newman, W.G.; Cuzick, J.; et al. A case-control evaluation of 143 single nucleotide polymorphisms for breast cancer risk stratification with classical factors and mammographic density. *Int. J. Cancer* **2020**, *146*, 2122–2129. [CrossRef]
56. Maurice, A.R.; Evans, D.G.R.; Shenton, A.; Ashcroft, L.; Baildam, A.; Barr, L.; Byrne, G.; Bundred, N.; Boggis, C.; Wilson, M.; et al. Howell A Screening younger women with a family history of breast cancer-does early detection improve outcome? *Eur. J. Cancer* **2006**, *42*, 1385–1390. [CrossRef] [PubMed]

57. Duffy, S.W. FH01 collaborative teams. Mammographic surveillance in women younger than 50 years who have a family history of breast cancer: Tumour characteristics and projected effect on mortality in the prospective, single-arm, FH01 study. *Lancet Oncol.* **2010**, *11*, 1127–1134. [CrossRef]
58. Evans, D.G.; Thomas, S.; Caunt, J.; Burch, A.; Brentnall, A.R.; Roberts, L.; Howell, A.; Wilson, M.; Fox, R.; Hillier, S.; et al. Final Results of the Prospective FH02 Mammographic Surveillance Study of Women Aged 35-39 at Increased Familial Risk of Breast Cancer. *EClinicalMedicine* **2019**, *7*, 39–46. [CrossRef]
59. Van den Ende, C.; Oordt-Speets, A.M.; Vroling, H.; van Agt, H.M.E. Benefits and harms of breast cancer screening with mammography in women aged 40-49 years: A systematic review. *Int. J. Cancer* **2017**, *141*, 1295–1306. [CrossRef] [PubMed]
60. Duffy, S.W.; Vulkan, D.; Cuckle, H.; Parmar, D.; Sheikh, S.; Smith, R.A.; Evans, A.; Blyuss, O.; Johns, L.; Ellis, I.O.; et al. Effect of mammographic screening from age 40 years on breast cancer mortality (UK Age trial): Final results of a randomised, controlled trial. *Lancet Oncol.* **2020**, *21*, 1165–1172. [CrossRef]
61. Shieh, Y.; Eklund, M.; Madlensky, L.; Sawyer, S.D.; Thompson, C.K.; Stover Fiscalini, A.; Ziv, E.; Van't Veer, L.J.; Esserman, L.J.; Tice, J.A.; et al. Breast Cancer Screening in the Precision Medicine Era: Risk-Based Screening in a Population-Based Trial. *J. Natl. Cancer Inst.* **2017**, *109*. [CrossRef]
62. UNICANCER (2018) My Personalized Breast Screening (myPeBS). Available online: https://clinicaltrials.gov/ct2/show/NCT0367233 (accessed on 12 October 2020).
63. Williams, M.; Woof, V.G.; Donnelly, L.S.; Howell, A.; Evans, D.G.; French, D.P. Risk stratified breast cancer screening: UK healthcare policy decision-making stakeholders' views on a low-risk breast screening pathway. *BMC Cancer* **2020**, *20*, 680. [CrossRef]
64. Ionescu, G.V.; Fergie, M.; Berks, M.; Harkness, E.F.; Hulleman, J.; Brentnall, A.R.; Cuzick, J.; Evans, D.G.; Astley, S.M. Prediction of reader estimates of mammographic density using convolutional neural networks. *J. Med. Imaging (Bellingham)* **2019**, *6*, 031405. [CrossRef]
65. Hopper, J.L.; Nguyen, T.L.; Schmidt, D.F.; Makalic, E.; Song, Y.M.; Sung, J.; Dite, G.S.; Dowty, J.G.; Li, S. Going Beyond Conventional Mammographic Density to Discover Novel Mammogram-Based Predictors of Breast Cancer Risk. *J. Clin. Med.* **2020**, *9*, 627. [CrossRef]
66. Evans, D.G.; Kesavan, N.; Lim, Y.; Gadde, S.; Hurley, E.; Massat, N.J.; Maxwell, A.J.; Ingham, S.; Eeles, R.; Leach, M.O.; et al. MRI breast screening in high-risk women: Cancer detection and survival analysis. *Breast Cancer Res. Treat.* **2014**, *145*, 663–672. [CrossRef]
67. Kuhl, C.K.; Schrading, S.; Leutner, C.C.; Morakkabati-Spitz, N.; Wardelmann, E.; Fimmers, R.; Kuhn, W.; Schild, H.H. Mammography, breast ultrasound, and magnetic resonance imaging for surveillance of women at high familial risk for breast cancer. *J. Clin. Oncol.* **2005**, *23*, 8469–8476. [CrossRef] [PubMed]
68. Kriege, M.; Brekelmans, C.T.; Boetes, C.; Besnard, P.E.; Zonderland, H.M.; Obdeijn, I.M.; Manoliu, R.A.; Kok, T.; Peterse, H.; Tilanus-Linthorst, M.M.; et al. Efficacy of MRI and mammography for breast-cancer screening in women with a familial or genetic predisposition. *N. Engl. J. Med.* **2004**, *351*, 427–437. [CrossRef] [PubMed]
69. Warner, E.; Plewes, D.B.; Hill, K.A.; Causer, P.A.; Zubovits, J.T.; Jong, R.A.; Cutrara, M.R.; DeBoer, G.; Yaffe, M.J.; Messner, S.J.; et al. Surveillance of BRCA1 and BRCA2 mutation carriers with magnetic resonance imaging, ultrasound, mammography, and clinical breast examination. *JAMA* **2004**, *292*, 1317–1325. [CrossRef] [PubMed]
70. Evans, D.G.; Harkness, E.; Howell, A.; Wilson, M.; Hurley, E.; Lim, Y.; Maxwell, A.; Moller, P. Intensive breast screening in BRCA2 mutation carriers is associated with reduced breast cancer specific and all cause mortality. *Hered. Cancer Clin. Pract.* **2016**, *14*, 8. [CrossRef]
71. Hopper, J.L.; Dite, G.S.; MacInnis, R.J. Age-specific breast cancer risk by body mass index and familial risk: Prospective family study cohort (ProF-SC). *Breast Cancer Res.* **2018**, *20*, 132. [CrossRef]
72. Arthur, R.S.; Wang, T.; Xue, X.; Kamensky, V.; Rohan, T.E. Genetic factors, adherence to healthy lifestyle behavior, and risk of invasive breast cancer among women in the UK Biobank. *J. Natl. Cancer Inst* **2020**, 893–901. [CrossRef]
73. Maas, P.; Barrdahl, M.; Joshi, A.D. Breast Cancer Risk from Modifiable and Nonmodifiable Risk Factors among White Women in the United States. *JAMA Oncol.* **2016**, *2*, 1295–1302. [CrossRef]
74. Behaviour Change Guidance PH6. 2007. Available online: https://www.nice.org.uk/Guidance/PH6 (accessed on 12 October 2020).

75. Wright, C.E.; Harvie, M.; Howell, A.; Evans, D.G.; Hulbert-Williams, N.; Donnelly, L.S. Beliefs about weight and breast cancer: An interview study with high risk women following a 12 month weight loss intervention. *Hered Cancer Clin. Pract* **2015**, *13*, 1. [CrossRef]
76. French, D.P.; Cameron, E.; Benton, J.S.; Deaton, C.; Harvie, M. Can Communicating Personalised Disease Risk Promote Healthy Behaviour Change? A Systematic Review of Systematic Reviews. *Ann. Behav. Med.* **2017**, *51*, 718–729. [CrossRef]
77. Cuzick, J.; Sestak, I.; Bonanni, B.; Costantino, J.P.; Cummings, S.; DeCensi, A.; Dowsett, M.; Forbes, J.F.; Ford, L.; LaCroix, A.Z.; et al. Selective oestrogen receptor modulators in prevention of breast cancer: An updated meta-analysis of individual participant data. *Lancet* **2013**, *381*, 1827–1834. [CrossRef]
78. Cuzick, J.; Sestak, I.; Cawthorn, S.; Hamed, H.; Holli, K.; Howell, A.; Forbes, J.F.; IBIS-I Investigators. Tamoxifen for prevention of breast cancer: Extended long-term follow-up of the IBIS-I breast cancer prevention trial. *Lancet Oncol.* **2015**, *16*, 67–75. [CrossRef]
79. Chlebowski, R.T.; Anderson, G.L.; Aragaki, A.K.; Manson, J.E.; Stefanick, M.L.; Pan, K.; Barrington, W.; Kuller, L.H.; Simon, M.S.; Lane, D.; et al. Association of Menopausal Hormone Therapy With Breast Cancer Incidence and Mortality During Long-term Follow-up of the Women's Health Initiative Randomized Clinical Trials. *JAMA* **2020**, *324*, 369–380. [CrossRef] [PubMed]
80. Donnelly, L.S.; Evans, D.G.; Wiseman, J.; Fox, J.; Greenhalgh, R.; Affen, J.; Juraskova, I.; Stavrinos, P.; Dawe, S.; Cuzick, J.; et al. Uptake of tamoxifen in consecutive premenopausal women under surveillance in a high-risk breast cancer clinic. *Br. J. Cancer* **2014**, *110*, 1681–1687. [CrossRef] [PubMed]
81. Smith, S.G.; Sestak, I.; Forster, A.; Partridge, A.; Side, L.; Wolf, M.S. Factors affecting uptake and adherence to breast cancer chemoprevention: A systematic review and meta-analysis. *Ann. Oncol.* **2016**, *27*, 575–590. [CrossRef]
82. Fallowfield, L.; Fleissig, A.; Edwards, R.; West, A.; Powles, T.J.; Howell, A.; Cuzick, J. Tamoxifen for the prevention of breast cancer: Psychosocial impact on women participating in two randomized controlled trials. *J. Clin. Oncol.* **2001**, *19*, 1885–1892. [CrossRef]
83. Smith, S.G.; Sestak, I.; Howell, A.; Forbes, J.; Cuzick, J. Participant-Reported Symptoms and Their Effect on Long-Term Adherence in the International Breast Cancer Intervention Study I (IBIS I). *J. Clin. Oncol.* **2017**, *35*, 2666–2673. [CrossRef]
84. Sestak, I.; Smith, S.G.; Howell, A.; Forbes, J.F.; Cuzick, J. Early participant-reported symptoms as predictors of adherence to anastrozole in the International Breast Cancer Intervention Studies II. *Ann. Oncol.* **2018**, *29*, 504–509. [CrossRef]
85. DeCensi, A.; Puntoni, M.; Guerrieri-Gonzaga, A.; Caviglia, S.; Avino, F.; Cortesi, L.; Taverniti, C.; Pacquola, M.G.; Falcini, F.; Gulisano, M.; et al. Randomized Placebo Controlled Trial of Low-Dose Tamoxifen to Prevent Local and Contralateral Recurrence in Breast Intraepithelial Neoplasia. *J. Clin. Oncol.* **2019**, *37*, 1629–1637. [CrossRef]
86. Robertson, J.F.; Willsher, P.C.; Winterbottom, L.; Blamey, R.W.; Thorpe, S. Onapristone, a progesterone receptor antagonist, as first-line therapy in primary breast cancer. *Eur. J. Cancer* **1999**, *35*, 214–218. [CrossRef]
87. Nolan, E.; Vaillant, F.; Branstetter, D.; Pal, B.; Giner, G.; Whitehead, L.; Lok, S.W.; Mann, G.B.; Kathleen Cuningham Foundation Consortium for Research into Familial Breast Cancer (kConFab); Rohrbach, K.; et al. RANK ligand as a potential target for breast cancer prevention in BRCA1-mutation carriers. *Nat. Med.* **2016**, *22*, 933–939. [CrossRef]
88. Hartmann, L.C.; Schaid, D.J.; Woods, J.E.; Crotty, T.P.; Myers, J.L.; Arnold, P.G.; Petty, P.M.; Sellers, T.A.; Johnson, J.L.; McDonnell, S.K.; et al. Efficacy of bilateral prophylactic mastectomy in women with a family history of breast cancer. *N. Engl. J. Med.* **1999**, *340*, 77–84. [CrossRef] [PubMed]
89. Razdan, S.N.; Patel, V.; Jewell, S.; McCarthy, C.M. Quality of life among patients after bilateral prophylactic mastectomy: A systematic review of patient-reported outcomes. *Qual. Life Res.* **2016**, *25*, 1409–1421. [CrossRef] [PubMed]
90. Jakub, J.W.; Peled, A.W.; Gray, R.J.; Greenup, R.A.; Kiluk, J.V.; Sacchini, V.; McLaughlin, S.A.; Tchou, J.C.; Vierkant, R.A.; Degnim, A.C.; et al. Oncologic Safety of Prophylactic Nipple-Sparing Mastectomy in a Population With BRCA Mutations: A Multi-institutional Study. *JAMA Surg.* **2018**, *153*, 123–129. [CrossRef] [PubMed]
91. Shay, P.; Jacobs, J. Autologous reconstruction following nipple sparing mastectomy: A comprehensive review of the current literature. *Gland Surg.* **2018**, *7*, 316–324. [CrossRef] [PubMed]

92. Dave, R.V.; Vucicevic Al Highton, L.; Harvey, J.R.; Johnson, R.; Kirwan, C.C.; Murphy, J. Medium term outcomes following immediate prepectoral implant based breast reconstruction using acellular dermal matrix. *Br. J. Surg.* **2020**. [CrossRef]
93. Gandhi, A.; Barr, L.; Johnson, R. Bioprosthetics: Changing the landscape for breast reconstruction. *Eur. J. Surg. Oncol.* **2013**, *39*, 24–25. [CrossRef] [PubMed]
94. Groen, J.W.; Negenborn, V.L.; Twisk, D.J.W.R.; Rizopoulos, D.; Ket, J.C.F.; Smit, J.M.; Mullender, M.G. Autologous fat grafting in onco-plastic breast reconstruction: A systematic review on oncological and radiological safety, complications, volume retention and patient/surgeon satisfaction. *J. Plast. Reconstr. Aesthet. Surg.* **2016**, *69*, 742–764. [CrossRef]
95. Ingham, S.L.; Sperrin, M.; Baildam, A.; Ross, G.L.; Clayton, R.; Lalloo, F.; Buchan, I.; Howell, A.; Evans, D.G. Risk-reducing surgery increases survival in BRCA1/2 mutation carriers unaffected at time of family referral. *Breast Cancer Res. Treat.* **2013**, *142*, 611–618. [CrossRef]
96. Heemskerk-Gerritsen, B.A.M.; Jager, A.; Koppert, L.B.; Obdeijn, A.I.; Collée, M.; Meijers-Heijboer, H.E.J.; Jenner, D.J.; Oldenburg, H.S.A.; van Engelen, K.; de Vries, J.; et al. Survival after bilateral risk-reducing mastectomy in healthy BRCA1 and BRCA2 mutation carriers. *Breast Cancer Res. Treat.* **2019**, *177*, 723–733. [CrossRef]
97. Evans, D.G.; Howell, S.J.; Howell, A. Should unaffected female *BRCA2* pathogenic variant carriers be told there is little or no advantage from risk reducing mastectomy? *Fam. Cancer* **2019**, *18*, 377–379. [CrossRef]
98. Braude, L.; Kirsten, L.; Gilchrist, J.; Juraskova, I. A systematic review of women's satisfaction and regret following risk-reducing mastectomy. *Patient Educ. Couns.* **2017**, *100*, 2182–2189. [CrossRef] [PubMed]
99. French, D.P.; Astley, S.; Brentnall, A.R.; Cuzick, J.; Dobrashian, R.; Duffy, S.W.; Gorman, L.S.; Harkness, E.F.; Harrison, F.; Harvie, M.; et al. What are the benefits and harms of risk stratified screening as part of the NHS Breast Screening Programme? Study protocol for a multi-site non-randomised comparison of BC-Predict versus usual screening. *BMC Cancer* **2020**, *20*, 570. [CrossRef] [PubMed]
100. French, D.P.; Southworth, J.; Howell, A.; Harvie, M.; Stavrinos, P.; Watterson, D.; Sampson, S.; Evans, D.G.; Donnely, L.S. Psychological impact of providing women with personalized ten-year breast cancer risk estimates. *Br. J. Cancer* **2018**, *118*, 1648–1657. [CrossRef] [PubMed]
101. Sabatino, S.A.; McCarthy, E.P.; Phillips, R.S.; Burns, R.B. Breast cancer risk assessment and management in primary care: Provider attitudes, practices, and barriers. *Cancer Detect Prev.* **2007**, *31*, 375–383. [CrossRef] [PubMed]
102. Keogh, L.A.; Steel, E.; Weideman, P.; Butow, P.; Collins, I.M.; Emery, J.D.; Mann, G.B.; Bickerstaffe, A.; Trainer, A.H.; Hopper, L.J.; et al. Consumer and clinician perspectives on personalising breast cancer prevention information. *Breast* **2019**, *43*, 39–47. [CrossRef] [PubMed]
103. Archer, S.; Babb de Villiers, C.; Scheibl, F.; Carver, T.; Hartley, S.; Lee, A.; Cunningham, A.P.; Easton, D.F.; McIntosh, J.G.; Emery, J.; et al. Evaluating clinician acceptability of the prototype CanRisk tool for predicting risk of breast and ovarian cancer: A multi-methods study. *PLoS ONE* **2020**, *15*, e0229999. [CrossRef]
104. Hippisley-Cox, J.; Coupland, C. Development and validation of QMortality risk prediction algorithm to estimate short term risk of death and assess frailty: Cohort study. *BMJ* **2017**, *358*, j4208. [CrossRef]
105. Lo, L.L.; Collins, I.M.; Bressel, M.; Butow, P.; Emery, J.; Keogh, L.; Weideman, P.; Steel, E.; Hopper, J.L.; Trainer, A.H.; et al. The iPrevent Online Breast Cancer Risk Assessment and Risk Management Tool: Usability and Acceptability Testing. *JMIR Form Res.* **2018**, *2*, e24. [CrossRef]
106. Howell, A.; Anderson, A.S.; Clarke, R.; Duffy, S.W.; Evans, D.G.; Garcia–Closas, M.; Gescher, A.J.; Key, T.J.; Saxton, J.M.; Harvie, M.N. Risk Determination and Prevention of Breast Cancer. *Breast Cancer Res.* **2014**, *16*, 446. [CrossRef]

Publisher's Note: MDPI stays neutral with regard to jurisdictional claims in published maps and institutional affiliations.

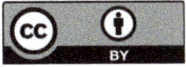

© 2020 by the authors. Licensee MDPI, Basel, Switzerland. This article is an open access article distributed under the terms and conditions of the Creative Commons Attribution (CC BY) license (http://creativecommons.org/licenses/by/4.0/).

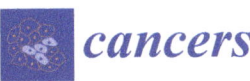

Article

Aberrant Dyskerin Expression Is Related to Proliferation and Poor Survival in Endometrial Cancer

Rafah Alnafakh [1,2,3], Gabriele Saretzki [4], Angela Midgley [5], James Flynn [6], Areege M. Kamal [2,7], Lucy Dobson [1,2], Purushothaman Natarajan [1,2], Helen Stringfellow [8], Pierre Martin-Hirsch [8], Shandya B. DeCruze [1], Sarah E. Coupland [9] and Dharani K. Hapangama [1,2,*]

1. Liverpool Women's Hospital NHS Foundation Trust, Member of Liverpool Health Partners, Liverpool L8 7SS, UK; R.A.A.Alnafakh@liverpool.ac.uk (R.A.); lucy.dobson@liverpool.ac.uk (L.D.); Puru.Natarajan@lwh.nhs.uk (P.N.); Bridget.Decruze@lwh.nhs.uk (S.B.D.)
2. Department of Women's and Children's Health, Institute of Life Course and Medical Sciences, University of Liverpool, Member of Liverpool Health Partners, Liverpool L8 7SS, UK; areegekamal@gmail.com
3. Department of Pathology, Al-Hilla Teaching Hospital, Babil, Iraq
4. Biosciences Institute, Campus for Ageing and Vitality, Newcastle University, Newcastle upon Tyne NE4 5PL, UK; gabriele.saretzki@newcastle.ac.uk
5. Experimental Arthritis Treatment Centre for Children, Institute in the Park, Department of Women's and Children's Health, University of Liverpool, Liverpool L12 2AP, UK; Angela.Midgley@liverpool.ac.uk
6. Illumina Inc., San Diego, CA 92122, USA; jflynn@illumina.com
7. Pathology Department, Oncology Teaching Hospital, Baghdad Medical City, Baghdad, Iraq
8. Lancashire Teaching Hospital NHS Trust, Preston PR2 9HT, UK; helen.stringfellow@lthtr.nhs.uk (H.S.); Pierre.Martin-Hirsch@lthtr.nhs.uk (P.M.-H.)
9. Molecular and Clinical Cancer Medicine, Institute of Systems, Molecular and Integrative Biology, University of Liverpool, Liverpool L7 8TX, UK; s.e.coupland@liverpool.ac.uk
* Correspondence: dharani@liverpool.ac.uk

Citation: Alnafakh, R.; Saretzki, G.; Midgley, A.; Flynn, J.; Kamal, A.M.; Dobson, L.; Natarajan, P.; Stringfellow, H.; Martin-Hirsch, P.; DeCruze, S.B.; et al. Aberrant Dyskerin Expression Is Related to Proliferation and Poor Survival in Endometrial Cancer. *Cancers* **2021**, *13*, 273. https://doi.org/10.3390/cancers13020273

Received: 1 November 2020
Accepted: 8 January 2021
Published: 13 January 2021

Publisher's Note: MDPI stays neutral with regard to jurisdictional clai-ms in published maps and institutio-nal affiliations.

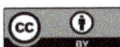

Copyright: © 2021 by the authors. Licensee MDPI, Basel, Switzerland. This article is an open access article distributed under the terms and conditions of the Creative Commons Attribution (CC BY) license (https://creativecommons.org/licenses/by/4.0/).

Simple Summary: Telomeres are the protective caps at the ends of chromosomes, and they are maintained by an enzyme called telomerase. Telomerase activity allows rapid reproduction of the cells (proliferation) of the lining of the womb (endometrium). Telomerase levels are high in cancers in general, including in endometrial cancer. Dyskerin is one of the main components of the telomerase enzyme. While the other main components of telomerase have been studied in endometrial cancer, there are no previous studies on dyskerin in the endometrium. Our study shows that dyskerin levels are significantly lower in endometrial cancer and levels are linked to the survival of women. Experimentally increasing dyskerin protein in endometrial cells in the laboratory reduces the rate of cell proliferation. Consequently, we propose that dyskerin may be a regulator of endometrial cancer cell proliferation, and further studies are required to test if it can be targeted to develop new therapies for endometrial cancer.

Abstract: Dyskerin is a core-component of the telomerase holo-enzyme, which elongates telomeres. Telomerase is involved in endometrial epithelial cell proliferation. Most endometrial cancers (ECs) have high telomerase activity; however, dyskerin expression in human healthy endometrium or in endometrial pathologies has not been investigated yet. We aimed to examine the expression, prognostic relevance, and functional role of dyskerin in human EC. Endometrial samples from a cohort of 175 women were examined with immunohistochemistry, immunoblotting, and qPCR. The EC cells were transfected with Myc-DDK-DKC1 plasmid and the effect of dyskerin overexpression on EC cell proliferation was assessed by flow cytometry. Human endometrium expresses dyskerin (*DKC1*) and dyskerin protein levels are significantly reduced in ECs when compared with healthy postmenopausal endometrium. Low dyskerin immunoscores were potentially associated with worse outcomes, suggesting a possible prognostic relevance. Cancer Genome Atlas (TCGA) ECs dataset (*n* = 589) was also interrogated. The TCGA dataset further confirmed changes in *DKC1* expression in EC with prognostic significance. Transient dyskerin overexpression had a negative effect on EC cell proliferation. Our data demonstrates a role for dyskerin in normal endometrium for the first time and confirms aberrant expression with possible prognostic relevance in EC. Interventions aimed at modulating dyskerin levels may provide novel therapeutic options in EC.

Keywords: dyskerin; *DKC1*; endometrial cancer; telomerase; proliferation; telomeres

1. Introduction

Telomeres are specialised nucleoprotein complexes consisting of tandem repeats of TTAGGG and associated specific shelterin proteins [1]. They prevent chromosomal ends from being identified as DNA damage and protect them from degradation and end to end fusion [2,3]. With each round of cell division, telomeric DNA is lost due to the end replication problem as well as oxidative stress [4,5]. In mitotic cells, critical shortening of telomeres induces apoptosis and senescence [6]. Telomerase is a specialised reverse-transcriptase which maintains and elongates telomeres [7] and is composed of: (i) the template-containing telomerase RNA component (TERC), (ii) the catalytic component of the enzyme, human telomerase reverse transcriptase (hTERT) and (iii) the protein dyskerin as one of the main core components [8]. In most human somatic cells, telomerase activity (TA) is either undetectable or very low [9]. However, human cells with high replicative demand such as lymphocytes [10] epithelial cells [11] and tissue stem cells have active or inducible telomerase [12]. The human endometrium is a highly regenerative tissue with a dynamic TA corresponding to epithelial proliferation [13]. Most cancer cells express constitutively high TA, providing them with an indefinite proliferative ability [14].

EC is the commonest gynaecological malignancy in developed countries, with an increasing incidence [15]. In an era of decreasing cancer-related deaths reported for most other cancers, mortality due to EC is expected to increase [16]. Therefore, novel biomarkers to stratify high-risk patients for therapy as well as novel therapeutic targets are urgently required to reduce the rising EC-associated mortality and morbidity.

High TA has been reported in over 90% of all ECs [17]. hTERT and hTERC expression levels and TA measured by Telomere Repeat Amplification Protocol (TRAP) assay have been previously reported in the healthy endometrium [13] and in ECs [17,18]. However, dyskerin, which forms the foundation of the H/ACA lobe structure of the telomerase holo-enzyme, has not been studied in normal or pathological endometrium. Dyskerin protein is encoded by the *DKC1* gene located on the X chromosome [19] and it stabilises hTERC and enhances TA [20]. Dyskerin also has an extra-telomerase function in ribosomal biogenesis [21,22].

Available evidence suggests either the gain or loss of dyskerin to be carcinogenic [23,24]. High dyskerin levels have been reported in breast and prostate cancers [21,25,26] while decreased levels of dyskerin had been linked to carcinogenesis in the pituitary gland [27]. Low dyskerin levels observed in dyskeratosis congenita (DC) [28] have also been associated with an increased cancer-susceptibility before the age of 30 due to prematurely shortened telomers [29]. This observation is also in agreement with the only available animal model, where half of the hypomorphic *DKC1* mutant (*DKC1m*) mice (with decreased *DKC1* expression) developed various malignancies [22]. We, therefore, aimed to explore the role of dyskerin in endometrial carcinogenesis.

2. Results

2.1. In Silico Interrogation of the Cancer Genome Atlas (TCGA) Endometrioid and Serous EC Dataset Demonstrates Dysregulation of DKC1 to Be Associated with Poor Survival

Analysis of the TCGA dataset demonstrated a more than 2-fold upregulation of DKC1 RNA levels in 69/477 (14.65%) of the endometrioid and serous ECs compared with a set of normal endometrial samples obtained from 35 EC patients, at 2–3 cm distance from the cancer margin [30]. High *DKC1* expression was significantly associated with poor prognosis ($p = 2 \times 10^{-5}$, Cox-regression = 0.91) (Figure 1).

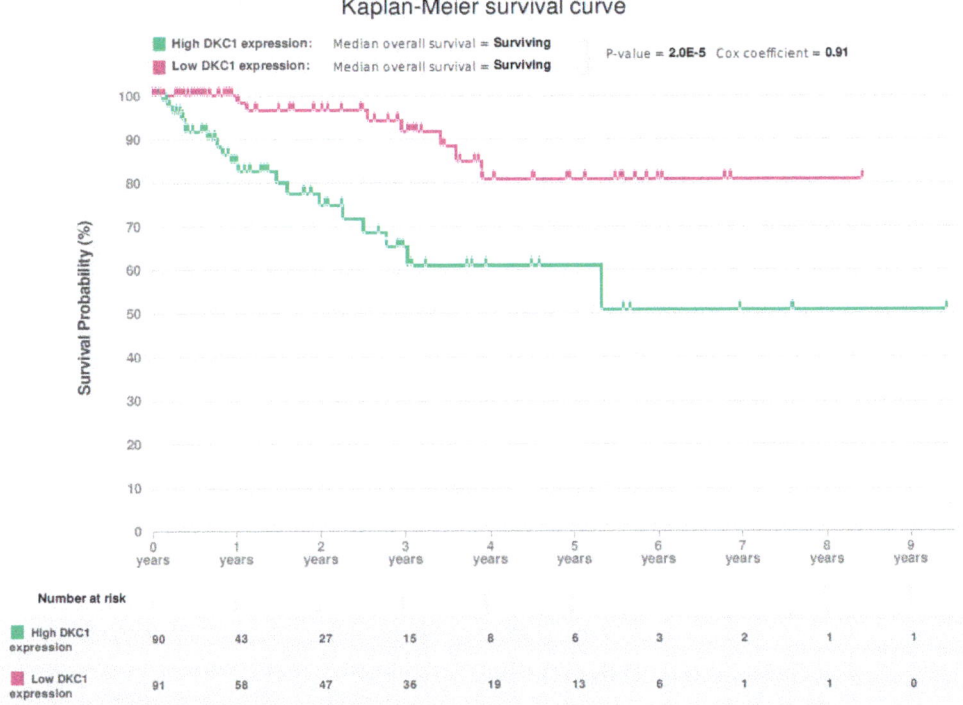

Figure 1. Kaplan-Meier survival curve for the association between DKC1 mRNA levels and overall survival ($p = 2 \times 10^{-5}$, Cox-regression = 0.91) in The Cancer Genome Atlas (TCGA) dataset (endometrioid and serous endometrial cancer) {$n = 477$}.

The mutation frequency of the *DKC1* gene in ECs was low (9/235, 3.69%) and consisted of mainly missense mutations that occurred without any *TERC* gene mutations (Figure S1).

Patients with ECs harboring a mutant *DKC1* gene seemed to have a better clinical outcome, compared with cancers carrying a wild-type *DKC1* gene (Figure S2). Twenty out of 464 (4.31%) ECs also demonstrated a copy number variation (mostly loss) of the *DKC1* gene. However, the TCGA dataset did not show a correlation of DKC1 RNA levels with the tumour grade ($r^2 = 0.19$, $p = 9.61 \times 10^{-23}$) or clinical stage ($r^2 = 0.02$, $p = 7.27 \times 10^{-4}$), (Figure S3A,B). Similarly, there was no correlation between RNA levels of *DKC1* with steroid receptor genes, *TERT* ($r^2 = 0.03$, $p = 3.43 \times 10^{-4}$), (Figure S4A) or *TERC* ($r^2 = 0.04$, $p = 1.62 \times 10^{-4}$), (Figure S4B). High DKC1 RNA levels were observed in *TP53* mutated ECs ($p = 1.23 \times 10^{-8}$) (Figure S5A) while in contrast, lower DKC1 RNA levels were observed in *FGFR2* ($p = 7.90 \times 10^{-3}$) (Figure S5B), *PTEN* ($p = 2.90 \times 10^{-6}$), *PIK3R1* ($p = 0.02$), (Figure S6A,B) and *CTNNB1* ($p = 1.67 \times 10^{-3}$) mutated ECs. No significant difference in *DKC1* RNA level was observed in *TERC, TERT, POLE, PIK3CA, KRAS,* and *ARID1A* mutated ECs compared with un-mutated EC samples.

2.2. Study Cohort

Patients' demographic details are detailed in Table 1. Women with high-grade EC (HGEC) were significantly older than those with low-grade EC (LGEC) and healthy postmenopausal (PM) women ($p < 0.001$, $p = 0.002$, respectively). A significantly higher body mass index (BMI) was observed in the endometrial hyperplasia with a cytological atypia (EHA) group compared with the healthy PM women ($p < 0.001$) and in the EC group. There was an apparent trend for the LGEC group to have a higher BMI compared with the HGEC group ($p = 0.06$).

Table 1. Demographic features of study groups.

Study Groups	No	%	* Age (Years)	** BMI (kg/m^2)
1. Healthy (total)	51			
• *Proliferative phase*	16		40 (30–57)	27 (18–41)
• *Postmenopausal*	35		63 (40–85)	26 (20–40)
2. Endometrial hyperplasia	15		55 (48–72)	36 (24–57)
3. Endometrial cancer (total)	109		68 (37–96)	30 (20–54)
LGEC	53	48.6	64 (37–89)	32 (21–54)
• *Endometrioid Grade 1*	34	31.2	64 (46–89)	33 (21–53)
• *Endometrioid Grade 2*	19	17.4	60 (37–78)	30 (22–54)
HGEC	56	51.4	73 (48–96)	30 (20–43)
• *Endometrioid Grade 3*	12	11	68 (54–96)	28 (24–43)
• *Serous*	12	11	76 (64–87)	29 (23–39)
• *Clear cell*	10	9.1	74 (48–82)	30 (27–39)
• *Carcinosarcoma*	19	17.4	78 (60–89)	26 (20–37)
• *Dedifferentiated*	1	0.9	79	32
• *Mixed cell adenocarcinoma*	2	1.8	63 & 66	
• *Metastatic EC*	34		68 (27–96)	28 (21–43)

Abbreviations: Body mass index (BMI); high-grade endometrial carcinoma (HGEC); low-grade endometrial cancer (LGEC); * Data expressed as median (range). ** BMI data were available for only 161 cases.

2.3. Dyskerin mRNA Was Lower in ECs Compared with Normal PM Endometrium

In contrast to the TCGA data in our patient samples, DKC1 mRNA levels showed a tendency towards downregulation in ECs in comparison with endometrium from healthy PM women ($p = 0.06$), (Figure 2A). No difference in the DKC1 mRNA level was observed between LGEC and HGEC.

2.4. Dyskerin Protein is Significantly Reduced in ECs When Compared with Healthy PM Control Endometrium

When EC samples were compared with healthy PM endometrium, immunoblotting demonstrated significantly reduced dyskerin protein levels (normalised to the epithelial marker pancytokeratin ($p = 0.02$, Figure 2B and Figure S7A), but significantly higher TA ($p = 0.009$, Figure 2C). IHC staining revealed the presence of dyskerin protein at a cellular level. In both epithelial and stromal cells of the healthy PP and PM endometrium, immunostaining was primarily localised in the nucleus and/or nucleolus (Figure 2D) and epithelial cells displayed stronger staining than the stroma. Dyskerin immunoscores were significantly lower in PP compared with PM ($p = 0.03$, Figure 2E). However, neither dyskerin quickscores nor DKC1 mRNA levels correlated with TA (Spearman r = -0.12, $p = 0.16$ and Spearman r = 0.04, $p = 0.77$, respectively).

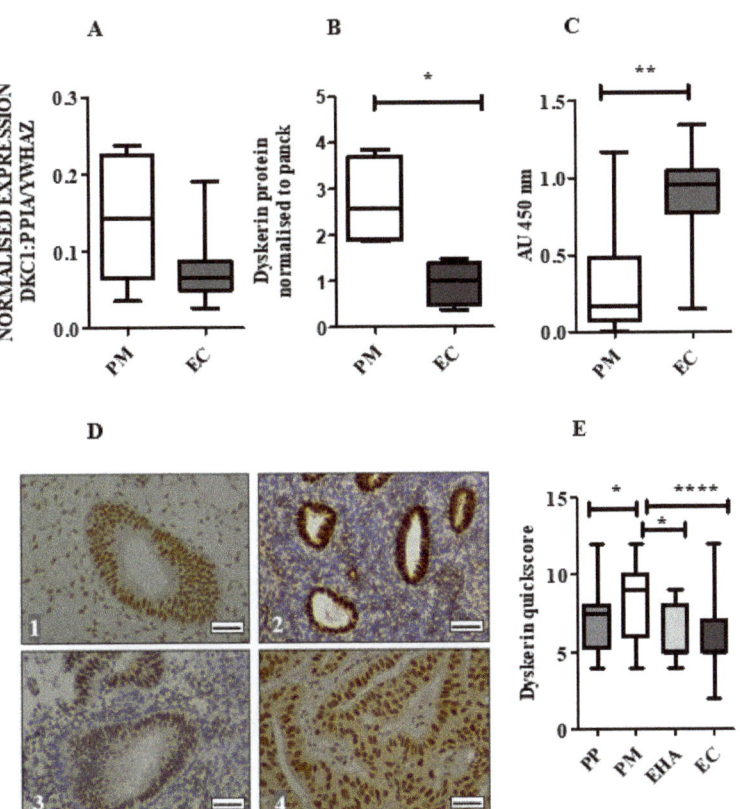

Figure 2. DKC1 mRNA and dyskerin protein in human endometrium. (**A**) DKC1 mRNA is normalised to geometric means of PPIA and YWHAZ and measured by qPCR in endometrial tissue samples: healthy postmenopausal (PM) ($n = 6$) and endometrial cancer (EC) ($n = 22$). Mann-Whitney test. (**B**) The amount of dyskerin protein was evaluated by immuno-blotting in healthy PM ($n = 4$) and EC ($n = 4$), Glyceraldehyde 3-Phosphate Dehydrogenase (GAPDH) was used to ensure equal loading of protein. Dyskerin protein levels in epithelial cells of tissue samples were analysed by normalising to pancytokeratin (panck). Mann-Whitney test, * $p < 0.05$. (**C**) Telomerase activity (TA) in healthy endometrial PM ($n = 6$) and EC ($n = 32$) was measured using a Telomere Repeat Amplification Protocol (TRAP) assay, Mann-Whitney test, ** $p < 0.01$. AU: arbitrary units (**D**) Representative microphotographs illustrating dyskerin IHC staining at the cellular level in endometrial samples in (**1**) normal proliferative phase (PP) endometrium, (**2**) healthy PM endometrium, (**3**) endometrial hyperplasia with cytological atypia (EHA) and (**4**) EC. Positive staining appears brown. Magnification 400×. Scale bar 50 μm. (**E**) Immunostaining quickscores for dyskerin protein in the human endometrium, healthy PP ($n = 16$), PM ($n = 30$), EHA ($n = 15$), EC ($n = 109$). Kruskal-Wallis test, * $p < 0.05$, **** $p < 0.0001$.

2.5. Loss of Dyskerin Was a Feature of Precancerous and Cancerous Endometrial Epithelial Cells

Dyskerin immunoscores were significantly lower in EHA and EC compared with normal PM endometrial epithelium ($p = 0.01$ and $p < 0.0001$, respectively, Figure 2E). All ECs in this cohort (Figure 3A) showed lower dyskerin scores compared with healthy PM endometrial tissue (Figure 3B), the difference was significant in endometrioid, carcinosarcoma and clear cell EC ($p < 0.0001$, $p < 0.0001$, and $p = 0.002$, respectively) and this reduction remained significant even when the histological LGEC ($p < 0.001$) and HGEC ($p < 0.001$) were considered separately (Figure 3C). There were no significant differences in dyskerin immunostaining among different EC subtypes or between LGEC and HGEC (Figure 3B,C). Metastatic lesions (Figure 4A) had significantly higher dyskerin immunoscores compared with their matched primary tumours ($p = 0.003$, Figure 4B), whereas ECs at advanced clinical stages (FIGO stages III&IV) had significantly lower dyskerin immunoscores compared with those at early stages (FIGO stages I&II, $p = 0.04$, Figure 4C).

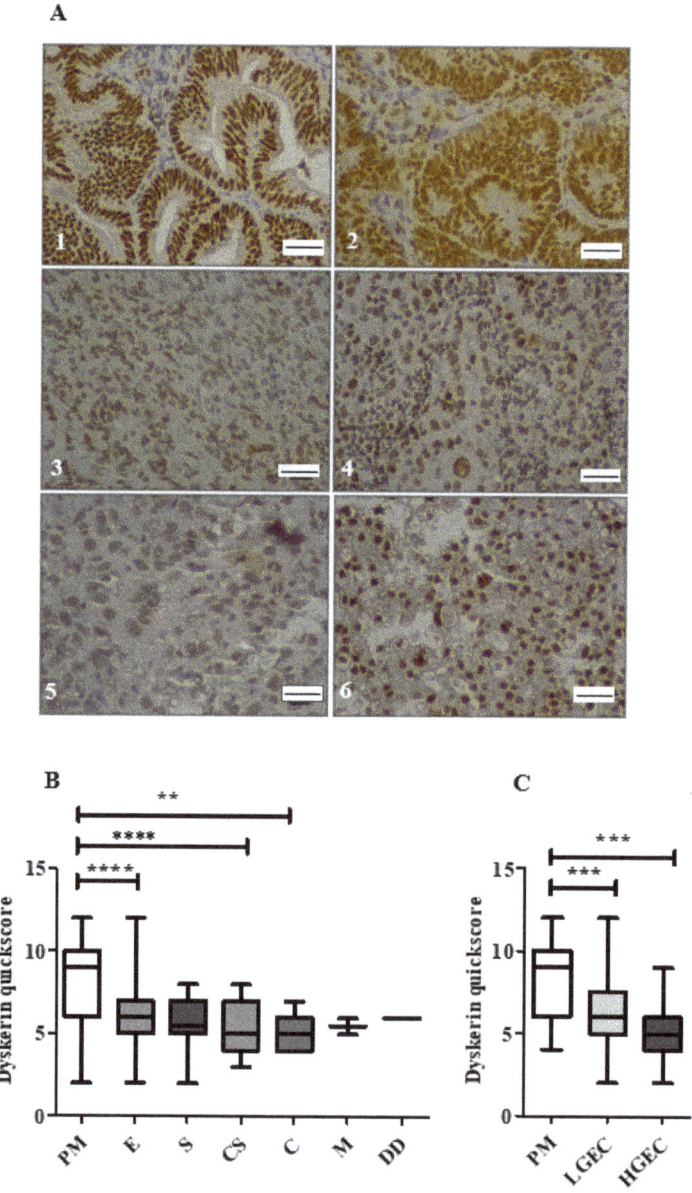

Figure 3. Immunostaining of dyskerin in endometrial cancer subtypes ($n = 109$). (**A**) Representative microphotographs of dyskerin in human ECs. (**1–3**) grade 1–3 endometrioid carcinoma, (**4**) serous subtype, (**5**) Carcinosarcoma and (**6**) clear cell carcinoma. Positive staining appears brown. Magnification 400×. Scale bar 50 μm. (**B**) Dyskerin immunoscores in healthy PM ($n = 30$) and various EC subtypes including endometrioid (E) ($n = 65$), Serous (S) ($n = 12$), carcinosarcoma (CS) ($n = 19$), clear cell carcinoma (**C**) ($n = 10$), mixed cell adenocarcinoma (M) ($n = 2$) and dedifferentiated EC (DD) ($n = 1$). ** $p < 0.01$, **** $p < 0.0001$. Kruskal-Wallis test. (**C**) Dyskerin immunoscores in human endometrial epithelium of healthy PM ($n = 30$), LGEC ($n = 53$) and HGEC ($n = 56$). *** $p < 0.001$. Kruskal-Wallis test.

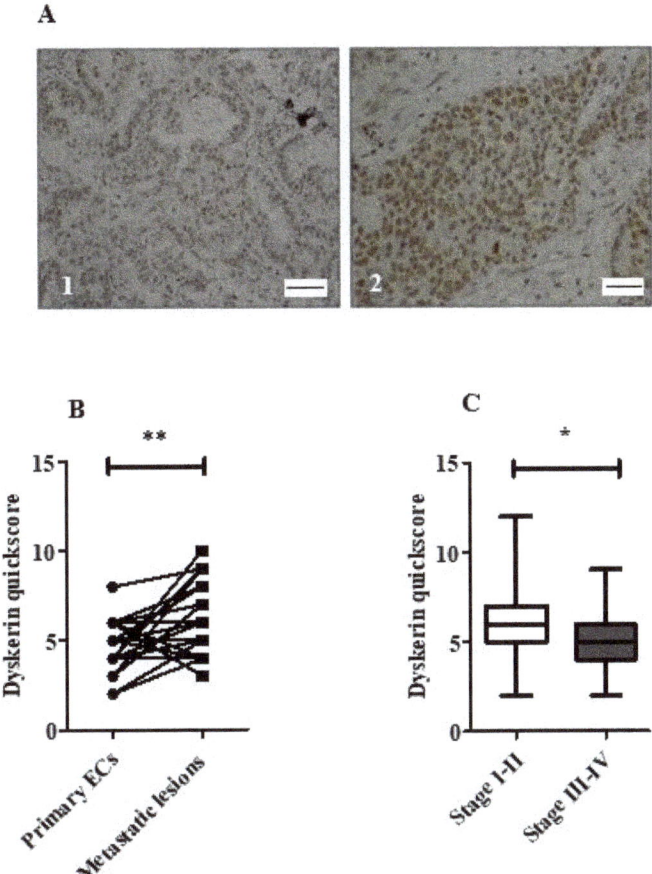

Figure 4. Dyskerin immunostaining in endometrial cancers. (**A**) Representative microphotographs illustrating dyskerin immunohistochemical staining in primary endometrial cancer (EC) (**1**) and matched metastatic lesion (**2**). Positive staining appears in brown. Magnification 400×, Scale bar 50 μm (**B**) Difference in dyskerin immunoscores in primary EC samples versus matched metastatic lesions (n = 30) each, ** p < 0.01. (**C**) Difference in dyskerin immunoscores between early-stage ECs (FIGO stage I–II) (n = 63) and advanced stage ECs (FIGO stage III–IV) (n = 43). Mann-Whitney test, * p < 0.05.

2.6. Endometrial Epithelial Dyskerin Immunoscores Correlate with ERβ Scores and Inversely with the Ki67 Proliferation Index (PI)

Dyskerin immunoscores in endometrial samples correlated with ERβ immunoscores (Spearman r = 0.46, p < 0.0001), while an inverse correlation was found with the Ki67 PI (Spearman r = −0.34, p < 0.0001). No correlation was identified with other steroid receptors' immunoscores (Table S1). Figure S7B shows immunostaining of dyskerin, Ki67 and steroid recepters.

2.7. Survival Analysis

According to the national guidance, patients were followed-up for at least 3 years after primary surgery in the two recruiting centers during the study period. By March 2020, follow-up data were available for 108 out of 109 women in our cohort [31]. During this follow-up period, there were 10 recurrent tumours and 38 deaths (27 as a result of disease progression and 11 from other causes). Worse outcomes were found in women with low dyskerin immunoscores. All outcomes analysed, including disease-free survival (DFS), cancer-specific survival (CSS), and overall survival (OS) suggested high dyskerin immunoscores to be potentially favourable ($p = 0.08$, $p = 0.07$, and $p = 0.06$, respectively, Figure 5A–C). For low dyskerin scores, the DFS hazard ratio (HR) = 1.92, 95% CI of HR (0.9200–4.006), CSS HR = 1.991, 95% CI of HR (0.9300–4.261), and OS HR = 1.841, 95% CI of HR (0.9667–3.506). When we only considered the endometrioid and serous ECs (similar to the selected TCGA EC dataset), low dyskerin immunoscores were still possibly suggestive of worse clinical outcomes with HR = 2.169, 95% CI of HR (0.7999–5.882), HR = 1.762, 95% CI of HR (0.5607–5.539) and HR = 1.698, 95% CI of HR (0.6925–4.165) for DFS, CSS, and OS, (Figure S7C–E), respectively. However, the p values were not significant (DFS, CSS, and OS; $p = 0.1$, $p = 0.3$, and $p = 0.2$, respectively) and confidence intervals were wide. These findings therefore need to be interpreted with caution and require future validation.

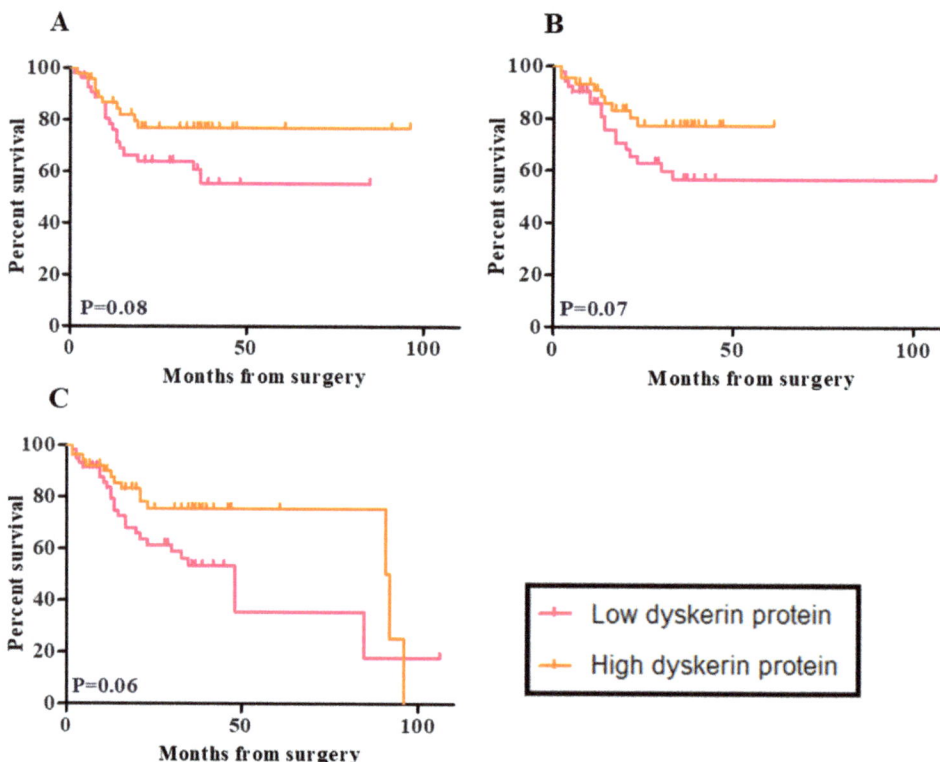

Figure 5. Kaplan Meier survival curves for the correlation between dyskerin immunoscores and patient outcome. (**A**) Disease-free survival (DFS), the median DFS time is undefined for low dyskerin and high dyskerin endometrial cancer groups. Hazard ratio (HR) = 1.92, 95% CI of the ratio (0.9200–4.006) (**B**) Cancer-specific survival (CSS), the median CSS time was undefined for low dyskerin and high dyskerin endometrial cancer groups. HR = 1.991, 95% CI of HR (0.9300–4.261) and (**C**) Overall survival (OS) in endometrial cancer samples (n = 109). Median OS time: Low dyskerin protein 8.00 months, High dyskerin protein 2.00 months. Low dyskerin/high dyskerin median survival Ratio: 0.5217, 95% CI of ratio (0.004444–1.039) HR = 1.841, 95% CI of HR (0.9667–3.506). A quickscore of 6 was chosen as the cut-off point. The p values relevant to the difference between low and high dyskerin protein levels in endometrial cancer groups that is visually represented in Kaplan Meier survival curves from the log-rank test.

When clinicopathological features were considered, dyskerin immunoscores inversely correlated with cervical invasion ($p = 0.01$, Table S2).

2.8. In Vitro Transient Transfection of ISK Cells with the DKC1 Gene Resulted in Successful Overexpression of Dyskerin Protein

A positive band corresponding to endogenous dyskerin was observed in negative controls (empty vector and non-transfected cells) and in transfected Ishikawa (ISK) cells at 6, 24, and 48 h after transfection (Figure 6A and Figure S8A). Exogenous dyskerin protein was first observed at 24 h and was still present at 48 h (although was decreased) in the DKC1 transfected cells (Figure 6A and Figure S8B).

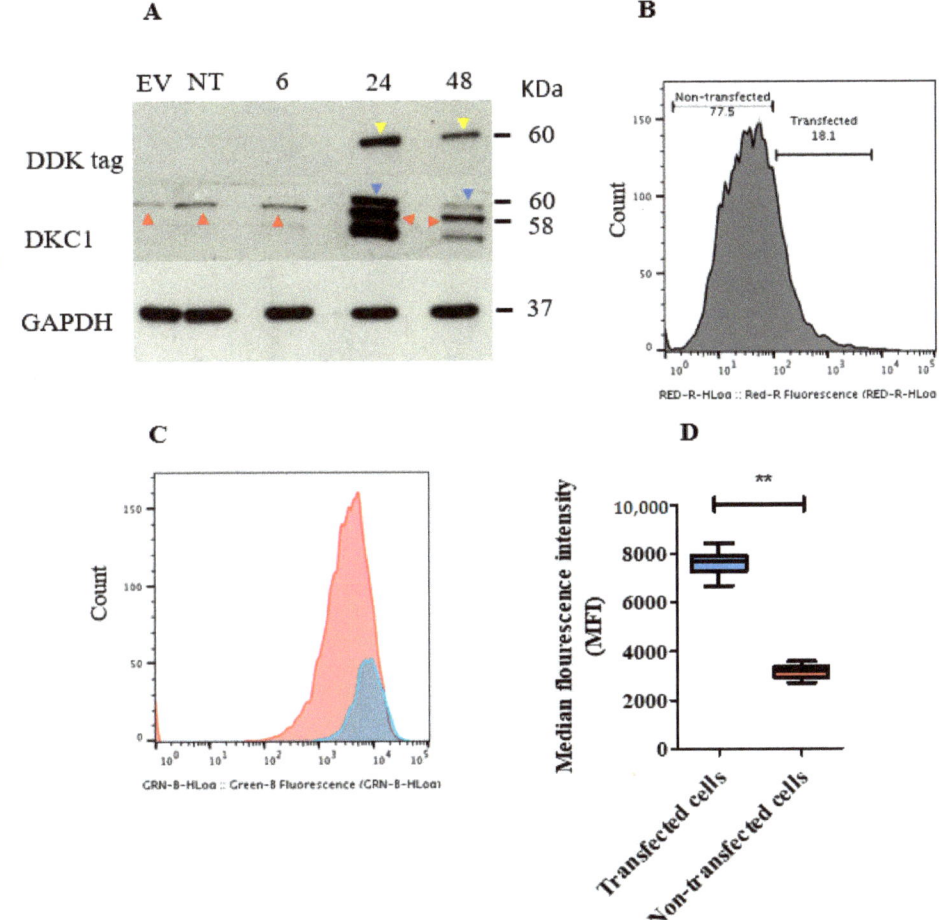

Figure 6. Transient overexpression of DKC1 in ISK cells. The plasmid and the empty vector (EV) used were tagged with the synthetic DYKDDDDK (DDK) protein to discern the transfected cells by using an anti-DDK antibody. (**A**) Immunoblot showing the level of dyskerin protein in DKC1 and EV transfected and non-transfected (NT) ISK cells. Cells were harvested 6, 24, and 48 h following transfection. Endogenous and exogenous dyskerin bands were present at the molecular weight of 58 and 60 KDa (red and blue arrows, respectively). DDK bands (yellow arrows) were observed at 60 KDa. Glyceraldehyde 3-Phosphate Dehydrogenase (GAPDH) bands were at 37 KDa. (**B**) Flow cytometric histogram showing the level of DDK tag protein in ISK cells. Cells positively stained with anti-DDK tag antibody represent transfected cells. (**C**) Cell proliferation was analysed using flow cytometry. ISK cells were stained with CellTrace Carboxyfluorescein Diacetate Succinimidyl Ester (CFSE) and fluorochrome-conjugated DDK Tag Antibody. Transfected cells (blue curve) and non-transfected cells (red curve). Higher proliferation is suggested when the curve was shifted to the left. (**D**) The difference in median fluorescence index (MFI) between transfected (T) and non-transfected ISK cells. ** $p < 0.01$, Wilcoxon signed-rank test.

A signal at the correct molecular weight (MW) demonstrates that the DDK tag peptide was present in transfected cells at 24 and 48 h only (Figure 6A and Figure S8C). Immunofluorescent staining with an anti-dyskerin antibody demonstrated the presence of endogenous dyskerin, characterised by a punctate pattern that was exclusively localised in the nuclei of all cells (cells transfected with *DKC1* and empty vector and in non-transfected cells) (Figure S8D) Exogenous dyskerin was located both in the nucleus and in the cytoplasm and observed only in *DKC1* transfected cells (Figure S8D).

Flow cytometric analysis of ISK cells 48 h after transfection revealed the transfection efficiency to be 18.1% in the dyskerin transfected cells (Figure 6B), 11% in the empty vector-transfected cells (Figure S9A), and 1.76% in the non-transfected control (false positive level) (Figure S9B). Figure S10 shows different negative staining controls used in the transient transfection experiment and Figure S11 shows the empty vector control map.

2.9. Transient Overexpression of the DKC1 Gene Reduced ISK Cell Proliferation In Vitro

Overexpression of *DKC1* reduced cellular proliferation rates (Figure 6C), as demonstrated by a significantly higher median fluorescence intensity (MFI) of Carboxyfluorescein Diacetate Succinimidyl Ester (CFSE) staining in *DKC1* transfected cells compared with the non-transfected cells ($p = 0.007$) (Figure 6D). Dyskerin transfected cells also have a lower proliferation rate compared with those transfected with the empty vector using an immune-staining method (Figure S12).

3. Discussion

To our knowledge, this is the first study to examine the expression of the telomerase core-component dyskerin in human endometrium. It validates the findings of our in silico interrogation of a published, large TCGA *DKC1* gene alteration profile of endometrioid and serous ECs, using a cohort of human ECs containing all histological EC-subtypes with transcriptional and protein data. We have demonstrated that healthy PP and PM endometrium express the *DKC1* gene and have detectable dyskerin protein levels. Importantly, EC samples have significantly lower dyskerin protein levels when compared with healthy PM controls. Our findings are important for the following reasons: (i) we examined the endometrial dyskerin protein levels with immunoblotting and at the cellular level with IHC for the first time; (ii) our local patient cohort consisted of all EC subtypes, including carcinosarcoma, dedifferentiated, mixed-cell adenocarcinoma and clear cell cancer types, precancerous EH samples and metastatic EC lesions, as well as external control healthy endometrium (both healthy PM and PP samples) to increase the generalisability of the data; (iii) Importantly, our data suggests a possible better clinical outcome in ECs containing high levels of dyskerin protein in comparison with those with lower dyskerin levels. Our data, therefore, fill the gaps in the current literature, including the TCGA dataset.

Sufficient dyskerin levels are required for competent TA to overcome telomere attrition [28]. *DKC1* dysregulation is associated with a high incidence of cancers in DC patients (reduced *DKC1*) and in *DKC1* hypomorphic mice [22], but no reports are available of DC associated with EC. Although high TA in over 90% of ECs had been reported, that is usually associated with short telomeres [32].

Examination of the TCGA dataset only identified *DKC1* out of the three core telomerase components to have an altered gene expression, with a prognostic relevance in ECs. Our data also suggests that dyskerin protein levels in ECs correlate with differences in patient outcomes. Variable dyskerin levels are also reported in other cancers [25,33]. Data from our cohort and the TCGA dataset jointly suggests a dysregulation of dyskerin in ECs. However, our cohort results differ from the TCGA data, and this discrepancy may be due to different "normal controls" used in the two studies and the fact that we examined protein rather than only mRNA levels. It is important to appreciate that endometrioid/serous ECs included in the TCGA data usually originate from a background of EHA or endometrial intraepithelial neoplasia (EIN). Thus, the normal tissue within 2 cm from the tumour included in the TCGA data as normal endometrium is likely to include hyperplastic tissue or EIN lesions. Our cohort data is more generalisable since we histologically confirmed our external healthy control tissue obtained from a well-characterised and age-matched population.

Many studies on different cancer types reported a high expression of the *DKC1* gene and dyskerin protein to be associated with poor prognosis [25,34]. For example, in contrast to our results on ECs, reports on prostate, hepatocellular carcinoma, and colorectal cancers showed that high *DKC1* is commonly associated with an extensive tumour growth pattern [25,34,35]. Recently, Elsharawy et al. showed that high DKC1 mRNA or protein levels in breast cancer associated with poor patient outcome and unfavourable clinicopathological characteristics [26]. In a recent study in breast cancer, *DKC1* over-expression associated with unfavourable clinicopathological characteristics and poor outcome [26]. Two publicly available "Breast Cancer Gene-Expression Miner v4.3" [26] and TCGA breast cancer datasets revealed high DKC1 mRNA levels to significantly correlate with larger tumour size, higher tumour grades, and poor prognosis. At the protein level, high dyskerin protein levels, whether in the nucleus and/or nucleoli, were reported to be associated with aggressive features in breast cancer [26]. In those tissues, however, carcinogenesis is associated with reactivation of TA compared with healthy tissues [36], whereas high TA is a feature of healthy PP endometrium [37]. Therefore, we suggest that ECs are different in this respect, and consequently, endometrial carcinogenesis seems to be associated with a reduction of dyskerin protein and *DKC1* gene expression.

Advanced primary ECs (stage-III and IV) had significantly lower dyskerin protein levels compared with early stages, suggesting that dyskerin protein may be useful in stratifying EC patients for further therapy after primary surgery. Prior reports have suggested metastatic EC lesions to demonstrate a regressed phenotype when compared with the matched primary tumour [38] which agrees well with our dyskerin data. The observed dyskerin loss we report may also produce a pro-oxidant environment in EC cells as demonstrated in other cancer cells [39]. Therefore, reduced dyskerin protein in the context of the excessive cellular division in ECs may contribute to genomic instability that is known to be present, particularly in more advanced ECs. Dyskerin deficiency may also contribute to carcinogenesis by adversely influencing the translational machinery via affecting the balance in ribosomal proteins [33] and by modifying the splicing of specific pre-mRNAs, or by altering the level of certain snoRNAs [40,41]. These mechanistic aspects need to be examined in future studies.

The healthy quiescent PM endometrium with absent cellular proliferative activity had high dyskerin levels. TA positively correlated with endometrial epithelial proliferation [13] and the downregulation of dyskerin protein in ECs in comparison with the healthy PM endometrium we observe, occurred in a background of high TA and Ki67 levels [18]. This suggests a tumour suppressor function [22] and an inhibitory effect on endometrial epithelial cell proliferation for dyskerin in ECs. Therefore, we sought to examine the functional consequence of overexpressing the *DKC1* gene on cell proliferation using a cell line that reflecting low grade ECs. Dyskerin knock-out is lethal, and thus all cells (independent of detectable TA) express the dyskerin gene/protein. The available *in vitro* *DKC1* gene manipulation studies had only examined knocking down of the *DKC1* gene [25] but not over-expression and they also did not examine cellular proliferation as an outcome. Knock-down studies in prostate carcinoma cells demonstrated dyskerin to be crucial in protein biosynthesis [25]. Both high and low dyskerin is associated with carcinogenesis [25], which fundamentally demonstrates the cardinal feature of excessive cellular proliferation. Our data demonstrates a consequential reduction in cell proliferation when dyskerin is overexpressed in the EC cell line, therefore establishing a functional effect of dyskerin on cell proliferation for the first time.

Reduction in dyskerin rendered human breast cancer cells to be more prone to incorrect codon recognition and induced a defect in rRNA uridine modification resulting in altered ribosome activity [42]. Low dyskerin expression levels correlated with poor overall survival of Chronic Lymphocytic Leukaemia (CLL) patients following chemotherapy [33].

The authors proposed that reduced dyskerin may cause a reduction of the synthesis of subsets of ribosomal proteins, and selectively alters the translatome of the cancer cells to increase their aggressiveness [33]. Loss of dyskerin dysregulates initiation of translation of tumour suppressor proteins such as p53 and p27 and thus may promote carcinogenesis [27,43]. In addition, dysregulation of p53 translation has been reported in DC patients with reduced dyskerin function via its internal ribosome entry segment being impaired resulting in increased cellular proliferation [44,45]. The exact mechanistic pathway by which dyskerin exerts this observed anti-proliferative effect on EC cells remains to be explored in future studies.

We used opportunistic recruitment and available archived samples in our study to answer our research question. This meant inclusion of retrospectively collected patient samples, and only a small proportion of cases seen in the centres over that time period were included in the study. Although this is a limitation of our study, since no previous data available for the levels of dyskerin protein in the EC, our study, which included a relatively sizeable EC cohort with associated important clinical details, fills the current gap in the literature, and provides significantly different results to inform sample sizes for adequately powered studies in the future.

Another limitation to our study is that we have included a similar number of LGEC and HGEC, meaning the stage distribution was skewed towards metastatic disease in the local cohort. This caused our sample to be deviated from the real incidence of non-endometrioid EC; however, this offers us a better assessment of HGECs, which are usually associated with poor prognosis. Although we have recruited women without known endometrial pathology as normal controls for EC samples, a potential limitation would be that all these control women were undergoing hysterectomy for a non-cancerous pathology, thus they may not represent asymptomatic and completely healthy normal women. Therefore, our findings require further validation in future prospective studies.

Endometrial TA and hTERT levels have been shown to be under hormonal regulation [13] and correspondingly, endometrial dyskerin immunoscores revealed a significant positive correlation with ERβ immunostaining. This may suggest dyskerin expression to be under estrogen regulation mainly via ERβ. ERβ is known to harness the estrogen-driven mitotic effect of ERα [46], therefore inducing dyskerin levels may also be a part of the ERβ-associated inhibition of the endometrial epithelial proliferation. Further studies are required to examine the hormonal regulation of dyskerin in human endometrium.

4. Materials and Methods

4.1. Study Groups:

4.1.1. TCGA Database Cohort

The publicly-available TCGA cohort of uterine cancers included data for RNA levels ($n = 477$), copy number variation ($n = 464$), and somatic mutation ($n = 235$); for *DKC1*, the data were interrogated using Illumina's Base Space Cohort Analyzer application (BSCA) [47] (Software; https://www.illumina.com/informatics/research/biological-data-interpretation/nextbio.html; Illumina, San Diego, CA, USA) [48]. The normal endometrial controls were obtained from 35 EC patients at 2–3 cm distance from the cancer margin [30].

4.1.2. Local Study Cohort

The study was performed in accordance with the Declaration of Helsinki. The Liverpool and Cambridge Adult Research Ethics Committees (LREC 09/H1005/55, 11/H1005/4 and CREC 10/H0308/75) approved the study. A total of 175 endometrial samples collected from women undergoing hysterectomy in the Liverpool Women's Hospital (LWH) and Lancashire Teaching Hospitals Trusts from 2009 to 2017 were included. Our cohort included a total of 15 endometrial samples with histological hyperplasia and cytological atypia were collected from patients undergoing hysterectomy at LWH. Out of these, three women had prior histological evidence of hyperplasia in an endometrial biopsy with ongoing symptoms of irregular or heavy menstrual bleeding; another 12 samples were from paraffin blocks of hyperplastic changes adjacent to EC that were retrieved from the Histopathology Department archive at the Royal Liverpool University Hospital.

Additionally, a total of 109 histologically confirmed EC samples from patients who underwent staging operations at LWH or at Lancashire Teaching Hospitals during the period between 2009 and 2017 were also recruited to the current study. Out of those 109 samples, 60 were pipelle biopsies collected at the time of their hysterectomy as part of their primary surgical treatment for EC. The remaining samples were paraffin blocks retrieved from the Histopathology Department archives at the Royal Liverpool University Hospital, or Lancaster Teaching Hospital. Paraffin blocks of 30 metastatic lesions from some of these women with ECs that were obtained during the same primary surgery were also studied. The sites of metastases were as follows: lymph nodes ($n = 11$), omentum ($n = 7$), parametrium ($n = 5$), soft tissue ($n = 4$), fallopian tube ($n = 1$), cervix ($n = 1$), and urinary bladder ($n = 1$).

None of the included EHA or EC patients had received hormonal treatment, chemotherapy, or pelvic radiation prior to surgery when the endometrial samples were harvested.

Demographic data are shown in Table 1. Experienced gynaecological pathologists confirmed the histological type and grade of EC specimens according to FIGO classification [49]. Considering the clinical relevant outcome, we further categorised the EC samples as low-grade (LGEC), consisting of grade 1 and grade 2 endometrioid EC or high-grade (HGEC), including grade 3 endometrioid, serous, clear cell carcinomas, carcinosarcoma, Mixed cell adenocarcinoma, and dedifferentiated ECs [43,50] as shown in Table 1. Healthy endometrial tissue specimens were collected from women undergoing hysterectomy for benign gynaecological pathologies such as prolapse or heavy bleeding without a known endometrial pathology (a full-thickness samples). Since EC is a disease mainly affecting postmenopausal (PM) women, 35 age-matched healthy endometrial tissue samples were included as an external control group. Some previous authors have suggested that the proliferative phase (PP) control samples were more suitable as a healthy comparator because EC is a proliferative disease; therefore, we also included a second external control group of 16 normal healthy premenopausal endometrial PP samples. Samples from healthy women were thus assigned to premenopausal (PP) and postmenopausal (PM) groups according to the last menstrual date and histological criteria [51].

4.2. Collection of Endometrial Samples

Once the uterus was removed at hysterectomy, in theatre, endometrial biopsies were collected by a trained member of the research team or the operating surgeon. Full-thickness endometrial biopsies were obtained from healthy women undergoing a hysterectomy, as previously described by cutting a thin slice of endometrium attached to underlying myometrium after opening the anterior uterine aspect in the coronal plane [52]. In order to avoid interference with pathological diagnosis and staging, samples from women undergoing primary surgery for EC were collected by using a pipelle suction curette (Laboratoire C.C.D., Paris, France). Each sample was split into two to three containers: (i) 15 mL 10% neutral buffered formalin (10% NBF) (Sigma, Dorset, UK) for immunohistochemistry study; (ii) 0.5 mL RNAlater (Sigma, Dorset, UK) for RNA extraction and PCR analysis; (iii) Immediately snap-frozen for immunoblotting and TRAP analysis.

4.3. Immunohistochemistry (IHC)

IHC was performed on 3 μm serial sections of formalin-fixed, paraffin-embedded endometrial tissue employing heat-induced antigen retrieval, and the ImmPRESS Polymerized Reporter Enzyme Staining System (Vector Laboratories, Peterborough, UK) as previously described [38]. The primary antibody sources, concentrations, and incubation conditions are detailed in Table S3.

Immunoreactivity for nuclear dyskerin was assessed using a modified quick score as previously described [53]. The four steroid receptors were evaluated semi-quantitatively using a four-tiered Liverpool endometrial steroid quick score (LESQS) as previously described [38]; the Ki67 proliferative index (PI) was evaluated as the percentage of positive cells of any intensity [38].

4.4. Real-Time qPCR

RNA was extracted, quantified, and reverse transcribed as previously described [53]. cDNA was amplified using iTaq universal SYBR Green supermix and CFX Connect Real-Time System (Bio-Rad, Hertfordshire, UK). Primers and reaction conditions are listed in Table S4 [35,54,55]. The $2^{-\Delta\Delta Ct}$ method was used to calculate relative transcript level. *DKC1* expression was normalised to *YWHAZ* and *PPIA* reference genes [56,57].

4.5. TRAP Assay

TA was measured using a TeloTAGGG™ TRAP assay (Sigma-Aldrich, Dorset, UK) according to the manufacturers' manual and as previously described [13]. Absorbance was measured at 450 nm in an Omega spectrophotometer (BMG, Labtech, UK) and presented as arbitrary units (AU). A total of 1 µg of protein was used per sample, and negative controls without protein were included and their absorption was subtracted from those of the samples.

4.6. Cell Culture

Cultured ISK cells were maintained in Dulbecco modified Eagle medium/F12 (DMEM/F12) supplemented with 10% (v/v) fetal bovine serum (FBS), L-glutamine, and penicillin/streptomycin at 37 °C in a 5% CO_2 atmosphere. All cell culture reagents were purchased from Sigma-Aldrich (Dorset, UK) as previously described [58].

4.7. Transient Transfection

Transfection of ISK cells was performed twenty-four hours after seeding cells on 6 well plates at a density of 0.5×10^6 cells/well by using a mixture of MYC-DDK tagged Dyskerin plasmid (OriGene Technologies, Rockville, MD, USA, 3 µL) with Lipofectamine 2000 (Thermo Fisher Scientific, Loughborough, UK, 9 µL). The plasmid or the Lipofectamine was diluted in 250 µL of Gibco Opti-MEM I (Thermo Fischer Scientific, Loughborough, UK). Empty vector (Myc-DDK tagged pCMV6-Entry) (OriGene Technologies, Rockville, MD, USA) and non-transfected cells were used as negative controls. The diluted plasmids and Lipofectamine were incubated for 20 min at room temperature. In the meantime, DMEM/F12 culture medium with supplements (FBS, L-glutamine and antibiotics) was replaced with the same medium but without antibiotics. A total of 4–6 h after transfection, the medium containing transfection reagents was removed and replaced with a fresh one supplemented with FBS, L-glutamine, and antibiotics. The cells were incubated at 37 °C, 5% CO_2. The plasmids used were tagged with the synthetic DYKDDDDK Tag (DDK) Tag protein to discern the transfected cells by using an anti-DDK antibody.

4.8. SDS-PAGE and Immunoblotting

Protein lysates from homogenised tissues and cultured cells were extracted using a Radioimmunoprecipitation assay (RIPA) buffer (Sigma-Aldrich, Dorset, UK) supplemented with protease inhibitor (Sigma-Aldrich, Dorset, UK) and phosphatase inhibitor (PhosSTOP, Roche Diagnostics Ltd., Burgess Hill, UK). Lysates were analysed by SDS-PAGE under reducing conditions on precast 12% gels (Mini-PROTEAN TGX, Bio-Rad, Hertfordshire, UK) and transferred to an Immune-Blot polyvinylidene difluoride (PVDF) membrane (Bio-Rad, Hertfordshire, UK). The primary antibody sources, concentrations, and incubation conditions are detailed in Table S3. Horseradish peroxidase (HRP)-linked secondary antibodies were from Thermo Fisher Scientific (Loughborough, UK). Signal detection was performed using SuperSignal West Dura Extended Duration chemiluminescent Substrate (Thermo Fisher Scientific, Loughborough, UK) and CL-Xposure film (Thermo Fisher Scientific, Loughborough, UK).

4.9. Immunofluorescence

In order to differentiate between endogenous dyskerin and exogenous overexpressed protein, immunofluorescent staining of dyskerin was performed, allowing examination of their respective location within ISK cell. Rabbit anti-dyskerin antibody (Santa Cruz Biotechnology, Dallas, TX, USA, 1:200) was added to the fixed cells, which were seeded onto coverslips in a 6 well plate. The secondary antibody was Alexa Fluor Anti-rabbit IgG (H + L), (Alexa Fluor 488 Conjugate), (Cell Signalling Technology, London, UK, 1:1000). The cells were mounted in DAPI containing medium (Vector Laboratories, Peterborough, UK,). Fluorescence was visualised with a Nikon Eclipse 50i microscope using NIS elements F software (Nikon, Tokyo, Japan). Rabbit and mouse isotype control antibodies were used as negative controls. Antibody details are provided in Table S3.

4.10. CFSE Labelling and Flow Cytometry

ISK Cells were initially labelled with CellTrace CFSE (Thermo Fisher Scientific, Loughborough, UK) according to manufacturers' guidelines, then fixed, permeabilised, and labelled with fluorochrome-conjugated primary antibody (anti-DYKDDDDK (DDK) Tag antibody [iFluor 647], Genscript, Piscataway, NJ, USA) and the corresponding fluorochrome-conjugated isotype control antibody (Alexa Fluor 647 antibody, Biolegend, UK). The cells were then incubated (1 h at 37 °C in the dark). A Guava EasyCyte flow cytometer (Millipore, Watford, UK) was used to perform flow cytometry and FlowJo v10 (Becton Dickinson, Franklin Lakes, NJ, USA) was used for data analysis.

4.11. Statistical Analysis

Statistical differences between groups were calculated by non-parametric tests (Kruskal–Wallis or Mann-Whitney U-test) using the Statistical Package for the Social Sciences (SPSS) version 24 (IBM Corp, Armonk, NY, USA). Descriptive values were presented as median and range. Graphs were plotted using GraphPad prism 5 (GraphPad Software, San Diego, CA, USA). The correlation between immunostaining scores was determined with a Spearman test and the association between dyskerin immunoscores and the multiple clinicopathological parameters were evaluated by Pearson's Chi-square test. The duration of DFS was measured from the date of surgery to the date of EC recurrence or death from EC, while the CSS duration was calculated from the date of surgery to the date of death from EC. OS duration was measured from the date of surgery to the date of death caused by any reason. All the observations were censored at the last date at which the patient was seen. Kaplan-Meier survival curves were constructed. Cumulative proportions of survivors in the high and low level of dyskerin protein were compared using Log-rank test. A significant difference between groups was only achieved with p value < 0.05. Significance values have been adjusted by Bonferroni correction for multiple tests.

5. Conclusions

Taking these observations together, we concluded that dyskerin protein and the *DKC1* gene are expressed in healthy endometrium [59] and in ECs. Low dyskerin immunoscores were potentially associated with worse outcomes, suggesting a possible prognostic relevance. Furthermore, increased dyskerin protein levels in ISK cells seem to inhibit cell proliferation, and therefore, the observed loss of dyskerin in endometrial cancer tissue may contribute to the increased cell proliferation and the progression of these ECs.

The detailed role of dyskerin in normal endometrial regeneration as well as in pathological conditions such as EC in the context of telomerase biology is yet to be determined. Since TA is known to play an intricate role in endometrial epithelial cellular proliferation, further studies elucidating the associated telomerase and other functions of dyskerin in the human endometrium and in EC are warranted.

Supplementary Materials: The following are available online at https://www.mdpi.com/2072-6694/13/2/273/s1, Table S1: Correlation between dyskerin quick scores with steroid receptors immunoscores and Ki67 proliferative index (PI) in endometrial samples. Table S2: Association between dyskerin protein immunoscores and clinicopathological parameters in EC samples. Table S3: Primary antibodies and conditions for IHC, immuno blotting and immunofluorescence. Table S4: Primer sequences used for qPCR amplification. Figure S1: Multi co-occurrence plot of somatic mutation, RNA level and copy number variation of *DKC1, TERT, and TERC* genes. Figure S2: Kaplan-Meier survival curve for the association between mutation status of the DKC1 gene and overall survival in endometrial cancers (ECs). Figure S3: Violin plot demonstrating the correlation between DKC1 RNA levels with tumour grades and stages. Figure S4: DKC1 RNA levels correlation with TERT and TERC RNA levels in The Cancer Genome Atlas (TCGA) dataset (endometrioid and serous endometrial cancers). Figure S5: Violin plot showing the association between DKC1 RNA levels with the mutation status: normal, mutant, or wild type + silence of TP53 and FGFR2 genes. Figure S6: Violin plot showing the association between DKC1 RNA levels and mutation status: normal, mutant or wildtype + silenceof PTEN and PIK3R1genes. Figure S7: Whole immunoblots, dyskerin, Ki67, and steroid receptors' immunohistochemical staining and the association of dyskerin immunoscores with survival outcome in endometrioid and serous EC samples {n = 77}. Figure S8: Transient overexpression of *DKC1* gene in ISK (Ishikawa) cells (Immunoblotting and immunofluorescence experiments). Figure S9: Negative controls used in the transient transfection experiment. Figure S10: Negative staining controls used in transient transfection experiment. Figure S11: pCMV6-Entry vector map. Figure S12: Transient overexpression of DKC1 in ISK cells.

Author Contributions: D.K.H. and P.M.-H. obtained the Ethical approval, and D.K.H. conceived the study design. D.K.H., R.A., and G.S. formulated experiments, analysed and interpreted data, produced figures, and produced the first draft. J.F. conducted the in silico study. Experimental data were produced by R.A., A.M., A.M.K., and G.S. with support from D.K.H. and S.E.C. The samples and outcome data were collected by D.K.H., L.D., P.N., S.B.D., P.M.-H., and H.S. All authors have read and agreed to the published version of the manuscript.

Funding: The authors would like to acknowledge the support from Wellbeing of Women project grant RG1487 and RG2137 (DKH) and Higher Committee for Education Development in Iraq (R.A.).

Institutional Review Board Statement: The study was performed in accordance with the Declaration of Helsinki. The Liverpool and Cambridge Adult Research Ethics Committees (LREC 09/H1005/55, 11/H1005/4 and CREC 10/H0308/75) approved the study.

Informed Consent Statement: Informed consent was obtained from all subjects involved in the study.

Data Availability Statement: Data is contained within the article or supplementary material.

Acknowledgments: The authors are grateful for Steven Lane for statistical advice, Josephine Drury and Kishen Popat for their help with immunohistochemistry, Stuart Ruthven of Royal Liverpool Hospital with supporting sample procurement, Helen Cox and Sarah Northey for assistance in preparing tissue sections, Lisa Heathcote for assistance with the BCA protein assay, Dada Pisconti for assistance with transient transfection, Phil Rudland, Stephane Gross, and Anthony Valentijn for assistance with immunoblotting, and Meera Adishesh for help with patient outcome data.

Conflicts of Interest: The authors declare no conflict of interest.

References

1. De Lange, T. Shelterin: The protein complex that shapes and safeguards human telomeres. *Genes Dev.* **2005**, *19*, 2100–2110. [CrossRef]
2. Griffith, J.D.; Comeau, L.; Rosenfield, S.; Stansel, R.M.; Bianchi, A.; Moss, H.; De Lange, T. Mammalian Telomeres End in a Large Duplex Loop. *Cell* **1999**, *97*, 503–514. [CrossRef]
3. Van Steensel, B.; Smogorzewska, A.; de Lange, T. TRF2 protects human telomeres from end-to-end fusions. *Cell* **1998**, *92*, 401–413. [CrossRef]
4. Levy, M.Z.; Allsopp, R.C.; Futcher, A.; Greider, C.W.; Harley, C.B. Telomere end-replication problem and cell aging. *J. Mol. Biol.* **1992**, *225*, 951–960. [CrossRef]
5. Von Zglinicki, T.; Saretzki, G.; Döcke, W.; Lotze, C. Mild hyperoxia shortens telomeres and inhibits proliferation of fibroblasts: A model for senescence? *Exp. Cell Res.* **1995**, *220*, 186–193. [CrossRef] [PubMed]

6. Campisi, J.; di Fagagna, F.D.A. Cellular senescence: When bad things happen to good cells. *Nat. Rev. Mol. Cell Biol.* **2007**, *8*, 729–740. [CrossRef] [PubMed]
7. Blackburn, E.H.; Greider, C.W.; Henderson, E.; Lee, M.S.; Shampay, J.; Shippen-Lentz, D. Recognition and elongation of telomeres by telomerase. *Genome* **1989**, *31*, 553–560. [CrossRef] [PubMed]
8. Cohen, S.B.; Graham, M.E.; Lovrecz, G.O.; Bache, N.; Robinson, P.J.; Reddel, R.R. Protein Composition of Catalytically Active Human Telomerase from Immortal Cells. *Science* **2007**, *315*, 1850–1853. [CrossRef]
9. Kim, N.W.; Piatyszek, M.A.; Prowse, K.R.; Harley, C.B.; West, M.D.; Ho, P.L.C.; Coviello, G.M.; Wright, W.E.; Weinrich, S.L.; Shay, J.W. Specific association of human telomerase activity with immortal cells and cancer. *Science* **1994**, *266*, 2011–2015. [CrossRef]
10. Liu, K.; Schoonmaker, M.M.; Levine, B.L.; June, C.H.; Hodes, R.J.; Weng, N.-P. Constitutive and regulated expression of telomerase reverse transcriptase (hTERT) in human lymphocytes. *Proc. Natl. Acad. Sci. USA* **1999**, *96*, 5147–5152. [CrossRef]
11. Yasumoto, S.; Kunimura, C.; Kikuchi, K.; Tahara, H.; Ohji, H.; Yamamoto, H.; Ide, T.; Utakoji, T. Telomerase activity in normal human epithelial cells. *Oncogene* **1996**, *13*, 433–439. [PubMed]
12. Hiyama, E.; Hiyama, K. Telomere and telomerase in stem cells. *Br. J. Cancer* **2007**, *96*, 1020–1024. [CrossRef] [PubMed]
13. Valentijn, A.J.; Saretzki, G.; Tempest, N.; Critchley, H.O.D.; Hapangama, D.K. Human endometrial epithelial telomerase is important for epithelial proliferation and glandular formation with potential implications in endometriosis. *Hum. Reprod.* **2015**, *30*, 2816–2828. [CrossRef] [PubMed]
14. Khattar, E.; Kumar, P.; Liu, C.Y.; Akıncılar, S.C.; Raju, A.; Lakshmanan, M.; Maury, J.J.P.; Qiang, Y.; Li, S.; Tan, E.Y.; et al. Telomerase reverse transcriptase promotes cancer cell proliferation by augmenting tRNA expression. *J. Clin. Investig.* **2016**, *126*, 4045–4060. [CrossRef] [PubMed]
15. Mistry, M.; Parkin, D.M.; Ahmad, A.S.; Sasieni, P. Cancer incidence in the United Kingdom: Projections to the year 2030. *Br. J. Cancer* **2011**, *105*, 1795–1803. [CrossRef]
16. CRUK. Uterine Cancer Statistics. Available online: http://www.cancerresearchuk.org/health-professional/cancer-statistics/statistics-by-cancer-type/uterine-cancer (accessed on 4 January 2020).
17. Kyo, S.; Kanaya, T.; Ishikawa, H.; Ueno, H.; Inoue, M. Telomerase activity in gynecological tumors. *Clin. Cancer Res.* **1996**, *2*, 2023–2028.
18. Ebina, Y.; Yamada, H.; Fujino, T.; Furuta, I.; Sakuragi, N.; Yamamoto, R.; Katoh, M.; Oshimura, M.; Fujimoto, S. Telomerase activity correlates with histo-pathological factors in uterine endometrial carcinoma. *Int. J. Cancer* **1999**, *84*, 529–532. [CrossRef]
19. Marrone, A.; Mason, P.J. Dyskeratosis congenita. *Cell Mol. Life Sci.* **2003**, *60*, 507–517. [CrossRef]
20. Montanaro, L.; Calienni, M.; Ceccarelli, C.; Santini, N.; Taffurelli, M.; Pileri, S.; Treré, D.; Derenzini, M. Relationship between Dyskerin Expression and Telomerase Activity in Human Breast Cancer. *Cell. Oncol.* **2008**, *30*, 483–490.
21. Montanaro, L.; Brigotti, M.; Clohessy, J.; Barbieri, S.; Ceccarelli, C.; Santini, D.; Taffurelli, M.; Calienni, M.; Teruya-Feldstein, J.; Treré, D.; et al. Dyskerin expression influences the level of ribosomal RNA pseudo-uridylation and telomerase RNA component in human breast cancer. *J. Pathol.* **2006**, *210*, 10–18. [CrossRef]
22. Ruggero, D.; Grisendi, S.; Piazza, F.; Rego, E.; Mari, F.; Rao, P.H.; Cordon-Cardo, C.; Pandolfi, P.P. Dyskeratosis Congenita and Cancer in Mice Deficient in Ribosomal RNA Modification. *Science* **2003**, *299*, 259–262. [CrossRef] [PubMed]
23. Alawi, F.; Lin, P. Dyskerin is required for tumor cell growth through mechanisms that are independent of its role in te-lomerase and only partially related to its function in precursor rRNA processing. *Mol. Carcinog.* **2011**, *50*, 334–345. [CrossRef] [PubMed]
24. Alnafakh, R.A.A.; Adishesh, M.; Button, L.; Saretzki, G.; Hapangama, D.K. Telomerase and Telomeres in Endometrial Cancer. *Front. Oncol.* **2019**, *9*, 344. [CrossRef] [PubMed]
25. Sieron, P.; Hader, C.; Hatina, J.; Engers, R.; Wlazlinski, A.; Müller, M.; Schulz, W.A. DKC1 overexpression associated with prostate cancer progression. *Br. J. Cancer* **2009**, *101*, 1410–1416. [CrossRef] [PubMed]
26. ElSharawy, K.A.; Mohammed, O.J.; Aleskandarany, M.A.; Hyder, A.; El-Gammal, H.L.; Abou-Dobara, M.I.; Green, A.R.; Dalton, L.W.; Rakha, E.A. The nucleolar-related protein Dyskerin pseudouridine synthase 1 (DKC1) predicts poor prognosis in breast cancer. *Br. J. Cancer* **2020**, *123*, 1543–1552. [CrossRef]
27. Bellodi, C.; Krasnykh, O.; Haynes, N.; Theodoropoulou, M.; Peng, G.; Montanaro, L.; Ruggero, D. Loss of function of the tumor suppressor DKC1 perturbs p27 translation control and contributes to pituitary tumorigenesis. *Cancer Res.* **2010**, *70*, 6026–6035. [CrossRef] [PubMed]
28. Parry, E.M.; Alder, J.K.; Lee, S.S.; Phillips, J.A.; Loyd, J.E.; Duggal, P.; Armanios, M. Decreased dyskerin levels as a mechanism of telomere shortening in X-linked dyskeratosis congenita. *J. Med. Genet.* **2011**, *48*, 327–333. [CrossRef]
29. Alter, B.P.; Giri, N.; Savage, S.A.; Rosenberg, P.S. Cancer in dyskeratosis congenita. *Blood* **2009**, *113*, 6549–6557. [CrossRef] [PubMed]
30. Huang, X.; Stern, D.F.; Zhao, H. Transcriptional Profiles from Paired Normal Samples Offer Complementary Information on Cancer Patient Survival—Evidence from TCGA Pan-Cancer Data. *Sci. Rep.* **2016**, *6*, 20567. [CrossRef]
31. Sundar, S.; Balega, J.; Crosbie, E.; Drake, A.; Edmondson, R.; Fotopoulou, C.; Gallos, I.; Ganesan, R.; Gupta, J.; Johnson, N.; et al. BGCS uterine cancer guidelines: Recommendations for practice. *Eur. J. Obs. Gynecol. Reprod. Biol.* **2017**, *213*, 71–97. [CrossRef]
32. Wang, S.-J.; Sakamoto, T.; Yasuda, S.-I.; Fukasawa, I.; Ota, Y.; Hayashi, M.; Okura, T.; Zheng, J.-H.; Inaba, N. The Relationship between Telomere Length and Telomerase Activity in Gynecologic Cancers. *Gynecol. Oncol.* **2002**, *84*, 81–84. [CrossRef]

33. Sbarrato, T.; Horvilleur, E.; Pöyry, T.; Hill, K.; Chaplin, L.C.; Spriggs, R.V.; Stoneley, M.; Wilson, L.; Jayne, S.; Vulliamy, T.; et al. A ribosome-related signature in peripheral blood CLL B cells is linked to reduced survival following treat-ment. *Cell Death Dis.* **2016**, *7*, e2249. [CrossRef] [PubMed]
34. Liu, B.; Zhang, J.; Huang, C.; Liu, H. Dyskerin Overexpression in Human Hepatocellular Carcinoma Is Associated with Advanced Clinical Stage and Poor Patient Prognosis. *PLoS ONE* **2012**, *7*, e43147. [CrossRef] [PubMed]
35. Turano, M.; Angrisani, A.; De Rosa, M.; Izzo, P.; Furia, M. Real-time PCR quantification of human DKC1 expression in colorectal cancer. *Acta Oncol.* **2008**, *47*, 1598–1599. [CrossRef]
36. Chen, C.-H.; Chen, R.-J. Prevalence of Telomerase Activity in Human Cancer. *J. Med. Assoc.* **2011**, *110*, 275–289. [CrossRef]
37. Tanaka, M.; Kyo, S.; Takakura, M.; Kanaya, T.; Sagawa, T.; Yamashita, K.; Okada, Y.; Hiyama, E.; Inoue, M. Expression of telomerase activity in human endometrium is localized to epithelial glandular cells and regu-lated in a menstrual phase-dependent manner correlated with cell proliferation. *Am. J. Pathol.* **1998**, *153*, 1985–1991. [CrossRef]
38. Kamal, A.M.; Bulmer, J.N.; DeCruze, S.B.; Stringfellow, H.F.; Martin-Hirsch, P.; Hapangama, D.K. Androgen receptors are acquired by healthy postmenopausal endometrial epithelium and their subsequent loss in endometrial cancer is associated with poor survival. *Br. J. Cancer* **2016**, *114*, 688–696. [CrossRef] [PubMed]
39. Ibáñez-Cabellos, J.S.; Pérez-Machado, G.; Seco-Cervera, M.; Berenguer-Pascual, E.; García-Giménez, J.L.; Pallardó, F.V. Acute telomerase components depletion triggers oxidative stress as an early event previous to telomeric shortening. *Redox Biol.* **2018**, *14*, 398–408. [CrossRef]
40. Angrisani, A.; Vicidomini, R.; Turano, M.; Furia, M. Human dyskerin: Beyond telomeres. *Biol. Chem.* **2014**, *395*, 593–610. [CrossRef]
41. Dos Santos, P.C.; Panero, J.; Stanganelli, C.; Nagore, V.P.; Stella, F.; Bezares, R.; Slavutsky, I. Dysregulation of H/ACA ribonucleo-protein components in chronic lymphocytic leukemia. *PLoS ONE* **2017**, *12*, e0179883. [CrossRef]
42. Penzo, M.; Rocchi, L.; Brugiere, S.; Carnicelli, D.; Onofrillo, C.; Couté, Y.; Brigotti, M.; Montanaro, L. Human ribosomes from cells with reduced dyskerin levels are intrinsically altered in translation. *FASEB J.* **2015**, *29*, 3472–3482. [CrossRef] [PubMed]
43. Montanaro, L.; Calienni, M.; Bertoni, S.; Rocchi, L.; Sansone, P.; Storci, G.; Santini, D.; Ceccarelli, C.; Taffurelli, M.; Carni-celli, D.; et al. Novel Dyskerin-Mediated Mechanism of p53 Inactivation through Defective mRNA Translation. *Cancer Res.* **2010**, *70*, 4767–4777. [CrossRef] [PubMed]
44. Carrillo, J.; González, A.; Manguán-García, C.; Pintado-Berninches, L.; Perona, R. p53 pathway activation by telomere attrition in X-DC primary fibroblasts occurs in the absence of ribosome biogenesis failure and as a consequence of DNA damage. *Clin. Transl. Oncol.* **2013**, *16*, 529–538. [CrossRef]
45. Bellodi, C.; Kopmar, N.; Ruggero, D. Deregulation of oncogene-induced senescence and p53 translational control in X-linked dyskeratosis congenita. *EMBO J.* **2010**, *29*, 1865–1876. [CrossRef] [PubMed]
46. Hapangama, D.K.; Kamal, A.; Bulmer, J. Estrogen receptor β: The guardian of the endometrium. *Hum. Reprod. Updat.* **2015**, *21*, 174–193. [CrossRef] [PubMed]
47. Kupershmidt, I.; Su, Q.J.; Grewal, A.; Sundaresh, S.; Halperin, I.; Flynn, J.; Shekar, M.; Wang, H.; Park, J.; Cui, W.; et al. Ontology-Based Meta-Analysis of Global Collections of High-Throughput Public Data. *PLoS ONE* **2010**, *5*, e13066. [CrossRef]
48. Robinson, M.D.; McCarthy, D.J.; Smyth, G.K. edgeR: A Bioconductor package for differential expression analysis of digital gene expression data. *Bioinformatics* **2009**, *26*, 139–140. [CrossRef] [PubMed]
49. Zaino, R.J.; Kurman, R.J.; Diana, K.L.; Paul Morrow, C. The utility of the revised International Federation of Gynecology and Obstetrics histologic grading of endometrial adenocarcinoma using a defined nuclear grading system. A Gynecologic Oncology Group study. *Cancer* **1995**, *75*, 81–86. [CrossRef]
50. Vossa, M.A.; Ganesan, R.; Ludeman, L.; McCarthy, K.; Gornall, R.; Schaller, G.; Wei, W.; Sundar, S. Should grade 3 endometrioid endometrial carcinoma be considered a type 2 cancer-a clinical and patholog-ical evaluation. *Gynecol. Oncol.* **2012**, *124*, 15–20. [CrossRef]
51. Noyes, R.W.; Hertig, A.T.; Rock, J. Dating the endometrial biopsy. *Am. J. Obs. Gynecol.* **1975**, *122*, 262–263. [CrossRef]
52. MacLean, A.; Kamal, A.M.; Adishesh, M.; Alnafakh, R.; Tempest, N.; Hapangama, D.K. Human Uterine Biopsy: Research Value and Common Pitfalls. *Int. J. Reprod. Med.* **2020**, *2020*, 9275360. [CrossRef] [PubMed]
53. Mathew, D.; Drury, J.A.; Valentijn, A.J.; Vasieva, O.; Hapangama, D.K. In silico, in vitro and in vivo analysis identifies a potential role for steroid hormone regulation of FOXD3 in endometriosis-associated genes. *Hum. Reprod.* **2016**, *31*, 345–354. [PubMed]
54. Jacob, F.; Guertler, R.; Naim, S.; Nixdorf, S.; Fedier, A.; Hacker, N.F.; Heinzelmann-Schwarz, V. Careful selection of reference genes is required for reliable performance of RT-qPCR in human normal and cancer cell lines. *PLoS ONE* **2013**, *8*, e59180. [CrossRef] [PubMed]
55. Marullo, M.; Zuccato, C.; Mariotti, C.; Lahiri, N.; Tabrizi, S.J.; Di Donato, S.; Cattaneo, E. Expressed Alu repeats as a novel, reliable tool for normalization of real-time quantitative RT-PCR data. *Genome Biol.* **2010**, *11*, R9. [CrossRef]
56. Romani, C.; Calza, S.; Todeschini, P.; Tassi, R.A.; Zanotti, L.; Bandiera, E.; Sartori, E.; Pecorelli, S.; Ravaggi, A.; Santin, A.D.; et al. Identification of optimal reference genes for gene expression normalization in a wide cohort of endometri-oid endometrial carcinoma tissues. *PLoS ONE* **2014**, *9*, e113781. [CrossRef]

57. Sadek, K.H.; Cagampang, F.R.; Bruce, K.D.; Shreeve, N.; Macklon, N.; Cheong, Y. Variation in stability of housekeeping genes in endometrium of healthy and polycystic ovarian syndrome women. *Hum. Reprod.* **2011**, *27*, 251–256. [CrossRef]
58. Parkes, C.; Kamal, A.; Valentijn, A.J.; Alnafakh, R.; Gross, S.R.; Barraclough, R.; Moss, D.; Kirwan, J.; Hapangama, D.K. Assessing Estrogen-Induced Proliferative Response in an Endometrial Cancer Cell Line Using a Universally Applicable Methodological Guide. *Int. J. Gynecol. Cancer* **2018**, *28*, 122–133. [CrossRef]
59. Alnafakh, R.; Choi, F.; Bradfield, A.; Adishesh, M.; Saretzki, G.; Hapangama, D.K. Endometriosis Is Associated with a Significant Increase in hTERC and Altered Telomere/Telomerase Associated Genes in the Eutopic Endometrium, an Ex-Vivo and In Silico Study. *Biomedicines* **2020**, *8*, 588. [CrossRef]

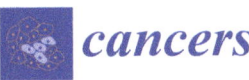

Article

Metabolomic Biomarkers for the Detection of Obesity-Driven Endometrial Cancer

Kelechi Njoku [1,2,3], Amy E. Campbell [3], Bethany Geary [3], Michelle L. MacKintosh [1,2], Abigail E. Derbyshire [1,2], Sarah J. Kitson [1,2], Vanitha N. Sivalingam [1,2], Andrew Pierce [4], Anthony D. Whetton [3,4,*,†] and Emma J. Crosbie [1,2,*,†]

1. Division of Cancer Sciences, Faculty of Biology, Medicine and Health, University of Manchester, 5th Floor Research, St Mary's Hospital, Oxford Road, Manchester M13 9WL, UK; kelechi.njoku@manchester.ac.uk (K.N.); michelle.mackintosh@mft.nhs.uk (M.L.M.); abiderbyshire@doctors.org.uk (A.E.D.); sarah.kitson@manchester.ac.uk (S.J.K.); vanitha.sivalingam@manchester.ac.uk (V.N.S.)
2. Department of Obstetrics and Gynaecology, Manchester Academic Health Science Centre, Manchester University NHS Foundation Trust, Manchester M13 9WL, UK
3. Stoller Biomarker Discovery Centre, Division of Cancer Sciences, Faculty of Biology, Medicine and Health, University of Manchester, Manchester M13 9PL, UK; amy.campbell@manchester.ac.uk (A.E.C.); bethany.geary@manchester.ac.uk (B.G.)
4. Wolfson Molecular Imaging Centre, Division of Cancer Sciences, University of Manchester, Palatine Road, Manchester M20 3LJ, UK; andrew.pierce@manchester.ac.uk
* Correspondence: tony.whetton@manchester.ac.uk (A.D.W.); emma.crosbie@manchester.ac.uk (E.J.C.); Tel.: +44-161-275-0038 (A.D.W.); +44-161-701-6942 (E.J.C.)
† These authors contributed equally to this paper as senior authors.

Citation: Njoku, K.; Campbell, A.E.; Geary, B.; MacKintosh, M.L.; Derbyshire, A.E.; Kitson, S.J.; Sivalingam, V.N.; Pierce, A.; Whetton, A.D.; Crosbie, E.J. Metabolomic Biomarkers for the Detection of Obesity-Driven Endometrial Cancer. *Cancers* 2021, *13*, 718. https://doi.org/10.3390/cancers13040718

Academic Editor: Eduardo Nagore
Received: 30 December 2020
Accepted: 6 February 2021
Published: 10 February 2021

Publisher's Note: MDPI stays neutral with regard to jurisdictional claims in published maps and institutional affiliations.

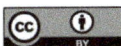

Copyright: © 2021 by the authors. Licensee MDPI, Basel, Switzerland. This article is an open access article distributed under the terms and conditions of the Creative Commons Attribution (CC BY) license (https://creativecommons.org/licenses/by/4.0/).

Simple Summary: Endometrial cancer is the commonest cancer of the female genital tract and obesity is its main modifiable risk factor. Over 80% of endometrial cancers develop in the context of obesity-induced metabolic changes. This study focuses on the potential of plasma-based metabolites to enable the early detection of endometrial cancer in a cohort of women with body mass index (BMI) ≥ 30 kg/m^2. Specific lipid metabolites including phospholipids and sphingolipids (sphingomyelins) demonstrated good accuracy for the detection of endometrial cancer, especially when combined in a diagnostic model. This study advances our knowledge of the role of metabolomics in endometrial cancer and provides a basis for the minimally invasive screening of women with elevated BMI.

Abstract: Endometrial cancer is the most common malignancy of the female genital tract and a major cause of morbidity and mortality in women. Early detection is key to ensuring good outcomes but a lack of minimally invasive screening tools is a significant barrier. Most endometrial cancers are obesity-driven and develop in the context of severe metabolomic dysfunction. Blood-derived metabolites may therefore provide clinically relevant biomarkers for endometrial cancer detection. In this study, we analysed plasma samples of women with body mass index (BMI) ≥ 30 kg/m^2 and endometrioid endometrial cancer (cases, $n = 67$) or histologically normal endometrium (controls, $n = 69$), using a mass spectrometry-based metabolomics approach. Eighty percent of the samples were randomly selected to serve as a training set and the remaining 20% were used to qualify test performance. Robust predictive models (AUC > 0.9) for endometrial cancer detection based on artificial intelligence algorithms were developed and validated. Phospholipids were of significance as biomarkers of endometrial cancer, with sphingolipids (sphingomyelins) discriminatory in postmenopausal women. An algorithm combining the top ten performing metabolites showed 92.6% prediction accuracy (AUC of 0.95) for endometrial cancer detection. These results suggest that a simple blood test could enable the early detection of endometrial cancer and provide the basis for a minimally invasive screening tool for women with a BMI ≥ 30 kg/m^2.

Keywords: endometrial cancer; obesity; metabolomics; liquid biopsy; mass spectrometry; plasma biomarkers; artificial intelligence

1. Introduction

Endometrial cancer is the most common gynaecological malignancy in the United Kingdom, where its incidence is rising in parallel with the obesity epidemic [1]. Obesity is the major risk factor for type I cancers of low-grade endometrioid morphology, with every 5 kg/m^2 increase in body mass index (BMI) linked to a 60% increased cancer risk [2]. Almost half of all endometrial cancers are attributed to overweight (BMI $\geq$ 25 kg/m^2) and obesity (BMI $\geq$ 30 kg/m^2) [3]. The strong dose–response relationship portends a 10–15% lifetime risk of endometrial cancer in women with class III obesity (BMI $\geq$ 40 kg/m^2) compared with a population average of 2% [4]. Whilst its aetiological importance is clear, the biology underpinning obesity-driven endometrial carcinogenesis is incompletely understood [5]. Adipose tissue is a rich source of oestrogens that stimulate endometrial proliferation, particularly when unopposed by progesterone in postmenopausal and anovulatory states [6]. Metabolically unhealthy obesity, rather than excess bodyweight per se, is of particular aetiological significance, with impaired glucose tolerance and chronic insulin resistance acting synergistically to increase endometrial cancer risk [7]. Type 2 diabetes mellitus is associated with a 62% upsurge [8], and uncontrolled diabetes mellitus a nearly five-fold greater susceptibility to endometrial cancer [9].

A recent study found occult endometrial abnormalities in 14% of women with class III obesity referred for weight loss management [10]. All but one had low-grade early-stage endometrial cancer or its precursor lesion, atypical hyperplasia. The early identification of these abnormalities in asymptomatic women could enable conservative management strategies that preserve fertility and/or reduce the morbidity of surgery [11,12]. Yet, no current screening programme exists for these high-risk women, partly because current diagnostics are invasive with low acceptability profiles and/or poor diagnostic accuracy [13]. A simple, minimally invasive endometrial cancer screening tool that can triage high-risk women for diagnostic workup, whilst safely reassuring those at low risk, would represent a major advance in the field [14,15].

High-throughput technologies and machine learning techniques have emerged as powerful tools for biomarker discovery and validation [15–19]. Metabolomics studies the downstream products of genomic, transcriptomic, and proteomic processes and best mirrors the human phenotype [20,21]. Thus, metabolomics has great potential to deliver clinically relevant biomarkers for endometrial cancer detection [22]. A blood-based test for cancer has broad appeal, being rated the second most important research priority for detecting cancer early in our recent James Lind Alliance Priority Setting Partnership [23]. A significant challenge is identifying cancer-relevant biomarkers within the context of severe metabolic dysfunction that characterises endometrial cancer risk. Here, we investigate the potential of plasma-based metabolites to detect endometrial cancer in a cohort of women with class III obesity, using a mass spectrometry-based metabolomics approach.

2. Materials and Methods

2.1. Study Population

This study included women with BMI $\geq$ 30 kg/m^2 participating in clinical research, who donated blood samples and gave written, informed consent for their pseudo-anonymised data to be used for future research. The primary research studies received approval from the North West and Cambridge East Research Ethics Committees and were conducted according to the principles of the Declaration of Helsinki. Cases and controls were recruited at Manchester University and Salford Royal NHS Foundation Trusts, United Kingdom. Cases were confirmed to have endometrioid endometrial cancer based on specialist histopathological assessment of biopsy and/or hysterectomy specimens [24,25]. Controls were women referred for weight loss management and confirmed to have normal histology on endometrial biopsy [10]. Clinicopathological data included age, BMI, smoking status, menopausal status, parity, type 2 diabetes mellitus status and medications used. All tissue specimens were assessed by at least two specialist gynaecological pathologists reporting according to UK Royal College of Pathology standards. Blood samples were collected following an overnight fast. Study investigators were blinded to the clinical information and biopsy results of subjects during acquisition of metabolomics data.

2.2. Metabolomic Profiling

Blood samples were collected in standard EDTA tubes, centrifuged at 2000 rpm for 10 min and the supernatant (plasma) was collected and stored at −80 °C. The samples were subsequently shipped to Metabolon Inc®, Durham, NC, USA, on dry ice and maintained at −80 °C until processed. Non-targeted MS metabolomic analysis was performed by Metabolon Inc®, according to company protocols and is summarised below.

2.2.1. Sample Preparation

Sample preparation was carried out using the automated MicroLab STAR® liquid handling system (Hamilton Company, Reno, NV, USA). Recovery standards were added to the samples prior to extraction for quality control purposes. To optimise the recovery of chemically diverse metabolites, proteins were removed by precipitation with methanol under vigorous shaking GenoGrinder 2000 by Glen Mills Inc., Clifton, NJ, USA) followed by centrifugation. The resulting extract was split into four aliquots and prepared for subsequent analysis using solvents compatible with the various separation and detection methods. Zymark TurboVap concentration evaporator (SOTAX AG, Aesch, Switzerland) was used to remove organic solvents.

2.2.2. Metabolite Separation and Detection

Multiple methods were used for metabolite separation and identification to maximise the number of metabolites detected. All methods were performed using a Waters ACQUITY ultra-performance liquid chromatography (UPLC) system (Waters Corporation, Milford, MA, USA) and a Thermo Scientific Q-Exactive high resolution/accurate mass spectrometer (ThermoFisher Scientific, Waltham, MA, USA). This was interfaced with a heated electrospray ionisation (HESI-II) source and Orbitrap mass analyzer operating at 35,000 mass resolution. Three sample extract aliquots were analysed using reversed phase UPLC with tandem mass spectrometry (RP UHPLCMS/MS). A positive ion mode electrospray ionisation (ESI) was used for two aliquots chromatographically optimised for more hydrophilic and more hydrophobic compounds, respectively, and a negative ion mode ESI for the third aliquot. The fourth aliquot was analysed using negative ion mode ESI following elution from a hydrophilic interaction liquid chromatography column (HILIC UPLCMS/MS). The chromatographic conditions used and optimised for the various metabolite species are summarised in Table S1.

2.2.3. Metabolite Identification

Raw data including molecular and fragment ions were searched against a reference library of over 14,000 metabolites based on authenticated standards. Metabolites were identified based on their chromatographic features (including MS/MS spectra), retention time/index (RI) and mass-to-charge ratio (m/z). The specific criteria used for biochemical identification included a retention index within a narrow window of the proposed identification and an accurate mass match to the library ± 10 ppm. MS/MS forward and reverse scores were used to control for false discovery rates. Ions that lacked a definite biochemical identity were given a numerical designation. Data curation was carried out by Metabolon, Inc, Durham, NC, USA data analysts to ensure accurate and consistent identification of metabolites as well as removal of artefacts, misassignments and background noise. Peak quantification was carried out using area under the curve analysis. Comparison of the peak area of a given metabolite in the sample to the peak area of a standard of known concentration was used to determine the metabolite concentration.

2.2.4. Data Pre-Processing

Metabolite concentrations were reported in the form of standardised intensities. Each metabolite concentration was rescaled to set the median equal to 1 (by dividing the concentration of each metabolite by the median). Thus, the concentration of a given metabolite in a given sample was made relative to the median concentration of all the samples processed as part of the study. The presence of missing values in this study was indicated by the concentration of a given metabolite falling below an assay's limit of detection (LOD). Missing metabolite concentrations were imputed with a standardised intensity set at the minimum detected value for that compound.

2.3. Data Analysis

All statistical analyses were performed using R version 3.2.5 (R Development Core Team, Vienna, Austria), STATA version 16, and MetaboAnalyst 4.0. The Shapiro–Wilk test was used to assess normality of continuous variables. Descriptive analyses of the study demographic data (continuous and categorical) were performed using means ($\pm$standard deviations) and counts (%), respectively, with differences between groups assessed using Student's t-test for continuous variables and the chi-square test for categorical variables. The majority of the metabolite concentrations (median scaled standardised intensity) were not normally distributed. As such, non-parametric tests were used in subsequent analysis. Specifically, the Mann–Whitney U test was used to compare metabolite concentrations in the cancer group versus control group and for other group comparisons made. We applied a false discovery rate adjustment for multiple testing using the Benjamini–Hochberg correction method (q = 0.05). A computation of the ratio of metabolite concentrations in cases and controls was used to identify the direction and degree of fold change and allowed for the identification of the groups of metabolites with unidirectional alterations. Principal component analysis (PCA) and t-distributed stochastic neighbour embedding (t-SNE) plots were used to assess degree of separation between groups. Random forest modelling was used to identify the best-performing biomarkers and to develop predictive models for the detection of endometrial cancer. Eighty per cent of the samples were randomly selected to serve as a "training set" and the remaining 20% were used to test the model. Heat maps were generated based on hierarchical clustering of the top discriminatory metabolites using the Euclidean distance measure and the Ward algorithm. Row scaling (heat maps) was performed for each metabolite by the subtraction of the mean from each feature and then dividing by the standard deviation. Area under the receiver-operator characteristic curves (AUC) and the 95% confidence intervals were computed for both metabolites and metabolomics signatures. The selection of cut-off points was based on the Youden Index (J = max {Sensitivity + Specificity $-$ 1}).

An overview of the study workflow is summarised in Figure S1.

3. Results

3.1. Participant Demographics

The study comprised 136 women with BMI $\geq$ 30kg/m^2 of whom 67 had endometrioid endometrial cancer (cases) and 69 had histologically normal endometrium (controls). The median age and BMI for the cohort was 54 years (IQR 43, 65) and 46 kg/m^2 (IQR 39, 52) respectively. Cases were older and more likely to be post-menopausal and nulliparous while controls were more obese. The majority of the endometrial cancers were low-grade (91.0% grades I/II), early-stage (88.0% stage I) cancers with lymphovascular space invasion occurring in only 12 women (18.0% of cases) (Table 1). Participant demographics and clinicopathological characteristics are summarised in Table 1.

Table 1. Clinicopathological characteristics of the cohort.

Participant Characteristics	Total Cohort (n = 136)	Cases (n = 67)	Controls (n = 69)	p-Value
Age (years) median(IQR)	54 (43,65)	63 (54,69)	46 (39,53)	<0.001
BMI (kg/m^2) median (IQR)	46 (39,52)	40 (34,46)	50 (46,55)	<0.001
White ethnicity	121 (89.0%)	59 (88.1%)	62 (89.9%)	0.888
Ever smokers	50 (36.8%)	23 (34.3%)	27 (39.1%)	0.833
Nulliparity	48 (35.3%)	37 (55.2%)	11 (15.9%)	<0.001
Post-menopausal	77 (56.6%)	56 (83.6%)	21 (30.4%)	<0.001
History of diabetes mellitus	46 (33.8%)	17 (25.4%)	29 (42.0%)	0.04
Tumour Characteristics				
FIGO (2009)				
Grade 1	-	47 (70.2%)	-	-
Grade 2	-	14 (20.9%)	-	-
Grade 3	-	6 (9.0%)	-	-
FIGO (2009)				
Stage 1	-	59 (88.0%)	-	-
Stage 2	-	2 (3.0%)	-	-
Stage 3	-	6 (9.0%)	-	-
Myometrial invasion ≥50%	-	12 (18.0%)	-	-
Presence of LVSI	-	12 (18.0%)	-	-

3.2. Metabolomic Analysis of Plasma Samples

A total of 1137 metabolites were quantified in the study plasma samples of which 733 (64.5%) were biochemically defined. These included amino acids, fatty acids, biogenic amines, sphingolipids, steroids, hexoses, nucleotides, phospholipids, vitamins and xenobiotics. The remaining 35.5% were unnamed biochemical entities, the pathways of which are unknown. We performed classical univariate ROC curve analyses of individual biomarkers to identify putative biomarkers for the discrimination of endometrial cancer from controls (Figure 1). In this analysis, 1-Lignoceroyl GPC (24:0), 1-(1-enyl-stearoyl)-2-linoleoyl-GPE (P-18:0/18:2) and 1-linolenoyl-GPC (18:3) were the most discriminatory biomarkers with AUCs of 0.91 (95%CI 0.86–0.95), 0.85 (95%CI 0.78–0.91) and 0.84 (95% CI 0.78–0.91), respectively. Phosphatidylcholines (PCs) thus feature as potentially important biomarkers. Other discriminatory biomarkers included 3-hydroxylbyryl carnitine and 3-hydroxybutyrate with AUCs of 0.83 and 0.82, respectively (see Figures 1 and 2). Principal component analysis (PCA) and t-distributed stochastic neighbour embedding (t-SNE) were employed and showed some discrimination between cancers and controls (Figure 3a,b). Random forest machine learning was then applied and identified the top 20 discriminatory biomarkers. These were ranked by their contributions to the classification accuracy based on the mean decrease accuracy metric and the mean decrease gini index (Figure 4). A PCA and t-SNE plot based on the top ten discriminatory biomarkers showed a strong degree of separation between cancers and controls (Figure 3c,d). Hierarchical clustering was subsequently performed based on the top 10 discriminatory biomarkers and a heat map was generated (Figure 5). The random forest algorithm was used to split the samples 80:20, 80% for the training set and 20% for testing. The algorithm demonstrated an accuracy of 86.2% (OOB error rate of 13.76%) in the training set, 92.6% prediction accuracy in the testing set and an AUC of 0.95 for endometrial cancer detection (Tables 2 and 3). Biochemical identities, super-pathways and sub-pathways of discriminatory metabolites for EC detection are summarized in Table S2. ROC curves based on the Random Forest diagnostic algorithms are shown in Figure S2.

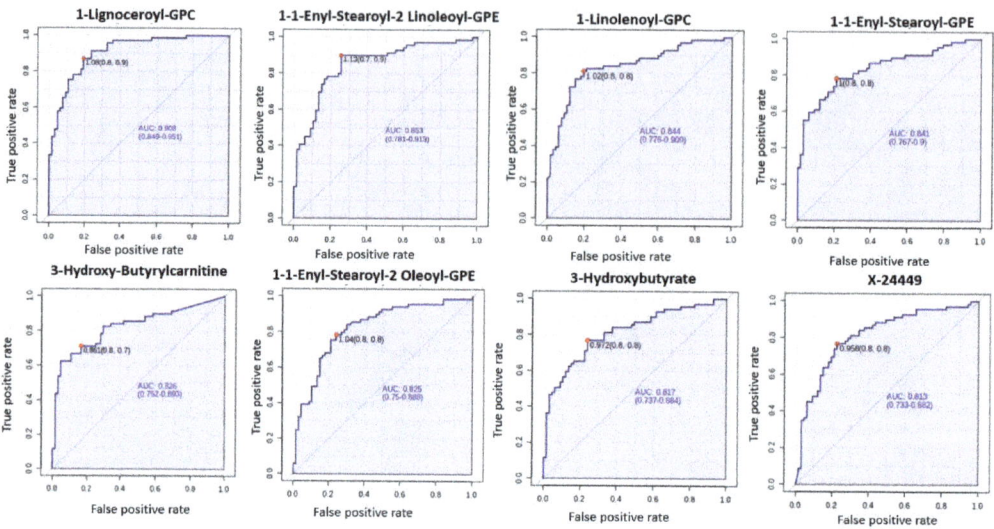

Figure 1. Receiver operating characteristic (ROC) curves of the promising endometrial cancer diagnostic biomarkers from different classes based on the area under the curve (AUC) analyses of $n = 67$ cancers and $n = 69$ controls. The optimal cut-off was based on the closest to the top left corner principle and is indicated by the red dot in the ROC curves. Metabolites starting with X are unnamed; the pathways of these are unknown. GPC—Glycerophosphocholine. GPE—Glycerophosphoethanolamine.

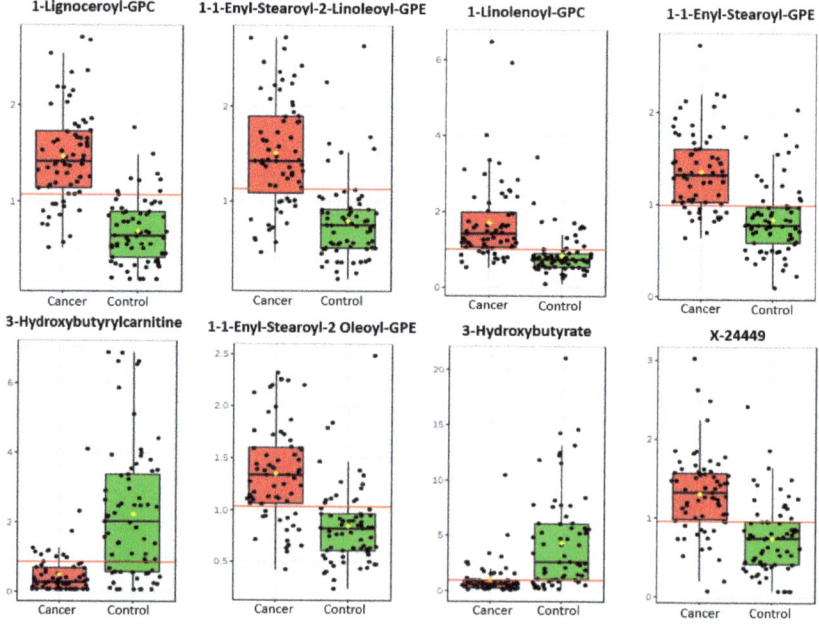

Figure 2. Box plot distribution of promising endometrial cancer diagnostic metabolites based on analyses of $n = 67$ cancers and $n = 69$ controls. The black dots along the Y axis in the box plots represent the concentrations of each metabolite while the yellow diamond represents the mean concentration for the group. The notch represents the 95% confidence interval around the median of each group. The horizontal red lines represent the optimal cut-off. Metabolites starting with X are unnamed; the pathways of these are unknown.

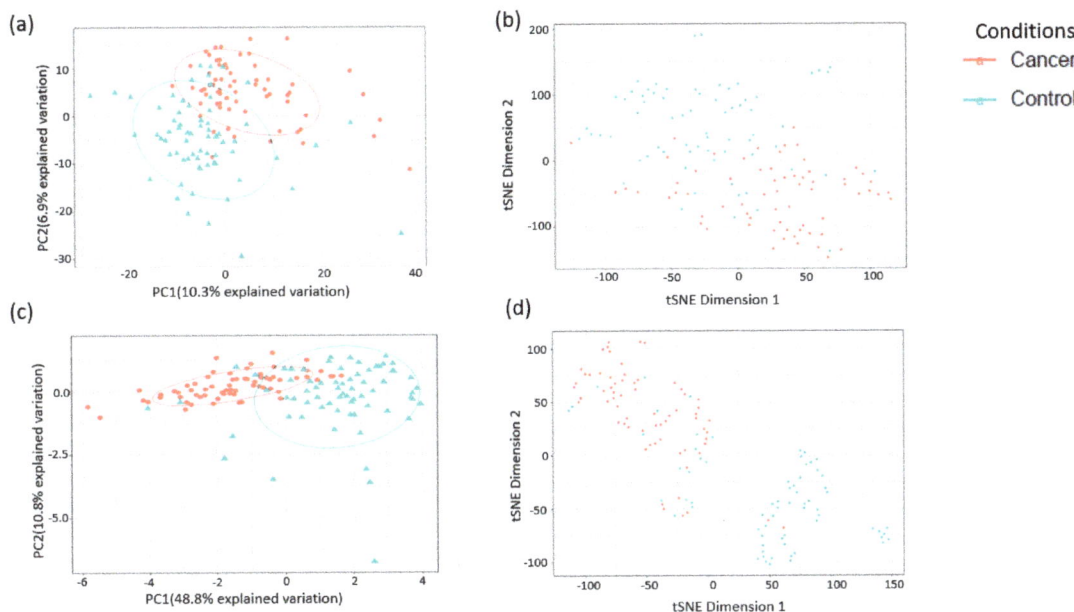

Figure 3. Analysis of sample separation using the training set (n = 109, cancers = 54, controls = 55) based on principal component (PCA) (**a,c**) and t-distributed stochastic neighbour embedding (t-SNE) (**b,d**) analyses using all identified metabolites (**a,b**) and the top 10 discriminatory metabolites (**c,d**) identified by random forest machine learning technique. t-SNE (perplexity: 5, iteration: 10,000).

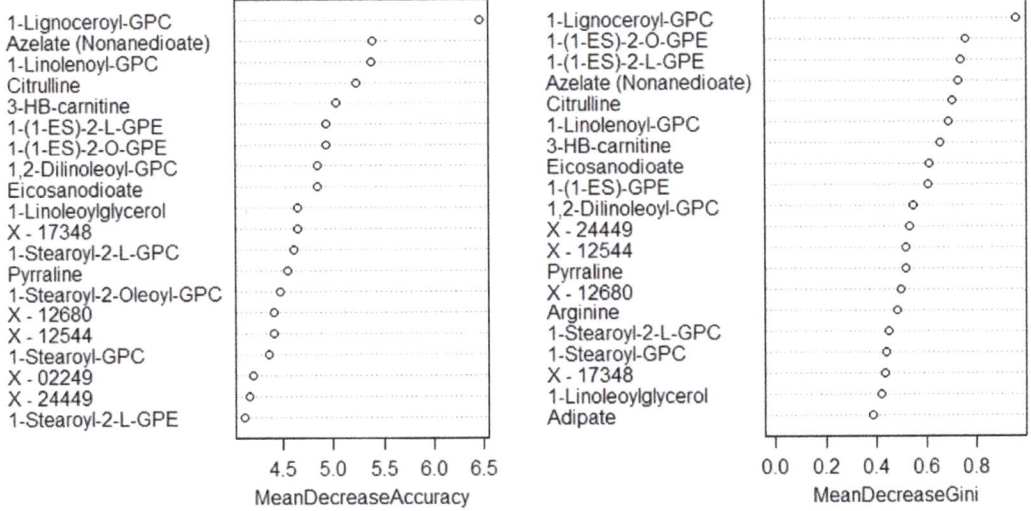

Figure 4. Top 20 discriminatory metabolites identified by random forest machine learning technique and ranked by their contribution to classification accuracy using mean decrease accuracy and mean decrease gini index (node impurity) based on the training set (n = 109, cancers = 54, controls = 55). Metabolites starting with X are unnamed; the pathways of these are unknown.

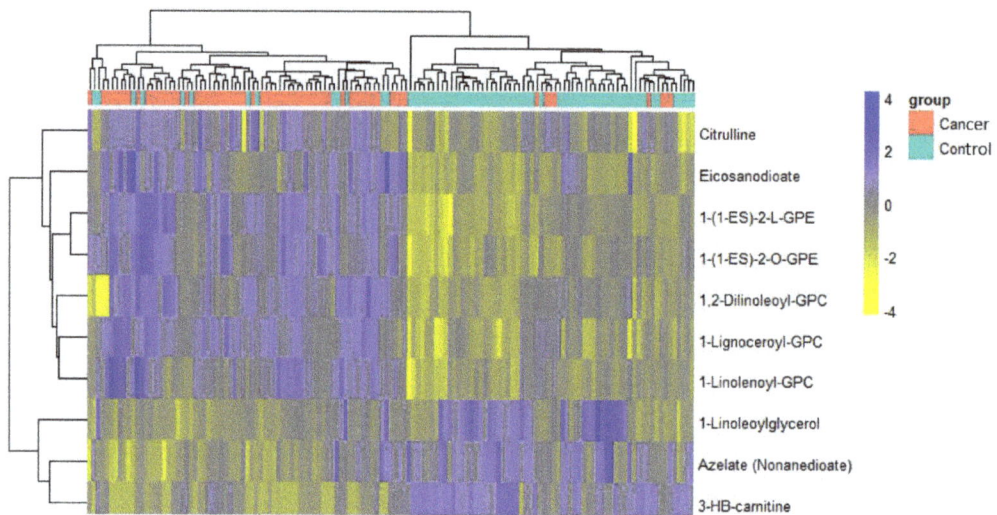

Figure 5. Hierarchical clustering using the top 10 discriminatory metabolites in the training set ($n = 109$, cancers = 54, controls = 55) based on mean decreasing accuracy. The difference in intensities of the top 10 metabolites by cancer-control status is shown. Each coloured cell in the map represents scaled/relative concentration of indicated metabolite. Metabolites are clustered along the vertical axis while subjects are clustered along the horizontal axis. Hierarchical clustering was based on the Euclidean distance measure and the Ward algorithm.

Table 2. Random forest diagnostic accuracy based on the training set made from 80% cases and controls ($n = 109$, cancers = 54, controls = 55).

Actual Group	Predicted Group		
	Cancer	Control	Class Error
Cancer	48	6	0.11111
Control	9	46	0.16363

OOB Error rate: 13.76%. Number of Trees: 1000. Number of variables tried at each split: 33. Sensitivity: 88.9%, specificity: 83.6%.

Table 3. Random forest prediction accuracy applied on the testing set made from 20% of cases and controls ($n = 27$, cancers = 13, controls = 14).

Actual Group	Predicted Group		
	Cancer	Control	Class Error
Cancer	12	1	0.0769
Control	1	13	0.0714

OOB Error rate: 7.41%. Prediction accuracy: 92.6%. AUC: 0.95.

3.3. Metabolomic Analysis for the Detection of Early-Stage Endometrial Cancer

It is important that plasma metabolites used for the identification of endometrial cancer can detect early-stage, not just advanced-stage, disease. We therefore sought to identify metabolites able to distinguish stage 1 endometrial cancer ($n = 59$) from controls ($n = 69$). PCA and t-SNE analyses showed good discrimination between stage 1 disease and controls on all study metabolites (Figure 6a,b) and based on the top 10 metabolites identified using random forest modelling (Figure 6c,d). The top 20 metabolites that distinguished stage 1 endometrial cancer from controls based on random forest algorithm are summarised in Figure 7 and their contribution to the classification accuracy ranked by the mean decrease accuracy and mean decrease gini index. Glycerophospholipids remained important predictors of stage 1 disease, however, the top discriminatory metabolites were uncharacterised chemical entities. Hierarchical clustering using the top 10 metabolites was performed and the generated heat map presented in Figure 8. This showed good discrimination between stage 1 endometrial cancer and controls based on selected metabolites. The study samples were subsequently split 80:20 (80% training set and 20% testing set) using random forest algorithm. The diagnostic algorithm demonstrated an OOB error rate of 14.7% in the training set, a prediction accuracy of 84.6% in the testing set and an AUC of 0.98 for stage 1 endometrial cancer detection (Tables 4 and 5).

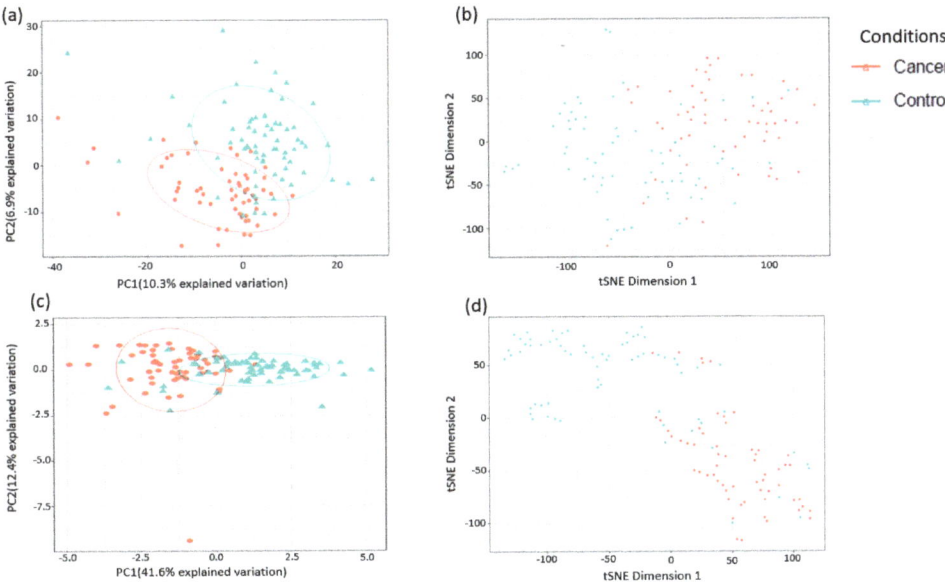

Figure 6. Analysis of sample separation (comparing early-stage (stage 1) endometrial cancer versus controls (*n* = 102, cancers = 47, controls = 55) based on PCA (**a,c**) and t-distributed stochastic neighbour embedding (t-SNE) (**b,d**) analyses using all identified metabolites (**a,b**) and the top 10 discriminatory metabolites (**c,d**) identified by random forest machine learning technique. t-SNE (perplexity: 5, iteration: 10,000).

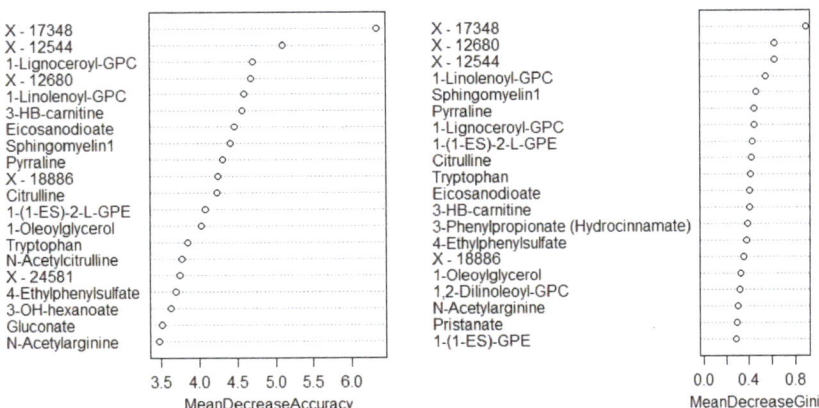

Figure 7. Top 20 discriminatory metabolites for the detection of early-stage endometrial cancer based on the training set (*n* = 102, cancers = 47, controls = 55) identified by random forest machine learning technique and ranked by their contribution to classification accuracy using mean decrease accuracy and mean decrease gini index. Metabolites starting with X are unnamed; the pathways of these are unknown.

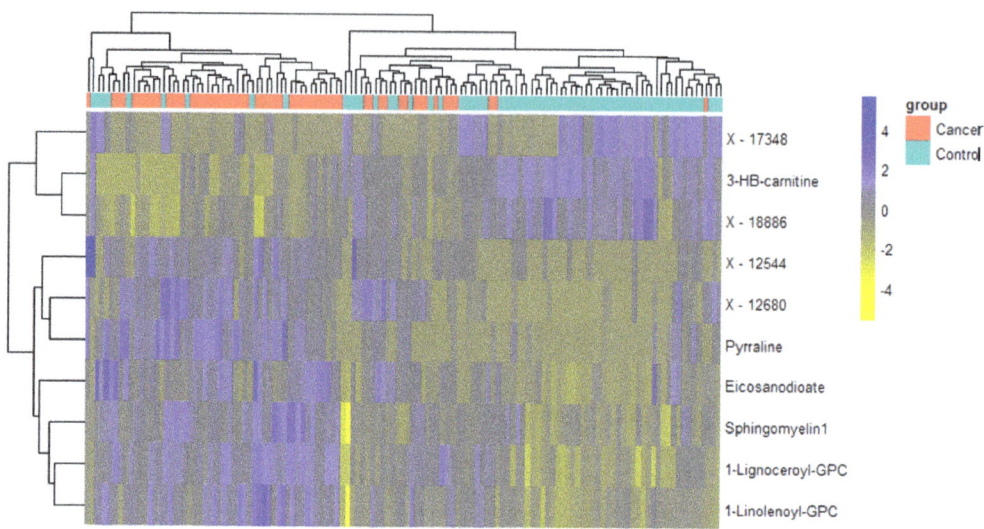

Figure 8. Hierarchical clustering using the top 10 discriminatory metabolites for the detection of early-stage endometrial cancer in the training set ($n = 102$, cancers = 47, controls = 55) based on mean decreasing accuracy using random forest classification algorithm. The difference in intensities of the top 10 metabolites by cancer-control status is shown. Each coloured cell in the map represents scaled/relative concentration of indicated metabolite. Metabolites are clustered along the vertical axis while subjects are clustered along the horizontal axis. Metabolites starting with X are unnamed; the pathways of these are unknown.

Table 4. Random forest diagnostic accuracy developed based on the training set made from 80% of stage 1 endometrial cancer cases and controls ($n = 102$, cancers = 47, controls = 55).

Actual Group	Predicted Group		
	Cancer	Control	Class Error
Cancer	41	6	0.1276
Control	9	46	0.16363

OOB Error rate: 14.71%. Number of Trees: 1000. Number of variables tried at each split: 22. Sensitivity: 87.2%, specificity: 83.6%.

Table 5. Random forest prediction accuracy applied on the testing set made from 20% of stage 1 endometrial cancer cases and controls ($n = 26$, cancers = 12, controls = 14).

Actual Group	Predicted Group		
	Cancer	Control	Class Error
Cancer	8	4	0.3333
Control	0	14	0.0000

OOB Error rate: 15.4%. Prediction accuracy: 84.6%.

3.4. Metabolomic Biomarkers for Predicting Deep Myometrial Invasion and LVSI

Lymphovascular space invasion (LVSI) and deep myometrial invasion are important endometrial cancer prognostic biomarkers. However, their characterisation in clinical practice is performed by histopathologists with moderate interobserver reproducibility. Metabolites with the potential to predict deep myometrial invasion and LVSI will significantly improve endometrial cancer prognostic characterisation. We therefore sought to identify metabolites that can predict LVSI ($n = 12$) and deep myometrial invasion ($n = 12$) in women with endometrioid endometrial cancer. We limited our analysis to univariate

ROC curve analysis and identified specific glycerophosphoethanolamines, glycerophosphocholines, heme and hydroxybutyrate as important predictors of LVSI with AUCs ranging from 0.75–0.83 (Figure 9). A number of unnamed metabolites were noted to predict deep myometrial invasion in addition to Homovanillate, 3-OH-isobutyrate and Tigloylglycine with AUCs ranging between 0.73 and 0.82 (Figure 10).

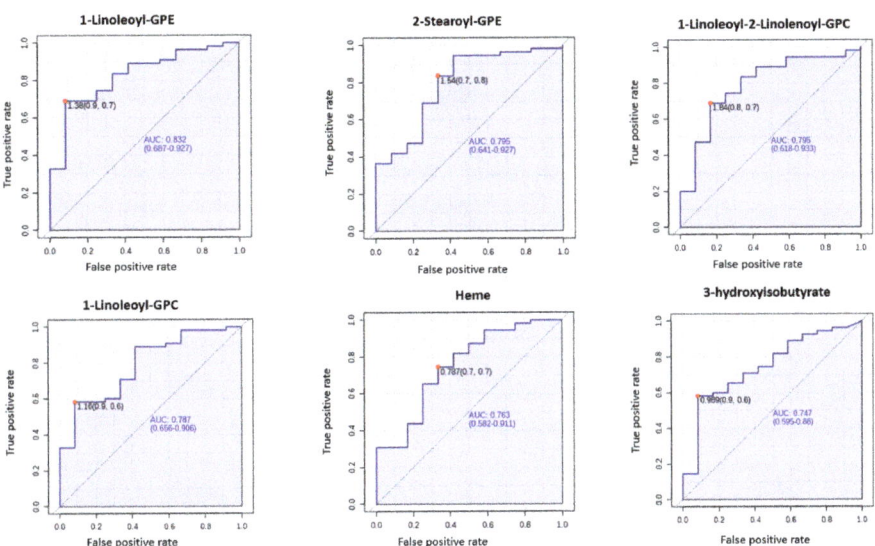

Figure 9. ROC curves of the promising biomarkers for the prediction of lymphovascular space invasion ($n = 12$) based on AUC analyses of $n = 67$ cancers. The optimal cut-off was based on the closest to the top left corner principle and is indicated by the red dot in the ROC curves. Metabolites starting with X are unnamed; the pathways of these are unknown.

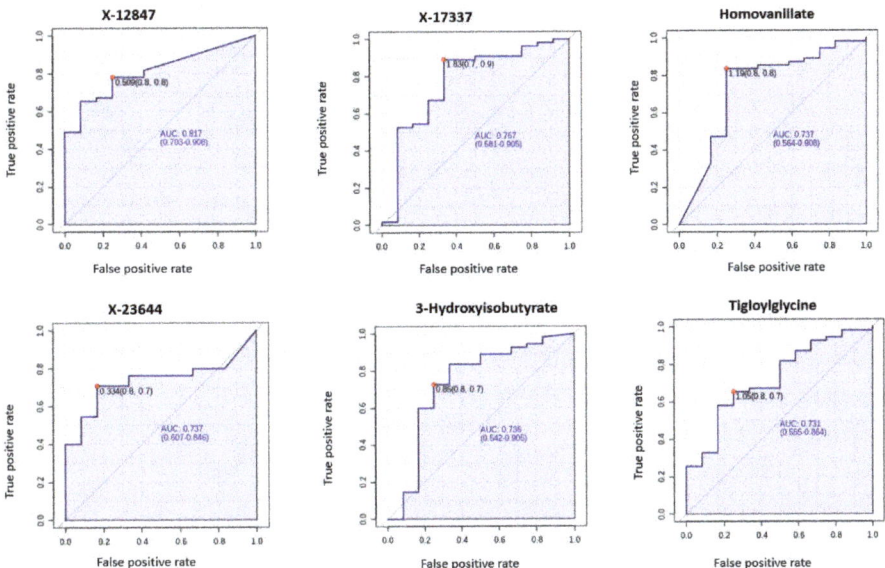

Figure 10. ROC curves of the promising biomarkers for the prediction of deep myometrial invasion ($n = 12$) based on AUC analyses of $n = 67$ cancers. The optimal cut-off was based on the closest to the top left corner principle and is indicated by the red dot in the ROC curves. Metabolites starting with X are unnamed; the pathways of these are unknown.

3.5. Consideration of Potential Confounding Factors

In order to confirm that the discriminatory power of the metabolite signature was due to the presence and absence of endometrial cancer and not confounding variables, we carried out further analyses, taking into consideration the effects of age, BMI, menopausal and diabetic status. First, we performed unsupervised exploratory analyses using score plots generated from PCAs to identify differences between groups (Figure 11). The PCA score plots showed a mild segregation pattern in the confounding factor comparisons suggesting that age, menopausal and diabetic status could potentially have influenced the diagnostic performance within groups of samples (Figure 11). However, these analyses were limited by small numbers within groups. Next, we performed pairwise Spearman's correlation analysis with Bonferroni correction looking at the correlation between age, BMI and selected metabolites (Table 6). There was no evidence of a strong correlation between the metabolite concentrations and age, BMI or parity. Correlation coefficients ranged between 0.25–0.45 for age-based comparisons, 0.33–0.58 for BMI-based comparisons and 0.21–0.32 for parity-based comparisons, suggesting weak correlations between age, BMI, parity and selected metabolite concentrations. While the glycerophospholipids (GPC, GPE) had a positive correlation with age and a negative correlation with BMI/parity, the reverse was the case for the hydroxybutyrates.

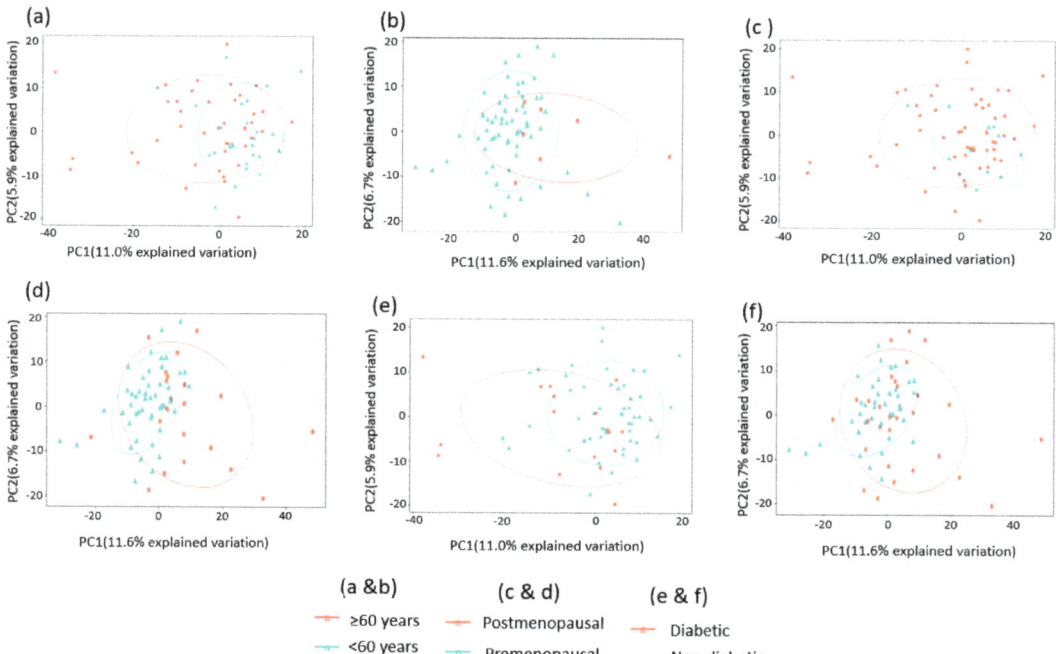

Figure 11. Score plots generated after unsupervised PCA to visualise differences and similarities according to confounding factors. (**a**,**b**) Score plots according to age (<60 years; ≥60 years) for cancers (**a**) and controls (**b**). (**c**,**d**) Score plots according to menopausal status for cancers (**c**) and controls (**d**). (**e**,**f**) Score plots according to diabetes (present; not present) for cancers (**e**) and controls (**f**).

Table 6. Pairwise correlation analysis for selected metabolites with age and BMI.

Correlation p-Value	Age	BMI	Parity	1-Lignoceroyl GPC	1-1 nyl-Steroyl-2-Linoleoyl-GPE	1-Linolenoyl GPC	1-1 Enyl-Steroyl GPE	3-OH-Butyryl Carnitine	1-1 EnylSteroyl-2-Oleoyl GPE	3-OH Butyrate	X-24449	Eicosanodiote	1-2-Dilinoleoyl GPC
Age	1.0000												
BMI		1.0000											
Parity			1.0000										
1-Lignoceroyl GPC	0.4427 * 0.0000	−0.5860 * 0.0000	−0.2802 * 0.0010	1.0000									
1-1 Enyl-Steroyl-2-Linoleoyl-GPE	0.3953 * 0.0001	−0.4879 * 0.0000	−0.3287 * 0.0001	0.7334 * 0.0000	1.0000								
1-Linolenoyl GPC	0.3881 * 0.0002	−0.4824 * 0.0000	−0.2581 * 0.0024	0.7474 * 0.0000	0.6760 * 0.0000	1.0000							
1-1Enyl-Steroyl GPE	0.4518 * 0.0000	−0.4846 * 0.0000	−0.3270 * 0.0001	0.6833 * 0.0000	0.7022 * 0.0000	0.6925 * 0.0000	1.0000						
3-OH-butyryl carnitine	−0.2566 0.1411	0.4438 * 0.0000	0.2164 * 0.0114	−0.6610 * 0.0000	−0.7025 * 0.0000	−0.6535 * 0.0000	−0.4620 * 0.0000	1.0000					
1-1EnylSteroyl-2-Oleoyl GPE	0.4278 * 0.0000	−0.4523 * 0.0000	−0.2680 * 0.0016	0.6379 * 0.0000	0.8935 * 0.0000	0.6511 * 0.0000	0.7199 * 0.0000	−0.5945 * 0.0000	1.0000				
3-OH butyrate	−0.3204 * 0.0079	0.3673 * 0.0000	0.2196 0.0102	−0.5891 * 0.0000	−0.6927 * 0.0000	−0.6334 * 0.0000	−0.5204 * 0.0000	0.8741 * 0.0000	−0.6605 * 0.0000	1.0000			
X-24449	0.4580 * 0.0000	−0.4386 * 0.0000	−0.2566 * 0.0026	0.6211 * 0.0000	0.5864 * 0.0000	0.4975 * 0.0000	0.5026 * 0.0000	−0.4870 * 0.0000	0.4886 * 0.0000	−0.4400 * 0.0000	1.0000		
Eicosanodiote	0.3294 * 0.0050	−0.3388 * 0.0000	−0.2135 * 0.0126	0.5632 * 0.0000	0.6889 * 0.0000	0.5576 * 0.0000	0.5017 * 0.0000	−0.5435 * 0.0000	0.6143 * 0.0000	−0.5169 * 0.0000	0.4147 * 0.0000	1.0000	
1-2-Dilinoleoyl GPC	0.3001 * 0.0212	−0.5158 * 0.0000	−0.3056 * 0.0003	0.7042 * 0.0000	0.7675 * 0.0000	0.6640 * 0.0000	0.5470 * 0.0000	−0.6416 * 0.0000	0.6019 * 0.0000	−0.5968 * 0.0000	0.5395 * 0.0000	0.5786 * 0.0000	1.0000

* p-value < 0.05. This was performed with pairwise correlation analysis with Bonferroni correction. There was no evidence of a strong correlation between age/BMI and selected metabolites.

We then applied an exclusion principle by eliminating women with type 2 diabetes mellitus, leaving 50 cancers and 40 controls. There was still a difference between cases and controls by menopausal status. The list of the top-performing metabolites remained largely similar (Figure 12) based on our machine learning (ML) approaches, suggesting that diabetic status did not significantly affect the diagnostic performance of the metabolites. A receiver characteristics curve analysis of these metabolites gave an AUC of 0.94, 0.90 and 0.89 for 1-Lignoceroyl GPC, 1-Steroyl GPC and 1-1 Enyl-Steroyl-2-Linoleoyl-GPE, respectively (Figure 13). The PCA analyses and heat maps also showed good discrimination between cancer cases and controls (Figures 14 and 15), confirming that diabetes status was not a significant confounder in the study analyses, especially with respect to the diagnostic performance of the glycerophospholipids. However, we noted that the hydroxybutyrates and their derivatives were no longer important discriminators of cancers from controls following exclusion of women with type 2 diabetes mellitus (Figure 12), suggesting that their diagnostic ability may be related to their association with diabetes mellitus. The samples of women with no clinical or biochemical evidence of diabetes mellitus were split 80:20 (80% training set and 20% testing set) with the training data used to build a model to separate cancers from controls. The random forest model had an OOB error rate of 11.1% and when tested using the remaining 20% data, it gave a prediction accuracy of 88.9% (Tables 7 and 8).

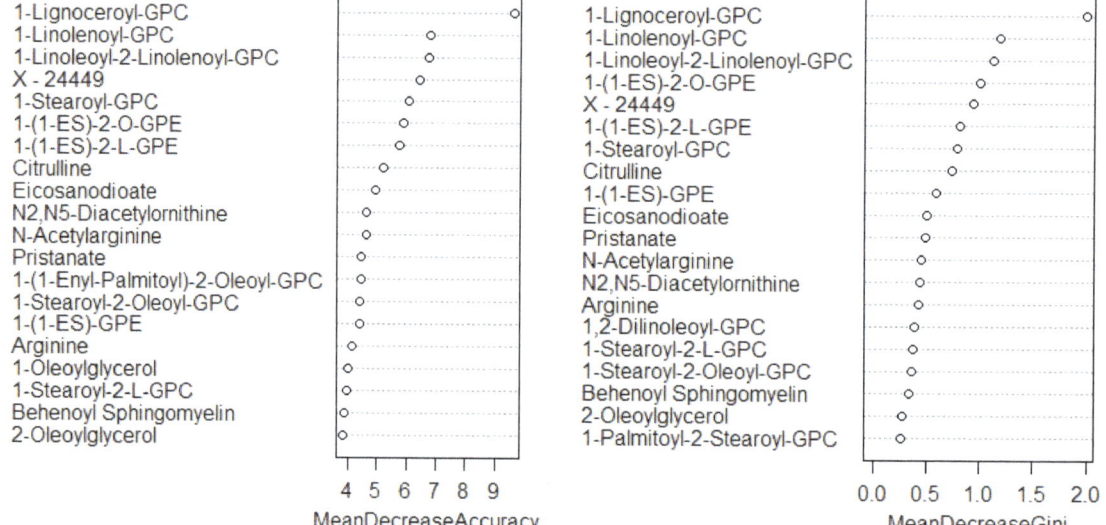

Figure 12. Top 20 discriminatory metabolites for the detection of endometrial cancer following exclusion of women with type 2 diabetes mellitus (training set: n = 72, cancers = 40, controls = 32) Metabolites were identified by random forest machine learning technique and ranked by their contribution to classification accuracy using mean decrease accuracy and mean decrease gini index. Metabolites starting with X are unnamed; the pathways of these are unknown.

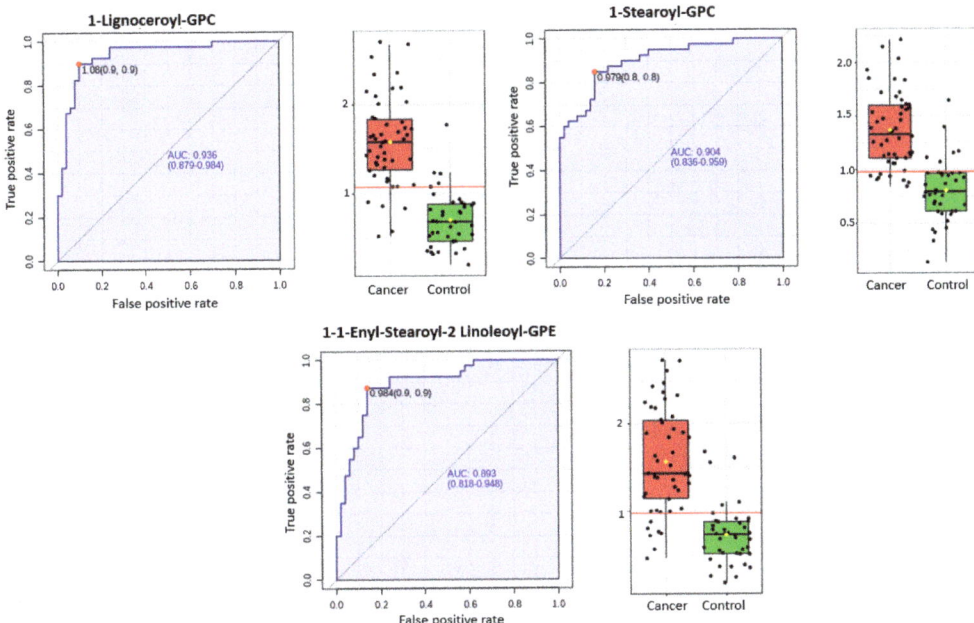

Figure 13. ROC curves of selected metabolites for endometrial cancer detection after exclusion of women with type 2 diabetes mellitus (n = 90, cases = 50, controls = 40) based on AUC analysis. The optimal cut-off was based on the closest to the top left corner principle and is indicated by the red dot in the ROC curves.

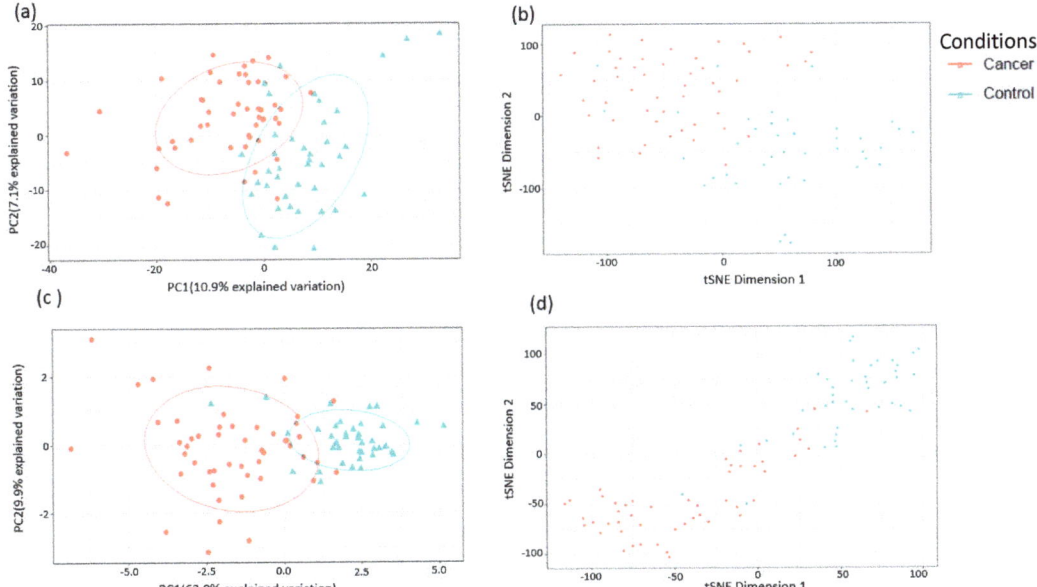

Figure 14. Analysis of sample separation after exclusion of women with type 2 diabetes mellitus (training set: n = 72, cancers = 40, controls = 32) based on PCA (**a**,**c**) and t-distributed stochastic neighbour embedding (t-SNE) (**b**,**d**) analyses using all identified metabolites (**a**,**b**) and the top 10 discriminatory metabolites (**c**,**d**) identified by random forest machine learning. t-SNE (perplexity: 5, iteration: 10,000).

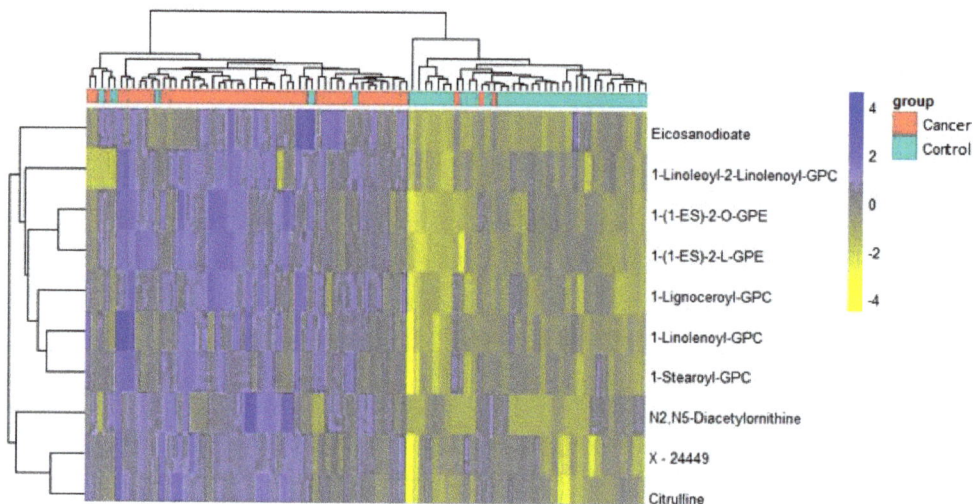

Figure 15. Hierarchical clustering using the top 10 discriminatory metabolites for the detection of endometrial cancer after exclusion of women with type 2 diabetes mellitus (training set: $n = 72$, cancers = 40, controls = 32). Discriminatory metabolites were based on mean decreasing accuracy metric from random forest analysis. The difference in intensities of the top 10 metabolites by cancer-control status is shown. Each coloured cell in the map represents the scaled/relative concentration of indicated metabolite. Metabolites are clustered along the vertical axis and subjects along the horizontal axis. Metabolites starting with X are unnamed with unknown pathways.

Table 7. Random forest diagnostic accuracy developed based on the training set made from 80% of endometrial cancer cases and controls after exclusion of those with type 2 diabetes mellitus ($n = 72$, cancers = 40, controls = 32).

Actual Group	Predicted Group		
	Cancer	Control	Class Error
Cancer	38	2	0.0500
Control	6	26	0.1875

OOB Error rate: 11.11%. Number of Trees: 1000. Number of variables tried at each split: 73. Sensitivity = 95%, Specificity = 81%.

Table 8. Random forest prediction accuracy applied on the testing set made from 20% of endometrial cancer cases and controls after exclusion of women with type 2 diabetes mellitus ($n = 18$, cancers = 10, controls = 8).

Actual Group	Predicted Group		
	Cancer	Control	Class Error
Cancer	8	2	0.200
Control	0	8	0.0000

OOB Error rate 11.11%. Prediction accuracy 88.9%.

Finally, we restricted the analysis to post-menopausal women ($n = 77$, cases = 56, controls = 21). There was still a difference according to diabetes status between cancers and controls in this cohort ($p = 0.001$). The PCA and t-SNE plots showed good discrimination between cancers and controls based on all study metabolites and on the top 10 discriminatory metabolites (Figure 16). The glycerophospholipids remained important predictors of endometrial cancer. The 3-hydroxybutyrate derivatives were also important predictors of endometrial cancer (ranked in the top 10 based on random forest mean decrease accuracy and mean decrease gini index) (Figure 17), confirming their likely association with type 2 diabetes mellitus. Importantly, we noticed the sphingolipids, specifically sphingomyelins, to be well represented in the top 10 discriminatory biomarkers in post-menopausal women (Figure 17). Tricosanoyl and Behenoyl sphingomyelins, in particular, demonstrated AUCs of 0.83 and 0.78, respectively (Figure 18). Hierarchical clustering also showed good discrimination based on the top 10 metabolites in this cohort (Figure 19).

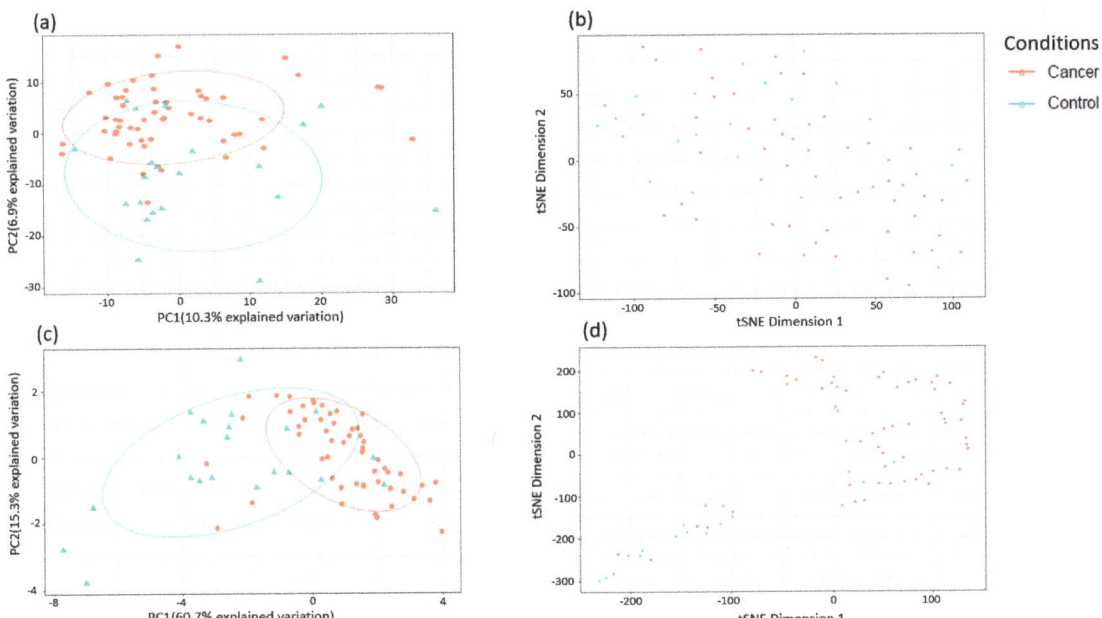

Figure 16. Analysis of sample separation for post-menopausal women (n = 77, cases = 56, controls = 21) based on PCA (**a,c**) and t-distributed stochastic neighbour embedding (t-SNE) (**b,d**) analyses using all identified metabolites (**a,b**) and the top 10 discriminatory metabolites (**c,d**) identified by random forest machine learning. t-SNE (perplexity: 5, iteration: 10,000).

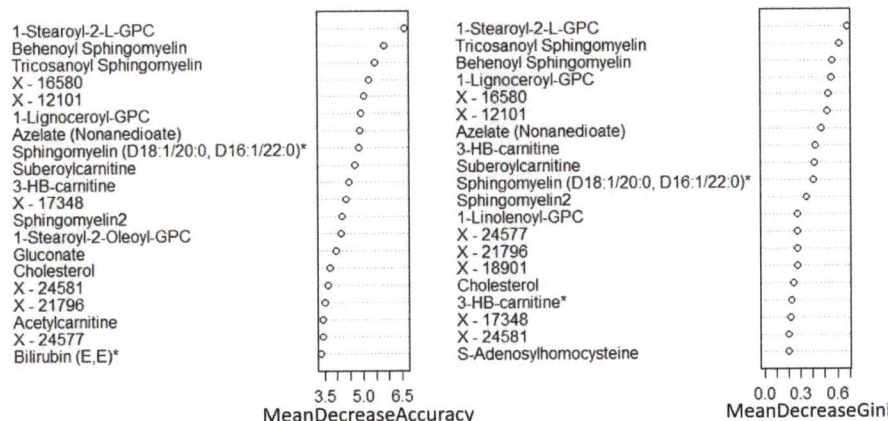

Figure 17. Top 20 discriminatory metabolites for the detection of endometrial cancer in post-menopausal women (n = 77, cases = 56, controls = 21). Metabolites were identified by random forest machine learning and ranked by their contribution to classification accuracy using mean decrease accuracy metric and mean decrease gini index. Metabolites starting with X are unnamed; the pathways of these are unknown.

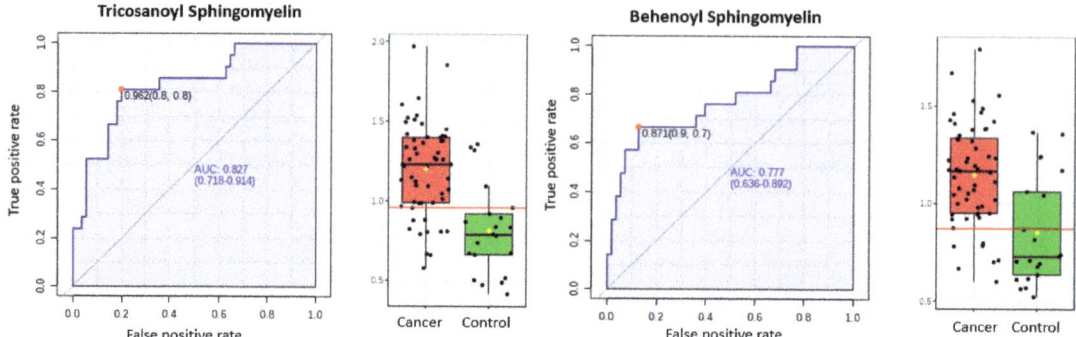

Figure 18. ROC and box-plot distributions of selected metabolites (sphingomyelins) for endometrial cancer detection in post-menopausal women ($n = 77$, cases = 56, controls = 21) based on AUC analysis. The optimal cut-off was based on the closest to the top left corner principle and is indicated by the red dot in the ROC figures. The black dots in the box plots represent the concentrations of each metabolite, while the red diamond represents the mean concentration for the group. The notch represents 95% confidence interval around the median of each group.

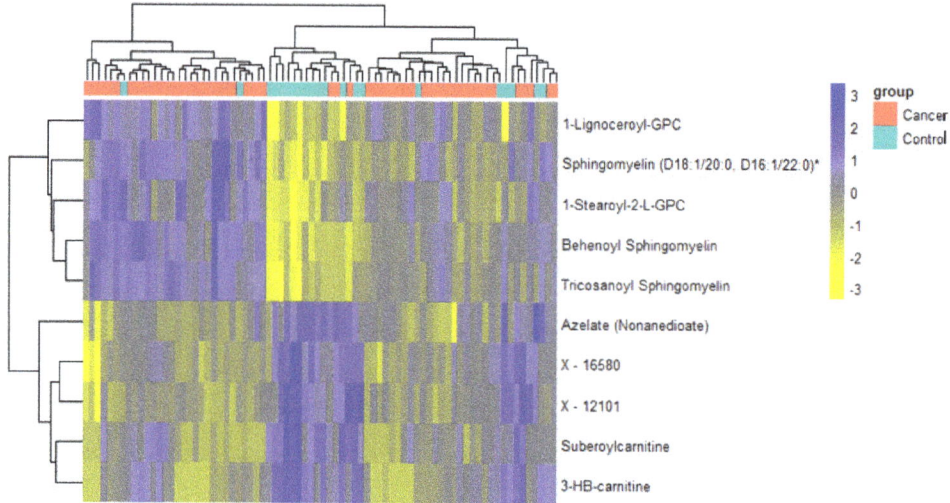

Figure 19. Hierarchical clustering using the top 10 discriminatory metabolites for the detection of endometrial cancer in post-menopausal women ($n = 77$, cases = 56, controls = 21). Discriminatory metabolites were based on mean decrease accuracy metric using random forest analysis. The difference in intensities of the top 10 metabolites by cancer-control status is shown. Each coloured cell in the map represents the scaled concentration of indicated metabolite. Metabolites are clustered along the vertical axis while subjects are clustered along the horizontal axis. Metabolites starting with X are unnamed; the pathways of these are unknown.

4. Discussion

In this study, we evaluated the potential of plasma-based metabolomic biomarkers to detect endometrial cancer in women with class III obesity. Top-performing metabolites, particularly glycerophospholipids and hydroxybutyrates, showed good accuracy for endometrial cancer detection, with AUCs > 0.80. An algorithm combining the ten most discriminatory metabolites was even more successful, with AUCs > 0.90. Potential sources of confounding, particularly age, BMI and diabetes status, did not demonstrate strong correlations with individual metabolites, with the exception of hydroxybutyrates and type

2 diabetes mellitus. These data suggest that a simple blood test could offer a minimally invasive endometrial cancer detection tool for women with class III obesity.

The rising prevalence of endometrial cancer has stimulated an interest in biomarker discovery alongside minimally invasive sampling technologies for its early detection [11]. Many studies have explored the possibility of detecting endometrial cancer in blood using genetic biomarkers (including tumour DNA [26], epigenetic modifications [27] and transcripts [28,29]), proteins [18,30] and metabolites [19,22] through genomic, epigenomic, transcriptomic, proteomic, spectroscopic and metabolomic approaches. The metabolome reflects the functional human phenotype and as such, has enormous potential to deliver clinically relevant biomarkers for endometrial cancer detection [20,31]. Indeed, metabolic reprogramming is a defining hallmark of carcinogenesis [32]. Pertubations in critical pathways involving fatty acid metabolism, choline metabolism, tricarboxylic acid cycle and glycolysis have all been described in the pathogenesis of cancer [21,33,34]. Metabolomic biomarkers have shown promise for the early detection of several cancers, including those of the breast [35], colon [36] and prostate [37], and may be particularly relevant in endometrial cancer, given its strong association with obesity, insulin resistance and type 2 diabetes mellitus [38].

Our finding that glycerophospholipids are important diagnostic biomarkers in endometrial cancer is consistent with published data [39–42]. Glycerophospholipids are the main components of biological membranes and, alongside fatty acids, glycerolipids, sphingolipids and sterols, have been linked to cancer development [43]. The upregulation of phospholipid biosynthetic pathways in cancer cells is a direct consequence of accelerated growth and enhanced membrane biosynthesis that accompanies tumorigenesis [44]. A recent systematic review by our group identified choline derivatives, specifically glycerophosphocholines and phosphocholines, as promising biomarkers for endometrial cancer detection [22]. Altered choline metabolism is a hallmark of carcinogenesis and is linked to mitogenic signal transduction, the regulatory mechanism that modulates cell proliferation, differentiation, metabolism and death [34,45,46]. Up-regulation of choline-containing precursors, including phosphocholines and total choline-containing compounds, is caused by the overexpression and activation of several key enzymes involved in choline metabolism by cancer cells. These processes are mediated by oncogenic signalling pathways, including RAS and PI3K-AKT [46,47]. Trousil and colleagues found that altered choline metabolism in endometrial cancer is caused by an overexpression of choline kinase alpha and hyperactivation of the deacylation pathway [48]. Choline derivatives are detectable in blood, tumour and vaginal fluid in women with endometrial cancer [39–41]. They have also been described in breast, prostate and other solid tumours [46]. 3-hydroxybutyrate and its derivatives have also shown promise for endometrial cancer detection [49,50]. Bahado-Singh found that 3-OH butyrate was an important endometrial cancer biomarker even after adjusting for diabetes [49]. In the current study, 3-OH butyrate and its derivatives did not significantly discriminate between cases and controls after excluding women with type 2 diabetes mellitus. This may relate to the strong association between 3-OH butyrate and diabetes, with multiple studies suggesting that 3-OH butyrate is an early marker of insulin resistance, even in non-diabetic populations [51–53]. 3-OH butyrate has also been identified as a potential biomarker of low-grade female papillary thyroid cancer [54] and high-grade serous carcinoma of the ovary [55]. Knapp and colleagues found sphinganine, sphingosine, dihydroceramide and ceramide levels to be significantly elevated in endometrial cancer tissue compared to healthy endometrium [56]. Audet-Delage and colleagues reported sphingolipids to be significantly elevated in the serum of women with recurrent non-endometrioid endometrial cancer [39]. Sphingolipids are involved in inflammation, proliferation, cell migration and apoptosis [57]. Here, we found tricosanoyl and behenoyl sphingomyelins to be upregulated in the plasma of post-menopausal women with endometrial cancer. Further studies are needed to validate the utility of these biomarkers for endometrial cancer detection.

Metabolomic biomarkers that can identify aggressive endometrial cancer phenotypes are important for directing therapy. Here, several metabolites were shown to have potential for establishing tumour stage, the presence of LVSI and deep myometrial invasion (Figures 9 and 10, respectively). Glycerophosphocholines, glycerophosphoethanolamines, heme and 3-OH butyrate were important predictors of LVSI while X-12847, X-17337, Homovanillate (HVA), X-23644, 3-OH butyrate and Tigloylglycine were important predictors of deep myometrial invasion. These results must be interpreted with caution given the small sample sizes. Heme, an iron-containing porphyrin, is an important source of electrons for electron transfer and has been shown to be elevated in the clinically aggressive type II endometrial cancer [39,58]. Homovanillate, a metabolite of dopamine, is a neurotransmitter originating from tyrosine [59]. We did not find any prior studies identifying HVA as a marker of deep myometrial invasion in endometrial cancer. These markers warrant validation in an independent cohort and their mechanistic links to endometrial cancer should be elucidated prior to clinical translation.

This study has several strengths. Our metabolomics methodology, using multiple approaches for metabolite separation and identification (Reverse Phase Liquid Chromatography and Hydrophilic Interaction Liquid Chromatography), helped maximise the number of metabolites identified. The use of artificial intelligence to select the best-performing metabolites and to qualify their performance in an independent sub-group of samples is a further strength, as this minimises the unwanted inflation of performance that occurs in the absence of independent testing. Identified metabolites showed sufficient accuracy for endometrial cancer detection (including early-stage tumours), especially when combined in a biomarker panel, and thus have good potential for clinical utility. Indeed, many of these metabolites have mechanistic links with the malignant transformation process. The use of obese controls maximises the chance that discriminatory metabolites are cancer-specific rather than obesity-related and sets our study apart from previous studies where apparently healthy controls (i.e., women with normal BMI) were used.

A limitation of our study design is that our metabolite panel may not identify non-endometrioid-/non-obesity-related tumours. It is also unclear how well the biomarkers will perform in other high-risk groups such as the elderly, those with postmenopausal bleeding or Lynch syndrome. The relatively small sample size and the attendant difficulty in controlling for potential confounding factors is another limitation. Several discriminatory metabolites could not be biochemically identified, which limits their clinical implementation.

5. Conclusions

We found specific plasma metabolites to have potential for the detection of endometrial cancer in a cohort of women with class III obesity. A metabolomic signature based on the top ten performing metabolites showed good promise. Glycerophospholipids, specifically glycerophosphocholines and glycerophosphoethanolamines, were particularly important in differentiating endometrioid endometrial cancer from controls. These findings suggest that a simple blood-based test has the potential to enable the early detection of endometrial cancer and provides a basis for a minimally invasive screening tool for women with class III obesity. Further studies are needed to validate the biomarker candidates and elucidate their role in endometrial carcinogenesis.

Supplementary Materials: The following are available online at https://www.mdpi.com/2072-6694/13/4/718/s1, Figure S1: Overview of study workflow, Figure S2: ROC curves based on Random Forest algorithms for the detection of endometrial cancer of all stages (a) and stage 1 endometrial cancer (b) using 80% of study samples and based on the top 10 discriminatory biomarkers, Table S1: Description of liquid chromatographic columns and mode of ionisation used in metabolite extraction based on protocols by Metabolon Inc, Table S2: Biochemical identities, super-pathways and sub-pathways of discriminatory metabolites for EC detection.

Author Contributions: K.N. analysed the data, carried out data interpretation and wrote the first draft of the manuscript including creation of figures. E.J.C. and A.D.W. conceptualised the study, supervised study execution, contributed to data interpretation and wrote the manuscript. A.E.C. and B.G. contributed to data analysis and interpretation. M.L.M., A.E.D., S.J.K., V.N.S. and E.J.C. recruited for the study and performed study procedures. A.P. contributed to data interpretation. E.J.C. and A.D.W. are Principal Investigators and obtained funding for the study. All authors provided critical comment. All authors have read and agreed to the published version of the manuscript.

Funding: K.N. is supported by Cancer Research UK (CRUK) Manchester Cancer Research Centre Clinical Research Fellowship and the Wellcome Trust Manchester Translational Informatics Training Scheme. S.J.K. and V.N.S. are supported by the National Institute for Health Research (NIHR) Academic Clinical Lectureship. The Stoller Biomarker Discovery Centre was established with an award from the Medical Research Council (MR/M008959/1). This work was supported by the CRUK Manchester Centre award (C5759/A25254) and Bloodcancer UK (Award 19007 to AP and ADW). ADW and EJC are supported by the National Institute for Health Research Manchester Biomedical Research Centre (IS-BRC-1215-20007).

Institutional Review Board Statement: PREMIUM study (North West Research Ethics Committee ref. 14/NW/1236), Weight loss study (North West Research Ethics Committee ref. 12/NW/0050), Metformin study (North West Research Ethics Committee ref. 11/NW/0442), and PROTEC study (Cambridge East Research Ethics Committee ref. 15/EE/0063).

Informed Consent Statement: Informed consent was obtained from all subjects involved in the study.

Data Availability Statement: Data are available through the corresponding author upon reasonable request.

Conflicts of Interest: The authors declare no conflict of interest.

References

1. Bray, F.; Ferlay, J.; Soerjomataram, I.; Siegel, R.L.; Torre, L.A.; Jemal, A. Global Cancer Statistics 2018: GLOBOCAN Estimates of Incidence and Mortality Worldwide for 36 Cancers in 185 Countries. *CA Cancer J. Clin.* **2018**, *68*, 394–424. [CrossRef]
2. Crosbie, E.J.; Zwahlen, M.; Kitchener, H.C.; Egger, M.; Renehan, A.G. Body Mass Index, Hormone Replacement Therapy, and Endometrial Cancer Risk: A Meta-Analysis. *Cancer Epidemiol. Prev. Biomark.* **2010**, *19*, 3119–3130. [CrossRef]
3. Onstad, M.A.; Schmandt, R.E.; Lu, K.H. Addressing the Role of Obesity in Endometrial Cancer Risk, Prevention, and Treatment. *J. Clin. Oncol.* **2016**, *34*, 4225. [CrossRef]
4. CRUK. Uterine Cancer Incidence Statistics. 2020. Available online: http://www.Cancerresearchuk.Org.Last (accessed on 1 June 2020).
5. Kitson, S.J.; Crosbie, E.J. Endometrial Cancer and Obesity. *Obstetrician Gynaecol.* **2019**, *21*, 237–245.
6. Kaaks, R.; Lukanova, A.; Kurzer, M.S. Obesity, Endogenous Hormones, and Endometrial Cancer Risk: A Synthetic Review. *Cancer Epidemiol. Prev. Biomark.* **2002**, *11*, 1531–1543.
7. Khandekar, M.J.; Cohen, P.; Spiegelman, B.M. Molecular Mechanisms of Cancer Development in Obesity. *Nat. Rev. Cancer* **2011**, *11*, 886–895. [CrossRef]
8. Saed, L.; Varse, F.; Baradaran, H.R.; Moradi, Y.; Khateri, S.; Friberg, E.; Khazaei, Z.; Gharahjeh, S.; Tehrani, S.; Sioofy-Khojine, A.-B. The Effect of Diabetes on the Risk of Endometrial Cancer: An Updated a Systematic Review and Meta-Analysis. *BMC Cancer* **2019**, *19*, 527. [CrossRef]
9. Zhang, Y.; Liu, Z.; Yu, X.; Zhang, X.; Lü, S.; Chen, X.; Lü, B. The Association between Metabolic Abnormality and Endometrial Cancer: A Large Case-Control Study in China. *Gynecol. Oncol.* **2010**, *117*, 41–46. [CrossRef]
10. MacKintosh, M.L.; Derbyshire, A.E.; McVey, R.J.; Bolton, J.; Nickkho-Amiry, M.; Higgins, C.L.; Kamieniorz, M.; Pemberton, P.W.; Kirmani, B.H.; Ahmed, B. The Impact of Obesity and Bariatric Surgery on Circulating and Tissue Biomarkers of Endometrial Cancer Risk. *Int. J. Cancer* **2019**, *144*, 641–650. [CrossRef] [PubMed]
11. Costas, L.; Frias-Gomez, J.; Guardiola, M.; Benavente, Y.; Pineda, M.; Pavón, M.Á.; Martínez, J.M.; Climent, M.; Barahona, M.; Canet, J. New Perspectives on Screening and Early Detection of Endometrial Cancer. *Int. J. Cancer* **2019**, *145*, 3194–3206. [CrossRef] [PubMed]
12. Njoku, K.; Abiola, J.; Russell, J.; Crosbie, E.J. Endometrial Cancer Prevention in High-Risk Women. *Best Pract. Res. Clin. Obstet. Gynaecol.* **2020**, *65*, 66–78. [CrossRef]
13. Gentry-Maharaj, A.; Karpinskyj, C. Current and Future Approaches to Screening for Endometrial Cancer. *Best Pract. Res. Clin. Obstet. Gynaecol.* **2020**, *65*, 79–97. [CrossRef]
14. Wan, Y.L.; Beverley-Stevenson, R.; Carlisle, D.; Clarke, S.; Edmondson, R.J.; Glover, S.; Holland, J.; Hughes, C.; Kitchener, H.C.; Kitson, S. Working Together to Shape the Endometrial Cancer Research Agenda: The Top Ten Unanswered Research Questions. *Gynecol. Oncol.* **2016**, *143*, 287–293. [CrossRef] [PubMed]

15. Njoku, K.; Chiasserini, D.; Jones, E.R.; Barr, C.E.; O'flynn, H.; Whetton, A.D.; Crosbie, E.J. Urinary Biomarkers and Their Potential for the Non-Invasive Detection of Endometrial Cancer. *Front. Oncol.* **2020**, *10*, 2420. [CrossRef]
16. Hasin, Y.; Seldin, M.; Lusis, A. Multi-Omics Approaches to Disease. *Genome Biol.* **2017**, *18*, 83. [CrossRef]
17. Rundle, A.; Ahsan, H.; Vineis, P. Better Cancer Biomarker Discovery through Better Study Design. *Eur. J. Clin. Investig.* **2012**, *42*, 1350–1359. [CrossRef] [PubMed]
18. Njoku, K.; Chiasserini, D.; Whetton, A.D.; Crosbie, E.J. Proteomic Biomarkers for the Detection of Endometrial Cancer. *Cancers* **2019**, *11*, 1572. [CrossRef]
19. Paraskevaidi, M.; Morais, C.L.M.; Ashton, K.M.; Stringfellow, H.F.; McVey, R.J.; Ryan, N.A.J.; O'Flynn, H.; Sivalingam, V.N.; Kitson, S.J.; MacKintosh, M.L. Detecting Endometrial Cancer by Blood Spectroscopy: A Diagnostic Cross-Sectional Study. *Cancers* **2020**, *12*, 1256. [CrossRef] [PubMed]
20. Tolstikov, V.; Moser, A.J.; Sarangarajan, R.; Narain, N.R.; Kiebish, M.A. Current Status of Metabolomic Biomarker Discovery: Impact of Study Design and Demographic Characteristics. *Metabolites* **2020**, *10*, 224. [CrossRef]
21. Pavlova, N.N.; Thompson, C.B. The Emerging Hallmarks of Cancer Metabolism. *Cell Metab.* **2016**, *23*, 27–47. [CrossRef]
22. Njoku, K.; Sutton, C.J.; Whetton, A.D.; Crosbie, E.J. Metabolomic Biomarkers for Detection, Prognosis and Identifying Recurrence in Endometrial Cancer. *Metabolites* **2020**, *10*, 314. [CrossRef] [PubMed]
23. Badrick, E.; Cresswell, K.; Ellis, P.; Crosbie, P.; Hall, P.S.; O'Flynn, H.; Martin, R.; Leighton, J.; Brown, L.; Makin, D. Top Ten Research Priorities for Detecting Cancer Early. *Lancet Public Health* **2019**, *4*, e551. [CrossRef]
24. Kitson, S.J.; Maskell, Z.; Sivalingam, V.N.; Allen, J.L.; Ali, S.; Burns, S.; Gilmour, K.; Latheef, R.; Slade, R.J.; Pemberton, P.W. PRE-Surgical Metformin In Uterine Malignancy (PREMIUM): A Multi-Center, Randomized Double-Blind, Placebo-Controlled Phase III Trial. *Clin. Cancer Res.* **2019**, *25*, 2424–2432. [CrossRef] [PubMed]
25. Sivalingam, V.N.; Kitson, S.; McVey, R.; Roberts, C.; Pemberton, P.; Gilmour, K.; Ali, S.; Renehan, A.G.; Kitchener, H.C.; Crosbie, E.J. Measuring the Biological Effect of Presurgical Metformin Treatment in Endometrial Cancer. *Br. J. Cancer* **2016**, *114*, 281–289. [CrossRef] [PubMed]
26. Cicchillitti, L.; Corrado, G.; De Angeli, M.; Mancini, E.; Baiocco, E.; Patrizi, L.; Zampa, A.; Merola, R.; Martayan, A.; Conti, L. Circulating Cell-Free DNA Content as Blood Based Biomarker in Endometrial Cancer. *Oncotarget* **2017**, *8*, 115230. [CrossRef]
27. Muraki, Y.; Banno, K.; Yanokura, M.; Kobayashi, Y.; Kawaguchi, M.; Nomura, H.; Hirasawa, A.; Susumu, N.; Aoki, D. Epigenetic DNA Hypermethylation: Clinical Applications in Endometrial Cancer. *Oncol. Rep.* **2009**, *22*, 967–972.
28. Laura, M.-R.; Carlos, C.-A.; Miguel, A. Liquid Biopsy in Endometrial Cancer: New Opportunities for Personalized Oncology. *Int. J. Mol. Sci.* **2018**, *19*, 2311. [CrossRef]
29. De Bruyn, C.; Baert, T.; Van den Bosch, T.; Coosemans, A. Circulating Transcripts and Biomarkers in Uterine Tumors: Is There a Predictive Role? *Curr. Oncol. Rep.* **2020**, *22*, 12. [CrossRef] [PubMed]
30. Moore, R.G.; Brown, A.K.; Miller, M.C.; Badgwell, D.; Lu, Z.; Allard, W.J.; Granai, C.O.; Bast Jr, R.C.; Lu, K. Utility of a Novel Serum Tumor Biomarker HE4 in Patients with Endometrioid Adenocarcinoma of the Uterus. *Gynecol. Oncol.* **2008**, *110*, 196–201. [CrossRef]
31. Bracewell-Milnes, T.; Saso, S.; Abdalla, H.; Nikolau, D.; Norman-Taylor, J.; Johnson, M.; Holmes, E.; Thum, M.-Y. Metabolomics as a Tool to Identify Biomarkers to Predict and Improve Outcomes in Reproductive Medicine: A Systematic Review. *Hum. Reprod. Update* **2017**, *23*, 723–736. [CrossRef]
32. Narayanan, S.; Santhoshkumar, A.; Ray, S.; Harihar, S. Reprogramming of Cancer Cell Metabolism: Warburg and Reverse Warburg Hypothesis. In *Cancer Cell Metabolism: A Potential Target for Cancer Therapy*; Springer: Berlin/Heidelberg, Germany, 2020; pp. 15–26.
33. Raffone, A.; Troisi, J.; Boccia, D.; Travaglino, A.; Capuano, G.; Insabato, L.; Mollo, A.; Guida, M.; Zullo, F. Metabolomics in Endometrial Cancer Diagnosis: A Systematic Review. *Acta Obstet. Gynecol. Scand.* **2020**, *9*, 1135–1146. [CrossRef]
34. Stewart, J.D.; Marchan, R.; Lesjak, M.S.; Lambert, J.; Hergenroeder, R.; Ellis, J.K.; Lau, C.-H.; Keun, H.C.; Schmitz, G.; Schiller, J. Choline-Releasing Glycerophosphodiesterase EDI3 Drives Tumor Cell Migration and Metastasis. *Proc. Natl. Acad. Sci. USA* **2012**, *109*, 8155–8160. [CrossRef]
35. Jasbi, P.; Wang, D.; Cheng, S.L.; Fei, Q.; Cui, J.Y.; Liu, L.; Wei, Y.; Raftery, D.; Gu, H. Breast Cancer Detection Using Targeted Plasma Metabolomics. *J. Chromatogr. B* **2019**, *1105*, 26–37. [CrossRef] [PubMed]
36. Farshidfar, F.; Weljie, A.M.; Kopciuk, K.A.; Hilsden, R.; McGregor, S.E.; Buie, W.D.; MacLean, A.; Vogel, H.J.; Bathe, O.F. A Validated Metabolomic Signature for Colorectal Cancer: Exploration of the Clinical Value of Metabolomics. *Br. J. Cancer* **2016**, *115*, 848–857. [CrossRef] [PubMed]
37. Kelly, R.S.; Vander Heiden, M.G.; Giovannucci, E.; Mucci, L.A. Metabolomic Biomarkers of Prostate Cancer: Prediction, Diagnosis, Progression, Prognosis, and Recurrence. *Cancer Epidemiol. Prev. Biomark.* **2016**, *25*, 887–906. [CrossRef] [PubMed]
38. Tokarz, J.; Adamski, J.; Lanišnik Rižner, T. Metabolomics for Diagnosis and Prognosis of Uterine Diseases? A Systematic Review. *J. Pers. Med.* **2020**, *10*, 294. [CrossRef]
39. Audet-Delage, Y.; Villeneuve, L.; Grégoire, J.; Plante, M.; Guillemette, C. Identification of Metabolomic Biomarkers for Endometrial Cancer and Its Recurrence after Surgery in Postmenopausal Women. *Front. Endocrinol.* **2018**, *9*, 87. [CrossRef]
40. Cheng, S.-C.; Chen, K.; Chiu, C.-Y.; Lu, K.-Y.; Lu, H.-Y.; Chiang, M.-H.; Tsai, C.-K.; Lo, C.-J.; Cheng, M.-L.; Chang, T.-C. Metabolomic Biomarkers in Cervicovaginal Fluid for Detecting Endometrial Cancer through Nuclear Magnetic Resonance Spectroscopy. *Metabolomics* **2019**, *15*, 146. [CrossRef]

41. Shi, K.; Wang, Q.; Su, Y.; Xuan, X.; Liu, Y.; Chen, W.; Qian, Y.; Lash, G.E. Identification and Functional Analyses of Differentially Expressed Metabolites in Early Stage Endometrial Carcinoma. *Cancer Sci.* **2018**, *109*, 1032–1043. [CrossRef] [PubMed]
42. Knific, T.; Vouk, K.; Smrkolj, Š.; Prehn, C.; Adamski, J.; Rižner, T.L. Models Including Plasma Levels of Sphingomyelins and Phosphatidylcholines as Diagnostic and Prognostic Biomarkers of Endometrial Cancer. *J. Steroid Biochem. Mol. Biol.* **2018**, *178*, 312–321. [CrossRef] [PubMed]
43. Huang, C.; Freter, C. Lipid Metabolism, Apoptosis and Cancer Therapy. *Int. J. Mol. Sci.* **2015**, *16*, 924–949. [CrossRef]
44. Casares, D.; Escribá, P.V.; Rosselló, C.A. Membrane Lipid Composition: Effect on Membrane and Organelle Structure, Function and Compartmentalization and Therapeutic Avenues. *Int. J. Mol. Sci.* **2019**, *20*, 2167. [CrossRef] [PubMed]
45. Sonkar, K.; Ayyappan, V.; Tressler, C.M.; Adelaja, O.; Cai, R.; Cheng, M.; Glunde, K. Focus on the Glycerophosphocholine Pathway in Choline Phospholipid Metabolism of Cancer. *NMR Biomed.* **2019**, *32*, e4112. [CrossRef]
46. Ackerstaff, E.; Glunde, K.; Bhujwalla, Z.M. Choline Phospholipid Metabolism: A Target in Cancer Cells? *J. Cell. Biochem.* **2003**, *90*, 525–533. [CrossRef]
47. Glunde, K.; Bhujwalla, Z.M.; Ronen, S.M. Choline Metabolism in Malignant Transformation. *Nat. Rev. Cancer* **2011**, *11*, 835–848. [CrossRef]
48. Trousil, S.; Lee, P.; Pinato, D.J.; Ellis, J.K.; Dina, R.; Aboagye, E.O.; Keun, H.C.; Sharma, R. Alterations of Choline Phospholipid Metabolism in Endometrial Cancer Are Caused by Choline Kinase Alpha Overexpression and a Hyperactivated Deacylation Pathway. *Cancer Res.* **2014**, *74*, 6867–6877. [CrossRef] [PubMed]
49. Bahado-Singh, R.O.; Lugade, A.; Field, J.; Al-Wahab, Z.; Han, B.; Mandal, R.; Bjorndahl, T.C.; Turkoglu, O.; Graham, S.F.; Wishart, D. Metabolomic Prediction of Endometrial Cancer. *Metabolomics* **2018**, *14*, 6. [CrossRef]
50. Troisi, J.; Sarno, L.; Landolfi, A.; Scala, G.; Martinelli, P.; Venturella, R.; Di Cello, A.; Zullo, F.; Guida, M. Metabolomic Signature of Endometrial Cancer. *J. Proteome Res.* **2018**, *17*, 804–812. [CrossRef]
51. Stephens, J.M.; Sulway, M.J.; Watkins, P.J. Relationship of Blood Acetoacetate and 3-Hydroxybutyrate in Diabetes. *Diabetes* **1971**, *20*, 485–489. [CrossRef]
52. Sheikh-Ali, M.; Karon, B.S.; Basu, A.; Kudva, Y.C.; Muller, L.A.; Xu, J.; Schwenk, W.F.; Miles, J.M. Can Serum β-Hydroxybutyrate Be Used to Diagnose Diabetic Ketoacidosis? *Diabetes Care* **2008**, *31*, 643–647. [CrossRef]
53. Gall, W.E.; Beebe, K.; Lawton, K.A.; Adam, K.-P.; Mitchell, M.W.; Nakhle, P.J.; Ryals, J.A.; Milburn, M.V.; Nannipieri, M.; Camastra, S. α-Hydroxybutyrate Is an Early Biomarker of Insulin Resistance and Glucose Intolerance in a Nondiabetic Population. *PLoS ONE* **2010**, *5*, e10883. [CrossRef]
54. Chen, J.; Hou, H.; Chen, H.; Luo, Y.; He, Y.; Zhang, L.; Zhang, Y.; Liu, H.; Zhang, F.; Liu, Y. Identification of β-Hydroxybutyrate as a Potential Biomarker for Female Papillary Thyroid Cancer. *Bioanalysis* **2019**, *11*, 461–470. [CrossRef]
55. Hilvo, M.; De Santiago, I.; Gopalacharyulu, P.; Schmitt, W.D.; Budczies, J.; Kuhberg, M.; Dietel, M.; Aittokallio, T.; Markowetz, F.; Denkert, C. Accumulated Metabolites of Hydroxybutyric Acid Serve as Diagnostic and Prognostic Biomarkers of Ovarian High-Grade Serous Carcinomas. *Cancer Res.* **2016**, *76*, 796–804. [CrossRef]
56. Knapp, P.; Baranowski, M.; Knapp, M.; Zabielski, P.; Błachnio-Zabielska, A.U.; Górski, J. Altered Sphingolipid Metabolism in Human Endometrial Cancer. *Prostaglandins Other Lipid Mediat.* **2010**, *92*, 62–66. [CrossRef]
57. Knapp, P.; Chomicz, K.; Świderska, M.; Chabowski, A.; Jach, R. Unique Roles of Sphingolipids in Selected Malignant and Nonmalignant Lesions of Female Reproductive System. *Biomed Res. Int.* **2019**, *2019*. [CrossRef]
58. Ponka, P. Cell Biology of Heme. *Am. J. Med. Sci.* **1999**, *318*, 241–256. [CrossRef]
59. Lionetto, L.; Lostia, A.M.; Stigliano, A.; Cardelli, P.; Simmaco, M. HPLC–Mass Spectrometry Method for Quantitative Detection of Neuroendocrine Tumor Markers: Vanillylmandelic Acid, Homovanillic Acid and 5-Hydroxyindoleacetic Acid. *Clin. Chim. Acta* **2008**, *398*, 53–56. [CrossRef]

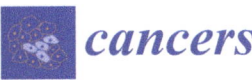

Article

Performance Characteristics of the Ultrasound Strategy during Incidence Screening in the UK Collaborative Trial of Ovarian Cancer Screening (UKCTOCS)

Jatinderpal Kalsi [1], Aleksandra Gentry-Maharaj [2], Andy Ryan [2], Naveena Singh [3], Matthew Burnell [2], Susan Massingham [2], Sophia Apostolidou [2], Aarti Sharma [4], Karin Williamson [5], Mourad Seif [6], Tim Mould [7], Robert Woolas [8], Stephen Dobbs [9], Simon Leeson [10], Lesley Fallowfield [11], Steven J. Skates [12], Mahesh Parmar [2], Stuart Campbell [13], Ian Jacobs [1,14], Alistair McGuire [15] and Usha Menon [2,*]

1 Department of Women's Cancer, Institute for Women's Health, University College London, London WC1E 6HU, UK; j.k.kalsi@ucl.ac.uk (J.K.); i.jacobs@unsw.edu.au (I.J.)
2 MRC Clinical Trials Unit at UCL, Institute of Clinical Trials & Methodology, London WC1V 6LJ, UK; a.gentry-maharaj@ucl.ac.uk (A.G.-M.); a.ryan@ucl.ac.uk (A.R.); m.burnell@ucl.ac.uk (M.B.); s.massingham@ucl.ac.uk (S.M.); s.apostolidou@ucl.ac.uk (S.A.); m.parmar@ucl.ac.uk (M.P.)
3 Department of Pathology, Barts and the London, London E1 2ES, UK; Naveena.Singh@bartshealth.nhs.uk
4 Department of Obstetrics and Gynaecology, University Hospital of Wales, Cardiff CF14 4XW, UK; Aarti.Sharma@wales.nhs.uk
5 Department of Gynaecological Oncology, Nottingham City Hospital, Nottingham NG5 1PB, UK; Karin.Williamson@nuh.nhs.uk
6 Division of Gynaecology and of Cancer Services, St. Mary's Hospital and University of Manchester, Manchester M13 9WL, UK; Mourad.Seif@mft.nhs.uk
7 Department of Gynaecological Oncology, University College London, London NW1 2BU, UK; tim.mould@uclh.nhs.uk
8 Department of Gynaecological Oncology, Queen Alexandra Hospital, Portsmouth PO6 3LY, UK; robert.woolas2@porthosp.nhs.uk
9 Department of Gynaecological Oncology, Belfast City Hospital, Belfast BT9 7AB, UK; Stephen.Dobbs@belfasttrust.hscni.net
10 Department of Obstetrics and Gynaecology, Ysbyty Gwynedd, Bangor, Gwynedd LL57 2PW, UK; simon.leeson@wales.nhs.uk
11 Cancer Research UK Sussex Psychosocial Oncology Group at Brighton & Sussex Medical School, University of Sussex, Falmer BN1 9PX, UK; L.J.Fallowfield@sussex.ac.uk
12 Massachusetts General Hospital, Harvard Medical School, Boston, MA 02115, USA; sskates@gmail.com
13 Create Fertility Clinic, London EC2V 6ET, UK; profscampbell@hotmail.com
14 Department of Women's Health, University of New South Wales, Australia, Sydney 2052, Australia
15 London School of Economics and Political Science, London WC2A 2AE, UK; A.J.Mcguire@lse.ac.uk
* Correspondence: u.menon@ucl.ac.uk; Tel.: +44-7670-4909

Simple Summary: The United Kingdom Collaborative Trial of Ovarian Cancer Screening was undertaken to assess whether screening postmenopausal women from the general population might result in detection of ovarian/tubal cancers at an earlier stage and thus save lives. One of the screening strategies tested was a yearly transvaginal ultrasound scan of the ovaries (USS). Following the initial screen, 44,799 of the 50,639 women in the USS group went on to have a further 280,534 annual scans during April 2002–December 2011. Abnormalities leading to surgery were detected in 960 women of whom 113 (80 invasive epithelial) had ovarian/tubal cancer. Ovarian/tubal cancer was missed in 52 (50 invasive epithelial) women. Of the screen-detected cancers, 37.5% and missed cancers 6% were early stage(I/II). The number (detection rate 61.5%; 80/130) and advanced stage of the missed invasive cancers suggests that a yearly ultrasound scan may not be suitable for screening average risk women for ovarian cancer.

Abstract: Randomised controlled trials of ovarian cancer (OC) screening have not yet demonstrated an impact on disease mortality. Meanwhile, the screening data from clinical trials represents a rich resource to understand the performance of modalities used. We report here on incidence screening in the ultrasound arm of UKCTOCS. 44,799 of the 50,639 women who were randomised to annual screening with transvaginal ultrasound attended annual incidence screening between 28 April 2002 and 31 December 2011. Transvaginal ultrasound was used both as the first and the second line test. Participants were followed up through electronic health record linkage and postal questionnaires. Out of 280,534 annual incidence screens, 960 women underwent screen-positive surgery. 113 had ovarian/tubal cancer (80 invasive epithelial). Of the screen-detected invasive epithelial cancers, 37.5% (95% CI: 26.9–49.0) were Stage I/II. An additional 52 (50 invasive epithelial) were diagnosed within one year of their last screen. Of the 50 interval epithelial cancers, 6.0% (95% CI: 1.3–16.5) were Stage I/II. For detection of all ovarian/tubal cancers diagnosed within one year of screen, the sensitivity, specificity, and positive predictive values were 68.5% (95% CI: 60.8–75.5), 99.7% (95% CI: 99.7–99.7), and 11.8% (95% CI: 9.8–14) respectively. When the analysis was restricted to invasive epithelial cancers, sensitivity, specificity and positive predictive values were 61.5% (95% CI: 52.6–69.9); 99.7% (95% CI: 99.7–99.7) and 8.3% (95% CI: 6.7–10.3), with 12 surgeries per screen positive. The low sensitivity coupled with the advanced stage of interval cancers suggests that ultrasound scanning as the first line test might not be suitable for population screening for ovarian cancer. Trial registration: ISRCTN22488978. Registered on 6 April 2000.

Keywords: ovarian cancer; screening; ultrasound; TVS; early detection; trial; randomised controlled trial; UKCTOCS

1. Introduction

Transvaginal ultrasonography (TVS) is considered the best modality for pelvic imaging, and is used routinely in the clinic for investigating women with suspected ovarian cancer. Based on its ability to assess ovarian volume and morphology, it has been used in large randomised trials of ovarian cancer screening as the primary screen. In the ovarian arm of the Prostate Lung Colorectal and Ovarian (PLCO) Cancer Screening trial [1], it was used in combination with the serum biomarker CA125 while in the ultrasound arm (USS) of the United Kingdom Collaborative Trial of Ovarian Cancer Screening (UKCTOCS), it was used as the sole primary screening test [2]. In both trials, there was no difference in the proportion of women detected with Stage I/II disease or deaths due to ovarian/tubal/peritoneal cancer between the ultrasound arm and the no screening (control) arm [2].

The data collected during these trials provides a rich resource to understand the performance characteristics of TVS in the setting of multicentre, general population screening. We have previously reported on the results of the initial (prevalence) USS screen [3]. We now report on the performance characteristics of USS screening in UKCTOCS during the 10 years of incidence screening.

2. Results

Following the initial (prevalence) screen, of the 50,639 women randomised to the USS arm 49,610 were eligible for incidence screening. Of them, 1029 were ineligible as both ovaries had been removed (896), death (131), moved away (2). Overall, 44,799 (88.5%) of those randomized to the USS arm underwent incidence screening (Figure 1).

In total the women underwent 280,534 annual incidence screens between 28 April 2002 and 31 December 2011. Of these screens, 257,337 (91.8%) were TVS, 20,707 (7.4%) transabdominal, 2309 (0.8%) both and for nine data on mode were missing. Individual women attended between 1 and 10 incidence screens with the median number per woman being 7 (IQR 5–8). The baseline characteristics of these women have been previously reported [2,3]. Median age of the women at the last annual incidence screen was 67 (IQR 62.6–72.0) years.

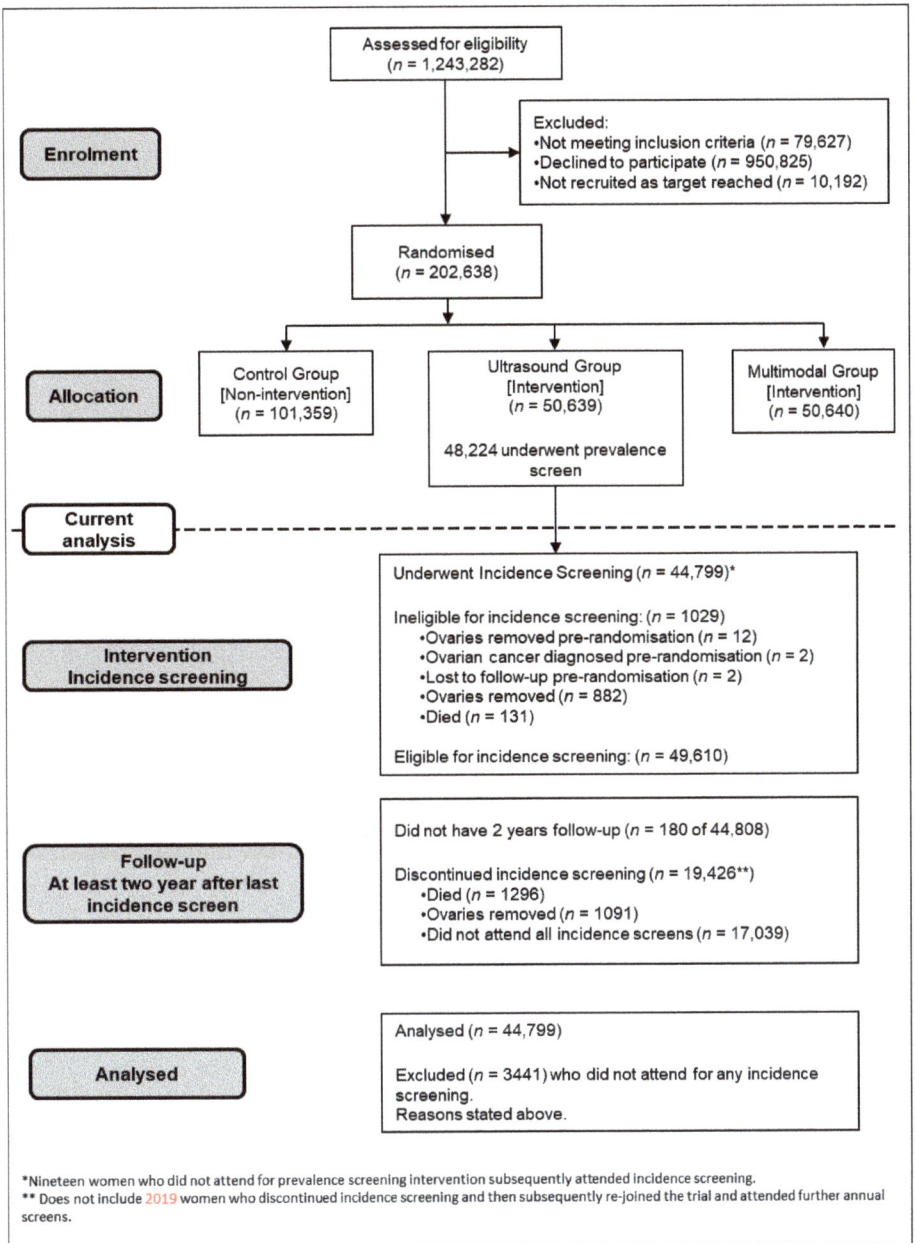

Figure 1. CONSORT diagram.

Overall, 99.4% (278,851/280,534) of the screens resulted in women being returned to annual screening. Two percent (5497/280,534) of screens involving 4256 (9.5%; 4256/44,799) women resulted in referral for clinical evaluation. Of these women 960 (0.34% of screens; 960/280,534) were screen positive and had surgery (Figure 2 and Table 1). This figure includes one woman with a simple ovarian cyst who underwent surgery against protocol recommendation.

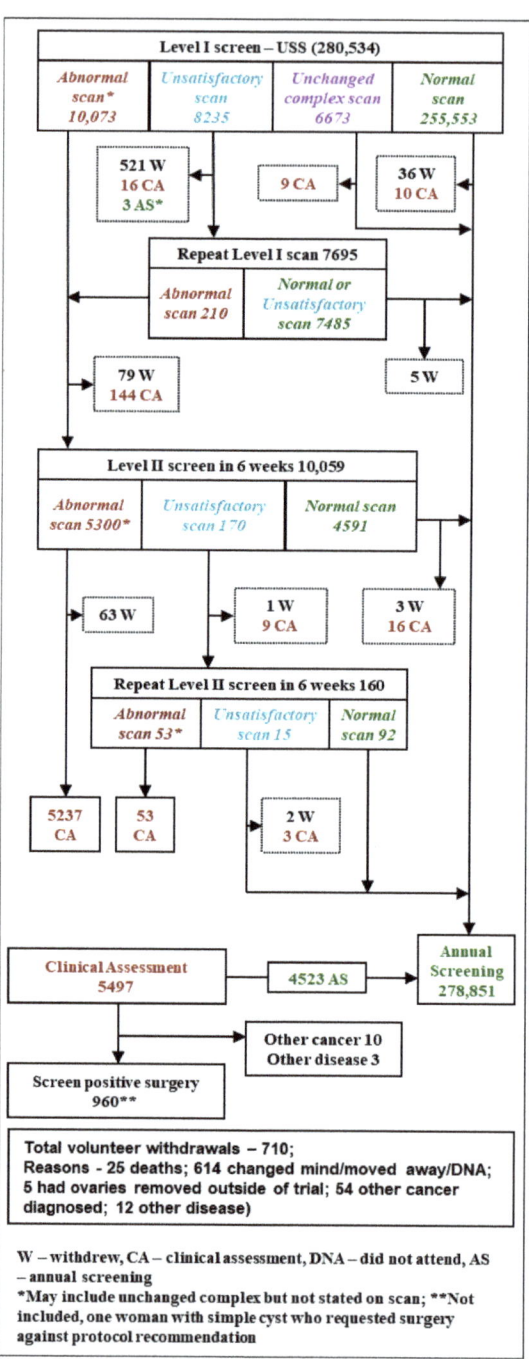

Figure 2. Ultrasound screening (USS) algorithm and outcome of incidence screening.

Table 1. Results of annual incidence screens performed in USS group.

Annual Incidence Screens	Women Years
No. of Level 1 Screens *	280,534 (100)
Normal Scan	262,227 (93.5)
Unsatisfactory Scan	8235 (2.9)
Abnormal Scan	10,072 (3.6)
No. who Underwent Repeat Level 1 Screen †	7695 (2.7)
Returned to annual screening	7485 (97.3)
Referred for Level 2 screen	210 (2.7)
No. Who Underwent Level 2 Screen †	10,060 (3.6)
Returned to annual screening	4591 (45.6)
Referred for clinical assessment	5299 (52.7)
Referred for Repeat Level 2 screen	170 (1.7)
No. Who Underwent Repeat Level 2 Screen †	160 (0.1)
Returned to annual screening	92 (57.5)
Referred for clinical assessment	68 (42.5)
No. Referred for Clinical Assessment †,‡	5495 (2.0)
No. Who Underwent Screen Positive Surgery †	960 (0.3)
Surgical Approach	
Diagnostic laparoscopy §	31 (3.2)
Operative laparoscopy	628 (65.4)
Combined laparoscopy and laparotomy	69 (7.2)
Laparotomy	214 (22.3)
Vaginal hysterectomy with BSO	3 (0.3)
Imaging guided cytology/biopsy	14 (1.5)
Missing data	1 (0.1)

Data is number (%). * Denominators for header rows are numbers of annual screens. Denominators for subsequent rows are number who underwent specific screen. † Difference in numbers between those recommended tests and number who underwent test is due to non-compliance. ‡ 123 women were clinically assessed following a level 1 screen. § Seven women went on to have laparotomy as a second procedure.

Of the 960 surgical procedures, 69% (662/960) were laparoscopic or vaginal. 113 (11.8%) women were diagnosed with ovarian/tubal cancers (Table 2). This included 80 (70.8%) invasive epithelial ovarian or tubal (iEOC), 29 (25.7%) borderline (low malignant potential) epithelial ovarian, and 4 (3.5%) non-epithelial ovarian cancers.

Table 2. Pathologic findings in screen positive women and those with interval cancers (screen negative).

Outcome of Screen Positive Surgery	All Women
Total *	960
Normal or benign pathology	831
Laparoscopy, ovaries normal, not removed	24
Normal ovaries	91
Benign ovarian pathology	716
Non-ovarian/tubal malignant neoplasms	13
Other non-ovarian cancer involving the ovaries (secondary ovarian neoplasm)	7 **
Other non-ovarian cancer not involving the ovaries	6
Screen Positive Women Diagnosed with Malignant Neoplasm of Ovary (ICD-C56) and Fallopian Tube (ICD-C57.0)	
Total	113
Non-epithelial neoplasm of ovary (ICD-C56)	4
Borderline epithelial neoplasm of ovary (ICD-C56)	29
Invasive epithelial neoplasm of tubo-ovarian origin (ICD-C56/C57.0)	80

Table 2. *Cont.*

Women with Screen Negative (Interval) Malignant Neoplasm of Ovary (ICD-C56) and Fallopian Tube (ICD-C57.0) Diagnosed within One Year of End of Screen	
Total	52
Borderline epithelial neoplasm of ovary (ICD-C56)	2
Invasive epithelial neoplasm of tubo-ovarian origin (ICD-C56/C57.0)	50

Data are numbers. * Includes one volunteer who withdrew consent for accessing medical records and two volunteers where the ovaries were not identified due to extensive adhesions arising from a previous hysterectomies. ** Cancers of colorectal (3) breast (1), stomach (1), lymphoma (1), carcinoid small bowel (1).

Of the 29 borderline epithelial ovarian cancers, 28 (96.5%) were Stage I/II as were 3 of 4 (75%) non-epithelial ovarian cancers. Of the screen detected iEOC, 37.5% (30/80) were Stage I/II (Table 3). Of the iEOC 80% (64/80) were Type II and 18.8% (15/80) were Type I. Majority (86.7%; 13/15) of Type I were Stage I/II. Of Type II, only 26.6% (17/64) were Stage I/II. The median time from Level 1 annual screen to surgery for screen detected iEOC was 12.6 weeks (IQR 8.7 to 20.5).

Table 3. Stage and type of invasive epithelial ovarian and tubal cancers as per WHO 2014 classification.

Characteristics	Positive	Negative
Total	80	50
	FIGO 2014 Stage	
I	18	2
II	12	1
III	45	26
IIIa	5	0
IIIb	13	3
IIIc	27	23
IV	5	21
Early (I/II) stage-%(95% CI)	37.5 (26.9, 49.0)	6.0 (1.3, 16.6)
	Morphology	
Type I iEOC (total)	**15 (18.8%)**	**1 (2.0%)**
Low grade serous	3	0
Endometrioid (low grade)	3	0
Clear cell	6	0
Mucinous	3	1
Type II iEOC (total)	**64 (80.0%)**	**42 (84.0%)**
High grade serous	53	36
High grade endometrioid	4	0
Carcinoma	4	6
Carcinosarcoma	3	0
Unclassified *	1 (1.3%)	7 (14.0%)

Date are numbers unless otherwise stated. * Morphology could not be determined as only peritoneal fluid cytology was undertaken.

Of the 960 women who had screen positive surgery, 831 had benign pathology or normal adnexa (Table 2). In this subgroup, 35 (4.2%) women had a major complication (with significant sequelae) (Table S1).

Median follow up from the end of incidence screening to cancer registration update in 2015 (25 March 2015 England and Wales, 15 April 2015 Northern Ireland) was 3.9 (IQR 3.6–5.0) years. Only 5 of 44,799 (0.01%) women had follow-up of less than 2 years after their last screen. An additional 52 women were diagnosed with ovarian/tubal cancer (screen negative/interval cancer) within 1 year of the last incidence screen scan (Table 2). This included 2 borderline and 50 iEOC. Of the latter, 6% (3/50) were diagnosed at Stage I/II (Table 3).

The sensitivity, specificity, and positive predictive values (PPV) were 68.5% (95% CI: 60.8–75.5), 99.7% (95% CI: 99.7–99.7), and 11.8% (95% CI: 9.814) respectively for all ovarian and tubal cancers with 8.5 operations per case detected during incidence screening. When the analysis was restricted to iEOC, sensitivity, specificity and positive predictive values were 61.5% (95% CI: 52.6–69.9); 99.7% (95% CI: 99.7–99.7); and 8.3% (95% CI: 6.7–10.3) with 12 surgeries per screen positive (Table 4).

Table 4. Performance characteristics of incidence USS screening for detection of ovarian and tubal cancers (WHO 2014 classification) within one year of screen.

Characteristics	No/% (95% CI)
Number of women screen years	280,534
Number of surgeries	960
Ovarian and Tubal Malignancies	
Screen positives	113
Screen negatives	52
Sensitivity	68.5% (60.8, 75.5)
Specificity	99.7% (99.7, 99.7)
Positive predictive value	11.8% (9.8, 14.0)
No. of operations per screen positive	8.5
Invasive Epithelial Ovarian and Tubal Malignancies *	
Screen positives	80
Screen negatives	50
Sensitivity	61.5% (52.6, 69.9)
Specificity	99.7% (99.7, 99.7)
Positive predictive value	8.3% (6.7, 10.3)
No. of operations per screen positive	12.0

Data are numbers or % (95% CI) * excludes non epithelial and borderline epithelial ovarian neoplasms).

Combining incidence and prevalence screening [3] of UKCTOCS, the sensitivity, specificity and positive predictive values were 72.3% (95% CI: 65.9–78.0), 99.5% (99.5–99.5), and 9.1% (95% CI: 7.8–10.5) for all ovarian and tubal cancers with 11.0 operations per case detected. When the analysis was restricted to iEOC, sensitivity, specificity, and positive predictive values were 63.3% (55.4, 70.6), 99.5% (95% CI: 99.5–99.5), and 5.8% (4.78–7) with 17.2 surgeries per screen positive.

3. Discussion

3.1. Principal Findings

The performance characteristics of ultrasound screening in the largest ovarian cancer screening trial suggests that USS may not be suitable as a first line test for population screening. While the PPV was significantly higher (11.8% vs. 5.3%; $p < 0.0001$) with fewer operations (8.5 vs. 18.8; $p < 0.0001$) required to detect an ovarian/tubal cancer during incidence screening compared to the prevalence [3], the sensitivity was lower (68.5% versus 84.9%; $p = 0.02$). For invasive epithelial cancers, while over one-third (38%) of the screen detected invasive cancers were early stage, the majority (94.0%) of the interval cancers were advanced (Stage III/IV). The latter, coupled with the low sensitivity (61.5%) resulted in no overall difference (24% USS versus 26% Control; $p = 0.57$) in low volume (Stage I, II, IIIa) invasive epithelial disease between USS and control arm on the previously reported intention to treat analysis [1,2].

3.2. Results in Context

While TVS is integral to all ovarian cancer screening strategies to date, its use as the primary screening test, as described here, has only been assessed in one other study, the University of Kentucky Ovarian Cancer Screening Trial (UKOCST). The latter study involved a slightly higher risk population with just under one fourth having a family history of ovarian and over 40% of breast cancer. It is a single arm single-centre prospective study and involved 46,101 women who underwent a mean of 6.5 annual screens [4]. Overall sensitivity for detecting ovarian cancers (85.5% vs. 72%) was higher than in the USS arm of our trial. TVS has a significant subjective component that is likely to be the key contributor to the differences noted. UKOCST involves a single centre, with all scans performed by a small group of highly experienced ultrasonologists. UKCTOCS involved over 200 Level I ultrasonologists [5] (certified sonographers or doctors with experience in gynaecological scanning in the National Health Service) across 13 centres undertaking ~45,000 scans every year. The latter is more akin to a general population screening programme which would require annual scans for millions of women.

The sensitivity in our USS arm was significantly higher than that sensitivity of TVS alone (44.6%; 33/74) noted during four rounds of screening in the PLCO trial [6]. In the latter trial, the overall sensitivity was higher as the annual screen involved CA125 in addition to a scan, with abnormalities in both tests triggering additional investigations (combined strategy).

In comparison to a CA125-based strategy, PPV of ultrasound screening is low. The number of operations per ovarian cancer decreased from 18.8 during prevalence screening in our USS arm to 8.5 during incidence screening. This latter is similar to the 7.4 operations per case reported in the Kentucky study [4]. It is not possible to calculate a comparable estimate in the PLCO trial as a combined strategy was used.

In our trial, 10,000 complex adnexal masses were detected during the annual incidence screen. Through a process of repeat scanning for persistence of lesion and evaluation of ultrasound features by Level 2 expert sonologists, we were able to restrict surgery to just below 1000 of these women. Both the Kentucky and International Ovarian Tumour Analysis (IOTA) groups have over the years developed increasingly sophisticated rules/scoring systems to improve risk stratification of these adnexal masses and encourage conservative management. In the most recent international IOTA5 study of women with adnexal masses, they were able to avoid surgery in one-third on the basis of low risk ultrasound features [7].

A key requirement to impact on the high ovarian cancer mortality is detection of invasive epithelial ovarian/tubal cancer at a sufficiently early stage. A similar proportion of screen detected ovarian cancers were invasive epithelial both in our analysis (71%: 80/113) and in the Kentucky study (75.5%; 71/94). However, only 37.5% (95% CI: 26.9, 49.0) of screen detected invasive epithelial cancers were early stage (I and II) in our trial compared to 51% (45/71; 95% CI: 51.1, 74.5) in the latest report of the Kentucky study [4]. In the latter, this together with increased sensitivity is likely responsible for the significantly higher 5-year disease-specific survival of women with ovarian (including interval) cancers in the screening group (79 ± 4%) compared to unscreened women with clinically detected epithelial ovarian cancer treated at the same centre during the same time period (45 ± 2%).

In comparison to a CA125 based approach [3], an ultrasound-based strategy detects a larger proportion of borderline ovarian cancers. This was similar in the Kentucky study (15.5%; 17/124, 95% CI: 9.3,23.6) and during incidence screening in UKCTOCS (18.8%; 29/165,95% CI: 13.1, 25.6). In our prevalence screen, it was higher (37.7%, 20/53, 95% CI: 24.7, 52.1). The lower incidence with time is likely due to increasing conservative management of less complex asymptomatic adnexal masses.

3.3. Clinical and Research Implications

The performance characteristics suggest that ultrasound as a first line test is not suitable for population ovarian cancer screening. The subjective nature of TVS, the challenges in identifying normal postmenopausal ovaries [8] that diminish in size with age and the low disease prevalence (1 in 2500) means that detection of disease early requires significant expertise coupled with constant attention to detail. In the course of the trial, we developed an accreditation programme for scanning postmenopausal ovaries [5]. However, our performance characteristics suggest that we were not able to replicate in the Level 1 ultrasonographers, the expertise available at a specialist centre such as Kentucky. The IOTA group have shown in multicentre studies that the performance of ultrasound prediction models/rules can be maintained in sonographers with varying levels of experience [9]. However, this is in the context of evaluation of adnexal masses, which is equivalent to a Level 2 rather than Level 1 screen during population screening. First line TVS screening of the population is always going to be a challenge given the size of the workforce required. The ideal is a less subjective, automated, and more reproducible test. In cervical screening, this has translated to HPV DNA testing increasingly replacing the older resource intensive and skill dependent cytology in many population-screening programmes.

Incidental adnexal findings are on the rise given the widespread use of ultrasound. The unnecessary surgery rates seen in our and the other ultrasound screening trials are relevant to the clinical management of these asymptomatic masses. Our findings suggest that many with low-risk features can be managed conservatively [10].

3.4. Strengths and Limitations

The key strengths of our study are the scale of the trial, high compliance with screening, the multicentre setting and detailed screening protocols and automated management algorithms, implemented by a dedicated central team. Completeness of data on screen-negative cancers was ensured by flagging of the trial cohort through cancer, death, and hospital administrative registries as well as postal follow-up of all women. All potential ovarian cancer cases were reviewed by an independent, blinded outcomes review committee.

A key limitation relates to use of self-reported visualisation of postmenopausal ovaries as a quality assurance measure during the trial. A retrospective audit of random, grey scale TVS images showed only moderate agreement for visualisation of normal ovaries between experts and sonographers and between expert reviewers alone [8]. This was despite a robust accreditation programme established within the trial for visualisation of postmenopausal ovaries. This again highlights the subjectivity of ultrasound scanning, use of video recordings of the ultrasound examination would probably have been a better-quality assurance measure. During the 14 years of trial, there have been significant advances in our understanding of the origin and heterogeneity of ovarian cancer. Our scanning protocol focused on evaluation of the ovary. However, we now know that at least half of high-grade serous cancers arise in the fallopian tube [11] making tubal evaluation critical. The Kentucky group has recently described and assessed such a protocol in older normal women and reported a 77% visualisation rate [12]. Furthermore, in the last decade, there has been significant improvement in the resolution of ultrasound machines and their ability to detect subtle changes as a result of advances in ultrasound transducer technology and electronics.

4. Materials and Methods

4.1. Ethical Approval

The trial (ISRCTN22488978, ClinicalTrials.gov NCT00058032) was approved by the UK North West Multicentre Research Ethics Committees (North West MREC 00/8/34) with site specific approval from the local regional ethics committees and the Caldicott guardians (data controllers) of the primary care trusts. All participants provided written consent.

4.2. Subjects and Screening Strategy

The trial design has been described previously [2,3,13]. Briefly, 202,638 postmenopausal women aged 50 to 74, from the general population were recruited through 13 regional trial centres located in NHS Trusts in England, Wales and Northern Ireland, between April 2001 and October 2005. Overall, 1.6% of women had a maternal history of ovarian cancer and 6.3% a maternal history of breast cancer [3]. Women at increased risk of familial ovarian cancer were excluded from the study. The participants were randomised 1:1:2 to annual screening (until 31 December 2011) with serum CA125 (MMS: 50, 640) or TVS (USS: 50, 639) or no screening (control C: 101, 359). The full trial protocol is accessible at http://ukctocs.mrcctu.ucl.ac.uk/media/1066/ukctocs-protocol_v90_19feb2020.pdf (accessed on 4 February 2021). In the USS arm, 48,230 women underwent an initial (prevalence) screen [3].

Scans were performed by trial sonographers, the majority of whom worked in the NHS providing gynaecological scanning. All trial sonographers underwent additional training for assessment of postmenopausal ovaries and from 2008, formal accreditation [5]. Annual (Level 1) scans were performed by Type 1 (certified sonographers, trained midwives, or doctors with experience in gynaecological scanning) or Type 2 (experienced gynaecologists/radiologists, or senior sonographers, usually superintendent grade with particular expertise in gynaecological scanning) ultrasonographers. Repeat scans on detection of an abnormality (Level 2 scans) were only undertaken by Type 2 sonographers. Most scans during 2002–2008 were done on a dedicated Kretz SA9900 ultrasound machine (Medison, Seoul, Korea) and from 2008–2011 on Acquvix (Medison, Seoul, Korea).

At the annual transvaginal scan (Level 1), ovarian morphology and dimensions were assessed, and ovarian volume calculated. Ovarian morphology was classified as normal, simple cyst (single, thin walled, anechoic cyst with no septa or papillary projections) or complex (ovary had any non-uniform ovarian echogenicity excluding single simple or inclusion cyst). The number and size of cysts, wall regularity, presence and thickness of septae, size of papillations, and echogenicity of the fluid contents were recorded. The cysts were initially classified using the Kentucky screening trial morphology index [14] and from 2003, the International Ovarian Tumour Analysis (IOTA) classification [15]. Where an ovary was not visualised, the sonographer documented 'good view' if 3–5 cms of iliac vessels with well-defined walls and a clear anechoic centre was seen or 'poor view' and stated the reason such as bowel, fibroids, pelvic varicosities, or other. Ascites was defined as a vertical pool of fluid measuring >10 mm in the Pouch of Douglas.

Ultrasound scans were classified based on the morphology of the adnexa and visualisation of the surrounding tissue as follows: (a) normal—where both ovaries had normal morphology or simple cysts were <60 cm^3, or were not visualised but a good view of the iliac vessels was obtained; (b) unsatisfactory—where one or both ovaries were not visualised due to a poor view); (c) abnormal—where one or both ovaries had complex morphology or simple cysts were >60 cm^3, or ascites was present. Based on these results the women were returned to annual screening (normal scan), repeat Level 1 scan (unsatisfactory scan) or Level 2 scan (abnormal scan). In women where adnexal masses had been previously managed conservatively and remained unchanged in morphology or volume (complex unchanged) on repeat annual screens, there was the option for clinical review of results and return to annual screening without undergoing Level 2. Women with an abnormal Level 2 scan were referred for clinical assessment.

This was undertaken at the regional centre by a designated trial clinician and included clinical evaluation and investigations as appropriate. Latter included serum CA125, repeat transvaginal scans and Doppler studies, CT/MRI of the abdomen and pelvis, and occasionally assessment of other tumour markers. A decision was made either to offer surgery or manage conservatively, taking into account the views of the woman, any significant comorbidity, morphological features of the ultrasound-detected lesion, previous hysterectomy, or major pelvic surgery that could contribute to false-positive ultrasound findings. The surgery in most cases involved removal of both ovaries and fallopian tubes using a laparoscopic approach where possible. If pelvic adhesions increased the risk of complications, the clinician could opt to remove only the 'abnormal' ovary. Hysterectomy was only undertaken where there was clear clinical indication. Women found to have ovarian or tubal cancer at a primary laparoscopic procedure underwent a subsequent staging procedure. Where there was high suspicion of ovarian cancer, laparotomy was undertaken. For those managed conservatively, the follow up plan usually involved a TVS and serum CA125 at 3 months with a possible repeat at 6 months, and return to annual screening if the findings were unchanged (unchanged complex).

4.3. Follow-Up

Follow up involved electronic health record linkage for cancer and death registration and hospital admissions using the NHS number through the appropriate national agencies. Cancer registrations received until 25 March 2015 (England and Wales) and 15 April 2015 (Northern Ireland) were used for this analysis. In addition, women were sent postal questionnaires, 3–5 years post randomisation, and again in April 2014 after the end of screening [2].

4.4. Confirmation of Diagnosis

Copies of medical notes were retrieved for all women who had surgery as a consequence of a positive screening test as previously described [2]. Where cancer was diagnosed, additional information e.g., multidisciplinary team meeting notes, discharge summaries, and other relevant correspondence was also collated. The above were also obtained for all women where a notification was received either through linked electronic health records, follow-up questionnaire, or personal communication of a possible ovarian/tubal/peritoneal cancer. The case notes of all of these individuals were reviewed by an Outcomes Review Committee blinded to the randomisation group. They confirmed primary site, stage, morphology, and—where possible—classified invasive epithelial cancer into Type I (low-grade serous, low-grade endometrioid, mucinous, and clear cell cancers) or Type II (high-grade serous, high-grade endometrioid, carcinosarcomas and undifferentiated carcinoma) cancers [16]. Primary site was originally classified according to WHO 2003 [17] and more recently revised using WHO 2014 classification [18]. As a result, cancers initially classified as peritoneal have been reclassified for this analysis as ovarian/tubal. Stage for all cases included in this analysis have been re-reviewed by the Outcomes Committee and assigned as per FIGO 2014 criteria [19].

4.5. Analysis

This analysis is limited to annual screens that followed the initial (prevalence screen). An annual screen as previously defined is a single or series of scans culminating in surgery (screen positive) or return to annual screening (screen negative). For this analysis, women were censored at one year following the last scan performed as part of their last screening episode on the trial. The primary outcome measure was ovarian or fallopian tube cancer as per WHO 2014 classification [18] diagnosed within 12 months of the last scan. Sensitivity (proportion of ovarian/tubal cancers diagnosed within one year that were detected by screening), specificity (proportion of those without ovarian/tubal cancer who had a negative screen) and positive predictive value (proportion with a positive test result who actually had ovarian/tubal cancer) of incidence screening was calculated. Subgroup analysis of invasive epithelial cancers (borderline epithelial and non-epithelial ovarian cancers were excluded) was undertaken. Proportion of cancers detected in early (I/II) stage were calculated.

5. Conclusions

The performance characteristics suggest that ultrasound as the first line test may not be suitable for population screening.

Supplementary Materials: The following table is available online at https://www.mdpi.com/2072-6694/13/4/858/s1, Table S1: Surgical complications in women with benign adnexal masses.

Author Contributions: Conceptualisation—I.J., U.M., S.C., L.F., S.J.S., M.P., and A.M.; Data curation—A.R. and U.M., Formal analysis—A.R., U.M., J.K., A.G.-M., and M.B.; Funding acquisition—I.J., U.M., M.P., L.F., S.J.S., S.C., and A.M.; Investigation—U.M., A.G.-M., A.R., A.S., K.W., M.S., T.M., R.W., S.D., S.L.; J.K., N.S., S.M., and S.A., Methodology—U.M., I.J., S.C., A.G.-M., A.R., and N.S., Project administration—U.M., J.K., A.G.-M., A.R., K.W., M.S., T.M., R.W., S.D., and S.L.; Resources—U.M., I.J., K.W., M.S., T.M., R.W., S.D., and S.L.; Software—U.M. and A.R.; Supervision—U.M., S.C., and I.J.; Validation—U.M., A.G.-M., A.R., S.M., A.S., and S.C.; Visualisation—A.R.; Writing—original draft

J.K., A.G.-M., A.R., and U.M.; Writing—review and editing—all. All authors have read and agreed to the published version of the manuscript.

Funding: The current analysis is supported by National Institute for Health Research (NIHR) HTA grant (16/46/01) and The Eve Appeal. UKCTOCS was funded by Medical Research Council (G9901012 and G0801228), Cancer Research UK (C1479/A2884), and the Department of Health, with additional support from The Eve Appeal. Researchers at UCL are supported by the NIHR University College London Hospitals (UCLH) Biomedical Research Centre and MRC CTU at UCL core funding (MR_UU_12023).

Institutional Review Board Statement: The trial was conducted according to the guidelines of the Declaration of Helsinki, and Good Clinical Practice. The trial was approved by the UK North West Multicentre Research Ethics Committees (North West MREC 00/8/34) on 21 June 2000 with site-specific approval from the local regional ethics committees and the Caldicott guardians (data controllers) of the primary care trusts. The current trial protocol is located at http://ukctocs.mrcctu.ucl.ac.uk/ukctocs/documents/ (accessed date 1 Feberuray 2021).

Informed Consent Statement: All trial participants provided written informed consent.

Data Availability Statement: The datasets used and/or analysed during the current study are available from the corresponding author on reasonable request.

Acknowledgments: The authors thank the volunteers without whom the trial would not have been possible and everyone involved in conduct and oversight, especially the Ultrasound Sub-Committee (http://ukctocs.mrcctu.ucl.ac.uk/ukctocs/committees/ (accessed date 1 Feberuray 2021)).

Conflicts of Interest: U.M. has stock ownership and has received research funding from Abcodia. I.J.J. reports personal fees from and stock ownership in Abcodia as the non-executive director and consultant. He has a patent for the Risk of Ovarian Cancer algorithm and an institutional license to Abcodia with royalty agreement. He is a trustee (2012–2014) and Emeritus Trustee (2015 to present) for The Eve Appeal. SJS reports personal fees from the LUNGevity Foundation and SISCAPA Assay Technologies as a member of their Scientific Advisory Boards, Abcodia as a consultant, and AstraZeneca as a speaker honorarium. He has a patent for the Risk of Ovarian Cancer algorithm and an institutional license to Abcodia. All other authors declare no competing interests.

Disclaimer: Views expressed in this publication are those of the authors and not necessarily those of the NHS, the NIHR or the Department of Health and Social Care.

References

1. Buys, S.S.; Partridge, E.; Black, A.; Johnson, C.C.; Lamerato, L.; Isaacs, C.; Reding, D.J.; Greenlee, R.T.; Yokochi, L.A.; Kessel, B.; et al. Effect of screening on ovarian cancer mortality: The Prostate, Lung, Colorectal and Ovarian (PLCO) Cancer Screening Randomized Controlled Trial. *JAMA* **2011**, *305*, 2295–2303. [CrossRef] [PubMed]
2. Jacobs, I.J.; Menon, U.; Ryan, A.; Gentry-Maharaj, A.; Burnell, M.; Kalsi, J.K.; Amso, N.N.; Apostolidou, S.; Benjamin, E.; Cruickshank, D.; et al. Ovarian cancer screening and mortality in the UK Collaborative Trial of Ovarian Cancer Screening (UKCTOCS): A randomised controlled trial. *Lancet* **2016**, *387*, 945–956. [CrossRef]
3. Menon, U.; Gentry-Maharaj, A.; Hallett, R.; Ryan, A.; Burnell, M.; Sharma, A.; Lewis, S.; Davies, S.; Philpott, S.; Lopes, A.; et al. Sensitivity and specificity of multimodal and ultrasound screening for ovarian cancer, and stage distribution of detected cancers: Results of the prevalence screen of the UK Collaborative Trial of Ovarian Cancer Screening (UKCTOCS). *Lancet Oncol.* **2009**, *10*, 327–340. [CrossRef]
4. van Nagell, J.R., Jr.; Burgess, B.T.; Miller, R.W.; Baldwin, L.; DeSimone, C.P.; Ueland, F.R.; Huang, B.; Chen, Q.; Kryscio, R.J.; Pavlik, E.J. Survival of Women With Type I and II Epithelial Ovarian Cancer Detected by Ultrasound Screening. *Obstet. Gynecol.* **2018**, *132*, 1091–1100. [CrossRef] [PubMed]
5. Sharma, A.; Burnell, M.; Gentry-Maharaj, A.; Campbell, S.; Amso, N.N.; Seif, M.W.; Fletcher, G.; Brunell, C.; Turner, G.; Rangar, R.; et al. Quality assurance and its impact on ovarian visualization rates in the multicenter United Kingdom Collaborative Trial of Ovarian Cancer Screening (UKCTOCS). *Ultrasound Obstet. Gynecol.* **2015**, *47*, 228–235. [CrossRef] [PubMed]
6. Partridge, E.E.; Kreimer, A.R.; Greenlee, R.T.; Williams, C.R.; Xu, J.-L.; Church, T.R.; Kessel, B.; Johnson, C.C.; Weissfeld, J.L.; Isaacs, C.; et al. Results From Four Rounds of Ovarian Cancer Screening in a Randomized Trial. *Obstet. Gynecol.* **2009**, *113*, 775–782. [CrossRef] [PubMed]
7. Froyman, W.; Landolfo, C.; De Cock, B.; Wynants, L.; Sladkevicius, P.; Testa, A.C.; Van Holsbeke, C.; Domali, E.; Fruscio, R.; Epstein, E.; et al. Risk of complications in patients with conservatively managed ovarian tumours (IOTA5): A 2-year interim analysis of a multicentre, prospective, cohort study. *Lancet Oncol.* **2019**, *20*, 448–458. [CrossRef]

8. Stott, W.; Gentry-Maharaj, A.; Ryan, A.; Amso, N.; Seif, M.; Jones, C.; Jacobs, I.; Parmar, M.; Menon, U.; Campbell, S.; et al. Audit of transvaginal sonography of normal postmenopausal ovaries by sonographers from the United Kingdom Collaborative Trial of Ovarian Cancer Screening (UKCTOCS). *F1000Research* **2018**, *7*, 1241. [CrossRef] [PubMed]
9. Sayasneh, A.; Wynants, L.; Preisler, J.; Kaijser, J.; Johnson, S.; Stalder, C.; Husicka, R.; Abdallah, Y.; Raslan, F.; Drought, A.; et al. Multi-centre external validation of IOTA prediction models and RMI by operators with varied training. *Br. J. Cancer* **2013**, *108*, 2448–2454. [CrossRef] [PubMed]
10. Sharma, A.; Apostolidou, S.; Burnell, M.; Campbell, S.; Habib, M.; Gentry-Maharaj, A.; Amso, N.; Seif, M.W.; Fletcher, G.; Singh, N.; et al. Risk of epithelial ovarian cancer in asymptomatic women with ultrasound-detected ovarian masses: A prospective cohort study within the UK collaborative trial of ovarian cancer screening (UKCTOCS). *Ultrasound Obstet. Gynecol.* **2012**, *40*, 338–344. [CrossRef] [PubMed]
11. Soong, T.R.; Howitt, B.E.; Horowitz, N.; Nucci, M.R.; Crum, C.P. The fallopian tube, "precursor escape" and narrowing the knowledge gap to the origins of high-grade serous carcinoma. *Gynecol. Oncol.* **2019**, *152*, 426–433. [CrossRef] [PubMed]
12. Lefringhouse, J.R.; Neward, E.; Ueland, F.R.; Baldwin, L.A.; Miller, R.W.; DeSimone, C.P.; Kryscio, R.J.; van Nagell, J.R.; Pavlik, E.J. Probability of fallopian tube and ovarian detection with transvaginal ultrasonography in normal women. *Womens Health* **2016**, *12*, 303–311. [CrossRef] [PubMed]
13. Menon, U.; Gentry-Maharaj, A.; Ryan, A.; Sharma, A.; Burnell, M.; Hallett, R.; Lewis, S.; Lopez, A.; Godfrey, K.; Oram, D.; et al. Recruitment to multicentre trials–lessons from UKCTOCS: Descriptive study. *BMJ* **2008**, *337*, a2079. [CrossRef] [PubMed]
14. van Nagell, J.R., Jr.; DePriest, P.D.; Ueland, F.R.; DeSimone, C.P.; Cooper, A.L.; McDonald, J.M.; Pavlik, E.J.; Kryscio, R.J. Ovarian cancer screening with annual transvaginal sonography: Findings of 25,000 women screened. *Cancer* **2007**, *109*, 1887–1896. [CrossRef] [PubMed]
15. Timmerman, D.; Valentin, L.; Bourne, T.H.; Collins, W.P.; Verrelst, H.; Vergote, I. International Ovarian Tumor Analysis (IOTA) Group. Terms, definitions and measurements to describe the sonographic features of adnexal tumors: A consensus opinion from the International Ovarian Tumor Analysis (IOTA) Group. *Ultrasound Obstet. Gynecol.* **2000**, *16*, 500–505. [CrossRef] [PubMed]
16. Kurman, R.J.; Shih, I.-M. The Dualistic Model of Ovarian Carcinogenesis: Revisited, Revised, and Expanded. *Am. J. Pathol.* **2016**, *186*, 733–747. [CrossRef] [PubMed]
17. Tavassoli, F.A.; Devilee, P. (Eds.) *Classification of Tumours, Pathology and Genetics: Tumors of the Breast and Female Genital Organs*; World Health Organization: Lyon, France, 2003.
18. Daya, D.; Cheung, A.N.; Khunamornpong, S. Tumors of the peritoneum: Epithelial tumors of Müllerian type. In *WHO Classification of Tumors of Female Reproductive Organs*, 4th ed.; Kurman, R.J., Carcangiu, M.L., Herrington, C.S., Young, R.H., Eds.; International Agency for Research on Cancer: Lyon, France, 2014; pp. 92–93.
19. Prat, J.; FIGO Committee on Gynecologic Oncology. Staging classification for cancer of the ovary, fallopian tube, and peritoneum. *Int. J. Gynecol. Obstet.* **2014**, *124*, 1–5. [CrossRef] [PubMed]

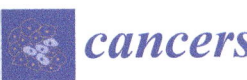

Article

Tumor Signature Analysis Implicates Hereditary Cancer Genes in Endometrial Cancer Development

Olga Kondrashova [1,†], Jannah Shamsani [1,†], Tracy A. O'Mara [1], Felicity Newell [1], Amy E. McCart Reed [2], Sunil R. Lakhani [2,3], Judy Kirk [4,5], John V. Pearson [1], Nicola Waddell [1,†] and Amanda B. Spurdle [1,*,†]

[1] Department of Genetics and Computational Biology, QIMR Berghofer Medical Research Institute, Brisbane 4006, Australia; olga.kondrashova@qimrberghofer.edu.au (O.K.); jannah@genieus.co (J.S.); Tracy.OMara@qimrberghofer.edu.au (T.A.O.); Felicity.Newell@qimrberghofer.edu.au (F.N.); John.Pearson@qimrberghofer.edu.au (J.V.P.); Nic.Waddell@qimrberghofer.edu.au (N.W.)

[2] UQ Centre for Clinical Research, Faculty of Medicine, The University of Queensland, Brisbane 4029, Australia; amy.reed@uq.edu.au (A.E.M.R.); s.lakhani@uq.edu.au (S.R.L.)

[3] Anatomical Pathology, Pathology Queensland, Brisbane 4029, Australia

[4] Familial Cancer Service, Crown Princess Mary Cancer Centre, Westmead Hospital, Sydney 2145, Australia; judy.kirk@sydney.edu.au

[5] Centre for Cancer Research, The Westmead Institute for Medical Research, Sydney Medical School, University of Sydney, Sydney 2145, Australia

* Correspondence: Amanda.Spurdle@qimrberghofer.edu.au; Tel.: +61-(73)-362-0371

† These authors contributed equally to the work.

Simple Summary: Women with a family history of cancer are at increased risk of cancer, including endometrial cancer (affecting the womb lining). In some of the women with such family history, the risk can be explained by deleterious changes in mismatch repair genes that cause Lynch syndrome. This study explored the role of other genes in risk of endometrial cancer, using several approaches. The number and type of changes in gene sequence information in women with endometrial cancer was compared to that from individuals in the general population. Gene sequence changes in endometrial cancer patients with a family history of cancer were also analyzed. Lastly, endometrial cancers from individuals with gene changes were examined for distinctive genomic patterns expected to be seen if a gene change was driving the cancer. This study has identified several additional genes for further exploration in relation to endometrial cancer risk and therapy.

Abstract: Risk of endometrial cancer (EC) is increased ~2-fold for women with a family history of cancer, partly due to inherited pathogenic variants in mismatch repair (MMR) genes. We explored the role of additional genes as explanation for familial EC presentation by investigating germline and EC tumor sequence data from The Cancer Genome Atlas (n = 539; 308 European ancestry), and germline data from 33 suspected familial European ancestry EC patients demonstrating immunohistochemistry-detected tumor MMR proficiency. Germline variants in MMR and 26 other known/candidate EC risk genes were annotated for pathogenicity in the two EC datasets, and also for European ancestry individuals from gnomAD as a population reference set (n = 59,095). Ancestry-matched case–control comparisons of germline variant frequency and/or sequence data from suspected familial EC cases highlighted *ATM*, *PALB2*, *RAD51C*, *MUTYH* and *NBN* as candidates for large-scale risk association studies. Tumor mutational signature analysis identified a microsatellite-high signature for all cases with a germline pathogenic MMR gene variant. Signature analysis also indicated that germline loss-of-function variants in homologous recombination (*BRCA1*, *PALB2*, *RAD51C*) or base excision (*NTHL1*, *MUTYH*) repair genes can contribute to EC development in some individuals with germline variants in these genes. These findings have implications for expanded therapeutic options for EC cases.

Keywords: endometrial cancer; genomic sequencing; tumor mutational signatures; hereditary cancer genes; mismatch repair; familial cancer

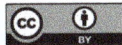

1. Introduction

Endometrial cancer (EC) is the most commonly diagnosed gynecological malignancy, with an increased prevalence rate in developed countries [1]. Modifiable factors such as obesity, lifestyle, and hormone levels are associated with increased risk of EC, and women with a family history of EC or other cancers, such as colorectal, are at ~2–3 fold increased risk of EC [2]. The genetic factors identified to date are either common low-risk cancer predisposition variants that act together to cause polygenic disease, or rare high-risk pathogenic variants in cancer syndrome genes generally present in patients with a monogenic disease phenotype [3].

The major known monogenic form of EC is Lynch syndrome, caused by germline pathogenic variants impacting the mismatch repair (MMR) genes *MLH1*, *MSH2*, *MSH6*, *PMS2*, as well as *EPCAM* deletions, which impact *MSH2* expression. Lynch syndrome accounts for approximately 3–5% of EC at the population level and an increased proportion in cases with family history of colorectal, endometrial and other cancers [4]. The lifetime cumulative risk of EC for women with Lynch syndrome is 40–70%, depending on which MMR gene is disrupted [5]. EC is also a spectrum cancer of Cowden syndrome, caused by the inheritance of pathogenic *PTEN* variants. The cumulative risk of EC for women up to 60 years of age with Cowden syndrome is around 20% [6]. Studies to date suggest that *PTEN* pathogenic variants are very rarely detected in the general population, and mostly in the context of clinical features of Cowden syndrome [7].

Results from a recent study assessing risk associated with reported family history of endometrial and other cancers, after considering proband MMR proficiency and MMR germline test results, indicate that the genetic basis for a substantial fraction of familial EC patients with MMR deficient and MMR proficient tumors remains unexplained [8].

Several genes involved in other hereditary cancer syndromes have been either directly or indirectly implicated in hereditary EC, but with insufficient or conflicting support that germline DNA gene testing would provide clinically useful information for genetic counseling [4]. These include established hereditary cancer syndrome genes, such as *POLE*, *POLD1*, *MUTYH*, *STK11*, *TP53*, *BRCA1* and *BRCA2* [9–21]. Additionally, germline alterations in a number of other known or candidate cancer risk genes have been identified in EC patients from clinical or research studies, including homologous recombination (HR) DNA repair pathway genes (reviewed in [4]). However, because of the paucity of studies focusing on EC and limitations due to study design, there is uncertainty regarding EC risk associated with variants in these genes [4,22].

To explore which genes may influence the EC risk beyond the well-recognized MMR genes, we assessed the frequency of pathogenic variants in a total of 30 known or candidate EC risk genes in publicly available EC and population data. To assist with the interpretation of the EC driver status of pathogenic variants, we performed tumor mutational signature analysis. We also sequenced and analyzed the germline exomes or whole genomes of 33 EC cases with reported family history of endometrial and other cancer types with no evidence of tumor MMR deficiency.

2. Materials and Methods

2.1. Study Participants and Data Resources

EC cases unselected for family history were accessed from The Cancer Genome Atlas Uterine Corpus Endometrial Carcinoma study (TCGA-UCEC; $n = 539$). Germline and tumor whole exome sequencing data was used. To align with the most recent NIH genomic data sharing policy, TCGA IDs have been de-identified. For case–control variant frequency comparison, the analysis was limited to individuals of European ancestry ($n = 308$; Table S1). Ancestry was determined from SNP arrays and classified as European or Non-European [23]. Where SNP-determined ancestry was not available, cases were selected by self-reported race.

GnomAD r2.1.1 database was used as a control population ($n = 15,708$ genomes and $n = 125,748$ exomes). To overcome issues around population stratification for case–control comparison, we limited our analysis to individuals of European ancestry (gnomAD—Non-Finnish Europeans; n = 95,095).

Suspected familial EC cases were selected from the Australian National Endometrial Cancer Study (ANECS), a population-based study of epidemiological and genetic risk factors for EC. Details of the ANECS study design, including recruitment and data collection, are described in detail in previous publications [8,24,25]. Cases were selected for this study if they met all of the following criteria: the case provided detailed cancer report information in first, second and selected third degree relatives by structured questionnaire and follow-up interview [8]; the case (or for one individual—endometrial cancer affected sister) had previously demonstrated tumor MMR proficiency using immunohistochemistry [24,25]; the case had reported at least one affected relative with a cancer diagnosis (excluding skin cancer due to the significant role of environmental factors in Australia, and excluding EC after a breast cancer diagnosis due to possible confounding by tamoxifen exposure); and there was a germline DNA sample (extracted from whole blood) available for analysis. Germline sequencing was undertaken for 33 unrelated EC cases. The clinical features of the cohort are summarized in Table S2. Participants self-reported British/Irish heritage, and/or were confirmed to have European heritage based on genetic markers.

2.2. Sequencing for Suspected Familial EC Cases

Genomic DNA was extracted from blood using a salting out method. DNA samples from 6 cases were sequenced using whole exome sequencing and 27 samples were sequenced using whole genome sequencing. Exome libraries were prepared using the Nextera Rapid Capture Exome Kit (Illumina) and sequencing was performed on the NextSeq500 (Illumina) using 2 × 150 bp reads with an average read depth of 75× (Table S3). Whole genome sequencing was performed using HiSeq X Ten (Illumina) with an average read depth of 36× (Table S3). Tumor DNA of one ANECS EC patient (case 28) carrying a germline *MUTYH* variant was extracted from Formalin-Fixed Paraffin-Embedded (FFPE) tissue using Qiagen DNeasy Blood and Tissue kit (Qiagen, Hilden, Germany). Tumor DNA whole genome sequencing was performed using HiSeq X Ten (Illumina, San Diego, CA, USA) to an average read depth of 12×.

2.3. Sequence Analysis

TCGA-UCEC sequencing data were downloaded as aligned reads (BAM format) and converted to FASTQ format for processing.

Sequencing reads were trimmed using Cutadapt (version 1.9) [26] and aligned to the reference genome (GRCh37) with BWA-MEM (version 0.7.13) [27]. Duplicate aligned reads were marked with Picard (version 1.141) (http://picard.sourceforge.net accessed on 17 November 2015) and sorted using samtools (version 1.3) [28]. Somatic and germline variants were identified by a dual calling strategy using qSNP [29] and GATK Haplotype caller [30], as previously described [31]. For the FFPE tumor sample (case 28), single nucleotide variants (SNVs) were annotated to identify overlapping reads to prevent overcalling due to DNA fragmentation from formalin fixation. SNVs with at least 5 alternate bases after removal of overlapping reads and those absent in dbSNP were kept for signature analysis.

Germline variants were annotated using the Ensembl Variant Effect Predictor (VEP) [32], with population allele frequency based on the Exome Aggregation Consortium (ExAC-nonTCGA v3). The *in silico* predictions were annotated using VEP-plugins: REVEL [33] and MaxEntScan [34]. Variants were also annotated for variant pathogenicity as submitted to ClinVar [35], if present in this database.

2.4. Variant Prioritization

Analysis was focused on rare germline variants (minor allele frequency (MAF) of less than 1% in any population in the ExAC-nonTCGA) in 30 genes of interest [4], including the four MMR genes and *EPCAM* (Table S4). In this study, we excluded from analysis any variants in exons 9 and 11–15 of *PMS2*, due to homology with the *PMS2L* pseudogene in these regions [36]. For *POLE* and *POLD1* genes, only missense variants were considered [37].

For the gnomAD and TCGA-UCEC dataset analysis, only pathogenic or likely pathogenic ClinVar variants or predicted truncating variants (termed as likely pathogenic in this study) were considered (Figure S1). The proportion of pathogenic/likely pathogenic carriers in TCGA and gnomAD datasets was calculated by dividing the number of observed pathogenic/likely pathogenic variants by the total number of individuals sequenced for that gene. For the gnomAD dataset, the number of individuals sequenced was calculated by halving the highest allele number for each gene.

For the familial EC dataset, variants present in three or more samples were excluded as common variants. The remaining variants were reviewed and included if they were: (i) predicted truncating variants (nonsense, frameshift indels, and splice donor or acceptor); (ii) predicted to be deleterious by *in silico* predictions using REVEL (cutoff of ≥ 0.5) or PROVEAN (cutoff of ≤ -2.5) [38]; (iii) predicted to disrupt native donor/acceptor site or create a de novo donor splice site (including synonymous) [34]; or (iv) annotated as pathogenic, likely pathogenic or uncertain significance (VUS), with supporting evidence provided, by multiple submitters in ClinVar database. All candidate variants identified in the familial EC samples were manually reviewed in the Integrated Genome Viewer (IGV) to eliminate any artefacts. Validation of the three prioritized variants was performed by Sanger sequencing.

2.5. Mutation Signature Analysis

At least 100 somatic SNVs per sample were required for signature analysis. SNV mutational signature analysis was performed using deconstructSigs and the COSMIC v2 signature catalogue with the minimum signature contribution set to 15% [39]. Default settings were used for the familial EC case 28 (whole-genome sequencing) and the exome settings for the TCGA-UCEC cohort. *De novo* signature analysis was previously performed using SigProfiler [40].

TCGA-UCEC data were assessed for tumor mutation burden (TMB), microsatellite instability (MSI) status, tumor enrichment of the germline variant in question and additional somatic variations in same gene for *POLE* and MMR genes. TMB was calculated as a number of all somatic mutations divided by the coverage (Mb) of capture kit used (hg18 Nimblegen v2—26.2 Mb, SureSelect All Exon—44 Mb, Nimblegen SeqCap EZ v2.0—36.5 Mb and Nimblegen SeqCap EZ v3.0—64 Mb). The level of MSI was assessed using MSIsensor (v0.2) on tumor-normal pairs [41]. The analysis was limited to the capture-covered regions. Samples with MSI scores ≥ 3.5 were classified as MSI-high. Germline variants were considered enriched in tumor if the percentage of sequence reads containing a variant was $\geq 60\%$ in the tumor sample.

POLE somatic mutation status for TCGA-UCEC samples was determined by checking for somatic missense *POLE* mutations in exons 9–14. MMR gene somatic mutation status for TCGA-UCEC samples was assessed using the same approach as for the germline variants. *MLH1* gene methylation and *MSH2* gene deletion (copy number-based) information for TCGA-UCEC (Firehose legacy) study [42] was downloaded from cBioPortal [43,44]. *MLH1* was classified as methylated if the beta-value was >0.3.

2.6. Code and Data Availability

Scripts used for TCGA and gnomAD data analysis are available on https://github.com/okon/EC_TCGA_vs_gnomAD. TCGA-UCEC data were downloaded from GDC data portal in October 2016. GnomAD variant files (r.2.1.1) were downloaded from the gnomAD portal in April 2019. ANECS sequencing data are available upon reasonable request and subject to ethics approval.

3. Results

3.1. Germline Variants in Data from Publicly Available EC Cases

We compared the frequency of germline variants between EC cases unselected for family history (TCGA-UCEC study) and the general population (gnomAD database) in a subset of 30 genes, previously highlighted as known or purported to be associated with risk of developing EC (Table S4) [4]. Pathogenic or likely pathogenic variants were selected based on ClinVar reports or predicted protein truncating effect, as outlined in Figure S1. We did not perform formal statistical comparisons because the EC cohort size (n = 308) was underpowered to detect significant differences for the expected rare observations, even for MMR genes.

A total of 19 distinct germline pathogenic or likely pathogenic variants were detected in 12 of 30 analyzed risk genes in 25 of 308 TCGA-UCEC cases (Table 1 and Table S5), similar to previous analyses [4,45]. The carrier frequency in the EC cases compared to the gnomAD population was more than double for three of the known MMR genes—*MSH6* (1.3% vs. 0.23%), *MSH2* (0.65% vs. 0.02%) and *PMS2* (0.32% vs. 0.13%), as well as for the HR repair genes *RAD51C* (0.97% vs. 0.1%), *PALB2* (0.32% vs. 0.14%) and *NBN* (0.32% vs. 0.15%). Pathogenic or likely pathogenic variants observed for other candidate EC risk genes occurred at less than 2-fold increased frequency or were found with a lower frequency in cases versus controls, namely: *BRCA1* (0.32% vs. 0.24%), *NTHL1* (0.65% vs. 0.45%), *FAN1* (0.32% vs. 0.31%), *SEC23B* (0.32% vs. 0.33%), *MUTYH* (1.62% vs. 1.73%) and *CHEK2* (0.97% vs. 1.86%).

3.2. Role of Germline Variants in Driving EC Development in TCGA-UCEC Cases

We explored the potential role of germline variants in known and candidate EC risk genes in cancer development by analyzing tumor sequencing data for evidence of tumor variant enrichment and presence of mutational signatures reflective of defective DNA repair pathways (e.g., HR pathway). We assessed 46 TCGA-UCEC cases, unselected by ancestry, with pathogenic or likely pathogenic germline variants (n = 31 distinct variants) in the 30 prioritized genes (Table S5).

Three of the eight cases with pathogenic or likely pathogenic germline variants in MMR genes had evidence of variant enrichment in tumor (one *MSH2* and two *MSH6* variants with >60% variant reads in the tumor sample; Figure 1). In three cases with *MSH2* or *MSH6* variants (one with germline variant enrichment in tumor), we detected a second somatic hit in the respective genes (Figure 1). While we did not observe tumor variant enrichment or second hits for the other three MMR-positive cases, all eight cases had high TMB (>10 Mut/Mb) indicative of MMR deficiency and MSI detected by MSIsensor. We also observed MMR-associated mutational signatures in all eight cases by *de novo* signature analysis (over 25% contribution; eight out of eight cases; Figure S2), and also by signature assignment to the 30 known COSMIC v2 signatures for two of the eight cases, further supporting the tumor driver role of MMR variants in these cases (Figure 1).

Nine cases with germline variants in HR-related genes *PALB2*, *BRCA1*, *RAD51C*, *FAN1* and *CHEK2* also showed evidence of enrichment of the germline variant in the tumor, while the other 12 cases with HR-related gene variants (seven *FAN1*, three *CHEK2*, one *BRIP1*, one *NBN*) did not (Figure 1). Using mutational signature assignment analysis, Signature 3—associated with HR deficiency, was detected in six of seven of tumors with *BRCA1*, *PALB2* and *RAD51C* variants. We did not observe Signature 3 in the other cases with germline alterations in HR-related genes, suggesting that they were HR pathway proficient.

One of two cases that harbored germline inactivating *NTHL1* variant (p.Gln9*) had evidence of tumor variant enrichment (Figure 1). This case showed high TMB and presence of Signature 30, characterized by the prevalence of C>T mutations and associated with deficiency in base excision repair expected due to *NTHL1* inactivation [46]. However, this case also showed high MSI and *MLH1* methylation. Finally, no cases with the germline pathogenic *MUTYH* variant (c.1187G>A, p.Gly396Asp) showed evidence of variant enrichment in the tumor nor presence of Signature 18, associated with *MUTYH* inactivation.

Of note, while three cases with *MUTYH* variants had high TMB, we attributed it to MMR deficiency in the tumor due to *MLH1* methylation or deletion of *MSH2*, supported by high MSI levels and MMR-deficient mutational signatures.

Table 1. Overall frequency of pathogenic and likely pathogenic variants in 30 known and candidate endometrial cancer (EC) risk genes in an EC sample set (TCGA-UCEC study) and the general population (gnomAD).

Gene	Endometrial Cancer Cases (TCGA-UCEC)				General Population (gnomAD)			
	Number of Carriers	Number of Homozygote Carriers	Number of Total Cases	Carrier Frequency (%)	Number of Carriers	Number of Homozygote Carriers	Number of Total Cases	Carrier Frequency (%)
MUTYH	5	0	308	1.62	1023	3	59,095	1.73
MSH6	**4**	**0**	**308**	**1.3**	**134**	**0**	**59,095**	**0.23**
CHEK2	3	0	308	0.97	1099	7	59,093	1.86
RAD51C	**3**	**0**	**308**	**0.97**	**61**	**0**	**59,093**	**0.1**
NTHL1	2	0	308	0.65	268	0	59,090	0.45
MSH2	**2**	**0**	**308**	**0.65**	**11**	**0**	**59,092**	**0.02**
SEC23B	1	0	308	0.32	197	0	59,094	0.33
FAN1	1	0	308	0.32	186	0	59,095	0.31
BRCA1	1	0	308	0.32	140	0	59,095	0.24
NBN	1	0	308	0.32	89	0	59,072	0.15
PALB2	1	0	308	0.32	85	0	59,094	0.14
PMS2	1	0	308	0.32	76	0	59,095	0.13
ATM	0	0	0	0	284	0	59,088	0.48
BRCA2	0	0	0	0	182	0	59,079	0.31
BRIP1	0	0	0	0	123	0	59,090	0.21
FANCC	0	0	0	0	104	0	59,095	0.18
RINT1	0	0	0	0	55	0	59,094	0.09
APC	0	0	0	0	50	0	59,090	0.08
MLH1	0	0	0	0	34	0	59,095	0.06
EPCAM	0	0	0	0	32	0	59,092	0.05
PTEN	0	0	0	0	27	0	59,095	0.05
SDHB	0	0	0	0	20	0	59,089	0.03
TP53	0	0	0	0	20	0	59,095	0.03
SDHC	0	0	0	0	14	0	59,093	0.02
SDHD	0	0	0	0	7	0	59,095	0.01
AKT1	0	0	0	0	4	0	59,094	0.01
PIK3CA	0	0	0	0	3	0	58,839	0.01
STK11	0	0	0	0	2	0	58,753	0
POLD1	0	0	0	0	0	0	59,092	0
POLE	0	0	0	0	0	0	59,095	0

Only cases with Non-Finnish European ethnicity were included. Genes highlighted in bold had a frequency of >2 times higher in TCGA-UCEC compared with gnomAD. Carrier frequency represents the sum of all (likely) pathogenic variants in that gene. Genes highlighted in bold had more than double variant carrier frequency in the EC cases compared to the gnomAD population.

3.3. Germline Variants in Suspected Familial EC Cases

To further explore which genes may explain the etiology of familial EC beyond the well-recognized MMR genes, we sequenced the germline exomes or whole genomes of 33 familial EC cases with no evidence of tumor MMR deficiency, and reported family history of endometrial or other cancer types. The analysis was focused on the same 30 genes as in the sections above (Table S4). Out of the 33 cases, we identified three cases with candidate variants in the prioritized genes. These were a frameshift deletion in *PALB2*:c.3116delA (p.Asn1039Ilefs), an in-frame deletion in *ATM*:c.7638_7646del (p.Arg2547_Ser2549del) and a missense pathogenic variant *MUTYH*:c.536A>G (p.Tyr179Cys).

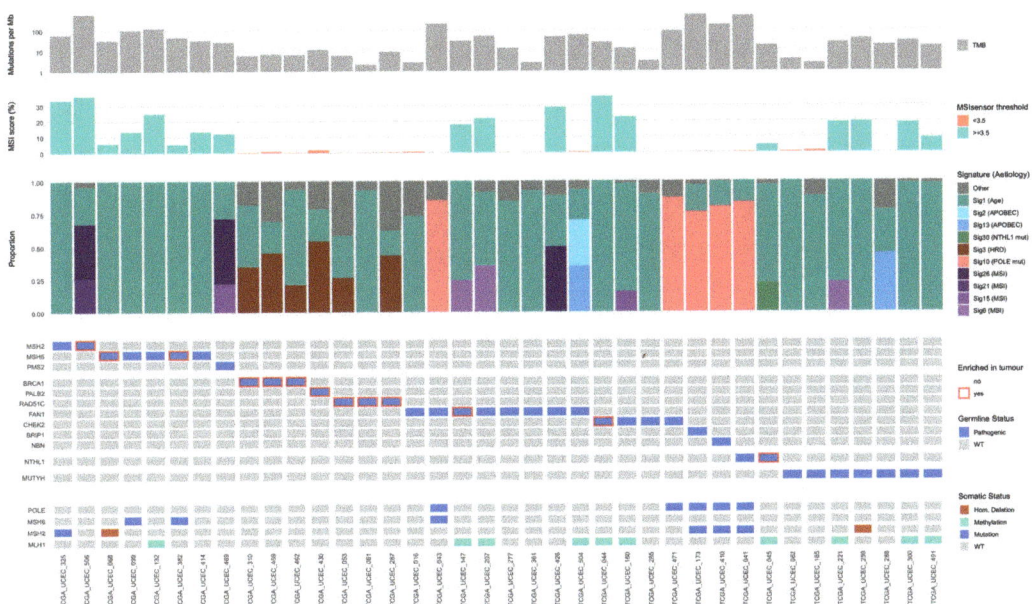

Figure 1. Somatic mutational signature analysis of the germline variant carriers in the TCGA-UCEC cohort. Tumor mutation burden (TMB), microsatellite instability (MSI) scores and mutational signatures observed in the TCGA-UCEC cases with pathogenic or likely pathogenic variants in DNA damage repair genes associated with specific mutational signatures.

The patient (case 2) carrying the pathogenic *PALB2* frameshift variant (c.3116delA, p.Asn1039Ilefs) was diagnosed with stage 1 endometrioid EC at age 70 years. She self-reported that 17 family members had been diagnosed with various types of cancer (Figure 2A), including two with EC—diagnosed at age 60 years (mother) and age 35 years (maternal aunt). Although DNA was not available from the EC-affected mother, the pedigree analysis indicates she is an obligate carrier; genotyping of three other relatives identified two carrying the *PALB2* variant, specifically a sister with colon cancer and maternal cousin with breast cancer (Figure 2A).

The in-frame deletion *ATM* variant (c.7638_7646del, p.Arg2547_Ser2549del) was predicted to be deleterious by PROVEAN and was classified as pathogenic for Ataxia-telangiectasia syndrome by multiple ClinVar submitters. The carrier (case 1) of this variant was diagnosed with stage 1 endometrioid EC at age 77 years. Two of the family members were also diagnosed with EC: mother at age 55 years and sister at age 54 years (Figure 2B). Other family members were affected with colorectal cancer at age 54 years (nephew) and cervical cancer at age 27 years (niece). DNA from relatives was not available for testing.

The missense heterozygous *MUTYH* variant (c.536A>G, p.Tyr179Cys) was identified in a female affected with grade 2 endometrioid EC at age 62 years (case 28). This *MUTYH* variant is a known common pathogenic missense variant known to cause MUTYH-associated polyposis (MAP) in Western populations when detected in homozygous or compound heterozygous state [47]. The proband reported seven family members affected with various cancers (Figure 2C), including a father diagnosed with melanoma, three relatives with breast cancer (maternal great aunt, paternal aunt, sister), two relatives affected with colorectal cancer (maternal grandfather, sister), and a maternal uncle with prostate cancer. A DNA sample was only available for the female sibling with breast cancer and we identified her to be a non-carrier of the *MUTYH* variant. Although no *MUTYH*-related cancers were reported for the parents of the proband, her maternal grandfather and female sibling were both affected with colorectal cancer at relatively young age, age 52 years and 39 years, respectively.

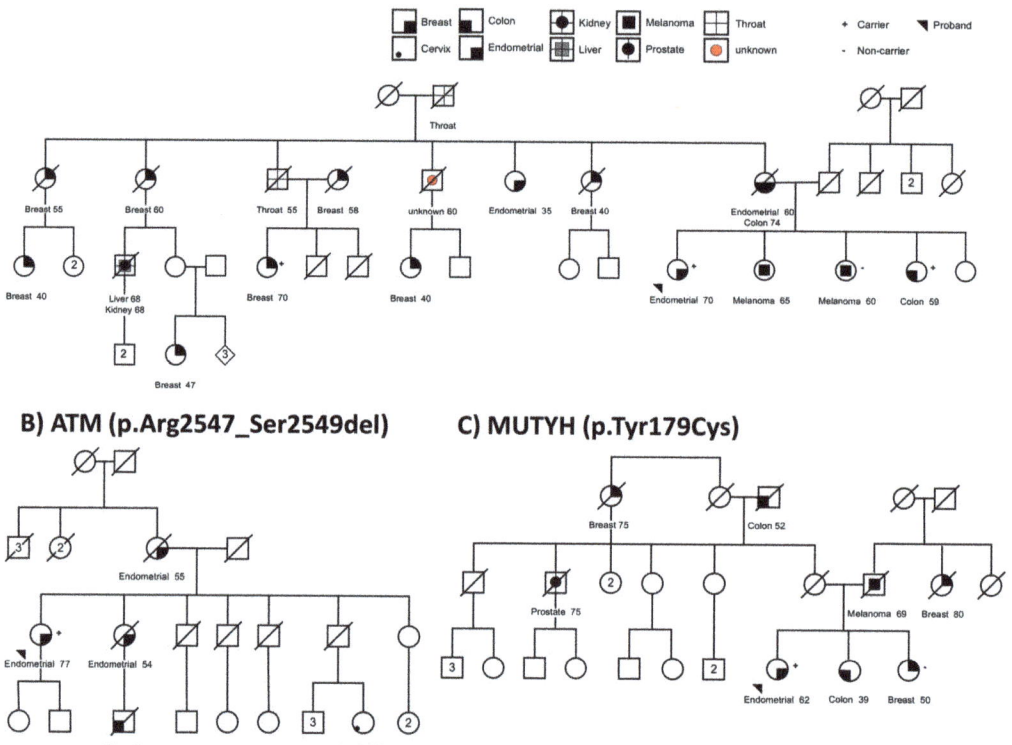

Figure 2. Pedigrees of families of the endometrial cancer cases carrying candidate variants. (**A**) Family pedigree of *PALB2* p.Asn1039Ilefs carrier. (**B**) Family pedigree of *ATM* p.Arg2547_Ser2549del carrier. (**C**) Family pedigree of the endometrial cancer case carrying candidate *MUTYH* p.Tyr179Cys. Squares symbolize males, circles symbolize females. Affected individuals are indicated by highlighted symbols, with cancer type and age at diagnosis noted below. Unaffected individuals are indicated by empty symbols. Endometrial cancer proband sequenced is indicated by black arrow below the symbol. Variant carriers are indicated by a (+) symbol and the non-carriers are indicated by a (−) symbol.

3.4. Tumor Sequencing to Assess Role of MUTYH Variant in a Suspected Familial EC Case

To explore the potential role of the germline heterozygous *MUTYH* variant in cancer development, we conducted tumor DNA sequencing of the heterozygous *MUTYH* variant carrier (case 28) to establish whether there was evidence of tumor variant enrichment and whether the *MUTYH*-associated mutational signature could be detected. We performed whole genome sequencing of an archival endometrial tumor block from the *MUTYH* carrier. The read depth was too low to accurately assess evidence of loss of heterozygosity at the *MUTYH* locus, although an increase in the percentage of variant reads from 43% in germline (16 of 37 reads) to 67% in the tumor (six of nine reads) was suggestive of tumor variant enrichment. The sequencing analysis also revealed a high proportion of C>T and C>A somatic mutations (Figure 3A). The pattern of C>T mutations is similar to COSMIC Signature 1, identified in many tumors and typically attributed to aging or deamination [48] and may be present due to formalin fixation. By performing signature assignment analysis we attributed 41% of all somatic single nucleotide variants to Signature 18 (Figure 3B), previously associated with inactivation of *MUTYH* in a series of familial colorectal cancer and adrenocortical carcinomas [49], indicating that the germline variant was driving the pattern of somatic mutations, and underlay development of EC in this individual.

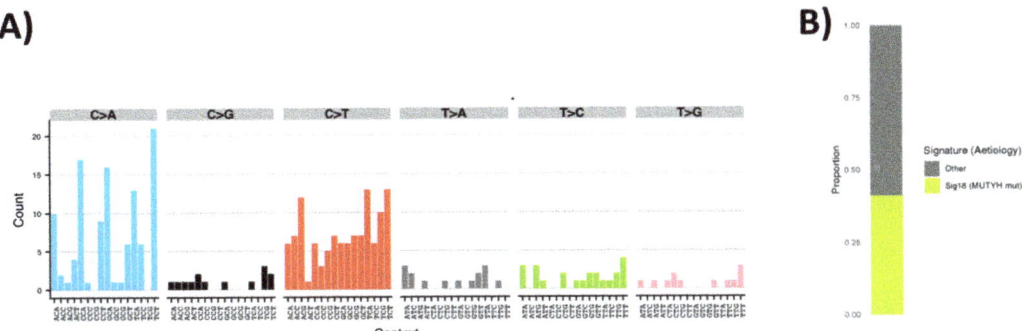

Figure 3. Somatic mutational signature analysis of the *MUTYH* germline variant carrier (suspected familial endometrial cancer cohort). (**A**) A total of 287 somatic single nucleotide variants (SNVs) identified in the endometrial tumor and used in signature analysis, plotted as counts in a 96 trinucleotide context. (**B**) The proportion of mutations in the tumor sample which were assigned to Signature 18.

4. Discussion

Based on the existing clinical management guidelines, a previous review suggested that only six genes currently have sufficient evidence of association with EC risk to be appropriate for hereditary EC diagnostic testing; these include the MMR genes (*MLH1*, *MSH2*, *MSH6* and *PMS2*), *EPCAM* (deletions due to their effect on *MSH2*) and *PTEN* [4]. We explored the role of candidate EC risk genes [4] beyond the MMR and *PTEN* genes, by analyzing an EC sample set unselected for family history and a cohort of familial EC cases. We also performed tumor sequencing analysis to explore whether these genes are cancer drivers associated with somatic mutagenesis in endometrial tumors.

The findings suggest that variation in the following genes should be considered in future studies of EC risk: *ATM*, *MUTYH*, *PALB2*, *RAD51C* and *NBN*. *PALB2* was highlighted by both case–control and suspected familial EC analysis. Tumor mutational signatures provided evidence that germline variation in *BRCA1*, *PALB2*, *RAD51C*, *MUTYH* and *NTHL1* can be (but is not always) associated with tumor mutational signatures consistent with a functional role of these genes in endometrial tumor development.

ATM encodes for a cell cycle checkpoint kinase that initiates DNA damage response via error-free repair pathway, HR, for double-stranded DNA breaks [50]. The *ATM* variant identified in a suspected familial EC case was classified as pathogenic for the rare autosomal recessive ataxia-telangiectasia syndrome by multiple submitters in ClinVar. The syndrome manifests a variety of phenotypic characteristics, including high incidence of cancer. Pathogenic variants in *ATM* are associated with increased breast cancer risk. Monoallelic c.7271T>G carriers are at a significantly increased risk, a 60% cumulative risk by age 80 years, similar to penetrance conferred by pathogenic germline variants in *BRCA2* [51]. Monoallelic carriers of other loss of function variants are reported to have a moderate increased risk of developing breast cancer (3-fold; 95% CI: 2.1–4.5) [52]. A number of *ATM* variants predicted to be deleterious to ATM protein function have been identified in EC cases, in unselected as well as a familial setting [7,53]. Another recent study [22] reporting results from germline panel testing of unselected EC cases identified *ATM* pathogenic variants as among the most common alterations observed (9/1170 cases), and estimated risk for *ATM* carriers to be OR 1.86 ($p = 0.07$) by comparison of case frequency to gnomAD non-Finnish European controls. Given that *ATM* loss of function variants are estimated to be associated with only a modest risk of breast cancer (OR 3.0, 95% CI 2.1–4.5) [52], larger well-designed studies will be required to determine if *ATM* variation confers a similar modest level of risk to EC.

PALB2 encodes for one of the key proteins involved in the HR DNA damage repair by recruiting BRCA2 to DNA breaks [54]. The *PALB2* truncating variant identified in our familial cohort has been classified as a pathogenic variant for familial breast cancer by multiple submitters to ClinVar. *PALB2* is emerging as a gene that confers a high risk of breast cancer, with data suggesting individuals with pathogenic variants in *PALB2* have a high lifetime risk of around 32% [55]. *PALB2* variants have also been associated with increased risk of ovarian and pancreatic cancers [56]. In our study, the EC patient carrying the *PALB2* variant had a strong family history of various cancers, with carrier or obligate carrier status confirmed for relatives with breast, colon and EC. EC has been reported in relatives of breast cancer patients known to carry loss of function variants in *PALB2* [57], but carrier status was not confirmed. *PALB2* loss of function variants have also been detected in EC patients in several previous studies [45,57–61]. The results to date indicate that the role of *PALB2* loss of function variants in conferring EC risk should be further explored.

Other HR pathway genes implicated in this study were *BRCA1*, *NBN* and *RAD51C*. Interestingly, while *NBN* and *RAD51C* had a more than 2-fold increased variant frequency in the EC sample set, *BRCA1* did not. To date, the role of *BRCA1* or *BRCA2* in EC risk has been much debated, with numerous conflicting reports [4]. Overall findings indicate that increased EC risk for *BRCA1/2* carriers has been associated with tamoxifen use for breast cancer prevention or treatment (since these genes confer high breast cancer risk) comparable to the risk observed in the general population [18,19]. There is also suggestive evidence that *BRCA1* pathogenic variants may confer a modest risk EC increase in the absence of tamoxifen exposure, particularly for serous and serous-like subtype cancers [62,63]. Unfortunately, the patient cancer history or tamoxifen exposure was not well documented for the TCGA-UCEC cancer cohort used in this study, hence we were unable to assess the possible contribution of tamoxifen for *BRCA1* or other genes that confer breast cancer risk. *RAD51C* has been recently shown to confer moderate risk for breast (relative risk (RR) = 1.99, 95% CI: 1.39–2.85) and high risk for ovarian cancers (RR = 7.55, 95% CI: 5.6–10.19) [64]; however, there have only been observational studies so far for EC [7,65]. Given the breast cancer risk, future studies on *RAD51C* and EC risk will need to account for tamoxifen exposure, same as for *BRCA1/2* genes. The role of *NBN* in EC risk has largely been unexplored. It is notable that while certain *NBN* variants have previously been reported to increase breast cancer risk [66], the most recent evidence from a large-scale case–control analysis refutes (OR 0.90, 95% CI 0.67–1.20) an association of truncating *NBN* variants with breast cancer risk [67].

In addition to considering a role of the above-mentioned HR-related genes in EC risk, we also investigated their potential role in EC development by analyzing tumor mutational signatures. We observed HR-associated mutational signature (Signature 3) in most tumors with *BRCA1*, *PALB2* and *RAD51C* pathogenic or likely pathogenic variants, but not in tumors with *BRIP1*, *CHEK2*, *FAN1* or *NBN* variants. This is consistent with previous reports in breast cancer and cell line experiments where Signature 3 was only detected for *BRCA1/2*, *PALB2* and *RAD51C* genes but not *ATM* or *CHEK2* [68,69]. The presence of Signature 3 in cases with *BRCA1*, *PALB2* and *RAD51C* variants, as well as tumor enrichment of these variants, suggest that these cancers are HR-deficient. Our observation is also supported by the report of tumor loss of heterozygosity in serous/serous-like EC with germline *BRCA1* mutations (two of three cases) [62].

Other genes implicated in this study included DNA base excision repair genes, *MUTYH* and *NTHL1*. Signature 36 (COSMIC v3), similar to Signature 18 detected in this study (COSMIC v2), has been associated with inactivation of *MUTYH* in MAP colorectal cancer [70] and observed in 5% of pancreatic neuroendocrine tumors that bore heterozygous germline *MUTYH* variants and subsequent loss of the wildtype allele in the tumor [71]. Together these observations indicate that oxidative DNA damage due to *MUTYH* inactivation may contribute to cancer etiology in several organs. In our study, a *MUTYH* variant considered pathogenic for MAP was likely enriched in the tumor of a suspected familial EC case, which presented with a tumor mutational signature consistent with the driver status of the *MUTYH* variant. However, *MUTYH* pathogenic variants were not more common in the TCGA unselected EC cohort relative to the population reference group (1.62% vs. 1.73%), and there was no evidence for tumor enrichment or appropriate tumor mutational signature in the TCGA cases. The majority of *MUTYH* pathogenic variants identified were two well recognized common pathogenic variants identified in the Western population to cause MAP (c.536A>G (p.Tyr179Cys), as detected in the suspected familial EC case; and c.1187G>A (p.Gly368Asp)) [47]. MAP is an autosomal recessively inherited predisposition to adenomatous polyposis and colorectal cancer [72]. The cumulative colorectal cancer risk to age 70 years for biallelic carriers is reported to be 75% (95% CI: 41–97%) for males and 72% (95% CI: 41–97%) for females, and for monoallelic carriers it is estimated to be 7% (95% CI: 5–11%) for males and 6% (95% CI: 4–9%) for females [73]. Indeed, the case reported here had a family history of colorectal cancer (in two relatives, ages 39 and 52). However, the risk of extracolonic cancers for *MUTYH* monoallelic pathogenic variant carriers with a family history of colorectal cancer is still uncertain, current evidence derived from a single study estimated cumulative risk of EC age 70 to be 4% (95% CI: 2–8%) for monoallelic *MUTYH* carriers [11], with an updated analysis of the same cohort [74] reporting a modest 2-fold EC risk for carriers (95% C.I 1.1–3.9). These previous findings suggest that, *MUTYH*-associated risk of EC, if validated, is likely to be extremely modest.

We have identified several genes in this study as possible additional EC risk genes; however, these results should be considered preliminary, and require further exploration in the follow-up studies. Although this study has not provided conclusive evidence regarding the role of the aforementioned genes in EC risk, results could nevertheless be of relevance as secondary findings for the patient and their relatives. We have shown that at least some germline carriers had a tumor mutational signature supportive of the driver role of the respective gene in cancer development. Overall, 28% of carriers of HR-related gene variants had a presence of HR-deficiency associated tumor mutational signature, which increased to 86% of carriers when only well-recognized HR genes (*BRCA1*, *PALB2* and *RAD51C*) were included [75]. This has implications for patient treatment decisions, since HR-deficient cancers are known to respond to PARP inhibitors [76]. Furthermore, cases with MMR-deficient or base excision repair-deficient (*MUTYH* or *NTHL1*-driven) tumors are likely to show hypermutated profiles, and thus would be good candidates for immunotherapy treatment, given the likely increase in neo-antigen production [77]. Our findings suggest potential value in secondary tumour profiling on identification of a germline gene alteration in EC patients, irrespective of a confirmed role of that gene in EC risk. Furthermore, somatic only changes would have the same implications for treatment decisions. It will thus be important to explore the overall proportion of EC cases with actionable tumor mutation profiles to determine the clinical value of unselected tumor mutational profiling.

5. Conclusions

We used genome sequencing and tumor mutational signature analysis to explore the role of purported EC risk genes in an EC sample set unselected for family history, and to identify candidate germline variants underlying the genetic cause of familial EC without MMR defects. Ancestry-matched case–control comparisons of germline variant frequency and/or sequence data from the suspected familial EC cases proposed several preliminary candidates for future risk association studies, with *PALB2* highlighted by both approaches. Tumor analysis highlighted germline variation in HR-related repair genes, particularly *BRCA1*, *PALB2* and *RAD51C*, to have a potential driver role in EC development based on the presence of mutational signature indicative of HR deficiency. For the heterozygous germline variants in other DNA damage repair genes, *MUTYH* and *NTHL1*, the mutational signature analysis indicates possible involvement in the etiology of EC, but only when there were indications of the germline variant being enriched in the tumor.

Inclusion of these highlighted genes in clinical testing panels for EC predisposition will require results from further large-scale studies, to assess the level of EC risk associated with loss of function variation in these genes. Such studies should preferably follow a population-based case–control design and consider the role of other genetic and environmental factors in disease penetrance, including previous exposure to tamoxifen. While we anticipate that genes outside of MMR pathway are unlikely to explain a large component of suspected familial EC, our results indicate that additional tumor signature analysis for individuals with a germline gene alteration has potential to impact therapeutic decisions.

Supplementary Materials: The following are available online at https://www.mdpi.com/article/10.3390/cancers13081762/s1, Figure S1: Variant filtering workflow used for germline pathogenic and likely pathogenic variants included in this study for TCGA-UCEC and gnomAD datasets, Figure S2: De novo mutational signature analysis in the TCGA-UCEC cases with pathogenic or likely pathogenic variants, Table S1: Subset of European TCGA-UCEC cases included in the variant frequency comparison with the gnomAD population of Non-Finnish Europeans, Table S2: Phenotypic characteristics of the familial endometrial cancer cases, Table S3: Summary of sequencing coverage and number of variants identified for each familial endometrial cancer case prior to filtering, Table S4: List of known and purported endometrial cancer risk genes, Table S5: List of pathogenic and likely pathogenic variants identified in the genes of interest in gnomAD (non-Finnish Europeans) and TCGA-UCEC cases.

Author Contributions: O.K. and J.S.: Designed the methods, carried out the analysis, interpreted the data and prepared the manuscript. A.B.S.: Conceived the study, designed the methods, and supervised the work. N.W.: Designed the methods, developed genomic analysis pipelines, supervised the work. T.A.O.: Designed the methods and supervised the work. F.N.: Carried out mutational analysis. A.E.M.R.: Reviewed and processed the tumor sample. S.R.L.: Reviewed the tumor sample and supervised the work. J.K.: Provided clinical input. J.V.P.: Managed the genomic data and developed the genomic pipelines for analysis. All authors read and approved the final manuscript.

Funding: J.S. is supported by a QIMR Berghofer PhD scholarship. N.W. is supported by a National Health and Medical Research Council (NHMRC) of Australia Senior Research Fellowship (APP1139071). A.B.S. was supported by NHMRC Funding (APP1061779, APP117524). T.A.O. was supported by NHMRC Funding (APP1111246, APP1173170). The Australian National Endometrial Cancer Study was supported by project grants from the NHMRC (Grant No. 339435); The Cancer Council Queensland (Grant No. 4196615); Cancer Council Tasmania (Grant No. 403031 and Grant No. 457636); the Cancer Australia Priority-driven Collaborative Cancer Research Scheme (#552468); Cancer Australia (Grant No. 1010859). The sequencing component of this study was funded by a "Rio Tinto Ride to Conquer Cancer & Weekend to End Women's Cancer Research Grant" administered by QIMR Berghofer Medical Research Institute.

Institutional Review Board Statement: Accessing TCGA-UCEC genome data and undertaking reanalysis to detect variants in the tumour and matching normal was performed with approval from the QIMR Berghofer Human Research Ethics Committee (HREC/P2905). Sequencing and analysis of familial EC patients was undertaken with approval from QIMR Berghofer Ethics Committee (HREC/P1051).

Informed Consent Statement: All ANECS participants provided informed written consent for participation in EC-related research, with overall study approval by the QIMR Berghofer Medical Research Institute Human Research Ethics Committee (P853), encompassing approvals from participating hospitals and cancer registries.

Data Availability Statement: TCGA-UCEC data were downloaded from GDC data portal in October 2016. GnomAD variant files (r.2.1.1) were downloaded from the gnomAD portal in April 2019. ANECS sequencing data are available upon reasonable request and subject to ethics approval.

Acknowledgments: We thank the individuals who participated in ANECS, the institutes and clinicians who contributed to recruitment and data collection (see website: www.anecs.org.au for the full list of contributors). We thank Sullivan Nicolaides Pathology for providing the archival tumor tissue for whole genome sequencing, and Stephen Kazakoff, Michael Bowman, Katia Nones, Ann-Marie Patch for helpful advice and contributions to data cleaning and processing. We thank Kathy Tucker for critique regarding interpretation and representation of clinical relevance of findings. The results shown here are in part based upon data generated by the TCGA Research Network: https://www.cancer.gov/tcga. Information about TCGA can be found at http://cancergenome.nih.gov. The TCGA dataset used in this study was accessed through dbGaP accession number phs000178.v11.p8.

Conflicts of Interest: O.K. has consulted for XING Technologies. N.W. and J.V.P. are co-founders and Board members of genomiQa. The other authors declare that they have no competing interests. The funders had no role in the design of the study; in the collection, analyses, or interpretation of data; in the writing of the manuscript, or in the decision to publish the results.

References

1. Zhang, S.; Gong, T.-T.; Liu, F.-H.; Jiang, Y.-T.; Sun, H.; Ma, X.-X.; Zhao, Y.-H.; Wu, Q.-J. Global, Regional, and National Burden of Endometrial Cancer, 1990–2017: Results from the Global Burden of Disease Study, 2017. *Front. Oncol.* **2019**, *9*, 1440. [CrossRef]
2. Win, A.K.; Reece, J.C.; Ryan, S. Family History and Risk of Endometrial Cancer. *Obstet. Gynecol.* **2015**, *125*, 89–98. [CrossRef]
3. O'Mara, T.A.; Glubb, D.M.; Kho, P.F.; Thompson, D.J.; Spurdle, A.B. Genome-Wide Association Studies of Endometrial Cancer: Latest Developments and Future Directions. *Cancer Epidemiol. Biomark. Prev.* **2019**, *28*, 1095–1102. [CrossRef]
4. Spurdle, A.B.; Bowman, M.A.; Shamsani, J.; Kirk, J. Endometrial Cancer Gene Panels: Clinical Diagnostic vs Research Germline DNA testing. *Mod. Pathol.* **2017**, *30*, 1048–1068. [CrossRef]
5. Randall, L.M.; Pothuri, B. The Genetic Prediction of Risk for Gynecologic Cancers. *Gynecol. Oncol.* **2016**, *141*, 10–16. [CrossRef]
6. Nieuwenhuis, M.H.; Kets, C.M.; Murphy-Ryan, M.; Yntema, H.G.; Evans, D.G.; Colas, C.; Møller, P.; Hes, F.J.; Hodgson, S.V.; Olderode-Berends, M.J.W.; et al. Cancer Risk and Genotype–Phenotype Correlations in PTEN Hamartoma Tumor Syndrome. *Fam. Cancer* **2014**, *13*, 57–63. [CrossRef] [PubMed]
7. Ring, K.L.; Bruegl, A.S.; Allen, B.A.; Elkin, E.P.; Singh, N.; Hartman, A.-R.; Daniels, M.S.; Broaddus, R.R. Germline Multi-Gene Hereditary Cancer Panel Testing in an Unselected Endometrial Cancer Cohort. *Mod. Pathol.* **2016**, *29*, 1381–1389. [CrossRef] [PubMed]
8. Johnatty, S.E.; Tan, Y.Y.; Buchanan, D.D.; Bowman, M.; Walters, R.J.; Obermair, A.; Quinn, M.A.; Blomfield, P.B.; Brand, A.; Leung, Y.; et al. Family History of Cancer Predicts Endometrial Cancer Risk Independently of Lynch Syndrome: Implications for Genetic Counselling. *Gynecol. Oncol.* **2017**, *147*, 381–387. [CrossRef]
9. Bellido, F.; Pineda, M.; Aiza, G.; Mas, R.M.V.; Navarro, M.; Puente, D.Á.; Pons, T.; González, S.; Iglesias, S.; Darder, E.; et al. POLE and POLD1 Mutations in 529 Kindred with Familial Colorectal Cancer and/or Polyposis: Review of Reported Cases and Recommendations for Genetic Testing and Surveillance. *Genet. Med.* **2016**, *18*, 325–332. [CrossRef] [PubMed]
10. Hu, R.; Hilakivi-Clarke, L.; Clarke, R. Molecular Mechanisms of Tamoxifen-Associated Endometrial Cancer (Review). *Oncol. Lett.* **2015**, *9*, 1495–1501. [CrossRef] [PubMed]
11. Win, A.K.; Cleary, S.P.; Dowty, J.G.; Baron, J.A.; Young, J.P.; Buchanan, D.D.; Southey, M.C.; Burnett, T.; Parfrey, P.S.; Green, R.C.; et al. Cancer Risks for Monoallelic MUTYH Mutation Carriers with a Family History of Colorectal Cancer. *Int. J. Cancer* **2010**, *129*, 2256–2262. [CrossRef] [PubMed]
12. Vogt, S.; Jones, N.; Christian, D.; Engel, C.; Nielsen, M.; Kaufmann, A.; Steinke, V.; Vasen, H.F.; Propping, P.; Sampson, J.R.; et al. Expanded Extracolonic Tumor Spectrum in MUTYH-Associated Polyposis. *Gastroenterology* **2009**, *137*, 1976–1985.e10. [CrossRef]
13. Giardiello, F.M.; Brensinger, J.D.; Tersmette, A.C.; Goodman, S.N.; Petersen, G.M.; Booker, S.V.; Cruz–Correa, M.; Offerhaus, J.A. Very High Risk of Cancer in Familial Peutz–Jeghers Syndrome. *Gastroenterology* **2000**, *119*, 1447–1453. [CrossRef] [PubMed]
14. Pennington, K.P.; Walsh, T.; Lee, M.; Ms, C.P.; Novetsky, A.P.; Bs, K.J.A.; Thornton, A.; Garcia, R.; Mutch, D.; King, M.-C.; et al. BRCA1, TP53, and CHEK2 Germline Mutations in Uterine Serous Carcinoma. *Cancer* **2013**, *119*, 332–338. [CrossRef] [PubMed]
15. Heitzer, E.; Lax, S.; Lafer, I.; Müller, S.M.; Pristauz, G.; Ulz, P.; Jahn, S.; Högenauer, C.; Petru, E.; Speicher, M.R.; et al. Multiplex Genetic Cancer Testing Identifies Pathogenic Mutations in TP53 and CDH1 in a Patient with Bilateral Breast and Endometrial Adenocarcinoma. *BMC Med. Genet.* **2013**, *14*, 129. [CrossRef]
16. Chao, A.; Lai, C.-H.; Lee, Y.-S.; Ueng, S.-H.; Lin, C.-Y.; Wang, T.-H. Molecular Characteristics of Endometrial Cancer Coexisting with Peritoneal Malignant Mesothelioma in LI-Fraumeni-like Syndrome. *BMC Cancer* **2015**, *15*, 8. [CrossRef] [PubMed]
17. Hornreich, G.; Beller, U.; Lavie, O.; Renbaum, P.; Cohen, Y.; Levy-Lahad, E. Is Uterine Serous Papillary Carcinoma a BRCA1-Related Disease? Case Report and Review of the Literature. *Gynecol. Oncol.* **1999**, *75*, 300–304. [CrossRef]
18. Duffy, D.L.; Antill, Y.C.; Stewart, C.J.; Young, J.P.; Spurdle, A.B. kConFab Report of Endometrial Cancer in Australian BRCA1 and BRCA2 Mutation-Positive Families. *Twin Res. Hum. Genet.* **2011**, *14*, 111–118. [CrossRef] [PubMed]
19. Segev, Y.; Iqbal, J.; Lubinski, J.; Gronwald, J.; Lynch, H.T.; Moller, P.; Ghadirian, P.; Rosen, B.; Tung, N.; Kim-Sing, C.; et al. The Incidence of Endometrial Cancer in Women with BRCA1 and BRCA2 Mutations: An International Prospective Cohort Study. *Gynecol. Oncol.* **2013**, *130*, 127–131. [CrossRef] [PubMed]

20. Bruchim, I.; Amichay, K.; Kidron, D.; Attias, Z.; Biron-Shental, T.; Drucker, L.; Friedman, E.; Werner, H.; Fishman, A. BRCA1/2 Germline Mutations in Jewish Patients with Uterine Serous Carcinoma. *Int. J. Gynecol. Cancer* **2010**, *20*, 1148–1153. [CrossRef]
21. Lavie, O.; Ben-Arie, A.; Segev, Y.; Faro, J.; Barak, F.; Haya, N.; Auslender, R.; Gemer, O. Brca Germline Mutations in Women with Uterine Serous Carcinoma—Still a Debate. *Int. J. Gynecol. Cancer* **2010**, *20*, 1531–1534. [PubMed]
22. Long, B.; Lilyquist, J.; Weaver, A.; Hu, C.; Gnanaolivu, R.; Lee, K.Y.; Hart, S.N.; Polley, E.C.; Bakkum-Gamez, J.N.; Couch, F.J.; et al. Cancer Susceptibility Gene Mutations in Type I and II Endometrial Cancer. *Gynecol. Oncol.* **2019**, *152*, 20–25. [CrossRef] [PubMed]
23. Carvajal-Carmona, L.G.; O'Mara, T.A.; Painter, J.N.; Lose, F.A.; Dennis, J.; Michailidou, K.; Tyrer, J.P.; Ahmed, S.; Ferguson, K.; Healey, C.S.; et al. Candidate Locus Analysis of the TERT–CLPTM1L Cancer Risk Region on Chromosome 5p15 Identifies Multiple Independent Variants Associated with Endometrial Cancer Risk. *Qual. Life Res.* **2014**, *134*, 231–245. [CrossRef] [PubMed]
24. Buchanan, D.D.; Tan, Y.Y.; Walsh, M.D.; Clendenning, M.; Metcalf, A.M.; Ferguson, K.; Arnold, S.T.; Thompson, B.A.; Lose, F.A.; Parsons, M.T.; et al. Tumor Mismatch Repair Immunohistochemistry and DNA MLH1 Methylation Testing of Patients with Endometrial Cancer Diagnosed at Age Younger Than 60 Years Optimizes Triage for Population-Level Germline Mismatch Repair Gene Mutation Testing. *J. Clin. Oncol.* **2014**, *32*, 90–100. [CrossRef] [PubMed]
25. Tan, Y.Y.; McGaughran, J.; Ferguson, K.; Walsh, M.D.; Buchanan, D.D.; Young, J.P.; Webb, P.M.; Obermair, A.; Spurdle, A.B. On Behalf of the ANECS Group Improving Identification of Lynch Syndrome Patients: A Comparison of Research Data with Clinical Records. *Int. J. Cancer* **2013**, *132*, 2876–2883. [CrossRef]
26. Martin, M. Cutadapt Removes Adapter Sequences from High-Throughput Sequencing Reads. *EMBnet. J.* **2011**, *17*, 10–12. [CrossRef]
27. Li, H. Aligning Sequence Reads, Clone Sequences and Assembly Contigs with BWA-MEM. *arXiv* **2013**, arXiv:1303.3997.
28. Li, H.; Handsaker, B.; Wysoker, A.; Fennell, T.; Ruan, J.; Homer, N.; Marth, G.; Abecasis, G.; Durbin, R. 1000 Genome Project Data Processing Subgroup. The Sequence Alignment/Map format and SAMtools. *Bioinformatics* **2009**, *25*, 2078–2079. [CrossRef]
29. Kassahn, K.S.; Holmes, O.; Nones, K.; Patch, A.-M.; Miller, D.K.; Christ, A.N.; Harliwong, I.; Bruxner, T.J.; Xu, Q.; Anderson, M.; et al. Somatic Point Mutation Calling in Low Cellularity Tumors. *PLoS ONE* **2013**, *8*, e74380. [CrossRef]
30. McKenna, A.; Hanna, M.; Banks, E.; Sivachenko, A.; Cibulskis, K.; Kernytsky, A.; Garimella, K.; Altshuler, D.; Gabriel, S.B.; Daly, M.J.; et al. The Genome Analysis Toolkit: A MapReduce Framework for Analyzing Next-Generation DNA Sequencing Data. *Genome Res.* **2010**, *20*, 1297–1303. [CrossRef]
31. Hayward, N.K.; Wilmott, J.S.; Waddell, N.; Johansson, P.A.; Field, M.A.; Nones, K.; Patch, A.-M.; Kakavand, H.; Alexandrov, L.B.; Burke, H.; et al. Whole-Genome Landscapes of Major Melanoma Subtypes. *Nat. Cell Biol.* **2017**, *545*, 175–180. [CrossRef]
32. McLaren, W.; Gil, L.; Hunt, S.E.; Riat, H.S.; Ritchie, G.R.S.; Thormann, A.; Flicek, P.; Cunningham, F. The Ensembl Variant Effect Predictor. *Genome Biol.* **2016**, *17*, 1–14. [CrossRef]
33. Ioannidis, N.M.; Rothstein, J.H.; Pejaver, V.; Middha, S.; McDonnell, S.K.; Baheti, S.; Musolf, A.; Li, Q.; Holzinger, E.; Karyadi, D.; et al. REVEL: An Ensemble Method for Predicting the Pathogenicity of Rare Missense Variants. *Am. J. Hum. Genet.* **2016**, *99*, 877–885. [CrossRef]
34. Shamsani, J.; Kazakoff, S.H.; Armean, I.M.; McLaren, W.; Parsons, M.T.; Thompson, B.A.; O'Mara, T.A.E.; Hunt, S.; Waddell, N.; Spurdle, A.B. A Plugin for the Ensembl Variant Effect Predictor That Uses MaxEntScan to Predict Variant Spliceogenicity. *Bioinformatics* **2019**, *35*, 2315–2317. [CrossRef] [PubMed]
35. Landrum, M.J.; Lee, J.M.; Riley, G.R.; Jang, W.; Rubinstein, W.S.; Church, D.M.; Maglott, D.R. ClinVar: Public Archive of Relationships among Sequence Variation and Human Phenotype. *Nucleic Acids Res.* **2014**, *42*, D980–D985. [CrossRef]
36. Chadwick, R.B.; Meek, J.E.; Prior, T.W.; Peltomaki, P.; de la Chapelle, A. Polymorphisms in a Pseudogene Highly Homolo-Gous To PMS2. *Hum. Mutat.* **2000**, *16*, 530. [CrossRef]
37. Mur, P.; Ms, S.G.-M.; Del Valle, J.; Ms, L.M.-P.; Vidal, A.; Pineda, M.; Cinnirella, G.; Ms, E.M.-R.; Pons, T.; López-Doriga, A.; et al. Role of POLE and POLD1 in familial cancer. *Genet. Med.* **2020**, *22*, 2089–2100. [CrossRef]
38. Choi, Y.; Chan, A.P. PROVEAN Web Server: A Tool to Predict the Functional Effect of Amino Acid Substitutions and Indels. *Bioinformatics* **2015**, *31*, 2745–2747. [CrossRef]
39. Rosenthal, R.; McGranahan, N.; Herrero, J.; Taylor, B.S.; Swanton, C. Deconstructsigs: Delineating Mutational Processes in Single Tumors Distinguishes DNA Repair Deficiencies and Patterns of Carcinoma Evolution. *Genome Biol.* **2016**, *17*, 31. [CrossRef]
40. Bonazzi, V.F.; Kondrashova, O.; Smith, D.; Nones, K.; Sengal, A.T.; Ju, R.; Packer, L.M.; Koufariotis, L.T.; Kazakoff, S.H.; Davidson, A.L.; et al. Genomic analysis of patient-derived xenograft models reveals intra-tumor heterogeneity in endometrial cancer and can predict tumor growth inhibition with talazoparib. *bioRxiv* **2021**. [CrossRef]
41. Niu, B.; Ye, K.; Zhang, Q.; Lu, C.; Xie, M.; McLellan, M.D.; Wendl, M.C.; Ding, L. MSI Sensor: Microsatellite Instability Detection Using Paired Tumor-Normal Sequence Data. *Bioinformatics* **2014**, *30*, 1015–1016. [CrossRef]
42. Levine, D.A.; Network, C.G.A.R. Integrated Genomic Characterization of Endometrial Carcinoma. *Nature* **2013**, *497*, 67–73. [CrossRef] [PubMed]
43. Cerami, E.; Gao, J.; Dogrusoz, U.; Gross, B.E.; Sumer, S.O.; Aksoy, B.A.; Jacobsen, A.; Byrne, C.J.; Heuer, M.L.; Larsson, E.; et al. The cBio Cancer Genomics Portal: An Open Platform for Exploring Multidimensional Cancer Genomics Data. *Cancer Discov.* **2012**, *2*, 401–404. [CrossRef]
44. Gao, J.; Aksoy, B.A.; Dogrusoz, U.; Dresdner, G.; Gross, B.; Sumer, S.O.; Sun, Y.; Jacobsen, A.; Sinha, R.; Larsson, E. Integrative Analysis of Complex Cancer Genomics and Clinical Profiles Using the cBioPortal. *Sci. Signal.* **2013**, *6*, pl1. [CrossRef] [PubMed]

45. Huang, K.-L.; Mashl, R.J.; Wu, Y.; Ritter, D.I.; Wang, J.; Oh, C.; Paczkowska, M.; Reynolds, S.; Wyczalkowski, M.A.; Oak, N.; et al. Pathogenic Germline Variants in 10,389 Adult Cancers. *Cell* **2018**, *173*, 355–370.e14. [CrossRef]
46. Grolleman, J.E.; De Voer, R.M.; Elsayed, F.A.; Nielsen, M.; Weren, R.D.A.; Palles, C.; Ligtenberg, M.J.L.; Vos, J.R.; Broeke, S.W.T.; De Miranda, N.F.C.C.; et al. Mutational Signature Analysis Reveals NTHL1 Deficiency to Cause a Multi-Tumor Phenotype Including a Predisposition to Colon and Breast Cancer. *SSRN Electron. J.* **2018**, *35*, 256–266. [CrossRef]
47. Nielsen, M.; Van De Beld, M.C.J.-; Jones, N.; Vogt, S.; Tops, C.M.; Vasen, H.F.; Sampson, J.R.; Aretz, S.; Hes, F.J. Analysis of MUTYH Genotypes and Colorectal Phenotypes in Patients With MUTYH-Associated Polyposis. *Gastroenterology* **2009**, *136*, 471–476. [CrossRef]
48. Alexandrov, L.B.; Nik-Zainal, S.; Wedge, D.C.; Aparicio, S.A.J.R.; Behjati, S.; Biankin, A.V.; Bignell, G.R.; Bolli, N.; Borg, A.; Børresen-Dale, A.-L.; et al. Signatures of Mutational Processes in Human Cancer. *Nature* **2013**, *500*, 415–421. [CrossRef] [PubMed]
49. Pilati, C.; Shinde, J.; Alexandrov, L.B.; Assié, G.; André, T.; Hélias-Rodzewicz, Z.; Doucoudray, R.; Le Corre, D.; Zucman-Rossi, J.; Emile, J.-F.; et al. Mutational Signature Analysis Identifies MUTYH Deficiency in Colorectal Cancers and Adrenocortical Carcinomas. *J. Pathol.* **2017**, *242*, 10–15. [CrossRef]
50. Maréchal, A.; Zou, L. DNA Damage Sensing by the ATM and ATR Kinases. *Cold Spring Harb. Perspect. Biol.* **2013**, *5*, a012716. [CrossRef] [PubMed]
51. Goldgar, D.E.; Healey, S.; Dowty, J.G.; Da Silva, L.; Chen, X.; Spurdle, A.B.; Terry, M.B.; Daly, M.J.; Buys, S.M.; Southey, M.C.; et al. Rare Variants in the ATMgene and Risk of Breast Cancer. *Breast Cancer Res.* **2011**, *13*, R73. [CrossRef]
52. Van Os, N.; Roeleveld, N.; Weemaes, C.; Jongmans, M.; Janssens, G.O.R.J.; Taylor, A.; Hoogerbrugge, N.; Willemsen, M. Health Risks for Ataxia-Telangiectasia Mutated Heterozygotes: A Systematic Review, Meta-Analysis and Evidence-Based Guideline. *Clin. Genet.* **2016**, *90*, 105–117. [CrossRef] [PubMed]
53. Hu, C.; Hart, S.N.; Bamlet, W.R.; Moore, R.M.; Nandakumar, K.; Eckloff, B.W.; Lee, Y.K.; Petersen, G.M.; McWilliams, R.R.; Couch, F.J. Prevalence of Pathogenic Mutations in Cancer Predisposition Genes among Pancreatic Cancer Patients. *Cancer Epidemiol. Biomark. Prev.* **2016**, *25*, 207–211. [CrossRef] [PubMed]
54. Xia, B.; Sheng, Q.; Nakanishi, K.; Ohashi, A.; Wu, J.; Christ, N.; Liu, X.; Jasin, M.; Couch, F.J.; Livingston, D.M. Control of BRCA2 Cellular and Clinical Functions by a Nuclear Partner, PALB2. *Mol. Cell* **2006**, *22*, 719–729. [CrossRef] [PubMed]
55. Hu, C.; Hart, S.N.; Gnanaolivu, R.; Huang, H.; Lee, K.Y.; Na, J.; Gao, C.; Lilyquist, J.; Yadav, S.; Boddicker, N.J. A Popu-lation-Based Study of Genes Previously Implicated in Breast Cancer. *N. Engl. J. Med.* **2021**, *384*, 440–451. [CrossRef]
56. Yang, X.; Leslie, G.; Doroszuk, A.; Schneider, S.; Allen, J.; Decker, B.; Dunning, A.M.; Redman, J.; Scarth, J.; Plaskocinska, I.; et al. Cancer Risks Associated with Germline PALB2 Pathogenic Variants: An International Study of 524 Families. *J. Clin. Oncol.* **2020**, *38*, 674–685. [CrossRef]
57. Teo, Z.L.; Park, D.J.; Provenzano, E.; Chatfield, C.A.; Odefrey, F.A.; Nguyen-Dumont, T.; Dowty, J.G.; Hopper, J.L.; Winship, I.; Goldgar, D.E.; et al. Prevalence of PALB2 Mutations in Australasian Multiple-Case Breast Cancer Families. *Breast Cancer Res.* **2013**, *15*, R17. [CrossRef]
58. Susswein, L.R.; Marshall, M.L.; Nusbaum, R.; Postula, K.J.V.; Weissman, S.M.; Yackowski, L.; Vaccari, E.M.; Bissonnette, J.; Booker, J.K.; Cremona, M.L.; et al. Pathogenic and Likely Pathogenic Variant Prevalence among the First 10,000 Patients Referred for Next-Generation Cancer Panel Testing. *Genet. Med.* **2016**, *18*, 823–832. [CrossRef]
59. Fulk, K.; Milam, M.R.; Li, S.; Yussuf, A.; Black, M.H.; Chao, E.C.; LaDuca, H.; Stany, M.P. Women with Breast and Uterine Cancer Are More Likely to Harbor Germline Mutations Than Women with Breast or Uterine Cancer Alone: A Case for Expanded Gene Testing. *Gynecol. Oncol.* **2019**, *152*, 612–617. [CrossRef]
60. Heeke, A.L.; Pishvaian, M.J.; Lynce, F.; Xiu, J.; Brody, J.R.; Chen, W.-J.; Baker, T.M.; Marshall, J.L.; Isaacs, C. Prevalence of Homologous Recombination–Related Gene Mutations Across Multiple Cancer Types. *JCO Precis. Oncol.* **2018**, *2018*, 1–13. [CrossRef]
61. Chan, G.H.; Ong, P.Y.; Low, J.J.; Kong, H.L.; Ow, S.G.; Tan, D.S.; Lim, Y.W.; Lim, S.E.; Lee, S.-C. Clinical Genetic Testing Outcome with Multi-Gene Panel in Asian Patients with Multiple Primary Cancers. *Oncotarget* **2018**, *9*, 30649–30660. [CrossRef]
62. Shu, C.A.; Pike, M.C.; Jotwani, A.R.; Friebel, T.M.; Soslow, R.A.; Levine, D.A.; Nathanson, K.L.; Konner, J.A.; Arnold, A.G.; Bogomolniy, F.; et al. Uterine Cancer After Risk-Reducing Salpingo-oophorectomy Without Hysterectomy in Women with BRCA Mutations. *JAMA Oncol.* **2016**, *2*, 1434–1440. [CrossRef]
63. Thompson, D.; Easton, D.F. Cancer Incidence in BRCA1 Mutation Carriers. *Obstet. Gynecol. Surv.* **2003**, *58*, 27–28. [CrossRef]
64. Yang, X.; Song, H.; Leslie, G.; Engel, C.; Hahnen, E.; Auber, B.; Horváth, J.; Kast, K.; Niederacher, D.; Turnbull, C.; et al. Ovarian and Breast Cancer Risks Associated with Pathogenic Variants in RAD51C and RAD51D. *J. Natl. Cancer Inst.* **2020**, *112*, 1242–1250. [CrossRef] [PubMed]
65. Pelttari, L.; Shimelis, H.; Toiminen, T.; Kvist, A.; Törngren, T.; Borg, Å.; Blomqvist, C.; Bützow, R.; Couch, F.; Aittomäki, K. Gene-Panel Testing of Breast and Ovarian Cancer Patients Identifies a Recurrent RAD51C Duplication. *Clin. Genet.* **2018**, *93*, 595–602. [CrossRef] [PubMed]
66. Gao, P.; Ma, N.; Li, M.; Tian, Q.-B.; Liu, D.-W. Functional Variants in NBS1 and Cancer Risk: Evidence from a Meta-Analysis of 60 Publications with 111 Individual Studies. *Mutagenesis* **2013**, *28*, 683–697. [CrossRef]
67. Dorling, L.; Carvalho, S.; Allen, J.; González-Neira, A.; Luccarini, C.; Wahlström, C.; Pooley, K.A.; Parsons, M.T.; Fortuno, C.; Wang, Q. Breast Cancer Risk Genes-Association Analysis in More than 113,000 Women. *N. Engl. J. Med.* **2021**, *384*, 428–439.

68. Polak, P.; Kim, J.; Braunstein, L.Z.; Karlic, R.; Haradhavala, N.J.; Tiao, G.; Rosebrock, D.; Livitz, D.; Kübler, K.; Mouw, K.W.; et al. A Mutational Signature Reveals Alterations Underlying Deficient Homologous Recombination Repair in Breast Cancer. *Nat. Genet.* **2017**, *49*, 1476–1486. [CrossRef]
69. Póti, Á.; Gyergyák, H.; Németh, E.; Rusz, O.; Tóth, S.; Kovácsházi, C.; Chen, D.; Szikriszt, B.; Spisák, S.; Takeda, S. Correlation of Homologous Recombination Deficiency Induced Mutational Signatures with Sensitivity to Parp Inhibitors and Cytotoxic Agents. *Genome Biol.* **2019**, *20*, 240. [CrossRef]
70. Viel, A.; Bruselles, A.; Meccia, E.; Fornasarig, M.; Quaia, M.; Canzonieri, V.; Policicchio, E.; Urso, E.D.; Agostini, M.; Genuardi, M. A Specific Mutational Signature Associated with DNA 8-Oxoguanine Persistence in MUTYH-Defective Colo-Rectal Cancer. *EBioMedicine* **2017**, *20*, 39–49. [CrossRef]
71. Scarpa, A.; Chang, D.K.; Nones, K.; Corbo, V.; Patch, A.-M.; Bailey, P.; Lawlor, R.T.; Johns, A.L.; Miller, D.K.; Mafficini, A.; et al. Whole-Genome Landscape of Pancreatic Neuroendocrine Tumours. *Nat. Cell Biol.* **2017**, *543*, 65–71. [CrossRef] [PubMed]
72. Balaguer, F.; Leoz, M.L.; Carballal, S.; Moreira, L.; Ocaña, T. The Genetic Basis of Familial Adenomatous Polyposis and Its Implications for Clinical Practice and Risk Management. *Appl. Clin. Genet.* **2015**, *8*, 95–107. [CrossRef] [PubMed]
73. Win, A.K.; Dowty, J.G.; Cleary, S.P.; Kim, H.; Buchanan, D.D.; Young, J.P.; Clendenning, M.; Rosty, C.; MacInnis, R.J.; Giles, G.G.; et al. Risk of Colorectal Cancer for Carriers of Mutations in MUTYH, With and Without a Family History of Cancer. *Gastroenterology* **2014**, *146*, 1208–1211.e5. [CrossRef]
74. Win, A.K.; Reece, J.C.; Dowty, J.G.; Buchanan, D.D.; Clendenning, M.; Rosty, C.; Southey, M.C.; Young, J.P.; Cleary, S.P.; Kim, H.; et al. Risk of Extracolonic Cancers for People with Biallelic and Monoallelic Mutations inMUTYH. *Int. J. Cancer* **2016**, *139*, 1557–1563. [CrossRef]
75. Nguyen, L.; Martens, J.W.M.; Van Hoeck, A.; Cuppen, E. Pan-Cancer Landscape of Homologous Recombination Deficiency. *Nat. Commun.* **2020**, *11*, 5584. [CrossRef]
76. D'Andrea, A.D. Mechanisms of PARP Inhibitor Sensitivity and Resistance. *DNA Repair* **2018**, *71*, 172–176. [CrossRef]
77. Mouw, K.W.; Goldberg, M.S.; Konstantinopoulos, P.A.; D'Andrea, A.D. DNA Damage and Repair Biomarkers of Immu-Notherapy Response. *Cancer Discov.* **2017**, *7*, 675–693. [CrossRef]

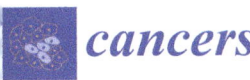

Article

Is Breast Cancer Risk Associated with Menopausal Hormone Therapy Modified by Current or Early Adulthood BMI or Age of First Pregnancy?

Eleni Leventea [1], Elaine F. Harkness [2,3,4], Adam R. Brentnall [5], Anthony Howell [2,4,6,7], D. Gareth Evans [2,4,6,8,9,10] and Michelle Harvie [2,4,6,7,*]

1. Department of Nutrition and Dietetics, Cambridge University Hospitals NHS Foundation Trust, Cambridge CB2 0QQ, UK; eleni.leventea@addenbrookes.nhs.uk
2. Nightingale Breast Screening Centre & Prevent Breast Cancer Unit, Wythenshawe Hospital, Manchester University NHS Foundation Trust, Manchester M23 9LT, UK; Elaine.F.Harkness@manchester.ac.uk (E.F.H.); Anthony.Howell@manchester.ac.uk (A.H.); Gareth.Evans@mft.nhs.uk (D.G.E.)
3. Centre for Imaging Science, Division of Informatics, Imaging and Data Science, Faculty of Biology, Medicine and Health, University of Manchester, Manchester Academic Health Science Centre, Manchester M23 9LT, UK
4. NIHR Manchester Biomedical Research Centre, Manchester M13 9WU, UK
5. Centre for Cancer Prevention, Wolfson Institute of Preventive Medicine, Barts and The London School of Medicine and Dentistry, Queen Mary University of London, London EC1M 6BQ, UK; a.brentnall@qmul.ac.uk
6. Manchester Breast Centre, The Christie Hospital, Manchester M23 9LT, UK
7. Division of Cancer Sciences, Medicine and Health, University of Manchester, Manchester Academic Health Science Centre, Manchester M23 9LT, UK
8. Manchester Centre for Genomic Medicine, Manchester University Hospitals NHS Foundation Trust, Manchester M23 9LT, UK
9. NW Genomic Laboratory Hub, Manchester Centre for Genomic Medicine, Manchester University Hospitals NHS Foundation Trust, Manchester M13 9WL, UK
10. Faculty of Biology, Division of Evolution and Genomic Sciences, School of Biological Sciences, Medicine and Health, University of Manchester, Manchester Academic Health Science Centre, Manchester M23 9LT, UK
* Correspondence: michelle.harvie@manchester.ac.uk

Simple Summary: Menopausal hormone therapy (MHT) increases risk of developing breast cancer (BC), and women are often advised to avoid its use for this reason. In this analysis we examined the size of this effect using data from a large cohort of women attending breast cancer screening in Manchester, UK. We additionally explored the extent to which risk from MHT might be modified by current BMI, early adulthood body mass index (BMI) (age 20 years), and age of first pregnancy. Identifying modifying effects would help enable better estimation of risk associated with MHT for an individual woman. Results indicated that women using combined oestrogen and progestagen MHT were at greater risk than those receiving oestrogen-only MHT. The Relative risk associated with MHT was less for obese women than non-obese women. After adjustment for current BMI, the effect of MHT did not appear to be substantially modified by early BMI or age of pregnancy.

Abstract: Menopausal hormone therapy (MHT) has an attenuated effect on breast cancer (BC) risk amongst heavier women, but there are few data on a potential interaction with early adulthood body mass index (at age 20 years) and age of first pregnancy. We studied 56,489 women recruited to the PROCAS (Predicting Risk of Cancer at Screening) study in Manchester UK, 2009-15. Cox regression models estimated the effect of reported MHT use at entry on breast cancer (BC) risk, and potential interactions with a. self-reported current body mass index (BMI), b. BMI aged 20 and c. First pregnancy >30 years or nulliparity compared with first pregnancy <30 years. Analysis was adjusted for age, height, family history, age of menarche and menopause, menopausal status, oophorectomy, ethnicity, self-reported exercise and alcohol. With median follow up of 8 years, 1663 breast cancers occurred. BC risk was elevated amongst current users of combined MHT compared to never users (Hazard ratioHR 1.64, 95% CI 1.32–2.03), risk was higher than for oestrogen only users (HR 1.03, 95% CI 0.79–1.34). Risk of current MHT was attenuated by current BMI (interaction HR 0.80, 95% CI 0.65–0.99) per 5 unit increase in BMI. There was little evidence of an interaction between MHT use, breast cancer risk and early and current BMI or with age of first pregnancy.

Citation: Leventea, E.; Harkness, E.F.; Brentnall, A.R.; Howell, A.; Evans, D.G.; Harvie, M. Is Breast Cancer Risk Associated with Menopausal Hormone Therapy Modified by Current or Early Adulthood BMI or Age of First Pregnancy? *Cancers* **2021**, *13*, 2710. https://doi.org/10.3390/cancers13112710

Academic Editor: Virgilio Sacchini

Received: 9 April 2021
Accepted: 25 May 2021
Published: 31 May 2021

Publisher's Note: MDPI stays neutral with regard to jurisdictional claims in published maps and institutional affiliations.

Copyright: © 2021 by the authors. Licensee MDPI, Basel, Switzerland. This article is an open access article distributed under the terms and conditions of the Creative Commons Attribution (CC BY) license (https://creativecommons.org/licenses/by/4.0/).

Keywords: menopausal hormone therapy; breast cancer risk; BMI; early BMI; age of pregnancy

1. Introduction

Approximately 80% of women going through the menopause experience symptoms [1]. Menopausal hormone therapy (MHT) is the most effective treatment option. MHT use halved in the early 2000s as a result of widely publicised associations between MHT use and increased risk of breast cancer and thromboembolism. Rates stabilised in the 2010s and currently there are an estimated one million MHT users in the UK each year, representing approximately 10% of women passing through the menopause [1]. A recent meta-analysis based on 58 prospective and retrospective studies, including 568,859 women and 143,887 breast cancer cases concluded that ever MHT use is associated with increased breast cancer risk (RR 1.26, 95% CI 1.24–1.28). Risk is higher for current compared to past users and increased with longer MHT use. Amongst current users, risk is greater with combined (oestrogen plus progestagen) MHT (RR for 5–14 years of use 2.08, 95% CI 2.02–2.15) compared to oestrogen only MHT (RR 1.33, 95% CI 1.28–1.37). Risk was attenuated amongst heavier women, particularly for oestrogen-only MHT, with little additional risk from oestrogen-only MHT in women who were obese [2].

MHT use increases breast cancer risk amongst women in the general population but also in women with increased risk due to familial cancer [3]. Many women, especially those at higher risk of breast cancer, are counselled to avoid or minimise MHT use [4]. Guidelines recommend an individual risk benefit assessment for prescribing MHT [5]. However there are limited data on whether MHT risk is modified by other patient characteristics which would help to inform this decision.

Increased body mass index (BMI) after the menopause (RR per 5 BMI units: 1.12, 95% CI 1.09–1.15) and weight gain throughout adult life after the age of 20 (RR per 5 kg: 1.06, 95% CI 1.05–1.08) are consistently associated with increased risk of postmenopausal breast cancer [6]. In contrast, higher weight during adolescence and early adulthood (age $\leq$30 years) are observed to have an inverse effect [7]. High body adiposity in early adulthood is associated with a reduced risk of postmenopausal (RR per 5 BMI units: 0.82, 95% CI 0.76–0.88) and premenopausal breast cancer (RR per 5 BMI units: 0.82, 95% CI 0.76–0.89) [6]. We recently reported higher BMI in early adulthood (>23.4 kg/m^2) negated the impact on risk of high later attained BMI [8].

Late age of first pregnancy (after the age of 30 years) and nulliparity are associated with increased risk of breast cancer. Women with first pregnancy after the age of 30 have approximately twice the risk of developing breast cancer compared to women with first pregnancy before the age of 20, and nulliparous women have a 30% increased risk compared to parous women [9]. Risks associated with attained adult and early adulthood weight and age of pregnancy are all in part mediated by different exposure to oestrogen and progesterone, and may alter the hormone responsiveness of the breast [10]. Thus they may modify the risk associated with MHT use.

Here we sought to examine the association between combined and oestrogen only MHT use and breast cancer risk in a cohort of women from the National Health Service Breast Screening Programme (NHSBSP), in Greater Manchester, UK. We examined whether BC risk associated with these types of MHT are modified by BMI at study entry (age 46–84 years) and/ or early adulthood BMI (age 20), or age at first pregnancy or nulliparity.

2. Methods

2.1. Population

The Predicting Risk of Cancer At Screening (PROCAS) study has been described in detail elsewhere. In total 57,902 women aged between 46 and 84 years in the National Health Service Breast Screening programme (NHSBSP) were recruited from five areas of Greater Manchester (Manchester, Oldham, Salford, Tameside and Trafford) between October 2009 and June 2015 [11]. Recruitment was carried out in two phases: initially all women who were invited for three-yearly breast screening (October 2009–October 2012) after which only women invited to their first screen in the area (mainly aged 46–53 years) were invited to participate in the study. Participants were invited once during the recruitment period. During the initial phase uptake to screening was 68% with uptake to PROCAS 37% of attendees, in the second phase screening uptake was 58% and uptake to PROCAS was 47% of attendees (screening uptake is lower in first time invitees).

2.2. Data Collection

Data collection was based on a two-page questionnaire, which was sent to participants with a consent form between their invitations to attend screening and scheduled screening appointment (Supplementary Materials).

The self-reported questionnaire gathered information on risk factors for breast cancer including: previous breast cancer diagnosis, breast or ovarian cancer in first and second degree relatives, hormonal risk factors, including age at menarche, oophorectomy and hysterectomy, menopausal status, age at menopause, parity and age at first pregnancy, physical activity levels, alcohol intake and ethnicity. Questions in relation to MHT use included name of preparation, duration of use and when MHT was last used (if no longer on MHT). Women were also asked to record their height, current weight and recalled weight at age 20 as a proxy of early adulthood BMI. Current BMI and BMI at 20 were calculated from these variables. Completed questionnaires were collated by the study team and entered into the study database.

2.3. Diagnosis of Breast Cancer

The primary outcome was diagnosis of a new breast cancer (invasive or ductal carcinoma in situ), from entry to PROCAS onwards, as identified through the NHSBSP and the Somerset and North West Cancer Intelligence services. Follow-up (median eight years) was censored at date of breast cancer diagnosis, date of death, date lost to follow-up, e.g., moving out of the area, or date cancer databases were last checked (April 2020). The current analysis excluded women with breast cancer diagnosed prior to study entry ($n = 895$).

2.4. MHT Use

MHT use was classed as never, current and former. Never users were women who indicated they had never been on MHT at any time. Current users were women who reported they were still on MHT and gave details about length of time on MHT but did not indicate a time of stopping. Former users were women who reported no longer using MHT but indicated how long they had been using MHT and time since stopping.

Where women did not provide an MHT name, it was assumed that those who had a hysterectomy had oestrogen only MHT, whereas women who did not have hysterectomy had combined (oestrogen plus progestagen) MHT. MHT status was missing for 514 women who were excluded from any further analyses (Figure 1).

The analyses included pre/peri and postmenopausal women enrolled in the PROCAS study. Women were considered postmenopausal if they indicated on the questionnaire they had been through the menopause (i.e., not had period for 12 months) or reported they had both ovaries removed (surgical menopause) or current use of MHT or age at menopause was unknown but age at time of questionnaire completion was 55 years or over as based on criteria defined by Phipps et al. [12].

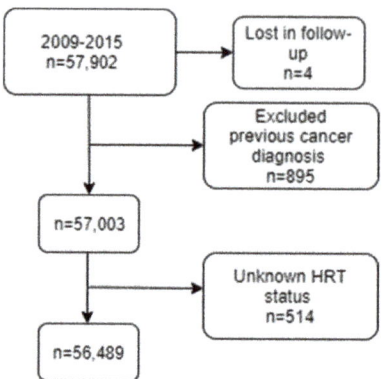

Figure 1. Flow diagram: Number of women in the cohort meeting the criteria for inclusion in the analysis.

2.5. BMI Data

We excluded attained BMI and early BMI values which were >60 or <16 kg/m^2. For current BMI, 3943 were unknown or beyond these cut-offs. For early BMI, 6300 values were unknown or beyond these cut-offs. Median value of the cohort was assumed for missing values (total 6.8% for current and 10.9% for BMI at age 20).

2.6. Statistical Analysis

Demographic Characteristics and Breast Cancer Risk Factors amongst MHT Users and Non-Users

Differences in demographic characteristics and breast cancer risk factors across MHT groups (never, current, former) were tested using one-way ANOVA and Chi-square tests where appropriate. Adjusted comparisons of continuous measure used linear regression (with covariates for age (years), current and early BMI (kg/m^2)).

2.7. MHT Use and BC Risk

Cox (or proportional hazards) regression was used to model the relationship between MHT use and diagnosis of breast cancer. Follow-up was censored at date of breast cancer, date of death or date of last follow-up (April 2020). Results were expressed as hazard ratios (HR) and 95% Wald confidence intervals (95% CI).

Fully adjusted Cox regression models included the following established risk factors for breast cancer: age (1 year), height (5 cm), BMI (5 units), early BMI (5 units), ethnicity (white/other), age at menarche (1 year), age at first pregnancy (<20, 20–24, 25–29, 30–34, ≥35) years, parity, age at menopause (1 year) menopausal status (pre/peri or postmenopausal), oophorectomy, self-reported exercise (1 h/week) and alcohol (1 unit/week), MHT status (current, former, never), MHT type (combined, oestrogen only) and family history (first or second degree). For the fully adjusted analysis, missing values were imputed as the median value of the cohort. We did not include the available mammographic density data in the models since there is some evidence this may be part of the pathway for reduced risk alongside higher early BMI [13]. The multiple deprivation score was not included since this was not associated with risk once the variables associated with this, such as age of pregnancy were included in the model (Table S1a, S1b).

2.8. MHT Use, Breast Cancer Risk and Effect Modification by Current BMI and Early BMI and Age of First Pregnancy

To assess whether current and early BMI modified the relationship between MHT and the risk of breast cancer the following two way interaction terms were also included in the fully adjusted models: current/ former MHT use* current BMI * (Table S2a) and current/

former MHT use* early BMI (Table S2b). We also tested the 3-way interactions: current/former MHT use*current BMI *early BMI (Table S2c).

For presentation the relationship between MHT use and BC risk was tabulated by stratifying above and below the median for current (26.4 kg/m^2) and early (21.6 kg/m^2) BMI. The reference group was never use of MHT, current BMI below the median and early BMI below the median. The median was used to dichotomise results and aid with interpretation (Table 1).

The relationship between late age at first pregnancy and nulliparity, MHT status and BC risk was assessed using analysis stratified by age at first pregnancy <30 years or a combined group which included women with first pregnancy ≥30 years or who were nulliparous (Table 2 and Table S5).

Due to previous known heterogeneity by type of MHT and subtype of breast cancer we also performed these analyses according to (i) MHT type (combined oestrogen and progestagen or oestrogen only) (Table 3) and (ii) oestrogen receptor positive breast cancer. (Table S1c).

Table 1. MHT and BC risk and current and early BMI.

A MHT use	BMI < 26.4 kg/m^2		BMI ≥ 26.4 kg/m^2	
	N (%) BC/ no BC	HR (95% CI)	N (%) BC/no BC	HR (95% CI)
Never	474 (2.5)/18,381 (97.5)	1.00 (Ref)	524 (3.2)/16016 (96.8)	1.44 (1.26–1.64)
Former	256 (3.2)/7858 (96.8)	1.12 (0.95–1.32)	251 (3.2)/7508 (96.8)	1.29 (1.09–1.53)
Current	101 (3.9)/2457 (96.1)	1.60 (1.28–1.98)	57 (3.2)/1725 (96.8)	1.45 (1.09–1.92)
B	BMI age 20 < 21.6 kg/m^2		BMI age 20 ≥ 21.6 kg/m^2	
	N (%) BC/noBC	HR (95% CI)	N (%)BC/no BC	HR (95% CI)
Never	439 (3.0)/14,292 (97.0)	1.00 (Ref)	559 (2.7)/20,105 (97.3)	0.85 (0.75–0.97)
Former	235 (3.3)/6878 (96.7)	0.98 (0.83–1.16)	272 (3.1)/8488	0.89 (0.75–1.05)
Current	80 (4.0)/1943 (96.0)	1.37 (1.08–1.75)	78 (3.4)/2239 (96.6)	1.11 (0.86–1.41)
C	BMI age 20 < 21.6 kg/m^2		BMI age 20 ≥ 21.6 kg/m^2	
	N (%) BC/no BC	HR (95% CI)	N (%) BC/no BC	HR (95% CI)
Never BMI < 26.4 kg/m^2	259 (2.6)/9737 (97.4)	1.00 (Ref)	139 (2.2)/6171 (97.8)	0.86 (0.70–1.06)
Never BMI ≥ 26.4 kg/m^2	180 (3.8)/4555 (96.2)	1.53 (1.26–1.85)	420 (2.9)/13,934 (97.1)	1.20 (1.02–1.40)
Former BMI < 26.4 kg/m^2	142 (3.2)/4249 (96.8)	1.12 (0.90–1.38)	83 (3.0)/2726 (97.0)	1.03 (0.80–1.33)
Former BMI ≥ 26.4 kg/m^2	93 (3.4)/2629 (96.6)	1.23 (0.97–1.57)	189 (3.2)/5762 (96.8)	1.17 (0.96–1.43)
Current BMI < 26.4 kg/m^2	54 (3.8)/1385 (96.2)	1.48 (1.10–2.00)	34 (4.0)/808 (96.0)	1.60 (1.12–2.30)
Current BMI ≥ 26.4 kg/m^2	558 (95.5)/26 (4.5)	1.84 (1.22–2.76)	1431 (97.0)/44 (3.0)	1.24 (0.90–1.71)

BC breast cancer; Units: age (1 year), BMI (5 BMI units), BMI at age 20 (5 BMI units), height (5 cm), age at menopause (1 year), exercise (1 h per week), alcohol (1 unit per week), age at menarche (1 year) BMI median: 26.4 kg/m^2, BMI20 median: 21.6 kg/m.

Table 2. MHT status and BC risk and age of pregnancy > 30 and nulliparity.

	Age at Pregnancy < 30		Age at Pregnancy ≥ 30	
	N (%) BC/ no BC	HR (95% CI)	N (%) BC/ no BC	HR (95% CI)
Never	670 (2.7)/24,126 (97.3)	1.00 (Ref)	328 (3.1)/10,271 (96.9)	1.20 (1.05–1.38)
Former	391 (3.1)/12,401 (96.9)	0.99 (0.86–1.13)	116 (3.8)/2965 (96.2)	1.25 (1.02–1.53)
Current	110 (3.5)/3076 (96.5)	1.31 (1.06–1.60)	48 (4.2)/1106 (95.8)	1.64 (1.22–2.20)
Oestrogen only				
	Age at Pregnancy < 30		Age at Pregnancy ≥ 30	
	N (%) BC/ no BC	HR (95% CI)	N (%) BC/ no BC	HR (95% CI)
Never	670 (2.7)/24,126 (97.3)	1.00 (Ref)	182 (3.2)/5465 (96.8)	1.28 (1.09–1.51)
Former	151 (2.7)/5399 (97.3)	0.89 (0.73–1.09)	14 (3.5)/390 (96.5)	1.22 (0.71–2.09)
Current	46 (2.6)/1715 (97.4)	0.96 (0.71–1.31)	9 (4.6)/187 (95.4)	1.81 (0.93–3.53)
Combined				
	Age at Pregnancy < 30		Age at Pregnancy ≥ 30	
	N (%) no BC/BC	HR (95% CI)	N (%) no BC/BC	HR (95% CI)
Never	670 (2.7)24,126 (97.3)	1.00 (Ref)	182 (3.2)/5465 (96.8)	1.29 (1.09–1.52)
Former	240 (3.3)/7002 (96.7)	1.07 (0.92–1.26)	41 (4.0)/984 (96.0)	1.36 (0.99–1.87)
Current	64 (4.5)/1361 (95.5)	1.74 (1.34–2.25)	16 (4.6)/331 (95.4)	1.90 (1.16–3.13)

BC breast cancer; Units: age (1 year), BMI (5 units), BMI at age 20 (5 units), height (5 cm), age at menopause (1 year), exercise (1 h per week), alcohol (1 unit per week), age at menarche (1 year).

Table 3. MHT type and BC risk and current and early BMI.

A				
	BMI < 26.4 kg/m^2		BMI ≥ 26.4 kg/m^2	
	N (%) BC/ no BC	HR (95% CI)	N (%) BC/ no BC	HR (95% CI)
Never	439 (3.0)/14,292 (97.0)	1.00 (Ref)	559 (2.7)/20,105 (97.3)	1.48 (1.29–1.69)
Former oestrogen only	79 (2.9)/2664 (97.1)	1.06 (0.81–1.38)	26 (2.1)/1199 (97.9)	1.23 (0.98–1.54)
Former combined	156 (3.6)/4214 (96.4)	1.17 (0.96–1.42)	52 (4.8)/1040 (95.2)	1.40 (1.15–1.69)
Current oestrogen only	37 (4.8)/984 (95.2)	1.29 (0.90–1.85)	112 (3.0)/3670 (97.0)	1.16 (0.79–1.70)
Current combined	43 (4.3)/959 (95.7)	1.86 (1.40–2.47)	160 (3.2)/4818 (96.8)	2.11 (1.53–2.92)
B				
	BMI age 20 < 21.6 kg/m^2		BMI age 20 ≥ 21.6 kg/m^2	
	N (%) BC / no BC	HR (95% CI)	N (%) BC/ no BC	HR (95% CI)
Never	439 (3.0)/14,292 (97.0)	1.00 (Ref)	559(2.7)/20,105 (97.3)	0.84 (0.74–0.96)
Former oestrogen only	79 (2.9)/2664 (97.1)	0.85 (0.66–1.10)	112 (3.0)/3670 (97.0)	0.83 (0.66–1.04)
Former combined	156 (3.6)/4214 (96.4)	1.04 (0.86–1.25)	160 (3.2)/4818 (96.8)	0.88 (0.73–1.06)
Current oestrogen only	37 (4.8)/984 (95.2)	1.23 (0.87–1.73)	26 (2.1)/1199 (97.9)	0.67 (0.45–1.00)
Current combined	43 (4.3)/959 (95.7)	1.47 (1.07–2.01)	52 (4.8)/1040 (95.2)	1.54 (1.15–2.06)

Table 3. Cont.

C

Oestrogen only MHT	BMI age 20 < 21.6 kg/m²		BMI age 20 ≥ 21.6 kg/m²	
	N (%) BC/ no BC	HR (95% CI)	N (%) BC/ no BC	HR (95% CI)
Never BMI < 26.4 kg/m²	259 (2.6)9737 (97.4)	1.00 (Ref)	6171 (97.8)/139 (2.2)	0.86 (0.70–1.05)
Never BMI ≥ 26.4 kg/m²	180 (3.8)/4555 (96.2)	1.54 (1.27–1.86)	420 (2.9)/13,934 (97.1)	1.20 (1.02–1.41)
Former BMI < 26.4 kg/m²	45 (2.9)/1484 (97.1)	1.05 (0.76–1.47)	30 (2.8)/1031 (97.2)	1.00 (0.67–1.48)
Former BMI ≥ 26.4 kg/m²	34 (2.8)/1180 (97.2)	1.04 (0.72–1.50)	82 (3.0)/2639 (97.0)	1.15 (0.87–1.50)
Current BMI < 26.4 kg/m²	23 (3.4)/663 (96.6)	1.33 (0.86–2.05)	11 (2.7)/395 (97.3)	1.06 (0.58–1.95)
Current BMI ≥ 26.4 kg/m²	14 (4.2)/321 (95.8)	1.68 (0.97–2.90)	15 (1.8)/804 (98.2)	0.75 (0.44–1.28)
Combined MHT	BMI age 20 < 21.6 kg/m²		BMI age 20 ≥ 21.6 kg/m²	
	N (%) BC/ no BC	HR (95% CI)	N (%) BC/ no BC	HR (95% CI)
Never BMI < 26.4 kg/m²	259 (2.6)9737 (97.4)	1.00 (Ref)	6171 (97.8)/139 (2.2)	0.86 (0.70–1.05)
Never BMI ≥ 26.4 kg/m²	180 (3.8)/4555 (96.2)	1.52 (1.25–1.84)	420 (2.9)13,934 (97.1)	1.19 (1.01–1.39)
Former BMI < 26.4 kg/m²	97 (3.4)/2765 (96.6)	1.14 (0.90–1.45)	53 (3.0)/1695 (97.0)	1.04 (0.77–1.40)
Former BMI ≥ 26.4 kg/m²	59 (3.9)/1449 (96.1)	1.36 (1.02–1.82)	107 (3.3)/3123 (96.7)	1.16 (0.92–1.47)
Current BMI < 26.4 kg/m²	31 (4.1)/722 (95.9)	1.60 (1.10–2.32)	23 (5.3)/413 (94.7)	2.08 (1.35–3.18)
Current BMI ≥ 26.4 kg/m²	12 (4.8)/237 (95.2)	1.96 (1.10–3.51)	29 (4.4)/627 (95.6)	1.80 (1.22–2.65)

BC breast cancer; Units: age (1 year), BMI (5 units), BMI at age 20 (5 units), height (5 cm), age at menopause (1 year), exercise (1 h per week), alcohol (1 unit per week), age at menarche (1 year); BMI median: 26.4 kg/m², BMI age 20 median: 21.6 kg/m².

3. Results

3.1. Flow Diagram

From the cohort of 57,902 women, 895 were diagnosed with breast cancer prior to study entry, 4 were lost to follow up and were excluded from the analysis. Women with unknown MHT use status were also excluded from the analysis (N = 514). The denominator for the main analysis was 56,489 with the endpoint being a new diagnosis of breast cancer (N = 1663, 3.2% of the cohort) (Figure 1).

3.2. Demographic Characteristics and Breast Cancer Risk Factors According to MHT Use

Demographic characteristics and BC risk factors according to MHT groups are shown in Table 4. Of those eligible for analysis 7.8% were current MHT users, 28.6% were former users and 63.6% had never used MHT. Across all MHT groups at study entry, 35.9% were in the underweight or normal BMI category range, 39.5% in the overweight, 24.6% in the obese BMI category, 3801 women had an unknown BMI. The median age at first pregnancy was 24 years (interquartile range [IQR] 21–28 years), 26.7% of women had their first pregnancy either at or after the age of 30 years. In total, 27.9% of women had a first or second degree family history of ovarian and/ or breast cancer.

When compared to never users, current MHT users had a higher percentage of oophorectomy (27.5% vs. 5.6%), lower BMI at study entry (median: 26.0 vs. 26.4 kg/m²), were less likely to have a family history of ovarian and/ or breast cancer (26.6% vs. 28.3%), a lower deprivation score (median: 17.6 vs. 19.4), and younger age of first pregnancy (median 23 vs. 24 years). As expected, former users were the oldest group, also reflected by the higher percentage of participants being postmenopausal.

Table 4. Baseline Characteristics of the 56,489 women in the PROCAS cohort (2009–2015).

		Status of MHT Use		
	Total	Never	Former	Current
Number of women (%)	56,489 (100)	35,933 (63.6)	16,149 (28.6)	4407 (7.8)
Ethnicity				
White	53,571 (94.8)	33,695 (93.8)	15,634 (96.8)	4242 (96.3)
Other	2918 (5.2)	2238 (6.2)	515 (3.2)	165 (3.7)
Unknown	1799	1027	648	124
Age at study entry				
Median (IQR)	56.9 (51.6–63.6)	53.9 (50.7–60.8)	62.9 (58.3–66.6)	55.2 (51.5–60.6)
Mean (SD)	57.8 (7.0)	56.0 (6.7)	62.3 (5.8)	56.4 (6.0)
Menopausal status				
premenopausal and perimenopausal	18,764 (33.2)	16,742 (46.6)	821 (5.1)	1201 (27.3)
postmenopausal	37,725 (66.8)	19,191 (53.4)	15,328 (94.9)	3206 (72.7)
Unknown	2831	2673	76	82
Age at menopause				
Median (IQR)	50.0 (46.0–53.0)	50.0 (48.0–53.0)	50.0 (45.0–53.0)	48.0 (44.0–51.0)
Mean (SD)	49.0 (5.6)	49.9 (4.7)	48.1 (6.4)	47.1 (6.6)
Unknown	46 (0.1)	29 (0.1)	15 (0.1)	2 (<0.1)
Age at menarche				
Median (IQR)	13.0 (12.0–14.0)	13.0 (12.0–14.0)	13.0 (12.0–14.0)	13.0 (12.0–14.0)
Mean (SD)	12.9 (1.6)	12.9 (1.6)	12.8 (1.6)	12.9 (1.6)
Unknown	1186 (2.1)	762 (2.1)	319 (2.0)	105 (2.4)
Parity and age at first pregnancy				
Nulliparous	7330 (13.0)	5028 (14.0)	1681 (10.4)	621 (14.1)
<30	41,408 (73.3)	25,259 (70.2)	13,013 (18.5)	3236 (73.4)
≥30	7751 (13.7)	5706 (15.8)	1455 (2.2)	550 (12.5)
Median age at first pregnancy (IQR)	24.0 (21.0–28.0)	24.0 (21.0–28.0)	23.0 (20.0–26.0)	23.0 (20.0–27.0)
Mean age at first pregnancy (SD)	24.4 (5.3)	25 (5.3)	23.5 (4.6)	24.1 (5.2)
Unknown	4 (<0.1)	3 (<0.1)	1 (<0.1)	0 (<0.1)
BMI				
Underweight or normal weight (<25 kg/m^2)	20,216 (35.9)	12,931 (36.1)	5486 (34.1)	1799 (41.0)
Overweight (25–29.9 kg/m^2)	22,249 (39.5)	13,813 (38.5)	6660 (41.4)	1776 (40.4)
Obese (≥30 kg/m^2)	13,868 (24.6)	9091 (25.4)	3959 (24.6)	818 (18.6)
Median (IQR)	26.4 (23.8–29.9)	26.4 (23.7–30.0)	26.4 (24.0–29.9)	26.0 (23.4–28.7)
Mean (SD)	27.4 (5.4)	27.5 (5.5)	27.4 (5.1)	26.5 (4.7)
Unknown	3801	2587	933	281
BMI at age 20				
Underweight or normal weight (<25 kg/m^2)	50,119 (88.8)	31,673 (88.2)	14,456 (89.6)	3990 (90.6)
Overweight (25–29.9 kg/m^2)	5105 (9.0)	3369 (9.4)	1388 (8.6)	348 (7.9)
Obese (≥30 kg/m^2)	1243 (2.2)	877 (2.4)	298 (1.8)	68 (1.5)
Median (IQR)	21.6 (20.3–23.0)	21.6 (20.3–23.2)	21.6 (20.2–23.0)	21.6 (20.0–22.8)
Mean (SD)	22.0 (3.1)	22.1 (3.1)	21.9 (2.9)	21.8 (2.9)
Unknown	6777	4694	1600	483
Mean Height (SD)	1.62 (0.07)	1.62 (0.07)	1.61 (0.06)	1.62 (0.06)
Median Height (IQR)	1.63 (1.57–1.65)	1.63 (1.57–1.65)	1.60 (1.57–1.65)	1.63 (1.57–1.68)
Unknown	1111	766	269	76
Oophorectomy				
Yes	6696 (12.0)	1999 (5.6)	3584 (22.2)	1213 (27.5)
No	49,693 (88.0)	33,934 (94.4)	12,565 (77.8)	3194 (72.5)
Unknown	8709	5183	2716	810
MHT type				
Oestrogen only	8895 (43.2)		6617 (41.0)	2278 (51.7)
Combined	11,661 (56.7)		9532 (59.0)	2129 (48.3)
Unknown	13,456		12,441	1015
Duration of MHT use (years)				
Median (IQR)	5 (2.0–10.0)		5 (2.0–10.0)	7 (2.5–13.0)
Mean (SD)	7.3 (4.6)		6.2 (5.4)	8.6 (7.2)
Unknown	2433		1178	1255
VAS Density				
Median (IQR)	24.8 (14.9–35.8)	24.8 (15.6–35.8)	22.4 (12.9–34.4)	29.5 (18.9–41.0)
Mean (SD)	27.1 (16.2)	27.5 (16.1)	25.3 (15.8)	31.3 (16.8)
Family History of Breast and/or Ovarian Cancer *				
Yes	15,738 (27.9)	10,185 (28.3)	4379 (27.1)	1174 (26.6)
No	40,748 (72.1)	25,748 (71.7)	11,768 (72.9)	3232 (73.4)
Median exercise hours per week (IQR)	3.5 (1.5–7.0)	3.5 (1.0–6.0)	3.5 (2.0–8.0)	3.5 (2.0–7.0)
Unknown	17,085	11,171	4630	1284
Median alcohol units per week (IQR)	4.0 (0.0–10.0)	4.0 (0.0–10.0)	4.0 (0.0–10.0)	4.0 (1.0–10.0)
Unknown	2512	1593	723	196
Median EIMD score 2010 (IQR) **	18.9 (10.4–35.1)	19.4 (10.5–35.4)	18.7 (10.6–34.9)	17.6 (9.7–32.5)
Unknown	312	176	111	25

BMI body mass index, SD standard deviation, IQR interquartile range; MHT hormonal replacement therapy, VAS visual analogue scale; EIMD English Index of multiple deprivation. * First or second degree relative with ovarian and/or breast cancer; ** Ever vs. never MHT EIMD 2010 $p = 0.002$, EIMD current vs. never $p < 0.001$, never vs. former $p = 0.444$; age adjusted comparisons: BMI current vs. never $p < 0.001$, never vs. former $p = 0.639$; age adjusted VAS current vs. never $p < 0.001$, never vs. former $p = 0.697$; age, menopausal status, BMI adjusted VAS current vs. never $p < 0.001$, never vs. former $p = 0.001$.

Compared with former users, current users were younger (median: 55.2 vs. 62.9 years), had longer use of MHT (median: 7 vs. 5 years), higher percentage use of oestrogen only

MHT (51.7% vs. 41.0%), lower BMI at entry (median: 26.0 vs. 26.4 kg/m^2), were less likely to have family history of breast and/ or ovarian cancer (26.6% vs. 27.1%), and lower deprivation score (median: 17.6 vs. 18.7). All differences cited have $p < 0.001$ due to large sample size. Women with known MHT status were lighter at entry to PROCAS, more likely to be white, and from less deprived backgrounds than those with unknown MHT status (Table S3).

3.3. MHT Use Status and Breast Cancer Risk

Median follow up from study entry was 8 years (IQR: 7–9, minimum 5 and maximum 12 years). Compared with never use, current MHT use was positively associated with breast cancer (HR 1.35, 95% CI 1.13–1.60), while there was little evidence of an association for former users (HR 1.03, 95% CI 0.91–1.17) (Table 5). The fully adjusted model fit is shown in Table S1b.

Table 5. MHT status and type of MHT and breast cancer risk.

MHT Use Status	N% BC/ N% no BC	HR (95% CI)	p-Value	HR (95% CI)	p-Value
Never	998 (2.8)/ 34,397 (97.2)	1.00		1.00	
Former	507 (3.2)/ 15,366 (96.8)	0.98 (0.88–1.10)	0.765	1.03 (0.91–1.17)	0.614
Current	158 (3.6)/ 4182 (96.4)	1.27 (1.07–1.50)	0.006	1.35 (1.13–1.60)	0.001
MHT type					
Never	998 (2.8)/ 34,397 (97.2)	1.00		1.00	
Former oestrogen only	191 (2.9)/ 6334 (97.1)	0.90 (0.76–1.05)	0.189	0.95 (0.79–1.14)	0.558
Former combined	316 (3.4)/ 9032 (96.6)	1.04 (0.91–1.19)	0.586	1.06 (0.93–1.22)	0.398
Current oestrogen only	63 (2.8)/ 2183 (97.2)	0.96 (0.74–1.24)	0.754	1.03 (0.79–1.34)	0.835
Current combined	95 (4.5)/ 1999 (95.5)	1.60 (1.30–1.98)	<0.001	1.64 (1.32–2.03)	<0.001

BC breast cancer, HR hazard ratio, CI confidence interval. Fully adjusted for age at consent (1 year), BMI (5 units), BMI at age 20 (5 units), height (5 cm), age at menarche (1 year), age at menopause (1 year), menopausal status (pre/perimenopausal vs. postmenopausal), ethnicity (white vs. other), alcohol consumption (1 unit/week), exercise (1 h/week), age at first pregnancy (<20, 20–24, 25–29, 30–34, ≥35), oophorectomy (yes vs. no), family history (yes vs. no).

Breast cancer risk was highest in current users of combined MHT ($n = 2129$) (HR 1.64, 95% CI 1.32–2.03), compared with never users. Risk amongst current users of oestrogen only was ($n = 2278$) (HR 1.03, 95% CI 0.79–1.34) compared with never users (Table 5).

Analysis was repeated for ER+ breast cancers only, which comprised 88% of breast cancer diagnoses in the cohort. Current MHT users (combined and oestrogen only) were at increased risk of an ER+ diagnosis BC (HR 1.45, 95% CI 1.20–1.74) (Table S1c).

3.4. Current BMI and MHT and Breast Cancer Risk

Current BMI was positively associated with breast cancer risk (adjusted HR 1.23 per 5 kg/m^2, 95% CI 1.16 to 1.30; Table S1). The effect of MHT in current users was attenuated by BMI (adjusted interaction 0.81, 95% CI 0.67 to 0.98; Table S1b). This is illustrated by the data in Table 1 Part A, where there is less difference in risk between never and current users of MHT in the higher BMI category than the lower BMI category.

3.5. Early Adulthood BMI and MHT and Breast Cancer Risk

BMI in young adulthood was inversely associated with breast cancer risk (adjusted HR 0.77 per 5 kg/m^2, 95% CI 0.69 to 0.87; Table S1b). BMI at age 20 did not attenuate risk of current MHT use (adjusted interaction 1.05, 95% CI 0.72 to 1.53; Table S1). Table 1 Part B shows high early BMI reduced risk across never, former and current users of MHT, MHT did however increase risk across women with early BMI above and below the median.

3.6. Combined Stratified Model with Current BMI, Early BMI and MHT and Breast Cancer Risk

Risk of breast cancer amongst MHT users was stratified for ≥ and < median for current BMI (26.4 kg/m^2) and ≥ and < median for BMI age 20 years (21.6 kg/m^2) (Table 1 Part C).

Higher BMI at age 20 appears to attenuate the effects of high current BMI on BC risk both amongst women who are not using MHT and amongst current MHT users (adjusted interaction BMI *BMI 20 HR 0.96, 95% CI 0.90–1.02; Table S1).

There is no specific interaction between MHT use, current BMI and early BMI (HR 0.99, 95% CI 0.74–1.31) (Table S2c). Risk was highest amongst MHT users with current BMI higher than the median and BMI at 20 less than the median (HR 1.84, 95% CI 1.22–2.76) (Table 1c). Analysis for ER+ breast cancer found comparable results to the overall analysis (Table S2d).

3.7. Effects of Oestrogen Only and Combined MHT and Current and Early BMI and Breast Cancer Risk

Current combined MHT use increased risk amongst women irrespective of their current and early adulthood BMI (Table 3 Part A). Oestrogen only MHT use did not significantly increase risk in current or former MHT users in any of the BMI groups (Table 3 parts A, B, and C). However, risk appeared lower amongst current users of oestrogen only MHT with early BMI > median (HR 0.67, 95% CI 1.45–1.00) compared to early BMI < median (HR 1.23, 95% CI 0.87–1.73) (Table 3 Part B). Attenuation of risk amongst current oestrogen only MHT users with current BMI > median is seen in women who also had early BMI > median (HR 0.75, 95% CI 0.44–1.28) compared to women with early BMI < median (HR 1.68, 95% CI 0.97–2.90) (Table 3 Part C).

3.8. MHT Use and Age at First Pregnancy

Women who had a late pregnancy had an increased risk of breast cancer (age of first pregnancy >35 years HR 1.38, 95% CI 1.08–1.76) (Table S1b). Late first pregnancy or nulliparity increased risk across MHT users and non-users (Table 2). There is no specific interaction between MHT use, age of pregnancy or nulliparity (HR 1.00, 95% CI 0.80–1.02) (Table S4).

3.9. Effects of Oestrogen Only and Combined MHT and Age of First Pregnancy

Risks were comparable with combined MHT use amongst women with age of first pregnancy <30 years (HR 1.74, 95% CI 1.34–2.25) and > age 30 or nulliparity (HR 1.90, 95% CI 1.16–3.13). However, risks appeared lower amongst current oestrogen only MHT users with age of first pregnancy <30 years (HR 0.96, 95% CI 0.71–1.31) compared to >age 30 or nulliparity (HR 1.81, 95% CI 0.93–3.53) (Table 2).

4. Discussion

In this cohort, women with a lower current BMI were more likely to be current MHT users compared to women with a higher BMI. We have confirmed that current use of MHT increases breast cancer risk with excess risk mainly attributed to use of combined MHT. Higher early adulthood BMI had a small reduction in risk across never, former and current MHT groups. Late first pregnancy or nulliparity increased risk across never, former and current use of MHT groups. Neither BMI at age 20 or late first pregnancy or nulliparity had a specific modifying effect on the breast cancer risk related to overall MHT use. Observations of lower risks with oestrogen only MHT amongst women with high early BMI and early age of first pregnancy are interesting and require further study in larger cohorts.

Previous studies have reported that women with higher BMI were less likely to have used MHT [14–16]. Possible reasons for less use of MHT by heavier women include: experiencing fewer menopausal symptoms although this seems unlikely as the majority of papers report increased vasomotor symptoms in heavier women [17,18]; reduced likelihood of heavier women engaging with health behaviours, and contra-indications to MHT prescription associated with higher risk of thrombosis [19].

Our findings of increased breast cancer risk with current combined MHT, particularly with ER+ cancers concur with those found by the Collaborative Group [2]. We did not however observe an increased breast cancer risk for former MHT users. There was no significant association with oestrogen only MHT and BC risk, however our reported confidence intervals of the HR for oestrogen only MHT overlap with that reported by the Collaborative Group, indicating the results are broadly similar.

In these analyses we observed that higher current BMI attenuates the BC risk associated with overall current (combined and oestrogen only) MHT use. The attenuation of BC risk associated with oestrogen only MHT amongst currently heavier women has previously been reported [2]. Postmenopausal oestrogen levels correlate with BMI since endogenous oestrogen synthesis occurs within adipose tissue. The observed attenuation of oestrogen MHT risk is thought to reflect that exogenous oestrogen do not further stimulate the breast tissue in heavier women. This is consistent with a previous stated model that proposes a threshold for free oestrogen concentration beyond which there is no additional risk of breast cancer [20].

The stratified analysis in the current study suggests the attenuation that effects of oestrogen only MHT amongst currently heavier women is mainly seen in women who were heavier at an early age, and are not seen in formerly lighter women. The confidence intervals of these associations are quite wide due to small numbers of current users. However this observation raises the possibility that the apparent attenuation of oestrogen only MHT breast cancer risk amongst currently heavier women may be related to early rather than current BMI effects. Previous reports summarised in the collaborative overview did not examine the effects of early BMI.

A previous analysis within the PROCAS cohort reported that for women with early adulthood BMI >23.4 kg/m^2 (top 25% centile) neither attained adult BMI nor adult weight gain was associated with breast cancer risk [8]. The observation that higher BMI in early adulthood attenuates the BC risk associated with later adiposity has been reported in a number of studies [21–23]. A significant part of BC risk associated with postmenopausal BMI is thought to be mediated by increased oestrogen levels and the associated stimulation of breast tissue proliferation [24]. Reduced breast tissue proliferation has been reported amongst pre and postmenopausal women who had been heavier at age 18 (BMI >22 kg/m^2) [25]. Higher early adulthood BMI may attenuate the proliferative response of breast tissue to endogenous (associated with current BMI) or exogenous (MHT) oestrogen through a number of mechanisms. These include reducing terminal end buds and ductal elongation, and an overall reduction in the number of cells within breast tissue [25–27] and decreased expression of genes involved with both oestrogen action, i.e., ESR1 and GATA3, and cell proliferation, i.e., RPS6KB1, in breast tissue [28]. Also, increased levels of bioavailable oestrogens in early adulthood (associated with insulin levels and decreased sex hormone binding globulin) [29] could induce earlier differentiation of mammary cells [30] and expression of the BRCA1 tumour suppressor gene [31]. Higher levels of insulin-like growth factor 1 (IGF-1) during childhood and adolescence are associated with lower levels in adulthood [32]. The synergistic effects and cross talk between IGF-1 and oestrogen and their receptors are well established [33]. In addition women who are heavier in early adulthood are likely to have greater numbers of adipocytes (a hyperplastic phenotype). In contrast formerly lean women who gain weight will develop adipose hypertrophy (few but large cells) which are associated with inflammation and dysregulated metabolism [34].

A prospective study among 483,241 women and 7656 breast cancers studied whether MHT-associated BC risk is modified by life course patterns of BMI. The study reported that current users of MHT who reported being overweight at the ages of 7 and 15 (self-identified as being heavier than their peers) were at higher risk (HR 1.68, 95% CI 1.32–2.14) compared to never users of MHT who were overweight as young. However, risks were higher amongst current MHT users who remained at normal weight throughout adult life (HR 2.25, 95% CI 1.93–2.62) or who had gained weight (HR 2.28, 95% CI 1.94–2.67) [35]. The authors reported these risks were higher than expected when adding the separate risks of BMI and MHT with respective relative excess risk due to the interaction scores of 0.52 (95% CI 0.09–0.95) and 0.37 (95% CI -0.07 – +0.08). They concluded that women who were overweight at a young age were less susceptible to the effects of MHT than women who remained a normal weight or who gain weight in adulthood. This effect was seen amongst the whole cohort (70% combined MHT and 23% oestrogen only) and within the combined only group. They did not report the associations amongst current oestrogen only MHT users. The findings from this large cohort are of interest, however the analyses of early weight did not adjust for current BMI. Since higher weight at a younger age is likely to result in a higher current BMI, this study may not distinguish any interactions between early weight and current BMI and the effects of MHT.

We found that late age at first pregnancy increased risk amongst never, current and former MHT users. Age at first pregnancy does not modify risk associated with overall MHT use and breast cancer. Oestrogen only MHT appeared to be associated with a greater risk amongst women with a late first pregnancy or nulliparity compared to women with age of first pregnancy <30. There was no modification of the risk of combined MHT.

Risk of late pregnancy relates to a prolonged duration of undifferentiated state of the mammary tissue [36]. Synergistic effects of nulliparity and high postmenopausal BMI on BC risk in women aged >70 years have been reported [37]. Murrow et al recently reported that parity and high BMI amongst premenopausal women both decreased the oestrogen and progesterone responsiveness of the breast. These effects were associated with respective reductions in hormone signalling in hormone responsive luminal cells and reductions in the proportion of hormone responsive luminal cells within the mammary epithelium [10]. This data suggests a common pathway that could be shared between early pregnancy and high young age adiposity that is protective against breast cancer.

Our stratified analysis aimed to study the independent and combined interactions of current BMI, early BMI, MHT use and BC risk. Also whether these interactions differed with combined and oestrogen only MHT. Our sample size limits the ability to study all of these relationships with sufficient power. The observed trends in higher early weight and early pregnancy reducing the risk of oestrogen only MHT breast cancer requires further investigation in larger cohort or consortium studies.

Strengths of this analysis are that it was conducted in a large UK population. Many confounders associated with breast cancer risk were taken into consideration. The independent effects of both current BMI and early adulthood BMI were elicited in the models by including BMI at two different time points. Additionally, detailed information regarding MHT use and type were collected and breast cancer diagnosis updated on a regular basis. Sensitivity analysis showed that the models were consistent.

All information used in this analysis were self-reported, including current weight, height, weight at age 20, age at first pregnancy, name of MHT, how long MHT was used for and when MHT was stopped for former users. It is well known that there is a bias of underreporting weight and over reporting height [38]. However validation studies show self-reported BMI is highly correlated with independently measured weight and the mean difference between self-reported and measured weight is minimal [8,39]. BMI at entry and at age 20 was missing for 7.0% and 12.4% of the study population respectively. Recall bias could also occur for variables such as MHT duration. We did not update HRT usage status during follow up, and so were unable to estimate any association between duration of HRT use and risk of BC. The median value of the cohort was assumed where data was missing, and other methods could be used to account for the missing values. Breast cancer risk varies across racial groups [40] and the majority of women in the study were Caucasian thus limiting generalization of the findings to other ethnic groups. Risk factor information was only collected at baseline and it is possible that MHT status, BMI and other risk factors changed for some women. Some current MHT users are likely to have become former users and premenopausal women who had not used MHT could have become postmenopausal and started using MHT during the eight years of follow up.

Implications for practice for this research include that clinical risk assessment of suitability of a woman to commence on MHT, should include consideration of their current BMI and potentially early adulthood BMI and the type of MHT to be prescribed. The findings of this study support recommendations to maintain a healthy weight across the life course. Breast cancer risk is similar among women with higher current BMI who never used MHT and women with lower BMI who use MHT. The smaller increase in risk with MHT amongst heavier women should not deter these women from losing weight. The highest BC risk is seen amongst current MHT users with a high current BMI, especially those with a low BMI at an early age. Women at increased weight taking MHT will have higher risks of other MHT associated adverse effects including venous thromboembolism, stroke and endometrial cancer [5]. Weight loss has been shown to decrease risk of other cancers including colorectal and endometrial cancer, and additionally might help manage menopausal symptoms [41].

Future studies need to investigate the associations between current and early BMI and age of pregnancy and MHT associated breast cancer risk. These studies could determine whether there are specific BMI ranges where these effects occur and whether the range is different within different ethnic groups.

5. Conclusions

Combined oestrogen and progestagen MHT was associated with the highest BC risk. This risk was not modified by early or current BMI and age of pregnancy. Exploratory analysis amongst oestrogen only MHT users showed an attenuation of risk with early BMI greater than or equal to the median compared to less than the median and with age of first pregnancy less than 30 years compared to equal or greater than age 30 or nulliparity which require further study. Identifying characteristics which modify a woman's MHT associated BC risk will allow their individual risks and benefits to be assessed and appropriate prescription of MHT to manage troublesome menopausal symptoms.

Supplementary Materials: The following are available online at https://www.mdpi.com/article/10.3390/cancers13112710/s1, Table S1a: MHT status and breast cancer risk model without BMI interactions, Table S1b: Type of MHT and breast cancer risk fully adjusted model, Table S1c: MHT status and breast cancer risk and ER+ breast cancer; Table S2a: MHT status and breast cancer risk fully adjusted model including current BMI interaction term, Table S2b: MHT status and breast cancer risk fully adjusted model including BMI at age 20 interaction term, Table S2c: MHT status and breast cancer risk fully adjusted, including MHT use* current BMI * BMI at age 20 interaction term, Table S3: characteristics of women with known and unknown MHT status; Table S4: MHT status and breast cancer risk fully adjusted with interaction term for age of first pregnancy.

Author Contributions: Conceptualization M.H., A.H., D.G.E., A.R.B., E.F.H.; Formal Analysis E.L.; Writing—Original Draft Preparation E.L., M.H.; Writing—Review & Editing E.L., M.H., A.H., D.G.E., A.R.B., E.F.H. All authors have read and agreed to the published version of the manuscript.

Funding: This research received no external funding.

Institutional Review Board Statement: The study was conducted according to the guidelines of the Declaration of Helsinki, and approved by the Central Manchester Research Ethics Committee (reference 09/H1008/81).

Informed Consent Statement: Informed consent was obtained from all subjects involved in the study.

Data Availability Statement: The dataset used and analysed during the current study is available from the corresponding author on reasonable request.

Acknowledgments: M.H.: D.G.E. and E.F.H. are supported by the NIHR Manchester Biomedical Research Centre (IS-BRC-1215-20007). This work is supported by the National Institute for Health Research (NF-SI-0513-10076 and IS-BRC-1215-20007 to D.G.E.). We thank all PROCAS researchers, clinicians, administrative staff and the individuals who contributed to our study. We thank Mary Pegington for proofreading.

Conflicts of Interest: The authors declare no conflict of interest. The funders had no role in the design of the study; in the collection, analyses, or interpretation of data; in the writing of the manuscript, or in the decision to publish the results.

References

1. Newson, L.R. Best practice for HRT: Unpicking the evidence. *Br. J. Gen. Pract.* **2016**, *66*, 597–598. [CrossRef]
2. Collaborative Group on Hormonal Factors in Breast Cancer Type and timing of menopausal hormone therapy and breast cancer risk: Individual participant meta-analysis of the worldwide epidemiological evidence. *Lancet* **2019**, *394*, 1159–1168. [CrossRef]
3. Marsden, J. British Menopause Society consensus statement: The risks and benefits of HRT before and after a breast cancer diagnosis. *Post Reprod. Health* **2019**, *25*, 33–37. [CrossRef] [PubMed]
4. NICE. *Familial Breast Cancer: Classification, Care and Managing Breast Cancer and Related Risks in People with a Family History of Breast Cancer*; NICE Clinical Guidelines: London, UK, 2013.
5. NICE. *Menopause: Diagnosis and Management*; NICE Clinical Guidelines: London, UK, 2015.
6. World Cancer Research Fund. *Diet, Nutrition, Physical Activity and Breast Cancer*; American Institute for Cancer Research: Washington, DC, USA, 2017.
7. Hidayat, K.; Yang, C.-M.; Shi, B.-M. Body fatness at a young age, body fatness gain and risk of breast cancer: Systematic review and meta-analysis of cohort studies. *Obes. Rev.* **2018**, *19*, 254–268. [CrossRef]
8. Renehan, A.G.; Pegington, M.; Harvie, M.N.; Sperrin, M.; Astley, S.M.; Brentnall, A.R.; Howell, A.; Cuzick, J.; Evans, D.G. Young adulthood body mass index, adult weight gain and breast cancer risk: The PROCAS Study (United Kingdom). *Br. J. Cancer* **2020**, *122*, 1552–1561. [CrossRef] [PubMed]
9. Al-Ajmi, K.; Lophatananon, A.; Ollier, W.; Muir, K.R. Risk of breast cancer in the UK biobank female cohort and its relationship to anthropometric and reproductive factors. *PLoS ONE* **2018**, *13*, e0201097. [CrossRef]
10. Murrow, L.M.; Weber, R.J.; Caruso, J.; McGinnis, C.S.; Borowsky, A.D.; Desai, T.A.; Thomson, M.; Tisty, T.; Gartner, Z.J. Pregnancy and obesity modify the epithelial composition and hormone signaling state of the human breast. *BioRxiv* **2020**. [CrossRef]
11. Evans, D.G.; Astley, S.; Stavrinos, P.; Harkness, E.; Donnelly, L.S.; Dawe, S.; Jackob, I.; Harvie, M.; Cuzick, J.; Brentall, A. Improvement in risk prediction, early detection and prevention of breast cancer in the NHS Breast Screening Programme and family history clinics: A dual cohort study. *Programm. Grants Appl. Res.* **2016**, *4*, 1–210. [CrossRef]
12. Phipps, A.I.; Ichikawa, L.; Bowles, E.J.; Carney, P.A.; Kerlikowske, K.; Miglioretti, D.L.; Buist, D.S. Defining menopausal status in epidemiologic studies: A comparison of multiple approaches and their effects on breast cancer rates. *Maturitas* **2010**, *67*, 60–66. [CrossRef] [PubMed]
13. Bertrand, K.A.; Baer, H.J.; Orav, E.J.; Klifa, C.; Shepherd, J.A.; Van Horn, L.; Snetselaar, L.; Stevens, V.J.; Hylton, N.M.; Dorgan, J.F. Body fatness during childhood and adolescence and breast density in young women: A prospective analysis. *Breast Cancer Res.* **2015**, *17*, 95. [CrossRef]
14. Adams, K.F.; Leitzmann, M.F.; Albanes, D.; Kipnis, V.; Mouw, T.; Hollenbeck, A.; Schatzkin, A. Body Mass and Colorectal Cancer Risk in the NIH-AARP Cohort. *Am. J. Epidemiol.* **2007**, *166*, 36–45. [CrossRef] [PubMed]
15. Hou, N.; Hong, S.; Wang, W.; Olopade, O.I.; Dignam, J.J.; Huo, D. Hormone Replacement Therapy and Breast Cancer: Heterogeneous Risks by Race, Weight, and Breast Density. *J. Natl. Cancer Inst.* **2013**, *105*, 1365–1372. [CrossRef] [PubMed]
16. McCullough, M.L.; Patel, A.V.; Patel, R.; Rodriguez, C.; Feigelson, H.S.; Bandera, E.V.; Gansler, T.; Thun, M.J.; Calle, E.E. Body Mass and Endometrial Cancer Risk by Hormone Replacement Therapy and Cancer Subtype. *Cancer Epidemiol. Biomark. Prev.* **2008**, *17*, 73–79. [CrossRef] [PubMed]
17. Daley, A.; MacArthur, C.; Stokes-Lampard, H.; McManus, R.; Wilson, S.; Mutrie, N. Exercise participation, body mass index, and health-related quality of life in women of menopausal age. *Br. J. Gen. Pract* **2007**, *57*, 130–135. [PubMed]
18. Koo, S.; Ahn, Y.; Lim, J.-Y.; Cho, J.; Park, H.-Y. Obesity associates with vasomotor symptoms in postmenopause but with physical symptoms in perimenopause: A cross-sectional study. *BMC Women's Health* **2017**, *17*, 126. [CrossRef] [PubMed]
19. Wu, O. Postmenopausal hormone replacement therapy and venous thromboembolism. *Gend. Med.* **2005**, *2*, S18–S27. [CrossRef]
20. Green, L.E.; Dinh, T.A.; Smith, R.A. An Estrogen Model: The Relationship between Body Mass Index, Menopausal Status, Estrogen Replacement Therapy, and Breast Cancer Risk. *Comput. Math. Methods Med.* **2012**, *2012*, 1–8. [CrossRef] [PubMed]
21. Canchola, A.J.; Anton-Culver, H.; Bernstein, L.; Clarke, C.A.; Henderson, K.; Ma, H.; Ursin, G.; Horn-Ross, P.L. Body size and the risk of postmenopausal breast cancer subtypes in the California Teachers Study cohort. *Cancer Causes Control* **2012**, *23*, 473–485. [CrossRef]
22. Eliassen, A.H.; Colditz, G.A.; Rosner, B.; Willett, W.C.; Hankinson, S.E. Adult Weight Change and Risk of Postmenopausal Breast Cancer. *JAMA* **2006**, *296*, 193–201. [CrossRef]
23. Neuhouser, M.L.; Aragaki, A.K.; Prentice, R.L.; Manson, J.E.; Chlebowski, R.T.; Carty, C.L.; Ochs-Balcom, H.M.; Thomson, C.A.; Caan, B.; Tinker, L.F.; et al. Overweight, Obesity, and Postmenopausal Invasive Breast Cancer Risk. *JAMA Oncol.* **2015**, *1*, 611–621. [CrossRef]
24. Endogenous Hormones Breast Cancer Collaborative Group. Body Mass Index, Serum Sex Hormones, and Breast Cancer Risk in Postmenopausal Women. *J. Natl. Cancer Inst.* **2003**, *95*, 1218–1226. [CrossRef]
25. Oh, H.; Eliassen, A.H.; Beck, A.H.; Rosner, B.; Schnitt, S.J.; Collins, L.C.; Connolly, J.L.; Montaser-Kouhsari, L.; Willett, W.C.; Tamimi, R.M. Breast cancer risk factors in relation to estrogen receptor, progesterone receptor, insulin-like growth factor-1 receptor, and Ki67 expression in normal breast tissue. *npj Breast Cancer* **2017**, *3*, 39. [CrossRef] [PubMed]
26. Olson, L.K.; Tan, Y.; Zhao, Y.; Aupperlee, M.D.; Haslam, S.Z. Pubertal exposure to high fat diet causes mouse strain-dependent alterations in mammary gland development and estrogen responsiveness. *Int. J. Obes.* **2010**, *34*, 1415–1426. [CrossRef]

27. Xu, J.; Fan, S.; Rosen, E.M. Regulation of the Estrogen-Inducible Gene Expression Profile by the Breast Cancer Susceptibility Gene BRCA1. *Endocrinology* **2005**, *146*, 2031–2047. [CrossRef]
28. Zhao, H.; Wang, J.; Fang, D.; Lee, O.; Chatterton, R.T.; Stearns, V.; Khan, S.A.; Bulun, S.E. Adiposity Results in Metabolic and Inflammation Differences in Premenopausal and Postmenopausal Women Consistent with the Difference in Breast Cancer Risk. *Horm. Cancer* **2018**, *9*, 229–239. [CrossRef]
29. Sørensen, K.; Andersson, A.M.; Skakkebæk, N.E.; Juul, A. Serum Sex Hormone-Binding Globulin Levels in Healthy Children and Girls with Precocious Puberty before and during Gonadotropin-Releasing Hormone Agonist Treatment. *J. Clin. Endocrinol. Metab.* **2007**, *92*, 3189–3196. [CrossRef] [PubMed]
30. Hilakivi-Clarke, L.; Forsén, T.; Eriksson, J.G.; Luoto, R.; Tuomilehto, J.; Osmond, C.; Barker, D.J.P. Tallness and overweight during childhood have opposing effects on breast cancer risk. *Br. J. Cancer* **2001**, *85*, 1680–1684. [CrossRef]
31. Magnusson, C.M.K.; Roddam, A.W. Breast cancer and childhood anthropometry: Emerging hypotheses? *Breast Cancer Res.* **2005**, *7*, 83. [CrossRef] [PubMed]
32. Poole, E.M.; Tworoger, S.; Hankinson, S.E.; Schernhammer, E.S.; Pollak, M.N.; Baer, H.J. Body Size in Early Life and Adult Levels of Insulin-like Growth Factor 1 and Insulin-like Growth Factor Binding Protein 3. *Am. J. Epidemiol.* **2011**, *174*, 642–651. [CrossRef] [PubMed]
33. Surmacz, E.; Bartucci, M. Role of estrogen receptor α in modulating IGF-I receptor signaling and function in breast cancer. *J. Exp. Clin. Cancer Res.* **2004**, *23*, 385–394.
34. Arner, P. Fat Tissue Growth and Development in Humans. Issues in Complementary Feeding. *Nestle Nutr. Inst. Workshop Ser.* **2018**, *89*, 37–45. [PubMed]
35. Sandvei, M.S.; Vatten, L.J.; Bjelland, E.K.; Eskild, A.; Hofvind, S.; Ursin, G.; Opdahl, S. Menopausal hormone therapy and breast cancer risk: Effect modification by body mass through life. *Eur. J. Epidemiol.* **2018**, *34*, 267–278. [CrossRef] [PubMed]
36. Dall, G.V.; Britt, K.L. Estrogen Effects on the Mammary Gland in Early and Late Life and Breast Cancer Risk. *Front. Oncol.* **2017**, *7*, 110. [CrossRef] [PubMed]
37. Opdahl, S.; Alsaker, M.D.K.; Janszky, I.; Romundstad, P.R.; Vatten, L.J. Joint effects of nulliparity and other breast cancer risk factors. *Br. J. Cancer* **2011**, *105*, 731–736. [CrossRef]
38. Merrill, R.M.; Richardson, J.S. Validity of self-reported height, weight, and body mass index: Findings from the national health and nutrition examination survey, 2001–2006. *Prev. Chronic. Dis.* **2009**, *6*, 4. Available online: http://www.cdc.gov/pcd/issues/2009/oct/08_0229.htm (accessed on 20 April 2021).
39. Rimm, E.B.; Stampfer, M.J.; Colditz, G.A.; Chute, C.G.; Litin, L.B.; Willett, W.C. Validity of Self-Reported Waist and Hip Circumferences in Men and Women. *Epidemiology* **1990**, *1*, 466–473. [CrossRef]
40. Evans, D.G.; Brentnall, A.R.; Harvie, M.; Astley, S.; Harkness, E.F.; Stavrinos, P.; Donnelly, L.; Sampson, S.; Idries, F.; Watterson, D.; et al. Breast cancer risk in a screening cohort of Asian and white British/Irish women from Manchester UK. *BMC Public Health* **2018**, *18*, 178. [CrossRef] [PubMed]
41. Kroenke, C.H.; Caan, B.; Stefanick, M.L.; Anderson, G.; Brzyski, R.; Johnson, K.C.; LeBlanc, E.; Lee, C.; La Croix, A.Z.; Park, H.L.; et al. Effects of a dietary intervention and weight change on vasomotor symptoms in the Women's Health Initiative. *Menopause* **2012**, *19*, 980–988. [CrossRef] [PubMed]

Article

The Relationship between Body Mass Index and Mammographic Density during a Premenopausal Weight Loss Intervention Study

Emma C. Atakpa [1], Adam R. Brentnall [1], Susan Astley [2,3,4], Jack Cuzick [1], D. Gareth Evans [2,3,5,6,7], Ruth M. L. Warren [8,9], Anthony Howell [2,3,10] and Michelle Harvie [2,*]

[1] Centre for Cancer Prevention, Wolfson Institute of Preventive Medicine, Barts and The London School of Medicine and Dentistry, Queen Mary University of London, London EC1M 6BQ, UK; e.c.atakpa@qmul.ac.uk (E.C.A.); a.brentnall@qmul.ac.uk (A.R.B.); j.cuzick@qmul.ac.uk (J.C.)
[2] Nightingale Breast Screening Centre & Prevent Breast Cancer Unit, Wythenshawe Hospital, Manchester University NHS Foundation Trust, Manchester M23 9LT, UK; Sue.astley@manchester.ac.uk (S.A.); Gareth.Evans@mft.nhs.uk (D.G.E.); anthony.howell@manchester.ac.uk (A.H.)
[3] Manchester Breast Centre, The Christie Hospital, Manchester M23 9LT, UK
[4] Division of Informatics, Imaging & Data Sciences, School of Health Sciences, Faculty of Biology, Medicine and Health, University of Manchester, Manchester M13 9PT, UK
[5] Manchester Centre for Genomic Medicine, Manchester University Hospitals NHS Foundation Trust, Manchester M23 9LT, UK
[6] Manchester Centre for Genomic Medicine, NW Genomic Laboratory Hub, Manchester University Hospitals NHS Foundation Trust, Manchester M13 9WL, UK
[7] Manchester Academic Health Science Centre, Division of Evolution and Genomic Sciences, Faculty of Biology, School of Biological Sciences, Medicine and Health, University of Manchester, Manchester M23 9LT, UK
[8] Cambridge Breast Unit, Addenbrooke's Hospital, Cambridge CB2 0QQ, UK; rmlw2@cam.ac.uk
[9] Girton College, University of Cambridge, Cambridge CB3 0JG, UK
[10] Manchester Academic Health Science Centre, Division of Cancer Sciences, Medicine and Health, University of Manchester, Manchester M23 9LT, UK
* Correspondence: michelle.harvie@manchester.ac.uk

Simple Summary: This study assessed the association between short-term weight change and mammographic density in premenopausal women losing weight through diet and exercise to reduce their risk of postmenopausal breast cancer. We aimed to understand whether a reduction in body mass index affects various components of the breast, which could indicate a potential pathway for the reduction in postmenopausal breast cancer risk seen with premenopausal weight loss. Understanding this pathway is useful for monitoring the effectiveness of prevention strategies based on lifestyle advice. We found that a short-term reduction in premenopausal body mass index through diet and exercise is associated with a reduction in breast fat, but it is unlikely to have a significant effect on the quantity of breast glandular tissue. Breast cancer risk determined by changes in breast density might not capture potential weight loss-induced breast cancer risk reduction, instead falsely ascribing an increased risk due to increased percent density.

Abstract: We evaluated the association between short-term change in body mass index (BMI) and breast density during a 1 year weight-loss intervention (Manchester, UK). We included 65 premenopausal women (35–45 years, ≥7 kg adult weight gain, family history of breast cancer). BMI and breast density (semi-automated area-based, automated volume-based) were measured at baseline, 1 year, and 2 years after study entry (1 year post intervention). Cross-sectional (between-women) and short-term change (within-women) associations between BMI and breast density were measured using repeated-measures correlation coefficients and multivariable linear mixed models. BMI was positively correlated with dense volume between-women ($r = 0.41$, 95%CI: 0.17, 0.61), but less so within-women ($r = 0.08$, 95%CI: −0.16, 0.28). There was little association with dense area (between-women $r = -0.12$, 95%CI: −0.38, 0.16; within-women $r = 0.01$, 95%CI: −0.24, 0.25). BMI and breast fat were positively correlated (volume: between $r = 0.77$, 95%CI: 0.69, 0.84, within $r = 0.58$, 95%CI: 0.36, 0.75; area: between $r = 0.74$, 95%CI: 0.63, 0.82, within $r = 0.45$, 95%CI: 0.23, 0.63). Multivariable models reported similar associations. Exploratory analysis suggested associations between BMI gain from 20 years and density measures (standard deviation change per +5 kg/m² BMI: dense area: +0.61 (95%CI: 0.12, 1.09); fat volume: −0.31 (95%CI: −0.62, 0.00)). Short-term BMI change is likely to be positively associated with breast fat, but we found little association with dense tissue, although power was limited by small sample size.

Keywords: mammographic density; body mass index; weight loss; breast cancer risk; breast cancer prevention; premenopausal

1. Introduction

Mammographic density (herein referred to as 'density') is an established risk factor for breast cancer. Women in the highest density category are at a 4- to 6-fold increased risk of breast cancer relative to those with little or no dense tissue [1]. When assessed by mammography, the breast is broadly characterised by two components: fibroglandular dense tissue and fatty non-dense tissue. Percent breast density is measured as the relative proportion of dense tissue in the breast, either in terms of area or volume depending on the measurement method. Visual assessment measures percent density with respect to the total breast area (TA) whilst automated and semi-automated methods can also measure the extent of dense and fatty tissue separately. Both absolute dense area (DA) and percentage dense area (PDA) are positively associated with risk of premenopausal (and postmenopausal) breast cancer [2–4], and absolute dense volume (DV) and percentage dense volume (PDV) have also shown positive associations [5,6]. Associations of breast fat area (FA) and volume (FV) with breast cancer risk are unclear, although there is some suggestion of an inverse relationship with premenopausal breast cancer risk [4,6].

In postmenopausal women, higher attained body mass index (BMI) is associated with a higher risk of breast cancer [7–9], with an estimated 40% increase in risk for every 10 kg/m² of BMI in never users of hormone replacement therapy [9]. This increase in risk is partly explained by increased aromatisation of androgens to oestrogen in peripheral adipose tissue, which promotes cell proliferation [10,11], carcinogenesis [10,11], and insulin resistance [12]. Whilst BMI is a widely accepted risk factor for breast cancer in postmenopausal women, there may be an inverse relationship in premenopausal women [13].

Weight gain across the premenopausal years has also been linked to an increased risk of postmenopausal breast cancer. Every 5 kg of adult weight gain is associated with an approximate 10% increase in risk amongst never or low-hormone replacement therapy users [14,15]. However, a number of studies (as summarised by Hardefeldt et al. [16]) suggest that these effects are reversible with efficient weight loss [16]. In particular, weight loss in the premenopausal years has been shown to reduce postmenopausal breast cancer risk [17,18]. Risk reductions of approximately 40% have also been seen with large weight losses as a result of bariatric surgery in populations of pre- and postmenopausal women [19].

The effects of short-term weight change on breast density are less well understood, particularly those as a result of dietary weight loss. Mammographic density is a dynamic phenotype and has the potential to respond to short-term weight changes, making density reduction a possible biomarker for reduction in risk as a result of weight loss. This study aims to explore the effect of short-term dietary weight change on density using both area-based and volumetric methods in a cohort of premenopausal women to ascertain whether the relationship between weight loss and reduced postmenopausal breast cancer risk could, in part, be mediated by reductions in mammographic tissue.

2. Materials and Methods

2.1. Study Design and Participants

The Lifestyle Study is a prospective non-randomised 1 year diet and exercise weight loss intervention study amongst 79 high-risk premenopausal women attending annual screening within the Breast Cancer Family History clinic at the Prevent Breast Cancer research unit at the Manchester University Hospital Foundation NHS Trust [20–23]. Attendees of our regional Family History Clinic, aged 35–45 years, received a mailed invitation to enter either a 12-month intensive diet and exercise weight loss programme or a usual care group receiving standard written advice only, depending on their proximity to the hospital. Eligibility required women to be premenopausal with regular menstrual cycles, non-smokers, have a self-reported adult weight gain ≥ 7 kg, and a sedentary lifestyle (<40 min moderate physical activity per week). All women had a family history of breast cancer (with lifetime risk 17–40% as assessed by the Tyrer–Cuzick model [24,25]), but were excluded if they had a known *BRCA1/2* mutation or a previous history of cancer. Women were also excluded if they were already successfully dieting or losing weight, were pregnant or planning to become pregnant over the next year, had used hormonal oral contraceptives in the last six months, or had psychiatric or physical co-morbidities that could affect their ability to take part in a diet and physical activity weight loss programme.

In the intervention group (n = 40), women followed a 12-month intensive supervised weight loss programme involving a 25% energy-restricted Mediterranean type diet and an individualised physical activity program (150 min moderate intensity physical activity and 40 min of resistance exercise per week). The usual care group (n = 39) received standard written advice about diet and physical activity but no additional support for weight loss. Women provided baseline information on alcohol intake (from a 4-day food diary) and physical activity (7-day recall from an interview questionnaire) at their baseline clinic visit. All subjects gave their informed consent for inclusion before they participated in the study. The study was conducted in accordance with the Declaration of Helsinki, and the protocol was approved by the South Manchester Ethics Committee (Reference no. 01/426).

The objective of this analysis was to assess the relationship between BMI and breast density in the entire cohort of women. All participants had changing BMI measures irrespective of the type of weight loss advice they received, hence the intervention and usual care groups were combined and treated as one cohort. Furthermore, to limit the effect of women contributing observations to an area-based measure or volumetric measure only, the cohort was restricted to those with both an area and volumetric density measurement at any one or more time points (n = 65, 82% of the cohort).

2.2. Mammographic Density

Mammographic films were digitised using a Kodak LS85 digitiser at a pixel size of 50 µm and with 12-bits (4096 grey levels) pixel depth. The images were then anonymised and randomised to ensure the radiologists remained unaware of the time point of each mammogram. Mammograms were analysed using three different methods: (1) a semi-automated area-based measure based on computer-assisted thresholding by a single expert user (Cumulus, Sunnybrook health sciences centre, Toronto, Canada, [26]); (2) an automated volumetric Stepwedge method developed at Manchester University [27]; and (3) a visual assessment score of percentage density read to the nearest 5% by two experienced readers and expressed as an average of the two scores to calculate PDA. Cumulus was used to calculate TA, DA, FA, and PDA, and the Manchester Stepwedge method calculated total volume (TV), DV, FV, and PDV. Density assessments were made at 3 time points: baseline, 1 year follow-up (at the end of the intervention) and 1 year after the end of the intervention. Baseline mammograms were taken at the point of entry to the study; for those women with a mammogram performed within one year of entry, their most recent mammogram within the last 12 months was used. Each woman had four mammographic views taken at each time point: Left Cranial-Caudal, Right Cranial-Caudal, Left Mediolateral-Oblique, and Right Mediolateral-Oblique, and a final mammographic score at each time point was calculated using an average of the four views. The main analysis refers to Cumulus measured area-based density and Stepwedge measured volumetric density only to assess the effects of BMI on dense and non-dense tissue separately. Visually-assessed density had similar results to Cumulus-assessed PDA, so was included as a secondary density measure only. Results for TA and TV are also reported as secondary density measures in the Supplementary Materials.

2.3. Body Weight and Body Composition

Weight, BMI, and a variety of different measures of body composition were assessed at baseline, 1 year follow-up (at the end of the intervention), and 1 year after the end of the intervention. Weight (kg) and height (m) were determined using a calibrated beam balance and stadiometer and used to calculate BMI (kg/m^2). Other body composition assessments were also made such as waist circumference; total body fat, fat free mass and % body fat (assessed using a DXA whole body scanner (Hologic Inc., Bedford, MA, USA) and bioelectrical impedance (Tanita TBF-300A, Tanita Europe B.V., Hoogoorddreef 56E, 1101 BE Amsterdam, The Netherlands)); and intra-abdominal and abdominal subcutaneous area (assessed using a magnetic resonance imaging (MRI) scan with a single transverse scan taken at the level of the intervertebral disc between the L2 and L3 vertebrae). Weight, BMI, waist circumference, and total body fat, fat free mass, and % body fat (impedance) were recorded at all three time points. Intra-abdominal area, abdominal subcutaneous area, and total body fat, fat free mass, and % body fat (DXA) were only measured at baseline and at 1 year. Weight at age 20 years was self-reported via questionnaire, and BMI at age 20 years was calculated using weight at age 20 years and height at study entry. Long-term adult BMI gain was calculated as the difference between baseline BMI and BMI at age 20 years. We discuss BMI as the measure of body weight throughout the main analysis because BMI is a commonly used adjustment for density and it is a well-established risk factor for breast cancer. Other body composition measures gave similar correlations with density to those of BMI and were highly correlated with BMI. Therefore, other body composition measures are included as secondary analyses in the Supplementary Materials. Weight gain during the intervention was defined as $\geq+3\%$ of baseline weight, weight loss was defined as $\leq-3\%$ of baseline weight, and a weight change $>-3\%$ to $<+3\%$ of the baseline weight was defined as a stable weight [28].

2.4. Statistical Analysis

Data were visualised using custom-made 'tadpole plots', where each tadpole represents a woman, the head plots the woman's BMI and density at her last time point, and the points on the tail plot her BMI and density at earlier time points. Correlation (r) between BMI and mammographic density was assessed on a cross-sectional basis (between women), and within women as their short-term BMI changed, using repeated measures methods that use all of the measurements at the same time [29,30]. Briefly, between women correlation was a weighted Pearson correlation coefficient [30], and within women correlation was based on the decomposition of sums of squares from an analysis of variance [29]. The 95% confidence intervals were estimated using an empirical bootstrap (10,000 resamples). The simultaneous association of between and within women correlations was tested using a linear mixed model adjusted for age [31] (Appendix A). To help with comparisons across different measures of breast density, the breast density values were first standardised (Appendix B). To make density measures more symmetric and approximately normally-distributed, they were transformed: a square root transformation for area measures and a cube root transformation for volumetric measures. An exploratory analysis was undertaken to assess the effect of adding BMI gain since 20 years of age to the model. An additional exploratory analysis tested whether there was an association between breast density and DXA bone density. A sensitivity analysis assessed repeated measures correlation coefficients for BMI and density stratified by intervention group.

Analysis used the statistical software R [32]. All tests were two-sided and considered significant at the 5% level.

3. Results

Baseline characteristics of the cohort are shown in Table 1. Median age was 41 years (interquartile range (IQR), 38–43 years), and the majority of women were Caucasian ($n = 60$, 92%) and parous ($n = 55$, 85%). At baseline, 27 women (42%) were classified as overweight (BMI ≥ 25 kg/m^2 and <30 kg/m^2), 20 (31%) were obese (BMI ≥ 30 kg/m^2), and 18 (28%) were in the normal BMI range (BMI ≥ 18.5 kg/m^2 and <25 kg/m^2). By the end of the 2 year study period (1 year post intervention), 22 women (34%) had lost weight, 16 (25%) had gained weight, and 26 (41%) maintained their original weight. Overall, women in the intervention group lost more weight than the usual care group (mean percentage of baseline weight at 1 year = −4.4% and 0.1%, respectively; mean percentage of baseline weight at 2 years = −2.9% and 2.0%, respectively).

Median PDA, DA, and FA of each woman's average density measure over the intervention were 37.1% (IQR, 2.5%–71.3%), 59.9 cm^2 (IQR, 5.8–158.4 cm^2) and 107.3 cm^2 (IQR, 23.6–405.1 cm^2), respectively. For Stepwedge measures, PDV, DV, and FV were 22.7% (IQR, 6.7%–69.4%), 191.5 cm^3 (IQR, 56.7–710.4 cm^3), and 573.0 cm^3 (IQR, 72.8–1992.1 cm^3), respectively. A flow chart detailing the availability of mammographic density measures across the intervention is shown in Figure S1 (all women had BMI available at all time-points except for one woman with missing BMI at 2 years—this data point was excluded from analyses involving BMI).

Table 2 shows the repeated measures correlations. DV was positively correlated with BMI between women ($r = 0.41$, 95%CI 0.17 to 0.61) but less so within women ($r = 0.08$, 95%CI −0.16 to 0.28). There was little association between DA and BMI (between women $r = −0.12$, 95%CI −0.38 to 0.16; within women $r = 0.01$, 95%CI −0.24 to 0.25). PDV was inversely associated with BMI between and within women (between $r = −0.48$, 95%CI −0.64 to −0.33; within $r = −0.36$, 95%CI −0.54 to −0.12), and PDA was inversely associated with BMI between women ($r = −0.58$, 95%CI −0.72 to −0.42), but less so within women ($r = −0.22$, 95%CI −0.44 to 0.01). FV and FA were positively correlated with BMI between and within women (volume: between $r = 0.77$, 95%CI 0.69 to 0.84, within $r = 0.58$, 95%CI 0.36 to 0.75; area: between $r = 0.74$, 95%CI 0.63 to 0.82, within $r = 0.45$, 95%CI 0.23 to 0.63). The magnitude of correlations was stronger between women than within women. These associations were also seen in Figure 1 when data were visually assessed using tadpole plots (trends in the tadpole heads represented the between women correlations and trends in the tadpole tails represented within women correlations).

Results for repeated measures correlation coefficients were similar when evaluated in a sensitivity analysis stratifying the cohort by intervention group. Within women associations for BMI and FA or FV were slightly stronger for women following the supervised weight loss programme compared with the usual care group, but there was little association (within women) for BMI and DA or DV in both intervention groups (Table S6).

Other body fat composition measures were highly correlated with BMI (Table S3), and the associations between breast density and other body fat compositions were similar to those with BMI (Tables S1 and S2). The correlations between various mammographic density measures are also reported in the Supplementary Materials (Table S4).

Table 1. Participant characteristics at study entry.

Characteristic	All	Intervention	Usual Care
Total	65	33	32
Age * (years)	41 (38–43)	41 (39–43)	40 (38–42)
Baseline BMI * (kg/m^2)	27.1 (24.7–33.4)	27.1 (25.1–31.9)	27.0 (24.4–34.0)
Baseline BMI categories [#] (kg/m^2)			
Normal ($\geq$18.5 to <25)	18 (28%)	7 (21%)	11 (34%)
Overweight ($\geq$25 to <30)	27 (42%)	16 (48%)	11 (34%)
Obese ($\geq$30)	20 (31%)	10 (30%)	10 (31%)
BMI gain since 20 years * (kg/m^2)	5.8 (4.7–9.4)	6.3 (4.7–10.0)	5.7 (4.6–8.9)
Height * (m)	1.64 (1.60–1.68)	1.63 (1.60–1.68)	1.65 (1.59–1.68)
Age at menarche * (years)	12 (12–13)	12 (12–13)	12 (12–13)
Number of live births [#]			
Nulliparous	10 (15%)	6 (18%)	4 (13%)
1–2	41 (63%)	20 (61%)	21 (66%)
3–4	12 (18%)	6 (18%)	6 (19%)
$\geq$5	2 (3%)	1 (3%)	1 (3%)
Age first live birth * (years)	27 (22–29)	27 (24–31)	26 (22–29)
Ethnicity [#] (% Caucasian)	60 (92%)	29 (88%)	31 (97%)
Previous smoker [#]			
Never	54 (83%)	29 (88%)	25 (78%)
Ever	11 (17%)	4 (12%)	7 (22%)
Previous oral contraception use [#]			
Never	5 (8%)	3 (9%)	2 (6%)
Ever	58 (89%)	29 (88%)	29 (91%)
Unknown	2 (3%)	1 (3%)	1 (3%)
Breastfed [#]			
Never	22 (34%)	12 (36%)	10 (31%)
Ever	41 (63%)	21 (64%)	20 (63%)
Unknown	2 (3%)	0 (0%)	2 (6%)
10-year Tyrer–Cuzick risk * (%)	4 (3–5)	5 (4–6)	3 (3–4)
Alcohol intake [a],* (units/week)	11 (3–24)	11 (3–22)	10 (1.5–26)
Physical activity [b],* ((kJ/kg)/week)	974 (945–999)	968 (941–999)	978 (953–1007)
Weight change from baseline to 1 year, categories [#]			
Loss	26 (40%)	20 (61%)	6 (19%)
Stable	27 (42%)	9 (27%)	18 (56%)
Gain	12 (18%)	4 (12%)	8 (25%)
Weight change from baseline to 1 year **	−2.2 (5.4)	−4.4 (5.0)	0.1 (4.8)
Weight change from baseline to 2 years, categories [#]			
Loss	22 (34%)	16 (48%)	6 (19%)
Stable	26 (41%)	13 (39%)	13 (42%)
Gain	16 (25%)	4 (12%)	12 (39%)
Weight change from baseline to 2 years **	−0.5 (7.1)	−2.9 (6.2)	2.0 (7.1)

BMI: Body mass index. [#] N (%); * Median (interquartile range); ** Mean (standard deviation) % of baseline weight (kg). [a] Alcohol from a 4-day food diary; [b] Physical activity from 7-day recall. Weight loss defined as $\leq$−3% of baseline weight (kg); Stable weight defined as >−3% to <+3% of baseline weight (kg); Weight gain defined as $\geq$+3% of baseline weight (kg).

Table 2. Repeated measures between women and within women correlations for mammographic density and body mass index.

Field	VAS (95%CI) (sqrt%)	PDA (95%CI) (sqrt%)	PDV (95%CI) (cbrt%)	FA (95%CI) (sqrt)	FV (95%CI) (cbrt)	DA (95%CI) (sqrt)	DV (95%CI) (cbrt)
Cross-sectional BMI (between women)	−0.62 (−0.74 to −0.47)	−0.58 (−0.72 to −0.42)	−0.48 (−0.64 to −0.33)	0.74 (0.63 to 0.82)	0.77 (0.69 to 0.84)	−0.12 (−0.38 to 0.16)	0.41 (0.17 to 0.61)
Short-term BMI change (within women)	−0.27 (−0.48 to −0.05)	−0.22 (−0.44 to 0.01)	−0.36 (−0.54 to −0.12)	0.45 (0.23 to 0.63)	0.58 (0.36 to 0.75)	0.01 (−0.24 to 0.25)	0.08 (−0.16 to 0.28)

VAS: Visual assessment score; PDA: percent dense area; PDV: percent dense volume; FA: fat area; FV: fat volume; DA: dense area; DV: dense volume; sqrt: square root transformed; cbrt: cube root transformed; BMI: body mass index; 95%CI: 95% confidence interval. Area-based measures from Cumulus; volumetric measures from Manchester Stepwedge. Within women correlations represent trends over the entire 2 year period.

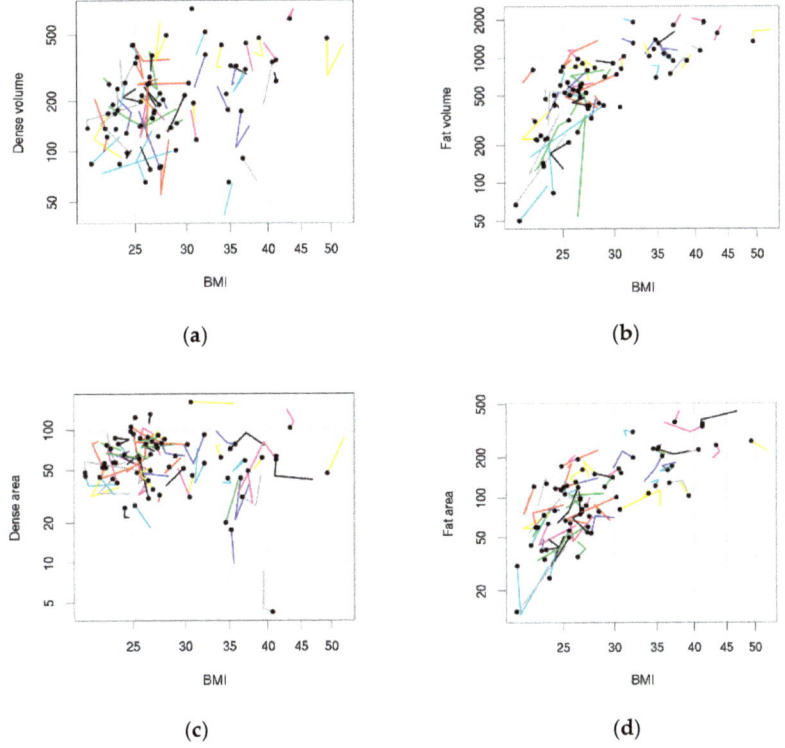

Figure 1. Tadpole plots showing body mass index (BMI) and density measures across the 2 year follow-up. Each tadpole represents a woman: the tadpole head shows BMI and density (if density is available) at her last follow-up and the points on the tail show BMI and density (if density is available) at her earlier follow-ups. (**a**) Dense volume; (**b**) Fat volume; (**c**) Dense area; (**d**) Fat area.

The between and within women associations for density and BMI measures were similar when estimated jointly in an age-adjusted linear mixed model (Table 3). In a sensitivity analysis, the same model was fit using weight instead of BMI, but it had a worse model fit for almost all density measures (Table S5).

Table 3. Multivariable linear mixed model fit results for mammographic density on body mass index (between and within women), adjusted for age (A1).

Density Outcome	Intercept (95%CI)	Age (95%CI) (Per 10 Years)	BMI (95%CI) [between] (Per 5 kg/m^2)	BMI (95%CI) [within] (Per 5 kg/m^2)
VAS (sqrt%)	3.75 (1.88 to 5.61)	−0.19 (−0.56 to 0.19)	−0.51 (−0.68 to −0.35)	−0.27 (−0.44 to −0.10)
PDA (sqrt%)	2.87 (0.57 to 5.17)	−0.05 (−0.53 to 0.43)	−0.46 (−0.63 to −0.30)	−0.32 (−0.59 to −0.05)
PDV (cbrt%)	1.73 (−1.07 to 4.53)	0.12 (−0.48 to 0.71)	−0.39 (−0.57 to −0.21)	−0.85 (−1.32 to −0.39)
FA (sqrt)	−3.63 (−5.25 to −2.02)	0.04 (−0.28 to 0.36)	0.60 (0.46 to 0.74)	0.43 (0.27 to 0.58)
FV (cbrt)	−3.46 (−5.27 to −1.64)	−0.04 (−0.42 to 0.34)	0.63 (0.50 to 0.76)	0.79 (0.56 to 1.03)
DA (sqrt)	0.57 (−2.13 to 3.27)	−0.03 (−0.59 to 0.53)	−0.08 (−0.28 to 0.11)	0.01 (−0.30 to 0.33)
DV (cbrt)	−2.39 (−5.11 to 0.33)	0.09 (−0.48 to 0.66)	0.35 (0.16 to 0.53)	0.16 (−0.24 to 0.55)

VAS: Visual assessment score; PDA: percent dense area; PDV: percent dense volume; FA: fat area; FV: fat volume; DA: dense area; DV: dense volume; sqrt: square root transformed; cbrt: cube root transformed; BMI: body mass index; 95%CI: 95% confidence interval. Area-based measures from Cumulus; volumetric measures from Manchester Stepwedge. Between women BMI calculated as the mean BMI for each woman; within women BMI calculated as the difference between each woman's BMI and her mean BMI. Density measures are standardised (see Appendix B). One woman with missing BMI at age 20 years excluded. Within women effects represent trends over the entire 2 year period.

When a term for BMI gain since age 20 years was added to the linear mixed model, the model fit improved for PDA, PDV, FV, and DA (all ΔLR-χ^2 $p < 0.05$) (Table 4). After including BMI gain since age 20 years, between women associations for BMI became more strongly inversely associated with percent density (approximately −0.5 to −0.8), more strongly positively associated with breast fat (approximately 0.6 to 0.8), more strongly inversely associated with DA (−0.1 to −0.5), and less strongly positively associated with DV (0.4 to 0.2). Within women effects of BMI on density were almost unchanged when including BMI gain since age 20 years. BMI gain from age 20 years (adjusted for attained BMI) was positively associated with DA, PDA, and PDV (5 kg/m^2 increase in BMI gain since age 20 years was associated with 0.61 (95%CI 0.12 to 1.09), 0.61 (95%CI 0.21 to 1.02), and 0.47 (95%CI 0.05 to 0.88) standard deviation increase in breast density (β), respectively), and inversely associated with FV ($\beta = -0.31$, 95%CI −0.62 to 0.00), but less association was seen with DV ($\beta = 0.15$, 95%CI −0.29 to 0.59) and FA ($\beta = -0.32$, 95%CI −0.67 to 0.03).

Finally, in tests of association between breast and bone density, there was some indication of a positive between women correlation for bone density and FV ($r = 0.26$, 95%CI, 0.00 to 0.50), DV ($r = 0.33$, 95%CI, 0.09 to 0.54), and TV ($r = 0.31$, 95%CI, 0.06 to 0.54) (Table S1), but we found little correlation within women (Table S2).

Table 4. Multivariable linear mixed model fit results for mammographic density on body mass index (between and within women) and body mass index gain since 20 years of age, adjusted for age (A2).

Density Outcome	Intercept (95%CI)	Age (95%CI) (Per 10 Years)	BMI (95%CI) (between) (Per 5kg/m^2)	BMI (95%CI) (within) (Per 5kg/m^2)	BMI Gain Since 20 Years of Age (95%CI) (Per 5kg/m^2)	ΔLR-χ^2 p-Value (A1 vs. A2)
VAS (sqrt%)	5.47 (3.34 to 7.60)	−0.25 (−0.61 to 0.12)	−0.92 (−1.23 to −0.62)	−0.27 (−0.45 to −0.10)	0.59 (0.20 to 0.97)	0.0031
PDA (sqrt%)	4.90 (2.34 to 7.46)	−0.16 (−0.63 to 0.31)	−0.89 (−1.22 to −0.57)	−0.32 (−0.59 to −0.06)	0.61 (0.21 to 1.02)	0.0033
PDV (cbrt%)	3.35 (0.30 to 6.40)	0.01 (−0.57 to 0.60)	−0.71 (−1.05 to −0.38)	−0.85 (−1.32 to −0.39)	0.47 (0.05 to 0.88)	0.0267
FA (sqrt)	−4.59 (−6.49 to −2.69)	0.08 (−0.24 to 0.40)	0.82 (0.54 to 1.10)	0.43 (0.28 to 0.59)	−0.32 (−0.67 to 0.03)	0.0704
FV (cbrt)	−4.42 (−6.44 to −2.40)	0.01 (−0.37 to 0.38)	0.84 (0.59 to 1.09)	0.79 (0.56 to 1.03)	−0.31 (−0.62 to 0.00)	0.0476
DA (sqrt)	2.58 (−0.48 to 5.64)	−0.14 (−0.70 to 0.41)	−0.51 (−0.90 to −0.12)	0.01 (−0.31 to 0.32)	0.61 (0.12 to 1.09)	0.0145
DV (cbrt)	−1.90 (−4.96 to 1.15)	0.06 (−0.51 to 0.64)	0.24 (−0.12 to 0.60)	0.16 (−0.24 to 0.55)	0.15 (−0.29 to 0.59)	0.4967

VAS: Visual assessment score; PDA: percent dense area; PDV: percent dense volume; FA: fat area; FV: fat volume; DA: dense area; DV: dense volume; sqrt: square root transformed; cbrt: cube root transformed; BMI: body mass index; 95%CI: 95% confidence interval. Area-based measures from Cumulus; volumetric measures from Manchester Stepwedge. Between women BMI calculated as the mean BMI for each woman; within women BMI calculated as the difference between each woman's BMI and her mean BMI; BMI gain from age 20 years calculated as the difference between each woman's BMI at baseline and her BMI at age 20 years. Density measures are standardised (see Appendix B). One woman with missing BMI at age 20 years excluded. ΔLR-χ^2 represents the difference in likelihood ratio for A1 versus A2. Within women effects represent trends over the entire 2 year period. All variables adjusted for each other in the multivariable model, therefore BMI gain since 20 years of age is adjusted for current BMI through the variable for between women BMI.

4. Discussion

The data in this study provide some support for the two main findings. First, it is possible that the higher a premenopausal woman's BMI, the higher her breast fat and dense tissue (in particular, dense volume), and the lower her percent density. Second, the data suggested that as a premenopausal woman loses weight, her breast fat reduces, dense tissue remains relatively unchanged, and percent dense tissue increases. Effective weight loss during premenopausal years has been associated with a reduced risk of postmenopausal breast cancer [16–18], but our study data suggest that risk reduction is unlikely to be mediated by a short-term reduction in dense breast tissue. This is likely to mean that incorporation of change in percent breast density into risk algorithms will not capture potential weight loss-induced breast cancer risk reduction and may falsely ascribe an increased risk due to increased percent density. Therefore, risk prediction models need to consider how best to incorporate changes in weight and mammographic density when predicting breast cancer risk.

The between women associations of attained premenopausal BMI and breast density observed in this study were consistent with previous studies. High BMI is associated with high dense volume [33–35], but the correlation between BMI and dense area is less strong, and often close to zero [36–39]. These differences are likely to be a result of volumetric measures representing breast tissue more accurately than area-based methods by accounting for breast thickness and overlapping tissue. Additionally, since the breast is a deposit for adipose tissue, high attained BMI is strongly associated with high levels of breast fat area [36–39] and breast fat volume [33,34], which in turn leads to an inverse association between BMI and both percent dense area [36–41] and percent dense volume [33–35,42,43].

There have been very few studies to assess the effect of dietary weight loss on breast density in premenopausal women. Boyd et al. reported reductions in total and dense area alongside modest weight change within an intervention trial of women on a 2-year low-fat, high-carbohydrate diet [44]. In particular, a 5.4% decrease in dense area was seen in premenopausal women in the low-fat diet group with a $0.1 kg/m^2$ BMI reduction ($n = 249$) compared with a 2.5% decrease in the control group with a $0.3 kg/m^2$ BMI gain ($n = 264$). These reductions may be associated with the large reductions in dietary fat (55 to 35 g/day) and saturated fat (19 to 12 g/day) rather than weight loss in this study. This was considerably higher than those advised and achieved in the current reported study (total fat reduced from 77 to 60 g/day and saturated fat reduced from 28 to 21 g/day). Other trials have also assessed the effect of lifestyle interventions for weight loss on breast density, although in postmenopausal women only. In the ALPHA trial, postmenopausal women on a 1-year aerobic exercise intervention lost on average 39 cm^3 more breast fat than the controls, but there was little difference in the change in dense tissue between the two groups [45]. Furthermore, the DAMA trial reported a reduction in volumetric percent density of approximately 14% for postmenopausal women following a 2-year diet or exercise intervention when compared with the controls [46]. Large weight loss with bariatric surgery is also associated with large reductions in breast fat alongside relatively smaller reductions in dense tissue, and an increase in percent density [47–49].

As an exploratory analysis, we also found an association between increased BMI gain since 20 years of age and higher dense tissue and percent density. It is possible that this is a pathway for the increased risk of postmenopausal breast cancer seen with adult weight gain [7,15,50–52]. However, this association is likely to reflect the inverse association seen in previous studies between adolescent body adiposity and dense tissue in later life [38,40,53–55], since, given the adjustment for current BMI, women with greater gain in BMI will have had lower BMI at 20 years of age. This interesting observation requires further investigation in larger datasets of women. Additionally, exploratory analysis of bone density found little association with breast density, which is in agreement with previous studies [56].

Strengths of this study include the various measures of breast density including Cumulus and the Stepwedge method, which allowed for the assessment of dense and fatty tissue separately as well as various measures of body weight to assess adiposity. The study also assessed breast density as an area-based measure and volumetrically; both of which have similar abilities for breast cancer risk prediction [57]. Additionally, all women were encouraged to lose weight, which produced data with large within women variation in BMI, in turn increasing the potential to see an effect of changing BMI on mammographic density. Furthermore, the Lifestyle Study provided a data source to assess premenopausal weight loss and density associations; something that is not possible in studies involving routine screening data. This also provided a greater ability to capture the effects of weight loss on density because this cohort of premenopausal women were likely to have had higher dense tissue at baseline (with greater ability to decrease) than screening populations involving postmenopausal women [58]. Finally, the use of repeated measures over a 2-year period allowed us to assess the association between BMI and breast density longitudinally, whilst making use of all available data simultaneously.

Limitations of the study include the small sample size, which limits statistical power. This is particularly relevant for volumetric measures, which had a moderate amount of missing data at the baseline. In addition, the study design was not powered for the analysis of mammographic density, which was a secondary analysis (the study was powered for salivary oestradiol). This was a relatively small study, and ideally, a larger study with sufficient power would be run to verify our evidence. Another limitation is the analysis of BMI gain since 20 years of age relies on self-reported information on weight at age 20 years. This may be less accurate than the measured values. However, validation studies show that self-reported BMI is highly correlated with independently measured BMI, and the mean difference between self-reported and measured weight is minimal [59,60]. Finally, breast thickness is likely to have changed whilst women lost weight during the intervention. Volumetric measures are influenced by breast thickness [61], hence there might have been larger variation in the serial compared with stable volumetric measurements, resulting in reduced ability to capture the within women effects of BMI on dense tissue volumetrically.

5. Conclusions

This study suggests that premenopausal weight loss reduces breast fat but that it does not reduce dense tissue. Short-term premenopausal weight loss is likely to be linked to lower postmenopausal breast cancer risk through reductions in adipose tissue, not fibroglandular tissue. This means that a potential breast cancer risk reduction as a result of weight loss might not be captured by changes in breast density, and the resulting increase in percent density may falsely ascribe an increase in risk. However, the study was limited by the small sample size, and more studies are required to provide evidence to confirm these results.

Supplementary Materials: The following are available online at https://www.mdpi.com/article/10.3390/cancers13133245/s1, Table S1: Complete results for repeated measures between women correlations for mammographic density and body composition measures; Table S2: Complete results for repeated measures within women correlations for mammographic density and body composition measures; Table S3: Complete results for repeated measures between women correlations for different body composition measures; Table S4: Complete results for repeated measures between women correlations for different mammographic density measures; Table S5: Multivariable linear mixed model fit results for A1 using either body mass index or weight; Table S6: Repeated measures between women and within women correlations for mammographic density and body mass index, stratified by intervention group; Figure S1: Flow chart of women included in the analysis and availability of mammographic density data.

Author Contributions: Conceptualization, A.H. and M.H.; Formal Analysis, E.C.A. and A.R.B.; Investigation, S.A., J.C., D.G.E., R.M.L.W., A.H., and M.H.; Data Curation, S.A., D.G.E., R.M.L.W., A.H., and M.H.; Writing—Original Draft Preparation, E.C.A., A.R.B., S.A., J.C., D.G.E., R.M.L.W., A.H., and M.H.; Writing—Review & Editing, E.C.A., A.R.B., S.A., J.C., D.G.E., R.M.L.W., A.H., and M.H. All authors have read and agreed to the published version of the manuscript.

Funding: E.C.A., A.R.B. and J.C. are supported by Cancer Research UK (C569/A16891 to J.C.); S.A., D.G.E., A.H., and M.H. are supported by the NIHR Manchester Biomedical Research Centre (IS-BRC-1215-20007 to D.G.E.). The funders had no role in the design of the study; in the collection, analysis and interpretation of data; in the writing of the manuscript, or in the decision to submit for publication.

Institutional Review Board Statement: The study was conducted according to the guidelines of the Declaration of Helsinki and was approved by the South Manchester Ethics Committee on 28 January 2002 (Reference no 01/426).

Informed Consent Statement: Informed consent was obtained from all subjects involved in the study.

Data Availability Statement: The dataset used and analysed during the current study is available from the corresponding author on reasonable request.

Acknowledgments: We thank Hilary Graff for contributions to the collection and assembly of data (University of Manchester). We are particularly grateful to the women who participated in this study and the entire medical and administrative staff who worked on the Lifestyle Study.

Conflicts of Interest: The authors declare no conflict of interest. The funders had no role in the design of the study; in the collection, analyses, or interpretation of data; in the writing of the manuscript, or in the decision to publish the results.

Abbreviations

DA	dense area
PDA	percent dense area
FA	fat area
TA	total area
DV	dense volume
PDV	percent dense volume
FV	fat volume
TV	total volume
BMI	body mass index
VAS	visual assessment score

Appendix A

Linear mixed model for mammographic density on body mass index and age. A linear mixed model was used to model density and body mass index (BMI) associations in Table 3. This model allows for repeated measures and uses all of the available data (missing pairs of density and BMI are excluded). Breast density y_{ij} for woman $i = 1, \ldots, n$ at time $j = \{1, 2, 3\}$ is modelled as:

$$y_{ij} = \alpha + \beta age_{ij} + \gamma \bar{x}_{i.} + \delta(x_{ij} - \bar{x}_{i.}) + u_i + e_{ij}; \tag{A1}$$

where α is an overall intercept; age_{ij} is the age at baseline for woman i at time j; β is the slope for age; $\bar{x}_{i.}$ is mean BMI for woman i; γ is the between women slope; x_{ij} is the BMI of woman i at time j; δ is the within women slope; and e_{ij} is an independent random error. Another term that allows for differences between women in their overall density level is the independent random intercept u_i for woman i. The model is completed by assuming normal distributions for u_i and e_{ij} with zero mean, unknown variances, and zero covariance. The model was fitted by maximum likelihood. To aid interpretation of the estimates across different measures of density, the density values were standardised (see Appendix B). To test $\gamma = 0$ (between women correlation) and $\delta = 0$ (within women correlation), a Wald test was applied.

The model was extended to consider BMI gain from age 20 years in Table 4:

$$y_{ij} = \alpha + \beta age_{ij} + \gamma \bar{x}_{i.} + \delta(x_{ij} - \bar{x}_{i.}) + u_i + \varepsilon z_i + e_{ij}; \tag{A2}$$

where z_i is the BMI gain since age 20 years for woman i: calculated as the difference between baseline BMI for woman i and BMI at age 20 years for woman i, and ε is the slope for BMI gain since age 20 years. To test $\varepsilon = 0$, a Wald test was applied.

Appendix B

Standardisation of each mammographic density measure:

$$\bar{x} = \frac{\sum_{i=1}^{n} \bar{x}_i}{n}$$

$$\sigma = \sqrt{\frac{\sum_{i=1}^{n} (\bar{x}_i - \bar{x})^2}{n-1}}$$

$$z_{ij} = \frac{d_{ij} - \bar{x}}{\sigma}$$

where $\bar{x}_i$ is the mean density for woman $i = 1, \ldots, n$; d_{ij} is the density measure for woman $i = 1, \ldots, n$ at time point $j = \{1, 2, 3\}$; and z_{ij} is the standardised density measure for woman i at time point j.

References

1. McCormack, V.A.; dos Santos Silva, I. Breast density and parenchymal patterns as markers of breast cancer risk: A meta-analysis. *Cancer Epidemiol. Biomark. Prev.* **2006**, *15*, 1159–1169. [CrossRef] [PubMed]
2. Boyd, N.F.; Byng, J.W.; Jong, R.A.; Fishell, E.K.; Little, L.E.; Miller, A.B.; Lockwood, G.A.; Tritchler, D.L.; Yaffe, M.J. Quantitative Classification of Mammographic Densities and Breast Cancer Risk: Results from the Canadian National Breast Screening Study. *J. Natl. Cancer Inst.* **1995**, *87*, 670–675. [CrossRef]
3. Byrne, C.; Schairer, C.; Wolfe, J.; Parekh, N.; Salane, M.; Brinton, L.A.; Hoover, R.; Haile, R. Mammographic Features and Breast Cancer Risk: Effects with Time, Age, and Menopause Status. *J. Natl. Cancer Inst.* **1995**, *87*, 1622–1629. [CrossRef] [PubMed]
4. Pettersson, A.; Hankinson, S.E.; Willett, W.C.; Lagiou, P.; Trichopoulos, D.; Tamimi, R.M. Nondense mammographic area and risk of breast cancer. *Breast Cancer Res.* **2011**, *13*, R100. [CrossRef]
5. Eng, A.; Gallant, Z.; Shepherd, J.; McCormack, V.; Li, J.; Dowsett, M.; Vinnicombe, S.; Allen, S.; Dos-Santos-Silva, I. Digital mammographic density and breast cancer risk: A case–control study of six alternative density assessment methods. *Breast Cancer Res.* **2014**, *16*, 439. [CrossRef] [PubMed]
6. Brentnall, A.R.; Cohn, W.F.; Knaus, W.A.; Yaffe, M.J.; Cuzick, J.; Harvey, J.A. A Case-Control Study to Add Volumetric or Clinical Mammographic Density into the Tyrer-Cuzick Breast Cancer Risk Model. *J. Breast Imaging* **2019**, *1*, 99–106. [CrossRef]
7. Kyrgiou, M.; Kalliala, I.; Markozannes, G.; Gunter, M.J.; Paraskevaidis, E.; Gabra, H.; Martin-Hirsch, P.; Tsilidis, K.K. Adiposity and cancer at major anatomical sites: Umbrella review of the literature. *BMJ* **2017**, *356*, j477. [CrossRef] [PubMed]
8. Renehan, A.G.; Tyson, M.; Egger, M.; Heller, R.F.; Zwahlen, M. Body-mass index and incidence of cancer: A systematic review and meta-analysis of prospective observational studies. *Lancet* **2008**, *371*, 569–578. [CrossRef]
9. Reeves, G.K.; Pirie, K.; Beral, V.; Green, J.; Spencer, E.; Bull, D. Cancer incidence and mortality in relation to body mass index in the Million Women Study: Cohort study. *BMJ* **2007**, *335*, 1134. [CrossRef]
10. Van Kruijsdijk, R.C.M.; Van Der Wall, E.; Visseren, F. Obesity and Cancer: The Role of Dysfunctional Adipose Tissue. *Cancer Epidemiol. Biomark. Prev.* **2009**, *18*, 2569–2578. [CrossRef]
11. Travis, R.C.; Key, T.J. Oestrogen exposure and breast cancer risk. *Breast Cancer Res.* **2003**, *5*, 239–247. [CrossRef] [PubMed]
12. Kim, B.-K.; Chang, Y.; Ahn, J.; Jung, H.-S.; Kim, C.-W.; Yun, K.E.; Kwon, M.-J.; Suh, B.-S.; Chung, E.C.; Shin, H.; et al. Metabolic syndrome, insulin resistance, and mammographic density in pre- and postmenopausal women. *Breast Cancer Res. Treat.* **2015**, *153*, 425–434. [CrossRef]
13. Schoemaker, M.J.; Nichols, H.B.; Wright, L.B.; Brook, M.N.; Jones, M.E.; O'Brien, K.M.; Adami, H.O.; Baglietto, L.; Bernstein, L.; Bertrand, K.A.; et al. Association of Body Mass Index and Age with Subsequent Breast Cancer Risk in Premenopausal Women. *JAMA Oncol.* **2018**, *4*, e181771. [CrossRef] [PubMed]
14. Amadou, A.; Ferrari, P.; Muwonge, R.; Moskal, A.; Biessy, C.; Romieu, I.; Hainaut, P. Overweight, obesity and risk of pre-menopausal breast cancer according to ethnicity: A systematic review and dose-response meta-analysis. *Obes. Rev.* **2013**, *14*, 665–678. [CrossRef] [PubMed]
15. Keum, N.; Greenwood, D.C.; Lee, D.H.; Kim, R.; Aune, D.; Ju, W.; Hu, F.B.; Giovannucci, E.L. Adult weight gain and adiposity-related cancers: A dose-response meta-analysis of prospective observational studies. *J. Natl. Cancer Inst.* **2015**, *107*, djv088. [CrossRef]
16. Hardefeldt, P.J.; Penninkilampi, R.; Edirimanne, S.; Eslick, G.D. Physical Activity and Weight Loss Reduce the Risk of Breast Cancer: A Meta-analysis of 139 Prospective and Retrospective Studies. *Clin. Breast Cancer* **2018**, *18*, e601–e612. [CrossRef] [PubMed]

17. Harvie, M.; Howell, A.; Vierkant, R.A.; Kumar, N.; Cerhan, J.R.; Kelemen, L.E.; Folsom, A.R.; Sellers, T.A. Association of Gain and Loss of Weight before and after Menopause with risk of postmenopausal breast cancer in the Iowa Women's Health Study. *Cancer Epidemiol. Biomark. Prev.* **2005**, *14*, 656–661. [CrossRef] [PubMed]
18. Trentham-Dietz, A.; Newcomb, P.A.; Egan, K.M.; Titus-Ernstoff, L.; Baron, J.A.; Storer, B.E.; Stampfer, M.; Willett, W.C. Weight change and risk of postmenopausal breast cancer (United States). *Cancer Causes Control* **2000**, *11*, 533–542. [CrossRef]
19. Winder, A.A.; Kularatna, M.; MacCormick, A.D. Does Bariatric Surgery Affect the Incidence of Breast Cancer Development? A Systematic Review. *Obes. Surg.* **2017**, *27*, 3014–3020. [CrossRef]
20. Harvie, M.; Cohen, H.; Mason, C.; Mercer, T.; Malik, R.; Adams, J.; Evans, D.G.R.; Hopwood, P.; Cuzick, J.; Howell, A. Adherence to a Diet and Exercise Weight Loss Intervention amongst Women at Increased Risk of Breast Cancer. *Open Obes. J.* **2010**, *2*, 71–80.
21. Graffy, H.; Harvie, M.; Warren, R.; Boggis, C.; Astley, S.; Evans, G.; Adams, J.; Howell, A. Abstract P4-13-09: The effect of weight change on breast adipose and dense tissue. *Poster Sess. Abstr.* **2012**, *72*, P4-13-09. [CrossRef]
22. Patel, H.G.; Astley, S.M.; Hufton, A.P.; Harvie, M.; Hagan, K.; Marchant, T.E.; Hillier, V.; Howell, A.; Warren, R.; Boggis, C.R.M. Automated breast tissue measurement of women at increased risk of breast cancer. In *Digital Mammography*; IWDM, 2006; Lecture Notes in Computer, Science; Astley, S.M., Brady, M., Rose, C., Zwiggelaar, R., Eds.; Springer: Heidelberg, Germany, 2006; Volume 4046.
23. Harvie, M.; Mercer, T.; Humphries, G.; Hopwood, P.; Adams, J.; Evans, G.; Sumner, H.; Astley, S.; Hayes, L.; Cooley, J.; et al. The effects of weight loss and exercise on biomarkers of breast cancer risk—Rationale and study design. *Recent Res. Dev. Nutr.* **2002**, *5*, 91–110.
24. Tyrer, J.; Duffy, S.W.; Cuzick, J. A breast cancer prediction model incorporating familial and personal risk factors. *Stat. Med.* **2004**, *23*, 1111–1130. [CrossRef]
25. IBIS Breast Cancer Risk Evaluation Tool. Available online: http://www.ems-trials.org/riskevaluator/ (accessed on 22 December 2020).
26. Byng, J.W.; Boyd, N.F.; Fishell, E.; Jong, R.A.; Yaffe, M.J. The quantitative analysis of mammographic densities. *Phys. Med. Biol.* **1994**, *39*, 1629–1638. [CrossRef] [PubMed]
27. Diffey, J.; Hufton, A.; Astley, S. A new step-wedge for the volumetric measurement of mammographic density. In *Digital Mammography*; IWDM, 2006; Lecture Notes in Computer, Science; Astley, S.M., Brady, M., Rose, C., Zwiggelaar, R., Eds.; Springer: Heidelberg, Germany, 2006; Volume 4046, pp. 1–9.
28. Stevens, J.; Truesdale, K.P.; McClain, J.E.; Cai, J. The definition of weight maintenance. *Int. J. Obes.* **2005**, *30*, 391–399. [CrossRef]
29. Bland, J.M.; Altman, D.G. Statistics notes: Calculating correlation coefficients with repeated observations: Part 1—correlation within subjects. *BMJ* **1995**, *310*, 446. [CrossRef]
30. Bland, J.M.; Altman, D.G. Statistics notes: Calculating correlation coefficients with repeated observations: Part 2—correlation between subjects. *BMJ* **1995**, *310*, 633. [CrossRef]
31. Crowder, M.J.; Hand, D.J. *Analysis of Repeated Measures*, 1st ed.; Monographs on Statistics and Applied Probability; Chapman & Hall: London, UK, 1990.
32. R Core Team. *R: A Language and Environment for Statistical Computing*; R Foundation for Statistical Computing: Vienna, Austria, 2015. Available online: https://www.r-project.org (accessed on 28 July 2019).
33. Hart, V.; Reeves, K.W.; Sturgeon, S.R.; Reich, N.G.; Sievert, L.L.; Kerlikowske, K.; Ma, L.; Shepherd, J.; Tice, J.; Mahmoudzadeh, A.P.; et al. The Effect of Change in Body Mass Index on Volumetric Measures of Mammographic Density. *Cancer Epidemiol. Biomark. Prev.* **2015**, *24*, 1724–1730. [CrossRef]
34. Alimujiang, A.; Appleton, C.; Colditz, G.A.; Toriola, A.T. Adiposity during early adulthood, changes in adiposity during adulthood, attained adiposity, and mammographic density among premenopausal women. *Breast Cancer Res. Treat.* **2017**, *166*, 197–206. [CrossRef]
35. Pereira, A.; Garmendia, M.L.; Uauy, R.; Neira, P.; Lopez-Arana, S.; Malkov, S.; Shepherd, J. Determinants of volumetric breast density in Chilean premenopausal women. *Breast Cancer Res. Treat.* **2017**, *162*, 343–352. [CrossRef] [PubMed]
36. Sung, J.; Song, Y.-M.; Stone, J.; Lee, K.; Kim, S.-Y. Association of Body Size Measurements and Mammographic Density in Korean Women: The Healthy Twin Study. *Cancer Epidemiol. Biomark. Prev.* **2010**, *19*, 1523–1531. [CrossRef] [PubMed]
37. Boyd, N.; Lockwood, G.; Byng, J.; Little, L.; Yaffe, M.; Tritchler, D. The relationship of anthropometric measures to radiological features of the breast in premenopausal women. *Br. J. Cancer* **1998**, *78*, 1233–1238. [CrossRef]
38. Harris, H.R.; Tamimi, R.M.; Willett, W.C.; Hankinson, S.E.; Michels, K.B. Body Size Across the Life Course, Mammographic Density, and Risk of Breast Cancer. *Am. J. Epidemiol.* **2011**, *174*, 909–918. [CrossRef] [PubMed]
39. Tseng, M.; Byrne, C. Adiposity, adult weight gain and mammographic breast density in US Chinese women. *Int. J. Cancer* **2011**, *128*, 418–425. [CrossRef] [PubMed]
40. Pollán, M.; Spain, D.; Lopez-Abente, G.; Miranda-García, J.; García, M.; Casanova, F.; Sánchez-Contador, C.; Santamariña, C.; Moreo, P.; Vidal, C.; et al. Adult weight gain, fat distribution and mammographic density in Spanish pre- and post-menopausal women (DDM-Spain). *Breast Cancer Res. Treat.* **2012**, *134*, 823–838. [CrossRef]
41. Samimi, G.; Colditz, G.A.; Baer, H.J.; Tamimi, R.M. Measures of energy balance and mammographic density in the Nurses' Health Study. *Breast Cancer Res. Treat.* **2008**, *109*, 113–122. [CrossRef]

42. Dorgan, J.F.; Klifa, C.; Shepherd, J.A.; Egleston, B.L.; Kwiterovich, P.O.; Himes, J.H.; Gabriel, K.P.; Van Horn, L.; Snetselaar, L.G.; Stevens, V.J.; et al. Height, adiposity and body fat distribution and breast density in young women. *Breast Cancer Res.* **2012**, *14*, R107. [CrossRef] [PubMed]
43. Jeffreys, M.; Warren, R.; Highnam, R.; Smith, G.D. Breast cancer risk factors and a novel measure of volumetric breast density: Cross-sectional study. *Br. J. Cancer* **2007**, *98*, 210–216. [CrossRef] [PubMed]
44. Boyd, N.F.; Greenberg, C.; Lockwood, G.; Little, L.; Martin, L.; Tritchler, D.; Byng, J.; Yaffe, M. Effects at Two Years of a Low-Fat, High-Carbohydrate Diet on Radiologic Features of the Breast: Results from a Randomized Trial. *J. Natl. Cancer Inst.* **1997**, *89*, 488–496. [CrossRef]
45. Woolcott, C.G.; Courneya, K.S.; Boyd, N.F.; Yaffe, M.J.; Terry, T.; McTiernan, A.; Brant, R.; Ballard-Barbash, R.; Irwin, M.L.; Jones, C.A.; et al. Mammographic Density Change with 1 Year of Aerobic Exercise among Postmenopausal Women: A Randomized Controlled Trial. *Cancer Epidemiol. Biomark. Prev.* **2010**, *19*, 1112–1121. [CrossRef]
46. Masala, G.; Assedi, M.; Sera, F.; Ermini, I.; Occhini, D.; Castaldo, M.; Pierpaoli, E.; Caini, S.; Bendinelli, B.; Ambrogetti, D.; et al. Can Dietary and Physical Activity Modifications Reduce Breast Density in Postmenopausal Women? The DAMA Study, a Randomized Intervention Trial in Italy. *Cancer Epidemiol. Biomark. Prev.* **2019**, *28*, 41–50. [CrossRef]
47. Hassinger, T.E.; Mehaffey, J.H.; Knisely, A.T.; Contrella, B.N.; Brenin, D.R.; Schroen, A.T.; Schirmer, B.D.; Hallowell, P.T.; Harvey, J.A.; Showalter, S.L. The impact of bariatric surgery on qualitative and quantitative breast density. *Breast J.* **2019**, *25*, 1198–1205. [CrossRef]
48. Williams, A.D.; So, A.; Synnestvedt, M.; Tewksbury, C.M.; Kontos, D.; Hsiehm, M.-K.; Pantalone, L.; Conant, E.F.; Schnall, M.; Dumon, K.; et al. Mammographic breast density decreases after bariatric surgery. *Breast Cancer Res. Treat.* **2017**, *165*, 565–572. [CrossRef] [PubMed]
49. Vohra, N.A.; Kachare, S.D.; Vos, P.; Schroeder, B.F.; Schuth, O.; Suttle, D.; Fitzgerald, T.L.; Wong, J.H.; Verbanac, K.M. The Short-Term Effect of Weight Loss Surgery on Volumetric Breast Density and Fibroglandular Volume. *Obes. Surg.* **2016**, *27*, 1013–1023. [CrossRef] [PubMed]
50. Magnusson, C.; Baron, J.; Persson, I.; Wolk, A.; Bergstrom, R.; Trichopoulos, D.; Adami, H.O. Body size in different periods of life and breast cancer risk in post-menopausal women. *Int. J. Cancer* **1998**, *76*, 29–34. [CrossRef]
51. Eliassen, A.H.; Colditz, G.; Rosner, B.; Willett, W.C.; Hankinson, S.E. Adult Weight Change and Risk of Postmenopausal Breast Cancer. *JAMA* **2006**, *296*, 193–201. [CrossRef]
52. Ahn, J.; Schatzkin, A.; Lacey, J.V.; Albanes, D.; Ballard-Barbash, R.; Adams, K.F.; Kipnis, V.; Mouw, T.; Hollenbeck, A.R.; Leitzmann, M.F. Adiposity, adult weight change, and postmenopausal breast cancer risk. *Arch. Intern. Med.* **2007**, *167*, 2091–2102. [CrossRef]
53. Bertrand, K.A.; Baer, H.J.; Orav, E.J.; Klifa, C.; Shepherd, J.A.; Van Horn, L.; Snetselaar, L.; Stevens, V.J.; Hylton, N.M.; Dorgan, J.F. Body fatness during childhood and adolescence and breast density in young women: A prospective analysis. *Breast Cancer Res.* **2015**, *17*, 1–10. [CrossRef] [PubMed]
54. Hopper, J.L.; Nguyen, T.L.; Stone, J.; Aujard, K.; Matheson, M.C.; Abramson, M.J.; Burgess, J.A.; Walters, E.H.; Dite, G.S.; Bui, M.; et al. Childhood body mass index and adult mammographic density measures that predict breast cancer risk. *Breast Cancer Res. Treat.* **2016**, *156*, 163–170. [CrossRef]
55. Boyd, N.F.; Martin, L.J.; Sun, L.; Guo, H.; Chiarelli, A.; Hislop, G.; Yaffe, M.; Minkin, S. Body Size, Mammographic Density, and Breast Cancer Risk. *Cancer Epidemiol. Biomark. Prev.* **2006**, *15*, 2086–2092. [CrossRef]
56. Lee, J.M.; Holley, S.; Appleton, C.; Toriola, A.T. Is There an Association Between Bone Mineral Density and Mammographic Density? A Systematic Review. *J. Women's Health* **2017**, *26*, 389–395. [CrossRef]
57. Astley, S.M.; Harkness, E.F.; Sergeant, J.C.; Warwick, J.; Stavrinos, P.; Warren, R.; Wilson, M.; Beetles, U.; Gadde, S.; Lim, Y.; et al. A comparison of five methods of measuring mammographic density: A case-control study. *Breast Cancer Res.* **2018**, *20*, 1–13. [CrossRef]
58. Burton, A.; Maskarinec, G.; Perez-Gomez, B.; Vachon, C.; Miao, H.; Lajous, M.; López-Ridaura, R.; Rice, M.; Pereira, A.; Garmendia, M.L.; et al. Mammographic density and ageing: A collaborative pooled analysis of cross-sectional data from 22 countries worldwide. *PLoS Med.* **2017**, *14*, e1002335. [CrossRef] [PubMed]
59. Renehan, A.G.; Pegington, M.; Harvie, M.N.; Sperrin, M.; Astley, S.M.; Brentnall, A.R.; Howell, A.; Cuzick, J.; Evans, D.G. Young adulthood body mass index, adult weight gain and breast cancer risk: The PROCAS Study (United Kingdom). *Br. J. Cancer* **2020**, *122*, 1552–1561. [CrossRef] [PubMed]
60. Rimm, E.B.; Stampfer, M.J.; Colditz, G.A.; Chute, C.G.; Litin, L.B.; Willett, W.C. Validity of Self-Reported Waist and Hip Circumferences in Men and Women. *Epidemiology* **1990**, *1*, 466–473. [CrossRef] [PubMed]
61. Diffey, J.; Hufton, A.; Beeston, C.; Smith, J.; Marchant, T.; Astley, S. Quantifying Breast Thickness for Density Measurement. In *Digital Mammography*; IWDM, 2008; Lecture Notes in Computer, Science; Krupinski, E.A., Ed.; Springer: Heidelberg, Germany, 2008; Volume 5116, pp. 651–658.

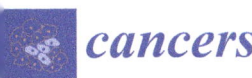

Article

Implementation of Multigene Germline and Parallel Somatic Genetic Testing in Epithelial Ovarian Cancer: SIGNPOST Study

Dhivya Chandrasekaran [1,2], Monika Sobocan [1,2,3], Oleg Blyuss [4,5,6], Rowan E. Miller [7], Olivia Evans [1], Shanthini M. Crusz [7], Tina Mills-Baldock [8], Li Sun [1,9], Rory F. L. Hammond [10], Faiza Gaba [1], Lucy A. Jenkins [11], Munaza Ahmed [11], Ajith Kumar [11], Arjun Jeyarajah [2], Alexandra C. Lawrence [2], Elly Brockbank [2], Saurabh Phadnis [2], Mary Quigley [8], Fatima El Khouly [8], Rekha Wuntakal [12], Asma Faruqi [10], Giorgia Trevisan [10], Laura Casey [10], George J. Burghel [13], Helene Schlecht [13], Michael Bulman [13], Philip Smith [13], Naomi L. Bowers [13], Rosa Legood [9], Michelle Lockley [14], Andrew Wallace [13], Naveena Singh [10], D. Gareth Evans [13] and Ranjit Manchanda [1,2,9,*]

1. Wolfson Institute of Population Health, Barts CRUK Cancer Centre, Queen Mary University of London, Charterhouse Square, London EC1M 6BQ, UK; d.chandrasekaran@qmul.ac.uk (D.C.); m.sobocan@qmul.ac.uk (M.S.); olivia.evans@nhs.scot (O.E.); li.sun1@lshtm.ac.uk (L.S.); f.gaba@qmul.ac.uk (F.G.)
2. Department of Gynaecological Oncology, Barts Health NHS Trust, London EC1 1BB, UK; arjun.jeyarajah@nhs.net (A.J.); alexandra.lawrence5@nhs.net (A.C.L.); elly.brockbank@nhs.net (E.B.); s.phadnis@nhs.net (S.P.)
3. Divison for Gynaecology and Perinatology, University Medical Centre Maribor, 2000 Maribor, Slovenia
4. School of Physics, Engineering and Computer Science, University of Hertfordshire, Hatfield AL10 9AB, UK; o.blyuss@qmul.ac.uk
5. Department of Paediatrics and Paediatric Infectious Diseases, Sechenov First Moscow State Medical University, Moscow 119991, Russia
6. World-Class Research Center "Digital Biodesign and Personalized Healthcare", Sechenov First Moscow State Medical University, Moscow 119991, Russia
7. Department of Medical Oncology, Barts Health NHS Trust, London EC1A 7BE, UK; rowan.miller2@nhs.net (R.E.M.); shanthini.crusz@nhs.net (S.M.C.)
8. Department of Medical Oncology, Barking, Havering & Redbridge University Hospitals, Essex RM7 0AG, UK; tinamills-baldock@nhs.net (T.M.-B.); mary.quigley5@nhs.net (M.Q.); fatima.el-khouly@nhs.net (F.E.K.)
9. Department of Health Services Research, Faculty of Public Health & Policy, London School of Hygiene & Tropical Medicine, London WC1H 9SH, UK; rosa.legood@lshtm.ac.uk
10. Department of Pathology, Barts Health NHS Trust, London E1 1FR, UK; r.f.l.hammond@smd14.qmul.ac.uk (R.F.L.H.); asma.faruqi@nhs.net (A.F.); giorgia.trevisan1@nhs.net (G.T.); laura.casey5@nhs.net (L.C.); naveenasingh7@gmail.com (N.S.)
11. North East Thames Regional Genetics Service, Great Ormond Street Hospital, London WC1N 3JH, UK; lucy.jenkins@gosh.nhs.uk (L.A.J.); munaza.ahmed@gosh.nhs.uk (M.A.); ajith.kumar@gosh.nhs.uk (A.K.)
12. Department of Gynaecology, Barking, Havering & Redbridge University Hospitals, Essex RM7 0AG, UK; r.wuntakal@nhs.net
13. Manchester Centre for Genomic Medicine, Saint Marys Hospital, Manchester M13 9WL, UK; george.burghel@mft.nhs.uk (G.J.B.); helene.schlecht@mft.nhs.uk (H.S.); michael.bulman@mft.nhs.uk (M.B.); philip.smith@mft.nhs.uk (P.S.); Naomi.Bowers@mft.nhs.uk (N.L.B.); andrew.wallace@mft.nhs.uk (A.W.); Gareth.Evans@mft.nhs.uk (D.G.E.)
14. Barts Cancer Institute, Queen Mary University of London, Charterhouse Square, London EC1M 6BQ, UK; m.lockley@qmul.ac.uk
* Correspondence: r.manchanda@qmul.ac.uk

Simple Summary: Multigene testing in ovarian cancer has received increased support due to its' applicability for cancer treatment and the impact it has on cancer prevention in families. This study shows that multi-gene germline and somatic testing uptake after counselling by a member of the multidisciplinary cancer clinical team in women with ovarian cancer, was high (97%). A total of 15.5% of women were identified to have germline *BRCA1/BRCA2* pathogenic variants and 7.8% had somatic *BRCA1/BRCA2* pathogenic variants. A total of 2.3% patients had *RAD51C/RAD51D/BRIP1* pathogenic variants. We found that 11% of germline pathogenic variants were large-genomic-rearrangements

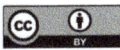

and were missed by somatic testing. Our findings support prospective parallel somatic-&-germline panel testing to maximize variant identification.

Abstract: We present findings of a cancer multidisciplinary-team (MDT) coordinated mainstreaming pathway of unselected 5-panel germline *BRCA1/BRCA2/RAD51C/RAD51D/BRIP1* and parallel somatic *BRCA1/BRCA2* testing in all women with epithelial-OC and highlight the discordance between germline and somatic testing strategies across two cancer centres. Patients were counselled and consented by a cancer MDT member. The uptake of parallel multi-gene germline and somatic testing was 97.7%. Counselling by clinical-nurse-specialist more frequently needed >1 consultation (53.6% (30/56)) compared to a medical (15.0% (21/137)) or surgical oncologist (15.3% (17/110)) ($p < 0.001$). The median age was 54 (IQR = 51–62) years in germline pathogenic-variant (PV) versus 61 (IQR = 51–71) in *BRCA* wild-type ($p = 0.001$). There was no significant difference in distribution of PVs by ethnicity, stage, surgery timing or resection status. A total of 15.5% germline and 7.8% somatic *BRCA1/BRCA2* PVs were identified. A total of 2.3% patients had *RAD51C/RAD51D/BRIP1* PVs. A total of 11% germline PVs were large-genomic-rearrangements and missed by somatic testing. A total of 20% germline PVs are missed by somatic first *BRCA*-testing approach and 55.6% germline PVs missed by family history ascertainment. The somatic testing failure rate is higher (23%) for patients undergoing diagnostic biopsies. Our findings favour a prospective parallel somatic and germline panel testing approach as a clinically efficient strategy to maximise variant identification. UK Genomics test-directory criteria should be expanded to include a panel of OC genes.

Keywords: ovarian cancer; *BRCA*; genetic testing; germline; somatic; *RAD51C*; *RAD51D*; *BRIP1*

1. Introduction

Ovarian cancer (OC) is the leading cause of deaths from gynaecological cancers, with 240,000 new cases and 152,000 deaths occurring worldwide annually [1]. GLOBOCAN data suggest the number of cases from OC will increase by 26% in the UK and 47% worldwide, respectively, over the next 20 years [1]. Standard treatment approaches have been associated with limited long-term OC survival of ~30% [2]. However, the progress over the last 10–15 years has provided the foundations for a precision medicine [3] approach for OC management, involving inherited cancer susceptibility genes. *BRCA1/BRCA2* pathogenic and likely pathogenic variants (henceforth termed 'pathogenic variants' or 'PVs') account for most of the known inheritable risk of OC. Around 11–18% of OC have germline *BRCA1/BRCA2* PV and another 6–9% have a somatic *BRCA1/BRCA2* PV in the tumour tissue alone which is not inherited. Women with germline *BRCA1/BRCA2* PVs have a cumulative risk by age 80 of 17–44% for developing EOC and 69–72% for developing breast cancer (BC) [4].

Genetic testing for OC susceptibility genes has recently received an impetus through increasing applicability for cancer treatment and eligibility for clinical trials. The proteins coded by *BRCA1/BRCA2* are essential in the homologous recombination repair (HRR) of double stranded DNA breaks, whilst PARP (poly ADP ribose polymerase) is an essential component of single-strand DNA repair. Inhibition of PARP increases double strand breaks and prevents HRR deficient (HRD) tumour cells from surviving chemotherapy induced DNA damage, leading to synthetic lethality [5]. Germline as well as somatic *BRCA* mutated OC have been shown to benefit from 'PARP inhibitor' (PARP-i) therapy with improved progression free survival at both recurrent and more recently primary settings [5–9]. Therefore, knowledge of *BRCA* status at the time of diagnosis has become pivotal in the guidance of treatment options. Genetic testing for germline *BRCA1/BRCA2* PVs in EOC was commissioned by NHS-England in 2015 [10], and has been recommended by other published guidelines over the last few years [11]. More recently, the American Society of Clinical Oncology (ASCO) [12], the British Gynaecological Cancer Society (BGCS) [13] and the European Society of Medical Oncology (ESMO) [14] have advocated for somatic testing too.

However, HRD can arise through somatic and germline PV in a wide range of OC susceptibility genes [15]. Approximately 50% of high-grade serous OC are characterised by HRD suggesting additional mechanisms other than *BRCA* mutations play a significant role [14]. HRD assays are now available and are beginning to be used in clinical practice [14]. Further moderate risk OC susceptibility genes in the HRR pathway, such as, *RAD51C*, *RAD51D* and *BRIP1* with lifetime OC-risks of 5.8 to 13% have been identified and their risks validated [16,17]. Testing for additional genes of clinical utility [18] can lead to wider therapeutic benefit. ASCO now recommends germline *BRCA* testing within the context of a multigene panel [12]. In addition to targeted therapy, identification of PVs offers opportunities for cancer surveillance and prevention for secondary cancers in index patients as well as cascade testing in relatives. Unaffected relatives with PVs can access relevant surgical prevention and screening options which have well established clinical benefit. This includes risk-reducing salpingo-oophorectomy (RRSO) to reduce their OC risk [19,20]; MRI/mammography screening, or risk reducing mastectomy (RRM) [21], or chemoprevention with selective oestrogen receptor modulators (SERM) to reduce their BC risk [22].

Over recent years, many models of care delivery for OC genetic testing have been implemented into clinical practice [23–25]. There has been great variation in these clinical pathways, with strategies varying with respect to (a) whom to test (unselected or restricted by histology such as for high-grade serous OC or restricted by age, such as under 70 years); (b) what to test (either germline only, or somatic only, or both) and (c) in which order to test (parallel or sequential); (d) which genes to test (*BRCA* only or multiple genes); and (e) who provides counselling and testing (genetics teams in genetics clinics, genetics professional embedded in oncology clinics, medical oncologists, surgical oncologists, or clinical nurse specialists (CNS)). Despite guidelines, historically, the overall uptake and access to genetic testing across health systems has remained poor, with only 20–30% eligible patients accessing testing [26,27]. Obstacles to introducing routine somatic testing at diagnosis have been attributed to reasons like cost, access/availability of validated somatic testing in a National Health Service (NHS) accredited laboratory and additional resources required to process tumour samples [28]. Most studies to date report clinical experience of implementing *BRCA* testing. Reports of systematic prospective parallel germline panel and somatic genetic testing are limited. We present our experience and findings of implementing a cancer multidisciplinary team (MDT) coordinated mainstreaming pathway of unselected 5-panel germline *BRCA1*, *BRCA2*, *RAD51C*, *RAD51D*, *BRIP1* and parallel somatic *BRCA1/BRCA2* testing in all women with high grade non-mucinous epithelial OC in the Systematic Genetic Testing for Personalised Ovarian Cancer Therapy (SIGNPOST) study (ISRCTN: 16988857) in women from North East London Cancer Network (NELCN). We report on the somatic testing success rates with different types of sample ascertainment. Moreover, importantly we highlight the discordance between germline and somatic testing strategies incorporating testing data from NELCN as well as the Manchester NHS Foundation trust.

2. Materials and Methods

2.1. Pre-Test Counselling and Recruitment

Women ≥18 years with high-grade non-mucinous epithelial OC, who were newly diagnosed or under follow-up in the NELCN, were offered parallel germline testing for *BRCA1*, *BRCA2*, *RAD51C*, *RAD51D*, *BRIP1* genes and concomitant *BRCA1/BRCA2* somatic genetic testing. This was undertaken through the SIGNPOST study (ISRCTN: 16988857). Newly diagnosed patients were identified from gynaecological oncology MDT meetings and consented for genetic testing during their primary treatment. Patients undergoing surveillance post-treatment, were identified through follow-up surgical and medical oncology clinics as well as pathology and clinical databases. Eligibility for genetic testing was established by the treating clinician. Patients received written pre-test education information regarding the advantages, disadvantages and implications of genetic-testing. Pre-test genetic counselling and consent was undertaken at routine clinic visits. This was led initially by medical and surgical oncology consultants, and subsequently also undertaken by cancer CNSs. Psychological support was offered by CNSs within the cancer services.

2.2. Germline and Somatic Testing

Testing was undertaken by clinically accredited NHS laboratories. A 4 mL EDTA blood sample was taken for germline genetic testing for *BRCA1*, *BRCA2*, *RAD51C*, *RAD51D* and *BRIP1*. Germline testing for NELCN samples was undertaken for *BRCA1*, *BRCA2*, *RAD51C*, *RAD51D* and *BRIP1* at the North East Thames Regional Genomics Laboratory (Great Ormond Street Hospital), while for Manchester samples testing for *BRCA1* and *BRCA2* was undertaken at the Genomic Diagnostic Laboratory at the North West Genomic Laboratory Hub. This was carried out using next generation sequencing (NGS; Agilent SureSelect and Illumina NextSeq) of the coding region, sequenced to a minimum depth of 30 reads, including intron/exon splice boundaries. Sanger sequencing was also carried out to confirm variants detected during the NGS screen. Additionally, exon deletions/duplications in *BRCA1* and *BRCA2* genes were detected using Exome Depth. Multiplex ligation-dependent probe amplification (MLPA; MRC Holland) kits P002-D1 and P090-C1, respectively.

Somatic testing was undertaken using formalin fixed paraffin embedded (FFPE) tissue specimen from diagnostic biopsies, or up front cytoreductive surgery or post-chemotherapy cytoreductive surgery as appropriate. FFPE blocks were reviewed by a consultant histopathologist to identify areas with >20% tumour content and therefore deemed suitable for somatic testing. The specimens were processed and sent as either 5 × 5 µM thick unstained sections, or as 3 mm core biopsies from paraffin blocks. Unstained slides were preferred for small volume diagnostic biopsies and in <20% neoplastic content. Tumour blocks were selected by the pathologist and graded as <20%, 20–50% and >50% neoplastic content. Testing was undertaken in two NHS accredited diagnostic laboratories. Majority NELCN and Manchester samples were analysed at the Manchester Genomics Laboratory while a few NELCN samples were also tested at the Royal Marsden Hospital laboratory. Detection of variants is dependent on the percentage of tumour infiltration, DNA input concentration and DNA quality. DNA extracted from FFPE tissue was analysed in the coding regions of *BRCA1* and *BRCA2*, using NGS and minimum variant allele depth was 10×. The analysis was performed with Molecular Diagnostics Information Management System v-4.0, based on genome hg19 or GeneRead DNAseq v2 Human Breast Cancer Panel (Qiagen) and Illumina NGS. Mutation and variant calling by custom bioinformatic analysis pipeline validated to detect SNVs and small insertion/deletion mutations (<40 bp) to 5% mutant allele frequency (MAF).

Variants were classified using the ACGS and CanVIG guidance in force (https://www.acgs.uk.com/quality/best-practice-guidelines/ (accessed on 5 January 2021)) [29,30]. Common, high frequency benign and likely benign variants were filtered bioinformatically from a curated list of variants whilst all other variants were assessed by a registered Clinical Scientist. In case of discordance between the germline and somatic samples, a further repeat analysis was undertaken and second report issued. Reports from both germline and somatic tests were sent to the referring clinician for disclosure to the patients.

Validation of 3 mm FFPE punch biopsies for high-volume somatic testing:

Somatic testing using NGS on FFPE specimens has been validated on 5 × 5 µM thick unstained sections. [31] In order to minimise delay without compromising DNA yield, particularly for archival FFPE tissue, 3 mm punch biopsies from FFPE tumour blocks were validated for diagnostic somatic testing. Following review by a gynaecological oncology histopathologist, a 5 mm area with high tumour content (>20%) was marked on the Haematoxylin and Eosin (H&E) stain slide. Keyes punch biopsy (routinely used for skin biopsy) was used to core out 3 mm sample from corresponding area in FFPE block.

Five 5 µM thick unstained sections were also cut from same block. Five matched 3 mm cores and unstained sections were compared for DNA yield.

2.3. Test Result Management

Most patients including all those diagnosed with a PV were given their test result and counselled in an outpatient clinic by their consenting and treating cancer clinician. A small proportion of patients on long-term follow up declined an additional hospital visit and were given the result by post. All patients with a PV were referred to North East Thames regional genetics service team for additional post-test genetic counselling and facilitating predictive testing in family members.

We report on testing undertaken between 01/05/2017 to 31/12/2019 across the NELCN, which provides cancer care to a ~1.7 M population covering six NHS hospitals. Patient demographic and clinical data were extracted from electronic patient records, and FH questionnaires completed by the patient. Positive (or strong) FH was defined as any index case of high-grade non-mucinous epithelial OC and breast cancer or epithelial OC in a first-degree or second-degree relative. Patients who had previously undergone genetic testing as they had been referred to clinical genetics in view of a strong FH, were excluded from mainstreaming, but are included in the analysis of prevalence estimates. For the analysis of discordance between germline and somatic *BRCA1/BRCA2* testing we also include data of 116 unselected OC cases from Manchester NHS Foundation trust who underwent parallel germline and somatic testing. The testing procedures and offer of testing was similarly undertaken in Manchester but germline testing was restricted to *BRCA1* and *BRCA2*.

Descriptive statistics were used for baseline characteristics. PV and wild type groups were compared for ethnicity, age, FH, histology, stage, timing of surgery, chemotherapy response score, and residual disease status. Variables associated with number of pre-test consultations (1 or >1) were explored for type of clinician undertaking counselling, disease status at time of counselling (new diagnosis or on follow up) and treatment status (whether undergoing active treatment or not).

Wilcoxon rank-sum test and Fisher's exact or Chi-square tests were used to test the difference in means and proportions correspondingly. Two-sided p-values were reported for all statistical tests. Statistical analysis was undertaken in R version 3.5.1 and SPSS version 26.

3. Results

Pathway Development

Development of the genetic testing pathway was preceded by a wide consultation with the regional clinical geneticists, genetic counsellors, surgical and medical oncologists, CNS, clinical scientists from genetic laboratories, patient representatives and *BRCA* charity leads. Patient representatives and charity leads expressed a preference for genetic testing to be provided at diagnosis, to be made available all patients including those remained under surveillance post-treatment, and for provision for adequate pre-test counselling and informed consent.

In preparation of a cancer MDT coordinated mainstreaming genetic testing service, all gynaecological cancer MDT members (surgical oncologists, medical oncologist, pathologist and CNS) attended small group teaching sessions led by the regional lead in clinical genetics and a gynaecological oncologist with a long-standing special interest and significant experience in cancer genetics, counselling and testing. This covered principles of Mendelian inheritance, OC susceptibility genes and associated cancer risks; the principles, structure and factors specific to genetic counselling; as well as the developed local testing and referral pathways. Knowledge questionnaires were completed by attendees to ensure appropriate understanding of issues. Following pathway implementation, ongoing professional support for the cancer MDT team was provided by gynaecological cancer precision prevention service, with support from the regional clinical genetics team. Pre-counselling written information was developed in collaboration with the major stakeholders and provided to all patients. Additionally, service management meetings across the broader group with representation from medical and surgical oncologist, lead clinical geneticist, clinical scientists from genetic laboratories, lead histopathologist were held every 6–9 months.

Counselling, Recruitment and Genetic Testing:

A total of 310 patients with high-grade non-mucinous epithelial OC who were eligible for genetic testing were identified across the NELCN. This included 188 newly diagnosed women and 122 patients on follow up post-treatment. Of these women seven were excluded: four died prior to commencing treatment, one was unable to consent due to dementia and learning difficulties and two declined genetic testing. The remainder 303 untested patients remained eligible for testing and received pre-test genetic counselling. Of these patients 7/122 (6%) under surveillance had previously undergone germline *BRCA1/BRCA2* mutation testing through clinical genetics due to a strong FH of BC or OC fulfilling prior standard clinical criteria for genetic testing. They were offered and underwent extended panel testing for *RAD51C, RAD51D* and *BRIP1* along-with somatic testing. Overall, we found a 97.7% uptake of parallel multi-gene germline and somatic testing via the cancer MDT mediated mainstreaming pathway.

All of the patients were counselled and consented by a member of the cancer MDT, with 45% (n = 137) by a medical oncology member, 36% (n = 110) by a surgical oncology member and 18% (n = 56) by a CNS. The majority required a single pre-test consultation (78%) prior to consenting, whereas 18% (n = 54) required two consultations, 4% (n = 13) required three and one patient required four consultations prior to decision to undergo testing (Table 1). The number of pre-test counselling sessions needed varied significantly depending on the clinical professional undertaking counselling. Counselling by CNS was more frequently associated with needing more than one consultation (53.6% (30/56)) compared to counselling by a medical oncologist (15.0% (21/137)) or a surgical gynae-oncologist (15% (17/110)) (p < 0.001). The number of consultations required did not significantly differ whether (a) the patient was newly diagnosed or under follow up; and (b) if they were undergoing active treatment or not (Table 1).

Table 1. Factors associated with number of pre-test consultations.

Variation	1 Consultation n (%)	>1 Consultation n (%)	p-Value *
Member of oncology team undertaking pre-test counselling			
Medical Oncologist	116/235 (49%)	21/68 (30%)	<0.001
Surgical Oncologist	93/235 (40%)	17/68 (22%)	
Clinical nurse specialist	26/235 (12%)	30/68 (48%)	
Disease status at the time of counselling			
New diagnosis of ovarian cancer	127/235 (54%)	40/68 (59%)	0.580
Under follow up	108/235 (46%)	28/68 (41%)	
Treatment status at the time of counselling			
Undergoing treatment	155/235 (66%)	50/68 (74%)	0.303
Not on treatment	80/235 (34%)	18/68 (26%)	

* Chi-square test comparing '1 consultation and >1 consultation groups' by variables of type of counselling clinician, disease status and treatment status at time of pre-test counselling.

Patient demographics and clinical characteristics are summarised in Table 2. The median age at OC diagnosis was 54 years (IQR 51–62) in germline PV compared with 61 (IQR 51–71) in *BRCA* wild type (*BRCA*-WT) (p = 0.001) patients. In germline *BRCA1/BRCA2/ RAD51C/RAD51D/BRIP1* PVs, 44.4% (24/54) had a positive FH compared to 11.3% (28/249) of sporadic tumours (p < 0.001) (Table 2). Thus 55.6% of PVs would have been missed by using FH alone. Only 2/7 of *RAD51C/RAD51D/BRIP1* PVs had a positive FH. Ethnicity of OC cases included 196 (64.7%) White, 28 (9.2%) Black, 52 (17.2%) South Asian and 27 (8.9%) were classed as 'other'. In women with somatic *BRCA1/BRCA2* PV, the median age at diagnosis was 61 (IQR 59–66) and 13% (2/15) had a positive FH. Most PVs had a high-grade serous (HGS) histology except one *BRCA1* with grade 3 endometrioid carcinoma and one *BRIP1* with mixed epithelial adenocarcinoma. There was no significant difference in distribution of PVs by ethnicity, stage at diagnosis, timing of surgery or resection status (Table 2). In post-chemotherapy cytoreductive surgery specimens, chemotherapy response score (CRS) of 3 (minimal residual disease) was recorded in 13/69 (18.8%) germline and somatic PVs compared to 13/234 (5.6%) of *BRCA*-WT tumours ($p = 0.025$).

Table 2. Demographic and clinical characteristics NELCN cohort.

Category	No Germline Pathogenic Variants	Germline Pathogenic Variants	Significance	
Total	249/303 (82.2%)	54/303 (17.8%)		
		Ethnicity		
White	164/249 (65.9%)	32/54 (59.3%)		
Black	23/249 (9.2%)	5/54 (9.3%)	$p = 0.515$	
South Asian	39/249 (15.7%)	13/54 (24.1%)		
Other	23/249 (9.2%)	4/54 (7.4%)		
		Age in years		
Median (IQR)	61 (51–71)	54 (51–62)	$p < 0.001$	
		Family History		
Positive	28/249 (11.2%)	24/54 (44.4%)	$p < 0.001$	
Negative	221/249 (88.8%)	30/54 (55.6%)		
		Histology		
HGSC	207/249 (83.1%)	52/54 (96.3%)	$p = 0.010$	
All others	42/249 (16.9%)	2/52 (3.7%)		
		Stage		
Early stage	57/249 (22.9%)	10/54 (18.5%)	$p = 0.589$	
Advanced stage	192/249 (77.1%)	44/54 (81.5%)		
	No Pathogenic Variants	Total Germline or Somatic Pathogenic Variants (PV)	Germline PV	Somatic PV
Total	234/303 (77.2%)	69/303 (22.8%) *	54/303 (17.8%)	15/232 (6.5%) *
		Timing of surgery		
Primary surgery	115/234 (49.1%)	30/69 (43.5%)	23/54 (42.6%)	7/15 (46.7%)
Interval surgery	69/234 (29.5%)	28/69 (40.6%)	23/54 (42.6%)	5/15 (33.3%)
Delayed surgery	12/234 (5.1%)	4/69 (5.8%)	2/54 (3.7%)	2/15 (13.3%)
no surgery	38/234 (16.1%)	7/69 (10.1%)	1/54 (1.9%)	1/15 (6.7%)
significance		$p = 0.307$		
		Disease status of ovarian cancer at time of counselling		
New diagnosis	126/234 (53.8%)	41/69 (59.4%)	35/54 (64.8%)	6/15 (40%)
Under follow up	108/234 (46.2%)	28/69 (40.6%)	19/54 (35.2%)	9/15 (60%)
significance		$p = 0.463$		
		Chemotherapy response score		
1	4/234 (1.7%)	0	0	0
2	52/234 (22.2%)	13/69 (18.8%)	12/54 (22.2%)	1/15 (6.7%)
3	13/234 (5.6%)	13/69 (18.8%)	9/54 (16.7%)	4/15 (26.7%)
Not applicable	165/234 (70.5%)	43/69 (60.0%)	33/54 (61.1%)	10/15 (66.7)
significance		$p = 0.025$		

Table 2. Cont.

Category	No Germline Pathogenic Variants	Germline Pathogenic Variants	Significance	
	Resection (residual disease) status post surgery			
R0	175/234 (74.8%)	54/69 (78.2%)	42/54 (77.8%)	12/15 (80%)
R1	14/234 (6.0%)	4/69 (5.8%)	3/54 (5.6%)	1/15 (6.7%)
R2	7/234 (3.0%)	5/69 (7.2%)	3/54 (5.6%)	2/15 (13.3%)
Not applicable	38/234 (16.2%)	6/69 (8.7%)	6/54 (11.1%)	0/15 (0%)
significance		$p = 0.276$		
	Mutation Prevalence NELCN Cohort			
	Gene	n	Pathogenic (%)	VUS (%)
	NELCN cohort			
Germline	BRCA1	303	33 (11%)	3 (1.0%)
	BRCA2	303	14 (4.6%)	7 (2.3%)
	RAD51C	303	2 (0.7%)	2 (0.7%)
	RAD51D	303	3 (1.0%)	2 (0.7%)
	BRIP1	303	2 (0.7%)	6 (2.0%)
	Total Germline PVs	303	54 (17.8%)	20 (6.6%)
	Sequence PVs	54	48 (88.9%)	-
	LGR PVs	54	6 (11.1%)	-
Somatic	BRCA1	232	11 (3.6%)	1 (3%)
	BRCA2	232	4 (1.3%)	4 (1.3%)
	Total Somatic PVs	232	15 (6.6%)	5 (2.2%)
Total PVs		303	69 (22.8%)	25 (8.3%)

Pathogenic variants = class 4/5 variant in BRCA1, BRCA2, RAD51C, RAD51D, BRIP1. Family history positive = first-degree or second degree relative with ovary and/or breast cancer. HGSC = high grade serous carcinoma. Early stage = stage 1–2; advanced stage = stage 3–4. R0 = zero or nil residual disease, R1 = ≤1 cm residual disease, R2 = >1 cm residual disease. IQR = inter quartile range, PV = Pathogenic variants, VUS = Variants of uncertain significance, LGR- large genomic rearrangements. This table describes outcomes by two groups: (a) with and (b) without germline/somatic pathogenic variants. Two-sided p-values were reported for statistical tests comparing these two groups * Results of somatic testing at time of analysis for 71 patients were unavailable (only 232 patients had paired samples). Of these 71 patients 9 had a germline PV.

Validation of 3 mm FFPE punch biopsies for somatic testing:

Analysis of 3 mm Keyes punch biopsy and 5 × 5 μM unstained sections from the same FFPE tumour block demonstrated comparable DNA concentration and yield; therefore, archived tumour samples of patients under follow-up were processed as 3 mm core which proved time-efficient, as it reduced consultant pathologist time needed for review, retrieval and marking of slides. This is therefore likely to be more cost-efficient (Table 3).

Table 3. Comparison of DNA concentration and yield from FFPE 3 mm core and unstained sections of tumour tissue.

Case ID	DNA Concentration (ng/μL)		DNA Yield (μg)	
	Slides	Punch	Slides	Punch
Case 1	69.35	176.4	6.94	17.64
Case 2	40.16	60.49	4.02	6.05
Case 3	25.12	69.64	2.51	6.96
Case 4	45.19	115.9	4.52	11.59
Case 5	54.02	41.93	5.40	4.19

Table 3 describes the validation data of DNA yield from FFPE 3 mm core biopsies and unstained sections of tumour tissue.

Tumour testing results were available for 232 NELCN cases. Of the 71 cases without tumour testing results, 40 cases lacked available archived tumour tissue for analysis (unable to retrieve from pathology archive or surgery at another cancer centre); and 25 archived cases lacked any tissue with adequate neoplastic content (minimal diagnostic biopsy or post-chemotherapy tumour necrosis leaving no viable sample for analysis); and six test results were awaited at the time of analysis (delays due to COVID pandemic). Of these 71 cases without a somatic result, nine had a PV on germline genetic testing (four *BRCA1*, three *BRCA2*, one *RAD51C*, one *RAD51D*). Of the 232 NELCN tumour samples that underwent testing, 19 (8.9%) failed analysis due to fragmented DNA or low neoplastic content. Of these failed 19 cases, one had a *BRCA1* PV and one a *RAD51D* PV on germline testing. Further details on tumour tissue processing are provided in Table 4. The failure rate was higher for diagnostic biopsies (22.9%; 11/48) compared to primary cytoreductive surgical specimens (5.4%; 6/110) and post-chemotherapy surgical specimens (2.7%; 2/74). Primary-surgery specimens that failed analysis were due to fragmented DNA. There were 11 (out of 232) samples categorised with <20% neoplastic content, of which five (45%) were subsequently found to be adequate for analysis (Table 4). A majority of the samples were sent for analysis as 3 mm core biopsies from paraffin blocks (174/232, 75%) and the rest as unstained slides (58/232, 25%). Failure rates were 3/174 (1.7%) in 3 mm cores and 16/58 (27.6%) in unstained slides, respectively. However, 6/16 failed analysis in the unstained slides group had <20% neoplastic content. In our centre, tissue was preferentially sent as unstained slides if neoplastic content was <20% or the sample was a small volume diagnostic biopsy.

Table 4. NELCN tumour tissue *BRCA1/BRCA2* next generation sequencing analysis.

Category	Successfully Reported (*n*,%)	Failed Analysis (*n*,%)
Total number of samples	213/232 (91.8%)	19/232 (8.9%) *
Type of tissue		
Pre-chemo diagnostic biopsy	37/48 (77.1%)	11/48 (22.9%)
Primary surgery	104/110 (94.5%)	6/110 (5.5%)
Post-chemo cytoreductive surgery	72/74 (97.3%)	2/74 (2.7%)
Type of tumour sample		
3 mm core from FFPE	171/174 (98.3%)	3/174 (1.7%)
5 × 5 µM unstained slides	42/58 (72.4%)	16/58 (27.6%)
Neoplastic content		
<20%	5/11 (45.5%)	6/11 (54.5%)
20–50%	33/40 (82.5%)	7/40 (17.5%)
>50%	175/181 (96.7%)	6/181 (3.4%)

This table describes the results of BRCA testing of tumour tissue in the NELCN cohort. Results are available for 232 cases. * Of the 19 failed analysis, one had a BRCA1 PV and one a RAD51D PV.

Genetic testing results:

Following multi-gene germline testing, 54 germline PVs were identified in 303 women from the NELCN cohort (Supplementary Table S1). Of these PVs, 33 (11%) were *BRCA1*; 14 (4.6%) *BRCA2*, 2 (0.7%) *RAD51C*, 3 (1.0%) *RAD51D* and 2 (0.7%) *BRIP1*). Six PVs were large genomic rearrangements (LGR) and detected by MLPA: four in *BRCA1*, one in *BRCA2* and one in *RAD51C*. The germline VUS rate in *BRCA1/BRCA2* was 3.3% (*n* = 10) and 3.3% (*n* = 10) in *RAD51C/RAD51D* and *BRIP1* (Table 5). Germline *BRCA1/BRCA2* testing in the Manchester cases identified 11 (9.5%) PVs, of which 8 (6.9%) were *BRCA1* and 3 (2.6%) were *BRCA2* PVs (Supplementary Table S1). Additionally, one *BRCA1* VUS was identified. The median age of the Manchester cohort was 63 years (IQR = 55–72). Overall, 14 Manchester patients had a strong FH of cancer. Four of the eleven germline PV had a strong FH, while seven lacked a strong FH and would have been missed without unselected testing. Combining data from NELCN and Manchester series, the total *BRCA1/BRCA2* germline PV rate was 15.5% (65/419) and *BRCA1/BRCA2* germline VUS rate was 2.6% (11/419).

Table 5. Mutation Prevalence (Manchester cohort).

	Gene	n	Pathogenic (%)	VUS (%)
Manchester Cohort				
Germline	BRCA1	116	8 (6.9%)	1 (0.9%)
	BRCA2	116	3 (2.6%)	
	Total Germline PVs		11 (9.5%)	
	Sequence PVs	11	10 (90.9%)	
	LGR PVs	11	1 (9.1%)	
Somatic	BRCA1	116	7 (6%)	1 (0.9%)
	BRCA2	116	5 (4.3%)	1 (0.9%)
	Total Somatic PVs		12 (10.3%)	2 (1.8%)
Total PVs		116	23 (19.8%)	

This table describes the prevalence of variants in the Manchester cohort. VUS—variants of uncertain significance. PV—pathogenic variants. LGR—Large genomic rearrangements.

A total of 232 tumour BRCA1/BRCA2 results were available at the time of analysis from NELCN cases. Somatic BRCA1/BRCA2 PVs were detected in 15 (6.6%) cases and the VUS rate was 2.2% (n = 5). Tumour BRCA1/BRCA2 testing in 116 Manchester cases identified 7 (6%) BRCA1 and 5 (4.3%) BRCA2 somatic PVs as well as 1 (0.9%) BRCA1 and 1 (0.9%) BRCA2 somatic VUS each (Table 5). The total BRCA1/BRCA2 somatic PV rate was 7.8% (27/348) and somatic VUS rate was 2% (7/348). A germline or somatic PV was identified in 22% (92/419) patients overall. The list of all the variants identified are detailed in Supplementary Table S1. PARP-i treatment was commenced in 49 (16%) NELCN women (27 following primary treatment and 22 following recurrence).

BRCA1/BRCA2 germline and somatic PV concordance:

Concordance of BRCA1/BRCA2 PV identified through germline and tumour testing was explored. This included 232 paired samples with results from NELCN and 116 paired samples with results from Manchester NHS Trust. There were six BRCA1/BRCA2 PVs that showed discordance between germline and tumour testing, five in the NELCN cases and one from the Manchester cases, comprising 10.3% of all germline PVs. Five of these six BRCA1/BRCA2 PVs were LGR that were not detected on somatic testing; one (3%) germline mutation (from NELCN cases) was initially reported in the somatic report but not in the germline. This mutation was then subsequently identified in the germline following re-analysis of the germline sample. The inability of routine somatic testing to reliably identify LGRs is an important finding with implications for those developing and/or implementing OC mainstreaming pathways and for those whose pathways currently use a somatic testing first triage mechanism. It is critical that patients with LGRs are not missed both from a cancer treatment perspective as well as for precision prevention in unaffected relatives with a PV identified through cascade testing.

Pathway improvements:

Changes to the NELCN pathway were incorporated over time to improve logistic efficiencies, communication between team members and timely communication of result to the patient. These included: agreement on a standardised format for reports received from genomic laboratories and omitting of reporting class-1 and class-2 variants. This improved interpretability by cancer clinicians and reduced unnecessary distress in patients.

Initially somatic reports were uploaded as supplementary reports to the original histology result but this caused delays in clinician receiving the information and communicating this to the patient. This was addressed by results being directly sent from the genomic laboratory creating to a shared email-box which was accessed by all members of the clinical team. Responsibility for monitoring and ensuring all results were actioned was subsequently undertaken by the lead medical oncologist.

Electronic communication with electronic request forms being sent directly to cellular pathology lead scientist rather than to the lead histopathologist, triggered the laboratory technician to pull the relevant blocks and slides for the attention of the gynaecological histopathologist, minimising the delay between clinician request and sample being sent to the genomic laboratory.

The NELCN has a Bengali speaking ethnic minority population, which varies from 3% to 33% depending on the borough. All patient facing documents were translated into Bengali to improve engagement and communication with Bengali patients and family members as well as improve decision making. Additionally, a Bengali-speaking clinical member of the extended team, acted as an advocate during genetic counselling.

4. Discussion

We demonstrate that unselected concomitant/parallel panel germline and somatic testing at OC diagnosis can be implemented within the NHS setting, and delivered by treating cancer clinicians/professionals through a cancer-MDT coordinated approach. Pre-test counselling was undertaken by all members of the cancer MDT team including medical oncologists, surgical oncologists and CNSs. Consistent with other reports of high uptake rates for *BRCA* testing [23,32–34], we showed this high acceptability extends to panel germline and somatic genetic testing too, with an uptake rate of 97%. PV carriers were younger, more likely to have a strong FH of cancer, HGSC histology and a CRS of 3 at histology. PV status was independent ethnicity, stage at diagnosis, timing of surgery or resection status. We undertook genetic testing prospectively for newly diagnosed patients and also for patients undergoing follow-up. Restricting this to prospective implementation of newly diagnosed cases alone (as has been implemented in some centres) would have missed 19 (19/54, 35.1%) germline PVs which were detected in the follow-up patients, thus significantly affecting screening/prevention options for these unaffected family members. A total of 56% of PVs would have been missed by using an FH based approach alone, reconfirming the importance of unselected testing and a mainstreaming approach. This is consistent with reports from others who also showed that around 50% PVs lacked a strong FH of BC or OC [23,33]. The *BRCA* PV prevalence in our NELCN cohort was higher than the Manchester cohort. Some boroughs in North East of London are known to have an Ashkenazi Jewish (AJ) population and the presence of AJ founder mutations in seven NELCN OC cases (Supplementary Table S1) is a contributory factor towards this as *BRCA* PV are commoner in AJ compared to non-AJ general population OC cases [35]. We found seven AJ BRCA founder mutations in the NELCN cohort but none of these patients self-reported Jewish ethnicity at recruitment. These patients may have had mixed parentage or grand-parentage and been unaware of their ethnicity or may have preferred not to report/disclose Jewish ethnicity. Additionally, NELCN includes 122 women who had previously been diagnosed and were alive at the time of commencement of the study. Although short term survival for *BRCA* PV carriers is higher, we did not find the sub-group of 122 women may be enriched for PV.

Our data show that over 1 in 5 (22%) patients have a PV which can affect their treatment, and 1 in 6 have a germline PV which can also affect predictive testing and screening and prevention in unaffected family members. This is consistent with some other reports in the literature [23,33,36,37]. Testing for a panel which includes *RAD51C, RAD51D, BRIP1* is not currently part of the NHS Genomics test directory and therefore not mandatory across the UK. However, it can if implemented identify an additional 13% (7/54) PVs, with a prevalence of 2.3% in OC patients, whose families can benefit from precision prevention. Rust et al. showed a slight increase in PVs detected with additional *RAD51C/RAD51D* testing but this was not completely unselected in their cohort and was undertaken either sequentially or in those with a strong FH [33]. Our data confirm the benefit of amending the UK test directory criteria to offer multi-gene panel testing to all UK women with OC. Our multi-gene germline test includes high- and intermediate risk genes which have already proven clinical utility [38]. A number of commercially available panels are available today which test for many more (30–100) genes. However, it is important that only genes of established clinical utility are tested for. We are against indiscriminate panel testing for genes without established clinical utility [39,40]. In addition to *RAD51C*, *RAD51D* and *BRIP1* genes, it would be appropriate for an OC panel to also include *PALB2* and Lynch Syndrome genes going forward. *PALB2* has recently been reported as a moderate risk OC gene [41] and Lynch Syndrome (MMR) genes may be found in another 1% OC patients [42–44]. Some initial reports suggest that cascade testing rates may be lower following mainstreaming compared to testing in clinical genetics [34]. However, all our patients with PVs are reviewed in clinical genetics teams, who are responsible for facilitating cascade testing. Additionally, cascade testing rates are likely to increase with longer follow up.

As multiple genes get incorporated into OC testing panels, the reported VUS rate will also increase. Our germline panel VUS rate was 6.6% and is comparable to that reported by others [45,46]. VUS reporting and subsequent management can pose challenges for counselling, variant monitoring and onwards risk management. This will become an increasingly important issue with widening of the panel of genes tested for [47]. Risk reducing surgery, chemoprevention, screening or downstream predictive testing for unaffected family members, is not recommended in individuals with a VUS. Our report also highlights the importance of uniform classification and standardised reporting of class 3 variants (VUS) across genetic laboratories, including the description in clinical reports issued. The Cancer Variant Interpretation Group UK (CanVIG-UK) now provides an exemplar of a multidisciplinary network addressing this nationally [30]. This improves interpretability of reports by cancer clinicians. Appropriate pre-test education of patients and providers is necessary to limit the harm that could result from VUS misinterpretation. While not of immediate direct relevance, a proportion of VUS will be reclassified in the future to PVs and then have implications for the patients and relatives. This reclassification rate has been reported as around 9% in a large cohort [48]. In our cohort, a germline mutation *BRCA1* c.442-22_442-13del reported in somatic but missed in initial germline (identified in re-analysis of germline) was initially reported as Class 3 VUS and subsequently a year on from testing, was re-classified as a PV.

Strengths of this study include prospective design and systematic approach to include all patients including those on follow up, as well as the high acceptability and uptake rates demonstrated with our pathway and testing process. The upfront staff training implemented across the pathway and continued support provided along-with broad stakeholder engagement contributed to improved patient experience and satisfaction. The extra efforts undertaken to engage with our ethnic minority Bengali population is another strength. In order to broaden access and informed decision making we translated information sheets into local Bengali language and trained a Bangladeshi oncology team member who was instrumental in engaging them in genetic counselling. Our analysis also demonstrates likely success rates for tumour testing for different types of samples which can be helpful for counselling patients and planning services. Limitations include lack of qualitative data and long term follow up data on patient outcomes. These are being collected.

Mainstreaming models such as ours delivered by the cancer MDT team enables implementation of large-scale genetic testing at cancer diagnosis. This approach too can encompass more than one pre-test counselling session where needed. A total of 22% women needed and received more than one pre-test counselling session in our study. Most other mainstreaming studies do not report on the number of pre-test counselling sessions needed or if multiple were offered. Our clinical nurse specialists favoured utilising more appointments/consultations prior to recruitment. While we did not undertake a formal quantitative assessment of reasons for multiple consultations, colleague feedback indicates these included, some patients needing more time to assimilate information and reflect on it before deciding and/or the need to discuss further with family before decision making; as well as a clinical assessment of not overloading the patient with too much information at the first setting especially if they were struggling with managing decision making and information related to their cancer care at the appointment. The issues of some initially long consultations and time pressures in a busy oncology clinic also contributed to this. Other examples of models used to deliver unselected genetic testing at OC diagnosis include a genetics team embedded in oncology clinics, [25] genetic nurse coordinated model [24] and medical oncology [32] delivered testing.

Validation and implementation of 3 mm cored biopsies from FFPE tumour blocks enabled time- and resource-efficient processing of archived samples. This is particularly suited for archived FFPE tissue (analysis of retrospective cases) and gave a comparable/higher DNA yield than that obtained through slides. Although, we were unable to test 21% of archived tumour samples, undertaking tumour testing at time of diagnosis for future cases will overcome this. Our pathway now incorporates pathology processing/preparation for genetic testing for all cases at the time of routine histopathology analysis of the initial diagnostic or surgical specimen itself. As a large proportion of failed analysis was pre-treatment diagnostic biopsies, we now routinely obtain additional tissue cores for all women suspected of advanced ovarian malignancy at the time of their diagnostic biopsy. This minimises additional pathology laboratory resources needed and is more cost and time efficient. We also provide estimates of failure rates of diagnostic biopsy (~23%), which is relevant for counselling and management of patients planned for neo-adjuvant chemotherapy. NHS Laboratory guidelines suggest the minimum tumour content for NGS somatic/tumour testing referrals should be 20% [13]. However, we showed benefit of undertaking tumour testing even with <20% content in 45% of such cases. Hence, tumour testing should not be held back in cases with low tumour content as it could be successful in almost half these cases, thus identifying additional women who may benefit from PARP-i treatment.

There has been debate whether both germline and somatic testing should be offered to all; whether unselected germline testing should be offered as first line, followed by somatic testing if germline is negative for PV; or whether reflex somatic testing should be done first, reserving germline if a somatic PV is identified. PVs caused by large genomic rearrangements (LGRs) are missed when PCR-based testing alone is used [49,50]. MLPA is a commonly/routinely used technique to detect LGRs and is found to be highly sensitive and inexpensive [51,52]. LGRs are far more prevalent in *BRCA1* than *BRCA2* genes and have been reported to account for a wide range of *BRCA1* (up to 27%) and *BRCA2* (up to 11%) PVs [53–55]. In a large study, LGRs were reported to constitute around 24% of *BRCA1/BRCA2* PVs in high-risk breast/ovarian cancer families, [55] while lower rates are reported in other series and in individuals without strong family histories [53,55,56]. Reports suggest significant ethnic variation in the presence of LGR-related PVs: [55] African (2.4%), Caribbean and Latin American (6.7%), Danish (9.2%) and Spanish ancestry (14.5%) [55–57]. A disadvantage of using an initial tumour/somatic testing triage strategy is the possibility of missing LGRs. The 11% LGR-rate in our cohort (6/54) is similar to the LGR rate reported in some high-risk breast and ovarian cancer families [54]. In the majority of diagnostic laboratories, NGS tumour/somatic *BRCA*-testing is not validated for detection of LGRs [50]. While sequential tumour/somatic followed by germline testing may be a less costly approach [58], this strategy runs the risk of missing some germline PVs, particularly LGRs. This can have significant consequences for cancer prevention in families which are missed. Additionally, although reflex tumour testing can identify PVs seen in the germline, up to 31% of patients found to have a PV in the tumour may not get referred for genetic counselling or germline testing [59]. This highlights a potential limitation of a somatic first strategy, and the need for more robust implementation pathways with built in quality control and fail-safe mechanisms.

In contrast to our findings, a few earlier reports suggest 100% concordance between somatic and germline testing [45,60,61]. However, the proportion of LGRs amongst the *BRCA* mutations reported in these studies is unknown, as these have not been described. It is probable/likely that these studies did not have any LGRs in their mutation spectrum. In our cohort, somatic *BRCA*-testing alone, would have missed 9.2% (4/54) of *BRCA1/BRCA2* germline PVs and seven PVs in *RAD51C/RAD51D* and *BRIP1*, which comprise 20% (11/54) of germline PVs detected from 5-gene panel testing, who can benefit from targeted therapy and downstream predictive testing.

Germline-testing alone would have missed 2% (1/54) germline *BRCA1/BRCA2* PVs, and 15 somatic PVs, comprising 23.1% (16/69) of all *BRCA1/BRCA2* PVs in this cohort, who can benefit from PARP-i treatment. The germline PV missed is an error, which is unlikely to be repeated. A germline first followed by a somatic testing strategy could be an alternative option, but this approach will lead to a longer delay in turn-around times and increase clinician counselling time for giving results as this will need to be done twice. It is also likely to increase the laboratory processing and reporting time and costs, as this is undertaken after initial diagnosis (not contemporaneously with diagnostic reporting). In our experience, a simultaneous or parallel somatic/tumour and germline strategy is a more efficient approach for patients.

5. Conclusions

We demonstrate successful implementation of unselected 5-panel germline and concomitant somatic *BRCA1/BRCA2* testing for patients with OC. *BRCA1/BRCA2* germline PVs were identified in 15.5% patients and *BRCA1/BRCA2* somatic PVs in 7.8%. *RAD51C/RAD51D/ BRIP1* PVs comprised 13% of PVs and were identified in an additional 2.3% patients. A total of 11% germline PVs are LGRs and are missed by a somatic first testing strategy. A total of 20% of germline PVs would be missed if somatic *BRCA*-testing alone was used to triage for germline testing. A total of 55.6% germline PVs would have been missed by using FH ascertainment alone. The somatic testing failure rate is higher (23%) for patients undergoing diagnostic biopsies. Retrospective archival FFPE tissue testing is feasible using 3 mm punch biopsies from tumour blocks. Our findings favour a prospective parallel somatic and germline panel testing approach as a clinically efficient strategy which maximises variant identification for clinical benefit. The UK Genomics test directory criteria should be expanded to include a panel of OC genes. Formal cost-effectiveness analysis for panel testing is needed and can facilitate wider clinical implementation.

Supplementary Materials: The following are available online at https://www.mdpi.com/article/10 .3390/cancers13174344/s1, Table S1: List of variants identified through germline and somatic testing.

Author Contributions: Conceptualization, R.M.; methodology, R.M., N.S., R.L., M.L. and D.G.E.; formal analysis, R.M., D.C., O.B. and D.G.E.; Implementation and Investigation, R.M., D.C., R.E.M., S.M.C., A.W., L.A.J., N.S., D.G.E., R.L., A.F., A.J., E.B., A.K., M.L., R.W. and M.Q.; resources, R.M., D.C., R.E.M., M.S., O.E., S.M.C., F.G., R.F.L.H., L.S., L.A.J., M.A., A.K., A.J., A.C.L., E.B., S.P., M.Q., T.M.-B., F.E.K., A.F., L.C., G.T., G.J.B., H.S., M.B., P.S., N.L.B., A.W., N.S. and D.G.E.; data curation, D.C., RM, O.B. and D.G.E.; writing—original draft preparation, R.M., M.S., D.C. and D.G.E.; writing—review and editing, All authors; supervision, R.M.; project administration, R.M., D.C. and M.S.; funding acquisition, R.M. All authors have read and agreed to the published version of the manuscript.

Funding: The study is funded by The Barts Charity, grant ECMG1B6R.

Institutional Review Board Statement: The study was conducted according to the guidelines of the Declaration of Helsinki, and approved by the Ethics Committee of London Riverside Ethics Committee (reference number 17/LO/0405).

Informed Consent Statement: Informed consent was obtained from all study participants.

Data Availability Statement: The data that support the findings of this study are available from the corresponding author, R.M. upon reasonable request.

Acknowledgments: D.G.E. is supported by the Manchester NIHR Biomedical Research Centre (IS-BRC-1215-20007). OB thanks the Ministry of Science and Higher Education of the Russian Federation within the framework of state support for the creation and development of World-Class Research Center „Digital biodesign and personalized healthcare" 075-15-2020-926.

Conflicts of Interest: R.M. declares research funding from Barts and the London Charity and Rosetrees Trust outside this work, an honorarium for grant review from Israel National Institute for Health Policy Research and honorarium for advisory board membership from AstraZeneca/MSD/GSK. R.M. is supported by an NHS Innovation Accelerator (NIA) Fellowship for population testing. The funders had no role in the design of the study; in the collection, analyses, or interpretation of data; in the writing of the manuscript, or in the decision to publish the results. FG declares research funding from The NHS Grampian Endowment Fund, Medtronic and Karl Storz outside this work.

References

1. International Agency for Research on Cancer. Cancer Tomorrow. In *A Tool That Predicts the Future Cancer Incidence and Mortality Burden Worldwide from the Current Estimates in 2018 Up Until 2040*; International Agency for Research on Cancer (IARC): Lyon, France, 2018.
2. CRUK. Ovarian cancer statistics. In *Ovarian Cancer Incidence*; Cancer Research UK: London, UK, 2017.
3. Collins, F.S.; Varmus, H. A new initiative on precision medicine. *N. Engl. J. Med.* **2015**, *372*, 793–795. [CrossRef] [PubMed]
4. Kuchenbaecker, K.B.; Hopper, J.L.; Barnes, D.R.; Phillips, K.A.; Mooij, T.M.; Roos-Blom, M.J.; Jervis, S.; van Leeuwen, F.E.; Milne, R.L.; Andrieu, N.; et al. Risks of Breast, Ovarian, and Contralateral Breast Cancer for BRCA1 and BRCA2 Mutation Carriers. *JAMA* **2017**, *317*, 2402–2416. [CrossRef] [PubMed]
5. Schettini, F.; Giudici, F.; Bernocchi, O.; Sirico, M.; Corona, S.P.; Giuliano, M.; Locci, M.; Paris, I.; Scambia, G.; De Placido, S.; et al. Poly (ADP-ribose) polymerase inhibitors in solid tumours: Systematic review and meta-analysis. *Eur. J. Cancer* **2021**, *149*, 134–152. [CrossRef] [PubMed]
6. Ledermann, J.; Harter, P.; Gourley, C.; Friedlander, M.; Vergote, I.; Rustin, G.; Scott, C.L.; Meier, W.; Shapira-Frommer, R.; Safra, T.; et al. Olaparib maintenance therapy in patients with platinum-sensitive relapsed serous ovarian cancer: A preplanned retrospective analysis of outcomes by BRCA status in a randomised phase 2 trial. *Lancet Oncol.* **2014**, *15*, 852–861. [CrossRef]
7. Moore, K.; Colombo, N.; Scambia, G.; Kim, B.G.; Oaknin, A.; Friedlander, M.; Lisyanskaya, A.; Floquet, A.; Leary, A.; Sonke, G.S.; et al. Maintenance Olaparib in Patients with Newly Diagnosed Advanced Ovarian Cancer. *N. Engl. J. Med.* **2018**, *379*, 2495–2505. [CrossRef]
8. Coleman, R.L.; Oza, A.M.; Lorusso, D.; Aghajanian, C.; Oaknin, A.; Dean, A.; Colombo, N.; Weberpals, J.I.; Clamp, A.; Scambia, G.; et al. Rucaparib maintenance treatment for recurrent ovarian carcinoma after response to platinum therapy (ARIEL3): A randomised, double-blind, placebo-controlled, phase 3 trial. *Lancet* **2017**, *390*, 1949–1961. [CrossRef]
9. Pujade-Lauraine, E.; Ledermann, J.A.; Selle, F.; Gebski, V.; Penson, R.T.; Oza, A.M.; Korach, J.; Huzarski, T.; Poveda, A.; Pignata, S.; et al. Olaparib tablets as maintenance therapy in patients with platinum-sensitive, relapsed ovarian cancer and a BRCA1/2 mutation (SOLO2/ENGOT-Ov21): A double-blind, randomised, placebo-controlled, phase 3 trial. *Lancet Oncol.* **2017**, *18*, 1274–1284. [CrossRef]
10. NHS England. *Clinical Commissioning Policy: Genetic Testing for BRCA1 and BRCA2 Mutations*; NHS England Specialised Services Clinical Reference Group for Medical Genetics: London, UK, 2015.
11. Practice Bulletin No 182: Hereditary Breast and Ovarian Cancer Syndrome. *Obstet. Gynecol.* **2017**, *130*, e110–e126. [CrossRef]
12. Konstantinopoulos, P.A.; Norquist, B.; Lacchetti, C.; Armstrong, D.; Grisham, R.N.; Goodfellow, P.J.; Kohn, E.C.; Levine, D.A.; Liu, J.F.; Lu, K.H.; et al. Germline and Somatic Tumor Testing in Epithelial Ovarian Cancer: ASCO Guideline. *J. Clin. Oncol.* **2020**, *38*, 1222–1245. [CrossRef]
13. Sundar, S.; Manchanda, R.; Gourley, C.; George, A.; Wallace, A.; Balega, J.; Williams, S.; Wallis, Y.; Edmondson, R.; Nicum, S.; et al. British Gynaecological Cancer Society/British Association of Gynaecological Pathology consensus for germline and tumour testing for BRCA1/2 variants in ovarian cancer in the United Kingdom. *Int. J. Gynecol. Cancer* **2021**, *31*, 272–278.
14. Miller, R.E.; Leary, A.; Scott, C.L.; Serra, V.; Lord, C.J.; Bowtell, D.; Chang, D.K.; Garsed, D.W.; Jonkers, J.; Ledermann, J.A.; et al. ESMO recommendations on predictive biomarker testing for homologous recombination deficiency and PARP inhibitor benefit in ovarian cancer. *Ann. Oncol.* **2020**, *31*, 1606–1622. [CrossRef]
15. Norquist, B.M.; Brady, M.F.; Harrell, M.I.; Walsh, T.; Lee, M.K.; Gulsuner, S.; Bernards, S.S.; Casadei, S.; Burger, R.A.; Tewari, K.S.; et al. Mutations in Homologous Recombination Genes and Outcomes in Ovarian Carcinoma Patients in GOG 218: An NRG Oncology/Gynecologic Oncology Group Study. *Clin. Cancer Res.* **2018**, *24*, 777–783. [CrossRef]
16. Ramus, S.J.; Song, H.; Dicks, E.; Tyrer, J.P.; Rosenthal, A.N.; Intermaggio, M.P.; Fraser, L.; Gentry-Maharaj, A.; Hayward, J.; Philpott, S.; et al. Germline Mutations in the BRIP1, BARD1, PALB2, and NBN Genes in Women With Ovarian Cancer. *J. Natl. Cancer Inst.* **2015**, *107*, djv214. [CrossRef] [PubMed]
17. Yang, X.; Song, H.; Leslie, G.; Engel, C.; Hahnen, E.; Auber, B.; Horvath, J.; Kast, K.; Niederacher, D.; Turnbull, C.; et al. Ovarian and breast cancer risks associated with pathogenic variants in RAD51C and RAD51D. *J. Natl. Cancer Inst.* **2020**, *112*, 1242–1250. [CrossRef] [PubMed]
18. Domchek, S.M.; Robson, M.E. Update on Genetic Testing in Gynecologic Cancer. *J. Clin. Oncol.* **2019**, *37*, 2501–2509. [CrossRef] [PubMed]
19. Finch, A.; Beiner, M.; Lubinski, J.; Lynch, H.T.; Moller, P.; Rosen, B.; Murphy, J.; Ghadirian, P.; Friedman, E.; Foulkes, W.D.; et al. Salpingo-oophorectomy and the risk of ovarian, fallopian tube, and peritoneal cancers in women with a BRCA1 or BRCA2 Mutation. *JAMA* **2006**, *296*, 185–192. [CrossRef]

20. Rebbeck, T.R.; Kauff, N.D.; Domchek, S.M. Meta-analysis of risk reduction estimates associated with risk-reducing salpingo-oophorectomy in BRCA1 or BRCA2 mutation carriers. *J. Natl. Cancer Inst.* **2009**, *101*, 80–87. [CrossRef]
21. Rebbeck, T.R.; Friebel, T.; Lynch, H.T.; Neuhausen, S.L.; van 't Veer, L.; Garber, J.E.; Evans, G.R.; Narod, S.A.; Isaacs, C.; Matloff, E.; et al. Bilateral prophylactic mastectomy reduces breast cancer risk in BRCA1 and BRCA2 mutation carriers: The PROSE Study Group. *J. Clin. Oncol.* **2004**, *22*, 1055–1062. [CrossRef]
22. Cuzick, J.; Sestak, I.; Bonanni, B.; Costantino, J.P.; Cummings, S.; DeCensi, A.; Dowsett, M.; Forbes, J.F.; Ford, L.; LaCroix, A.Z.; et al. Selective oestrogen receptor modulators in prevention of breast cancer: An updated meta-analysis of individual participant data. *Lancet* **2013**, *381*, 1827–1834. [CrossRef]
23. George, A.; Riddell, D.; Seal, S.; Talukdar, S.; Mahamdallie, S.; Ruark, E.; Cloke, V.; Slade, I.; Kemp, Z.; Gore, M.; et al. Implementing rapid, robust, cost-effective, patient-centred, routine genetic testing in ovarian cancer patients. *Sci. Rep.* **2016**, *6*, 29506. [CrossRef]
24. Plaskocinska, I.; Shipman, H.; Drummond, J.; Thompson, E.; Buchanan, V.; Newcombe, B.; Hodgkin, C.; Barter, E.; Ridley, P.; Ng, R.; et al. New paradigms for BRCA1/BRCA2 testing in women with ovarian cancer: Results of the Genetic Testing in Epithelial Ovarian Cancer (GTEOC) study. *J. Med. Genet.* **2016**, *53*, 655–661. [CrossRef]
25. Senter, L.; O'Malley, D.M.; Backes, F.J.; Copeland, L.J.; Fowler, J.M.; Salani, R.; Cohn, D.E. Genetic consultation embedded in a gynecologic oncology clinic improves compliance with guideline-based care. *Gynecol. Oncol.* **2017**, *147*, 110–114. [CrossRef] [PubMed]
26. Childers, C.P.; Childers, K.K.; Maggard-Gibbons, M.; Macinko, J. National Estimates of Genetic Testing in Women with a History of Breast or Ovarian Cancer. *J. Clin. Oncol.* **2017**, *35*, 3800–3806. [CrossRef]
27. Kurian, A.W.; Ward, K.C.; Howlader, N.; Deapen, D.; Hamilton, A.S.; Mariotto, A.; Miller, D.; Penberthy, L.S.; Katz, S.J. Genetic Testing and Results in a Population-Based Cohort of Breast Cancer Patients and Ovarian Cancer Patients. *J. Clin. Oncol.* **2019**, *37*, 1305–1315. [CrossRef] [PubMed]
28. Randall, L.M.; Pothuri, B.; Swisher, E.M.; Diaz, J.P.; Buchanan, A.; Witkop, C.T.; Bethan Powell, C.; Smith, E.B.; Robson, M.E.; Boyd, J.; et al. Multi-disciplinary summit on genetics services for women with gynecologic cancers: A Society of Gynecologic Oncology White Paper. *Gynecol. Oncol.* **2017**, *146*, 217–224. [CrossRef]
29. Ellard, S.; Baple, E.L.; Berry, I.; Forrester, N.; Turnbull, C.; Owens, M.; Eccles, D.M.; Abbs, S.; Scott, R.; Deans, Z.; et al. *ACGS Best Practice Guidelines for Variant Classification in Rare Disease 2020*; Association for Clinical Genomic Science (ACGS): London, UK, 2020. Available online: https://www.acgs.uk.com/quality/best-practice-guidelines/ (accessed on 1 May 2021).
30. Garrett, A.; Callaway, A.; Durkie, M.; Cubuk, C.; Alikian, M.; Burghel, G.J.; Robinson, R.; Izatt, L.; Talukdar, S.; Side, L.; et al. Cancer Variant Interpretation Group UK (CanVIG-UK): An exemplar national subspecialty multidisciplinary network. *J. Med. Genet.* **2020**, *57*, 829–834. [CrossRef] [PubMed]
31. Ellison, G.; Huang, S.; Carr, H.; Wallace, A.; Ahdesmaki, M.; Bhaskar, S.; Mills, J. A reliable method for the detection of BRCA1 and BRCA2 mutations in fixed tumour tissue utilising multiplex PCR-based targeted next generation sequencing. *BMC Clin. Pathol.* **2015**, *15*, 5. [CrossRef] [PubMed]
32. Rumford, M.; Lythgoe, M.; McNeish, I.; Gabra, H.; Tookman, L.; Rahman, N.; George, A.; Krell, J. Oncologist-led BRCA 'mainstreaming' in the ovarian cancer clinic: A study of 255 patients and its impact on their management. *Sci. Rep.* **2020**, *10*, 3390. [CrossRef] [PubMed]
33. Rust, K.; Spiliopoulou, P.; Tang, C.Y.; Bell, C.; Stirling, D.; Phang, T.; Davidson, R.; Mackean, M.; Nussey, F.; Glasspool, R.M.; et al. Routine germline BRCA1 and BRCA2 testing in patients with ovarian carcinoma: Analysis of the Scottish real-life experience. *BJOG* **2018**, *125*, 1451–1458. [CrossRef]
34. Flaum, N.; Morgan, R.D.; Burghel, G.J.; Bulman, M.; Clamp, A.R.; Hasan, J.; Mitchell, C.L.; Badea, D.; Moon, S.; Hogg, M.; et al. Mainstreaming germline BRCA1/2 testing in non-mucinous epithelial ovarian cancer in the North West of England. *Eur. J. Hum. Genet.* **2020**, *28*, 1541–1547. [CrossRef] [PubMed]
35. Modan, B.; Hartge, P.; Hirsh-Yechezkel, G.; Chetrit, A.; Lubin, F.; Beller, U.; Ben-Baruch, G.; Fishman, A.; Menczer, J.; Ebbers, S.M.; et al. Parity, oral contraceptives, and the risk of ovarian cancer among carriers and noncarriers of a BRCA1 or BRCA2 mutation. *N. Engl. J. Med.* **2001**, *345*, 235–240. [CrossRef]
36. Rahman, B.; Lanceley, A.; Kristeleit, R.S.; Ledermann, J.A.; Lockley, M.; McCormack, M.; Mould, T.; Side, L. Mainstreamed genetic testing for women with ovarian cancer: First-year experience. *J. Med. Genet.* **2019**, *56*, 195–198. [CrossRef] [PubMed]
37. Norquist, B.M.; Harrell, M.I.; Brady, M.F.; Walsh, T.; Lee, M.K.; Gulsuner, S.; Bernards, S.S.; Casadei, S.; Yi, Q.; Burger, R.A.; et al. Inherited Mutations in Women with Ovarian Carcinoma. *JAMA Oncol.* **2016**, *2*, 482–490. [CrossRef] [PubMed]
38. Manchanda, R.; Legood, R.; Antoniou, A.C.; Gordeev, V.S.; Menon, U. Specifying the ovarian cancer risk threshold of 'pre-menopausal risk-reducing salpingo-oophorectomy' for ovarian cancer prevention: A cost-effectiveness analysis. *J. Med. Genet.* **2016**, *53*, 591–599. [CrossRef]
39. CDC. ACCE Model Process for Evaluating Genetic Tests. In *Genomic Testing*; The Office of Public Health Genomics (OPHG), Centers for Disease Control and Prevention (CDC): Atlanta, GA, USA, 2010. Available online: http://www.cdc.gov/genomics/gtesting/ACCE/ (accessed on 1 January 2021).
40. Burke, W.; Zimmerman, R. *Moving beyond ACCE: An Expanded Framework for Genetic Test. Evaluation*; PHG Foundation: London, UK, 2007.

41. Yang, X.; Leslie, G.; Doroszuk, A.; Schneider, S.; Allen, J.; Decker, B.; Dunning, A.M.; Redman, J.; Scarth, J.; Plaskocinska, I.; et al. Cancer Risks Associated with Germline PALB2 Pathogenic Variants: An International Study of 524 Families. *J. Clin. Oncol.* **2020**, *38*, 674–685. [CrossRef]
42. Pal, T.; Akbari, M.R.; Sun, P.; Lee, J.H.; Fulp, J.; Thompson, Z.; Coppola, D.; Nicosia, S.; Sellers, T.A.; McLaughlin, J.; et al. Frequency of mutations in mismatch repair genes in a population-based study of women with ovarian cancer. *Br. J. Cancer* **2012**, *107*, 1783–1790. [CrossRef]
43. Song, H.; Cicek, M.S.; Dicks, E.; Harrington, P.; Ramus, S.J.; Cunningham, J.M.; Fridley, B.L.; Tyrer, J.P.; Alsop, J.; Jimenez-Linan, M.; et al. The contribution of deleterious germline mutations in BRCA1, BRCA2 and the mismatch repair genes to ovarian cancer in the population. *Hum. Mol. Genet.* **2014**, *23*, 4703–4709. [CrossRef]
44. Minion, L.E.; Dolinsky, J.S.; Chase, D.M.; Dunlop, C.L.; Chao, E.C.; Monk, B.J. Hereditary predisposition to ovarian cancer, looking beyond BRCA1/BRCA2. *Gynecol. Oncol.* **2015**, *137*, 86–92. [CrossRef] [PubMed]
45. Fumagalli, C.; Tomao, F.; Betella, I.; Rappa, A.; Calvello, M.; Bonanni, B.; Bernard, L.; Peccatori, F.; Colombo, N.; Viale, G.; et al. Tumor BRCA Test for Patients with Epithelial Ovarian Cancer: The Role of Molecular Pathology in the Era of PARP Inhibitor Therapy. *Cancers* **2019**, *11*, 1641. [CrossRef] [PubMed]
46. Zuntini, R.; Ferrari, S.; Bonora, E.; Buscherini, F.; Bertonazzi, B.; Grippa, M.; Godino, L.; Miccoli, S.; Turchetti, D. Dealing With BRCA1/2 Unclassified Variants in a Cancer Genetics Clinic: Does Cosegregation Analysis Help? *Front. Genet.* **2018**, *9*, 378. [CrossRef] [PubMed]
47. Eccles, D.M.; Mitchell, G.; Monteiro, A.N.; Schmutzler, R.; Couch, F.J.; Spurdle, A.B.; Gomez-Garcia, E.B.; Group, E.C.W. BRCA1 and BRCA2 genetic testing-pitfalls and recommendations for managing variants of uncertain clinical significance. *Ann. Oncol.* **2015**, *26*, 2057–2065. [CrossRef]
48. Mersch, J.; Brown, N.; Pirzadeh-Miller, S.; Mundt, E.; Cox, H.C.; Brown, K.; Aston, M.; Esterling, L.; Manley, S.; Ross, T. Prevalence of Variant Reclassification Following Hereditary Cancer Genetic Testing. *JAMA* **2018**, *320*, 1266–1274. [CrossRef]
49. Sluiter, M.D.; van Rensburg, E.J. Large genomic rearrangements of the BRCA1 and BRCA2 genes: Review of the literature and report of a novel BRCA1 mutation. *Breast Cancer Res. Treat.* **2011**, *125*, 325–349. [CrossRef] [PubMed]
50. Wallace, A.J. New challenges for BRCA testing: A view from the diagnostic laboratory. *Eur. J. Hum. Genet.* **2016**, *24* (Suppl. 1), S10–S18. [CrossRef] [PubMed]
51. Schouten, J.P.; McElgunn, C.J.; Waaijer, R.; Zwijnenburg, D.; Diepvens, F.; Pals, G. Relative quantification of 40 nucleic acid sequences by multiplex ligation-dependent probe amplification. *Nucleic Acids Res.* **2002**, *30*, e57. [CrossRef] [PubMed]
52. Bunyan, D.J.; Eccles, D.M.; Sillibourne, J.; Wilkins, E.; Thomas, N.S.; Shea-Simonds, J.; Duncan, P.J.; Curtis, C.E.; Robinson, D.O.; Harvey, J.F.; et al. Dosage analysis of cancer predisposition genes by multiplex ligation-dependent probe amplification. *Br. J. Cancer* **2004**, *91*, 1155–1159. [CrossRef]
53. Woodward, A.M.; Davis, T.A.; Silva, A.G.; Kirk, J.A.; Leary, J.A. Large genomic rearrangements of both BRCA2 and BRCA1 are a feature of the inherited breast/ovarian cancer phenotype in selected families. *J. Med. Genet.* **2005**, *42*, e31. [CrossRef]
54. James, P.A.; Sawyer, S.; Boyle, S.; Young, M.A.; Kovalenko, S.; Doherty, R.; McKinley, J.; Alsop, K.; Beshay, V.; Harris, M.; et al. Large genomic rearrangements in the familial breast and ovarian cancer gene BRCA1 are associated with an increased frequency of high risk features. *Fam. Cancer* **2015**, *14*, 287–295. [CrossRef]
55. Judkins, T.; Rosenthal, E.; Arnell, C.; Burbidge, L.A.; Geary, W.; Barrus, T.; Schoenberger, J.; Trost, J.; Wenstrup, R.J.; Roa, B.B. Clinical significance of large rearrangements in BRCA1 and BRCA2. *Cancer* **2012**, *118*, 5210–5216. [CrossRef] [PubMed]
56. Hansen, T.; Jonson, L.; Albrechtsen, A.; Andersen, M.K.; Ejlertsen, B.; Nielsen, F.C. Large BRCA1 and BRCA2 genomic rearrangements in Danish high risk breast-ovarian cancer families. *Breast Cancer Res. Treat.* **2009**, *115*, 315–323. [CrossRef]
57. del Valle, J.; Feliubadalo, L.; Nadal, M.; Teule, A.; Miro, R.; Cuesta, R.; Tornero, E.; Menendez, M.; Darder, E.; Brunet, J.; et al. Identification and comprehensive characterization of large genomic rearrangements in the BRCA1 and BRCA2 genes. *Breast Cancer Res. Treat.* **2010**, *122*, 733–743. [CrossRef]
58. Kwon, J.S.; Tinker, A.V.; Karsan, A.; Schrader, K.A.; Sun, S. Costs and benefits of tumor testing for mutations in high-grade serous ovarian cancer as a triage for confirmatory genetic testing. *Gynecol. Oncol.* **2019**, *154*, 5. [CrossRef]
59. Vlessis, K.; Purington, N.; Chun, N.; Haraldsdottir, S.; Ford, J.M. Germline Testing for Patients With BRCA1/2 Mutations on Somatic Tumor Testing. *JNCI Cancer Spectr.* **2020**, *4*, pkz095. [CrossRef]
60. de Jonge, M.M.; Ruano, D.; van Eijk, R.; van der Stoep, N.; Nielsen, M.; Wijnen, J.T.; Ter Haar, N.T.; Baalbergen, A.; Bos, M.; Kagie, M.J.; et al. Validation and Implementation of BRCA1/2 Variant Screening in Ovarian Tumor Tissue. *J. Mol. Diagn.* **2018**, *20*, 600–611. [CrossRef] [PubMed]
61. Hauke, J.; Hahnen, E.; Schneider, S.; Reuss, A.; Richters, L.; Kommoss, S.; Heimbach, A.; Marme, F.; Schmidt, S.; Prieske, K.; et al. Deleterious somatic variants in 473 consecutive individuals with ovarian cancer: Results of the observational AGO-TR1 study (NCT02222883). *J. Med. Genet.* **2019**, *56*, 574–580. [CrossRef] [PubMed]

MDPI
St. Alban-Anlage 66
4052 Basel
Switzerland
Tel. +41 61 683 77 34
Fax +41 61 302 89 18
www.mdpi.com

Cancers Editorial Office
E-mail: cancers@mdpi.com
www.mdpi.com/journal/cancers

www.ingramcontent.com/pod-product-compliance
Lightning Source LLC
LaVergne TN
LVHW070219100526
838202LV00015B/2065